Atlas of Ultrasound-Guided Central Venous Catheter Placement

Fernando Montes-Tapia

Atlas of Ultrasound-Guided Central Venous Catheter Placement

Neonatal and Pediatric Approach

Springer

Fernando Montes-Tapia
Pediatrics Department
Hospital Universitario "Dr. José Eleuterio González"
Universidad Autónoma de Nuevo Leon
Monterrey, Mexico

ISBN 978-3-031-61886-4 ISBN 978-3-031-61887-1 (eBook)
https://doi.org/10.1007/978-3-031-61887-1

This Springer imprint is published by the registered company Springer Nature Switzerland AG
The registered company address is: Gewerbestrasse 11, 6330 Cham, Switzerland

I wish to dedicate this book first to Him, for without His wisdom, this endeavor would not have been possible.

"A truly good wife is the most precious treasure a man can find! Her husband depends on her, and she never lets him down." Her name is Rosario; thank you.

To Félix and Fernando, I hope to have been a good steward.
To my parents, who gave me the chance to exist.
To my siblings, who are always here despite the distance.
To my in-laws, for welcoming me into their family.
To my patients, for whom I have always strived to provide a quality experience, especially warmth when a vascular access was required.

Foreword

Undoubtedly, the placement of a central venous catheter is an essential procedure in the management of hospitalized pediatric patients. Central venous catheters constitute a vital line for fluid volume management, venous access, medication infusion, and provide a safe and consistent means of monitoring the short-, medium-, and long-term treatment of critically ill patients.

Acquiring the skill to place a central venous catheter is therefore of paramount importance in clinical hospital training, both in infants and adults. In the specific case of pediatric patients, the size of the patient and the dimensions of the vessels to be cannulated are distinctive factors in the difficulty of the procedure, presenting an additional challenge to the patient's clinical condition. Evidently, the size and weight of pediatric patients can range widely from neonates to adolescents, making the learning and mastery of techniques across different pediatric ages highly relevant. Precision, assertiveness with the patient, and good judgment complement the operator's knowledge of regional anatomy, the venous system, and nerve branches. All of this must now be integrated with the ability to handle ultrasound equipment, which has facilitated the execution of this meticulous and indispensable procedure.

For the successful execution of this vascular access technique, the guidance, recommendation, and visual support from experienced practitioners are always welcome. This is where a work like the present *Atlas of Ultrasound-Guided Central Venous Catheter Placement: Neonatal and Pediatric Approach* shows its value and relevance. This atlas is a reliable guide that, step by step, image by image, illustrates the path that the operator must follow when placing a central venous catheter in neonates and pediatric patients. The guide in this vascular procedure is the pediatric surgeon Fernando Montes-Tapia, MD, PhD, professor in the Department of Pediatrics at the "Dr. José Eleuterio González" University Hospital of the Universidad Autónoma de Nuevo León, who, through his experience and collaboration with pioneers in pediatric catheterization like Antonio Rodríguez-Tamez, MD, has made the practice of ultrasound-guided vascular access a significant clinical science in hospital practice.

Professor Montes-Tapia guides the operator through the process of placing a central venous catheter, marking each step, each detail, and warning of possible difficulties and causes of errors throughout 23 chapters, organized by vascular access route. In these chapters, he provides a detailed and meticulous overview, supported by 469 photographs of patient positioning, procedures, anatomical access, and ultrasound transducer positioning. Additionally, through 472 ultrasound images parallel to the procedure photographs, he shows in a detailed and schematic manner the vascular structures, nerves, and tissues, presenting the catheter's position within the vascular pathway. In summary, the procedure is illustrated to be performed safely and expertly.

As the author rightly points out, this invasive medical procedure is not a minor one. It demonstrates not only the skills and competence of the individual operator but also the high quality and teamwork capabilities of the clinical services where it is performed. Under certain circumstances, achieving this can become a true challenge for the medical team.

It is a great satisfaction for me and for the academic medical community of the university hospital that our colleague, Dr. Montes-Tapia, publishes this atlas and makes it available to health professionals worldwide who need to perform vascular access from the neonatal stage to adolescence. I conclude by reiterating this atlas as a useful, relevant, accessible work with a didactic format for precise follow-up. Equally and fundamentally important, it will benefit patients undergoing this procedure under reliable and effective guidance.

Dean of the Faculty of Medicine and Hospital Universitario "Dr. Jose E. González"
Universidad Autónoma de Nuevo León
Monterrey, Nuevo León, Mexico

Oscar Vidal-Gutierrez

Preface

Central venous catheter (CVC) placement is the most frequently performed invasive procedure in pediatric and adult patients. The indications for a CVC include hemodynamic monitoring, administration of parenteral solutions, antibiotics, parenteral nutrition, among others.

Traditionally, vascular access is performed using anatomical guides; however, its effectiveness depends on the expertise of the operator. The success of the anatomical guide procedure decreases as the patient's age and weight decrease or the patient has had previous catheterizations or abnormal anatomy. In addition, the risk of associated complications such as hematomas, pneumothorax, cardiac tamponade, or deaths is reported when using this technique.

Ultrasound-guided central venous catheter placement is recognized by the National Institute for Clinical Excellence (2002) recommendations, which state that ultrasound guidance is the preferred method for elective CVC insertion in both adults and children. However, it has not yet become the standard due to lack of training or adequate equipment (ultrasound) to perform it.

This atlas aims to contribute to the development of the knowledge component and, potentially, facilitate the acquisition of skills through the photographic demonstration of techniques within the competence of performing ultrasound-guided vascular access procedures. This atlas is the first in the literature to present a graphic/clinical step-by-step format for each of the 23 types of vascular access in neonatal and pediatric ages.

The decision to share this knowledge stems from a commitment to improving the quality and safety of a procedure often minimized by many physicians as "just vein puncture." However, facing a 0.500 kg newborn or a 100+ kg adolescent presents challenges often associated with complications and fatal incidents.

More than 41 years ago, my mentor Dr. Antonio Rodríguez Taméz began with anatomical guide-based vascular accesses, quickly transitioning to ultrasound-guided placement with the first Site Rite® in Mexico in 1992. His expertise over the years and the use of various ultrasound devices made him a great expert. Thus, in 2002, I started my training in ultrasound-guided vascular access under my mentor, later learning other vascular accesses that I now share with him.

A competitive advantage of ultrasound-guided vascular access lies not only in its quality and safety but also in the psychological impact on the operator. Faced with patients who have multiple previous punctures, difficult vascular access due to weight, clinical condition, or congenital anomalies, the use of ultrasound provides fundamental confidence, ensuring the location of a suitable vein. This confidence gives the operator a decisive initial advantage, approaching the procedure with a mindset of assured success.

Regarding the chapters:

- When the venous access technique is applicable to both neonatal and pediatric stages, we dedicate a chapter to the puncture of the same vein in each age group, acknowledging their unique peculiarities. Conversely, if the technique is strictly for pediatric patients, the description will focus solely on this age group.
- We include chapters illustrating the venous puncture technique from both long-axis (LAX) and short-axis (SAX) views, allowing for the learning of both techniques, and giving the reader the freedom to choose the one they feel more comfortable with and can learn more effectively.

The atlas chapters start with the internal jugular vein access, which I recommend as the first to learn because it is easy to locate and has a direct path to the superior vena cava. In neonates, due to the neck size, the LAX view is impossible, making the SAX view optimal.

Regarding the SAX view technique, described as out of the plane, thus potentially puncturing unvisualized structures (out of the plane), this is mitigated by performing ultrasound-guided dynamic needle-tip positioning (DNTP) to guide the intravenous catheter puncture or the introducer needle; in other words, you must learn to perform a sweep down or up the transducer as you progress with the puncture, ensuring at all times that the needle does not puncture other structures.

We will then describe the puncture technique of the most used vein in my series, the subclavian vein via the infraclavicular route. The puncture is performed in LAX view, which is more difficult to learn, but mastering it will eliminate the major complication described as pneumothorax from my incident scenario. As I always say when teaching this approach, the major incident is not cannulating the vein, but the cervicothoracic region has other veins and other subclavian access routes, such as the supraclavicular route described next, which I only describe in the pediatric stage.

The technique for puncturing the extrathoracic subclavian vein, originally described for pacemaker placement, has a limited margin for location. Anatomically, the subclavian vein starts after the confluence of the cephalic vein with the axillary vein, located in the deltopectoral groove. Thus, there is a short segment of the extrathoracic subclavian vein between this junction and the clavicle before its subclavicular passage. In patients older than 8 years, this segment measures approximately 3 cm in length, increasing as the individual's weight and height increase. Furthermore, the closer the vein is to the clavicle, the larger its diameter. I propose puncturing this specific segment of the subclavian vein, not the axillary vein. Although you will see that the suggested reading for these two chapters only contains literature on pacemaker placement.

Another vein in the cervicothoracic region is the brachiocephalic vein, notable for being a large vessel even in the neonatal stage; I only describe the puncture technique in LAX view.

We continue with the demonstration of femoral vein puncture, particularly in neonatal patients of very low weight (less than 1.5 kg), where many punctures are performed on the iliac vein due to its larger caliber. It can be confirmed in LAX view that the puncture is executed above the femoral head.

Finally, I present the technique for puncturing the upper extremity veins such as the brachial, basilic, and cephalic veins. These are used for the placement of a peripherally inserted central catheter (PICC), which can be punctured using either SAX or LAX views, though I suggest starting with SAX view.

It is my hope that this atlas serves as your guide whenever you perform a venous puncture to place a central venous catheter and that you adopt ultrasound-guided puncture as your standard for quality and safety. Our patients, whom we are privileged to serve, deserve nothing less.

Monterrey, Mexico Fernando Montes-Tapia, MD PhD

Acknowledgments

I wish to express my gratitude to the Universidad Autónoma de Nuevo León, through the Hospital Universitario "Dr. José E. González", for providing the setting for most of my professional practice, a place I consider home. To Dr. Oscar Vidal Gutiérrez, for his trust and the anticipation of better things to come. To Dr. Antonio Rodríguez-Taméz, who is undoubtedly my mentor in the field of ultrasound-guided vascular access; without your expertise and, above all, your friendship, I would not have acquired this skill. To my colleagues Dr. Ulises Garza-Luna and Guillermo Martínez-Flores, for their invaluable support and experience in the field of pediatric surgery. To my fellow faculty members in the Department of Pediatrics for considering me a peer. To the various generations of residents from the Department of Pediatrics at the Hospital Universitario "Dr. José E. González", for their valuable assistance during "the catheter time." To my research interns, Antonio Castillo, Zelenia García-Alcudia, Madeline Nuñez-Ku, who inspired me to excel, Evelyn González and Emilia González for believing in my project, and Karen Cantú for continuing the legacy of her colleagues. To Berenice Ricardez, for her invaluable support in photography. To Sergio Lozano M.D., who assisted me in conveying the knowledge contained in this book in English.

About the Book

This atlas provides a detailed illustration of the venous puncture technique under real-time ultrasonographic guidance, specifically for neonatal and pediatric patients for the insertion of central venous catheters. Comprising 23 chapters, it thoroughly covers all documented venous accesses to date. Each chapter is enhanced with clinical images capturing each phase of the procedure, alongside their corresponding ultrasonographic images, offering a detailed, step-by-step guide for executing each technique.

Contents

About the Author

Fernando Montes-Tapia, MD PhD is a pediatric surgeon and chief of the Department of Pediatrics at the Hospital Universitario "Dr. José E. González and professor at the Faculty of Medicine, Universidad Autónoma de Nuevo León, Monterrey, Mexico. He teaches both undergraduate and graduate courses and is a researcher with National Council of Humanities, Science and Technology (Consejo Nacional de Humanidades, Ciencias y Tecnología - CONAHCYT). His research focuses on ultrasound-guided vascular accesses in neonatal and pediatric patients, for which he has won national research awards in this area. He has participated in multiple conferences to promote the use of ultrasound as the standard for vascular access and offers workshops on ultrasound-guided vascular accesses. He has received various grants for his research and the acquisition of ultrasound equipment (Rotary Club International).

Abbreviations

BCV	Brachiocephalic vein
CA	Carotid artery
CV	Cephalic vein
DNT	Dynamic needle tracking
DNTP	Dynamic needle-tip positioning
ETSCA	Extrathoracic subclavian artery
ETSCV	Extrathoracic subclavian vein
FV	Femoral vein
IJV	Internal jugular vein
IVC	Inferior vena cava
LAX	Long axis
LBCV	Left brachiocephalic vein
LBrV	Left brachial vein
LBV	Left basilic vein
LCA	Left carotid artery
LCV	Left cephalic vein
LETSCA	Left extrathoracic subclavian artery
LETSCV	Left extrathoracic subclavian vein
LFA	Left femoral artery
LFV	Left femoral vein
LIA	Left iliac artery
LIJV	Left internal jugular vein
LIV	Left iliac vein
LSCA	Left subclavian artery
LSCV	Left subclavian vein
RBcV	Right brachial vein
RBCV	Right brachiocephalic vein
RBV	Right basilic vein
RCA	Right carotid artery
RCV	Right cephalic vein
RETSCA	Right extrathoracic subclavian artery

RETSCV	Right extrathoracic subclavian vein
RFA	Right femoral artery
RFV	Right femoral vein
RIA	Right iliac artery
RIJV	Right internal jugular vein
RIV	Right iliac vein
RSCA	Right subclavian artery
RSCV	Right subclavian vein
SAT	Subcutaneous adipose tissue
SAX	Short axis
SCA	Subclavian artery
SCM	Sternocleidomastoid
SCV	Subclavian vein
SVC	Superior vena cava

Chapter 1
General Principles

Due to the nature of this atlas, indications and contraindications are not covered. However, every time a decision is made to perform vascular access, these details must be analyzed and discussed with the attending physician to evaluate the best venous access according to the intended use.

1.1 Informed Consent

- It should be obtained from all patients or legal guardians before performing the procedure.
- This process is carried out with each family member and patient who is mature enough to understand the purpose of the procedure and the benefits, risks, and complications according to the patient's clinical condition.

1.2 Universal Protocol

- Since it is an invasive procedure, all patients should be considered for the pre-procedure, time-out, and post-procedure evaluation.

F. Montes-Tapia, *Atlas of Ultrasound-Guided Central Venous Catheter Placement*, https://doi.org/10.1007/978-3-031-61887-1_1

1.3 Patient Monitoring

- Vascular access is an invasive and high-risk procedure which is performed in the operating room but that can be performed outside the operating room. Quality and safety during the procedure must be guaranteed, so all patients must have at least the following:
  - Cardiac monitoring.
  - Pulse oximeter.
  - Oxygen therapy.
  - Equipment for invasive airway management.

1.4 Sedation

- Our hospital protocol uses the following drugs: midazolam associated with ketamine, fentanyl, or propofol. The combination of these is administered according to the patient's clinical status.
- In infants and anxious patients, start with a dose of midazolam when starting positioning and pre-procedure scanning.
- In patients who do not have vascular access, sedation can be provided intranasally, intramuscularly, intraosseously, or with a combination of these routes, according to the biosorption of each drug.
- In our institution, more than 95% of vascular accesses are performed under sedation outside the operating room.

1.5 Sterile Procedure

- Antiseptic solutions such as chlorhexidine-alcohol or chlorhexidine are used to disinfect the area chosen for the procedure.
- Operator cap and mask.
- Operator handwashing.
- Sterile gown and gloves.
- Protection barriers such as sterile cloth or synthetic fiber fields. These should cover a large area so that they can be placed over a 50-cm guidewire.
- Central venous catheter placement kit: See Fig. 1.1.

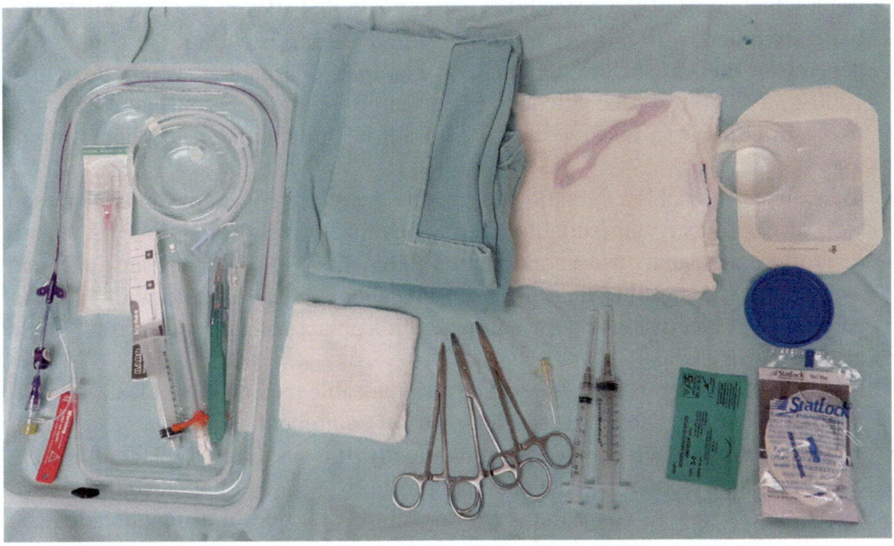

Fig. 1.1 The set we use at our institution

1.6 Anesthesia

- In all patients, local infiltration with 1% lidocaine is performed at the puncture site, catheter route, and fixation site. This procedure can be done under ultrasonographic guidance in real time or after previous ultrasound marking.
- In premature patients, local infiltration with lidocaine can cause a hyperechoic area in the tissues that later prevents visualization of the vessels or intravenous catheter below the infiltration. Therefore, the patient is sedated in these cases, and the vessel is punctured with a 24-G intravascular catheter. Once the vein is cannulated, and the guidewire is inserted into the vessel, lidocaine is infiltrated to perform the following steps, which are more painful, such as dilation of the trajectory and fixation with skin suture.

1.7 Ultrasound-Guided Vascular Access

- This atlas only presents the real-time ultrasound-guided vascular access technique.
- It is recommended to use a linear array probe, especially high frequency with a range of more than 10 Mhz. The high frequency allows the visualization of structures close to the skin with greater clarity. In this atlas, we used 13–6 MHz.
- Type of footprint (contact area of the transducer with the skin). There are different sizes according to the brand. The smallest is in the shape of a hockey stick

(with which most of the procedures presented in this atlas were performed), and there are others with a larger footprint of up to 6 cm. However, the choice will depend on the size of the patient. For example, if a patient weighs less than 1500 g, a 5-cm transducer would be too large for the neck or supraclavicular fossa. In contrast, a hockey stick would not be suitable for a teenager weighing 80 kg.

- Transducer and cable coverage equipment. There are covers designed for each type of transducer with suitable alternatives that each hospital designs. In our institution, we usually use a condom or a sterile glove to cover the transducer and a cloth or synthetic fiber field to cover the cable, which you hold with gauze or garters. The objective is that the equipment in contact with the sterile area should also be sterile.
- It is convenient to wash the transducer and the cable to keep them clean, according to the handling standards of each piece of equipment.
- The ultrasound screen is placed ergonomically. It is preferred to place it in front of the operator. Sometimes the patient's position does not allow it, so it is necessary to know how to adapt the screen position, so it does not impede adequate visualization and comfort for the procedure.
- In knobology, we must identify and know how to modify the following parameters:

  – *Position indicator or orientation marker* refers to a reference point on the body of the transducer that serves as a reference point to orient the image on the monitor, that is, which side of the transducer corresponds to the side of the monitor.

    In the procedures demonstrated in this atlas, the mark is placed on the left side of the screen, indicating the tip of the hockey stick probe or the mark on the linear transducer with the largest footprint. The mark on the screen can be of different types. In this atlas, with the equipment we use, it appears as an aqua-colored dot in the upper left corner (Fig. 1.2).
    Before starting to scan, the probe's orientation must be checked, placing gel on the transducer and moving it over the patient to confirm if it moves to our left or right. Another way is by touching one of the ends of the footprint and identifying if the left and right of the transducer correspond to the left or right of the screen and the right and left of the operator.

  – *Depth:* This parameter should allow the chosen vessel to be displayed as close to the top of the screen because the top of the screen is the patient's skin. When using the short-axis (SAX) view, the vessel to be punctured is intended to be displayed in the center of the screen. In the images in this atlas, which are ultrasound screen images, the depth in centimeters (1,9, 2,2, etc.) appears in the lower right corner (Fig. 1.2).

    Certain equipment has the zoom function. It is identified in the upper left of the monitor as an indicator on the side of the probe in the equipment we use for the procedures. In zoom mode, it is a "z" within an aqua circle (Fig. 1.3).

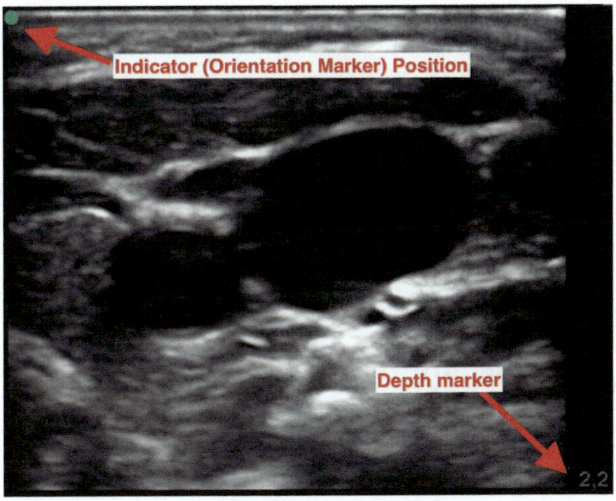

Fig. 1.2 Indicator position and depth marker

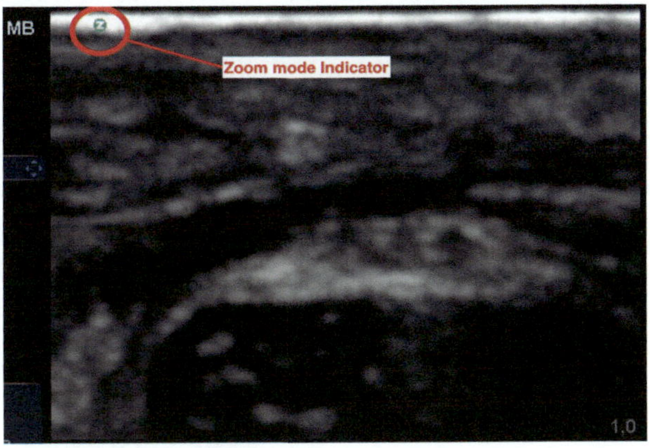

Fig. 1.3 Zoom mode indicator

Although zoom mode allows better visualization of vessels less than 0.5 cm, movements are also magnified, and it is necessary to know how to move when scanning. Movements and displacements must be short and slow.

– *Gain:* This will cause the scanned structures to appear darker in the monitor image (low gain) or the structures to be whiter (high gain).

This setting is important when the puncture is performed in the SAX view since the tip of a needle is normally displayed as hyperechoic. If we have a high gain (very white image), the tip of the intravenous catheter or the introducer needle will not be recognized. Therefore, the gain must be lowered (to see the image darker), and contrast the needle tip with the surrounding tissue to dynamic needle tip positioning (DNTP).

1.8 Pre-Procedure Scan

- The choice of the vein is made after performing:
  - Rapid central vein assessment (RaCeVA) of the cervicothoracic region for the jugular, subclavian, extrathoracic subclavian, or brachiocephalic veins.
  - RaCeVA of the brachial region for the basilic, brachial, or cephalic veins.
  - Rapid femoral vein assessment (RaFeVA) for the femoral/iliac vein.

1.9 Puncture Technique

- Non-sterile ultrasound gel is placed between the transducer and the sterile cover. Then, to achieve good contact with the skin, saline solution is used since, especially in patients punctured with a very small intravenous catheter, such as 24 G, it can become occluded with gel and obstruct the intravascular cannula.
- In-plane technique. The scan is performed in long-axis (LAX) view (Fig. 1.4); the vessel is visualized longitudinally (Fig. 1.5). In the puncture with this

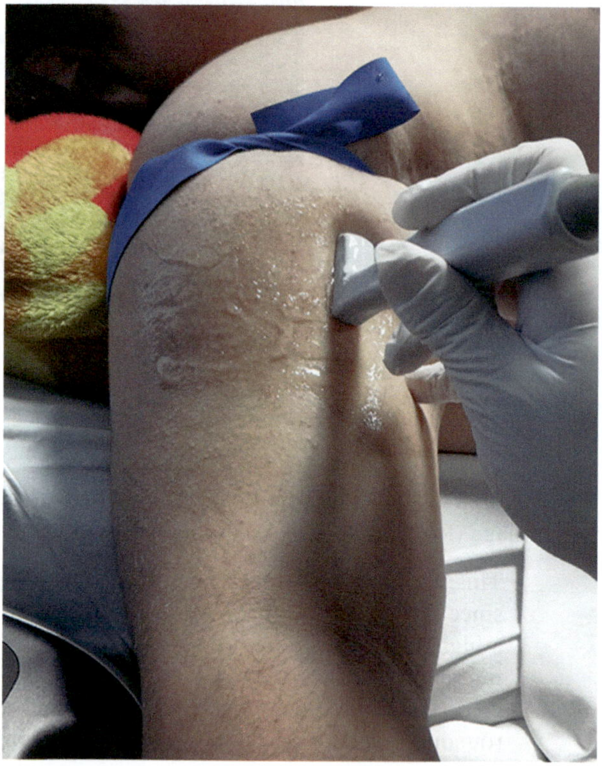

Fig. 1.4 Transducer in longitudinal position on the right arm

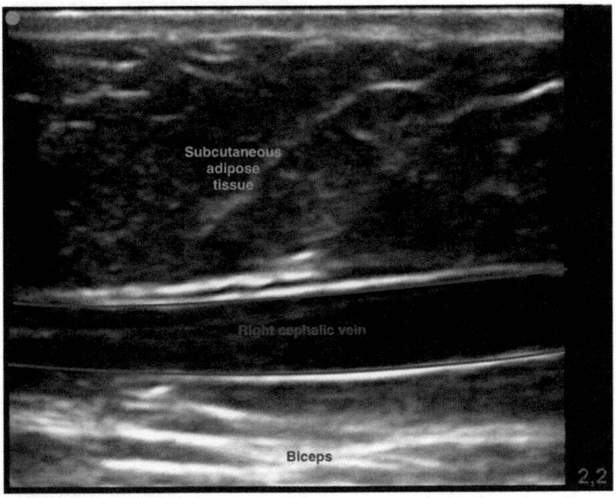

Fig. 1.5 The right cephalic vein in LAX view

technique, the needle is viewed longitudinally; the tip and body are visualized. However, this puncture technique is technically more difficult, but it avoids going beyond the posterior wall of the vessel if we reach it intravascularly.

- Out-of-the-plane technique is when the scan is performed in SAX view (Fig. 1.6); that is, the vessel is visualized in a cross-sectional or transverse cut (Fig. 1.7), and when the puncture is performed with this technique, only the needle tip is seen.
  - This technique requires less training; however, there is a greater risk of puncture to neighboring structures. This incident can be avoided by learning to perform dynamic needle tip positioning.
- *Dynamic needle tracking (DNT)*: to guide the puncture in real time.
- This technique involves viewing the tip and body of the needle longitudinally, throughout the entire penetration process from the skin to the vein. To achieve this, it is always necessary to keep the intravenous catheter or the introducer needle in the middle part of the thickness of the transducer; for this, the movements of the transducer will be lateral or medial to achieve adequate tracking.
- We can visualize this technique in the following figures and corresponding images of how the introducer needle progressively penetrates and its ultrasonographic visualization in LAX view (Figs. 1.8, 1.9, 1.10, 1.11, 1.12 and 1.13).
- *Dynamic needle tip positioning (DNTP)*: to guide the puncture in real time.
- This technique involves recognizing the needle tip that is visualized as a hyperechogenic point. It can be followed as it advances through the tissues since the punctures are usually oblique; that is, the transducer must progressively advance into the skin as the puncture depth increases and the needle tip penetrates deeper.
- We can visualize this technique in the following figures and corresponding images of how the intravascular catheter progressively penetrates and its ultrasonographic visualization in SAX view (Figs. 1.14, 1.15, 1.16, 1.17, 1.18 and 1.19).

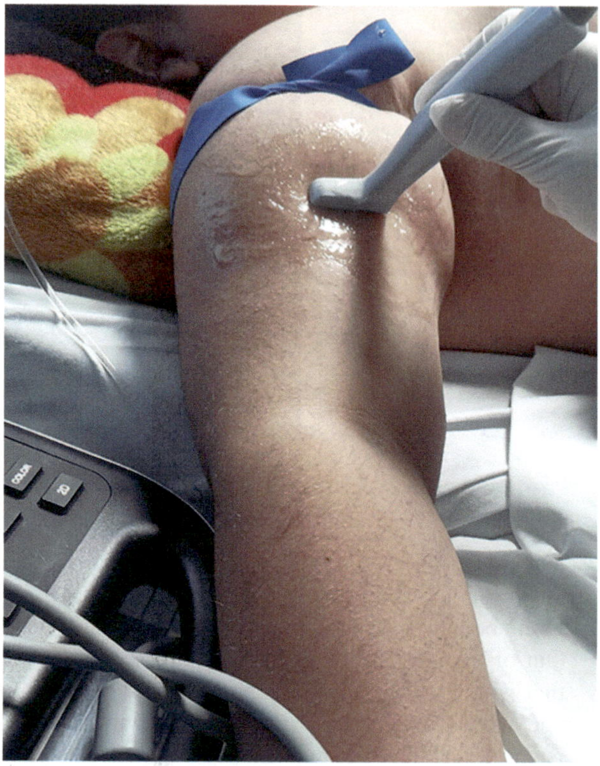

Fig. 1.6 Transducer in transverse position on the right arm

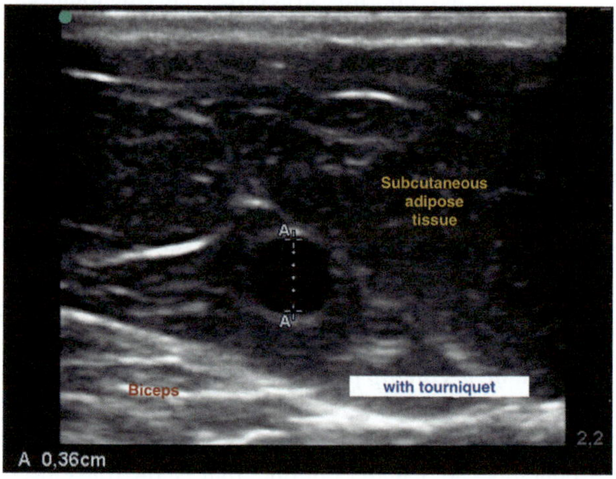

Fig. 1.7 The right cephalic vein in SAX view

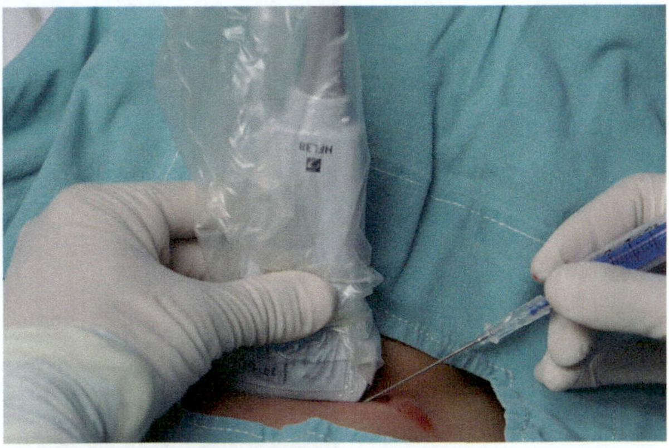

Fig. 1.8 Beginning of the DNT technique

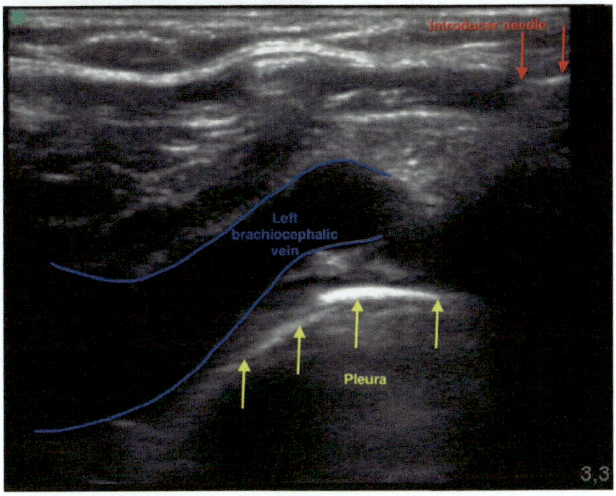

Fig. 1.9 LAX view of the beginning of the penetration of the introducer needle

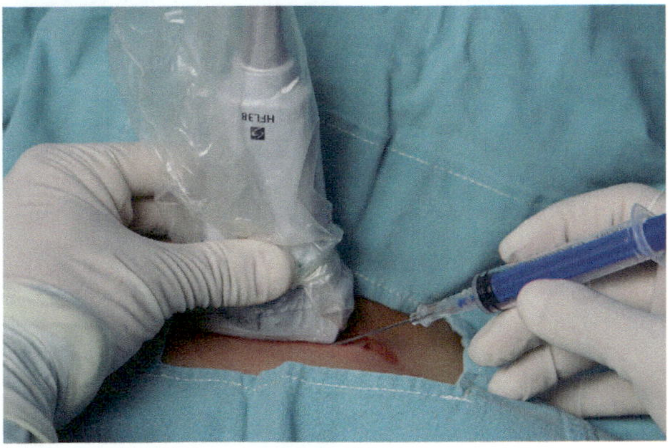

Fig. 1.10 Progression of the puncture keeping the transducer and introducer needle in the middle part of the thickness of the transducer and having the needle in the insonation area

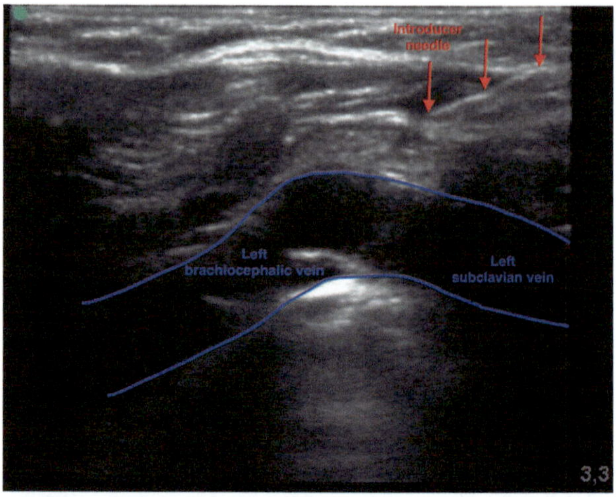

Fig. 1.11 LAX view of the inserting needle approaching the chosen vein. You can also see the two walls of the needle

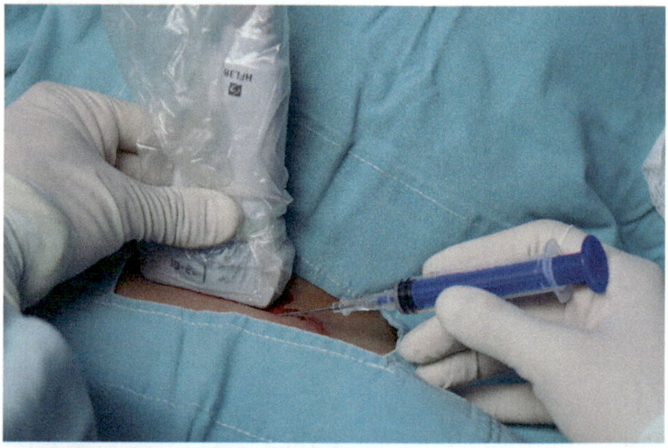

Fig. 1.12 Always keep the needle under the insonation area; sometimes, it requires moving the transducer medially or laterally, and if the needle penetrates further, you can slide the transducer to follow the trajectory of the puncture

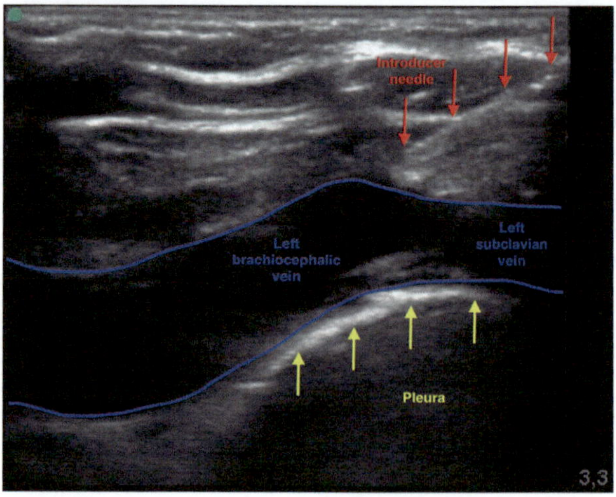

Fig. 1.13 LAX view of the tip and body of the introducer needle

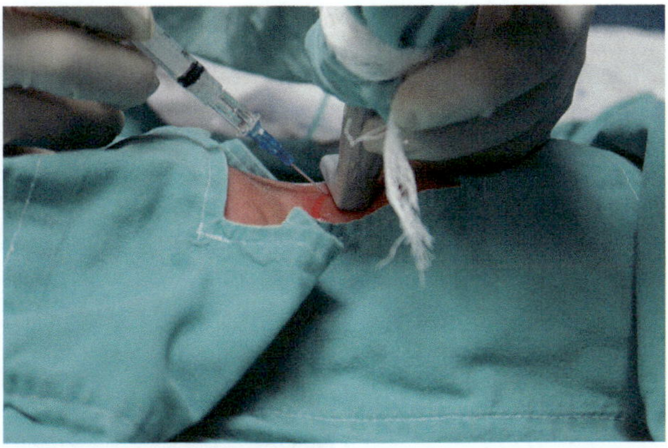

Fig. 1.14 Beginning of the DNTP technique

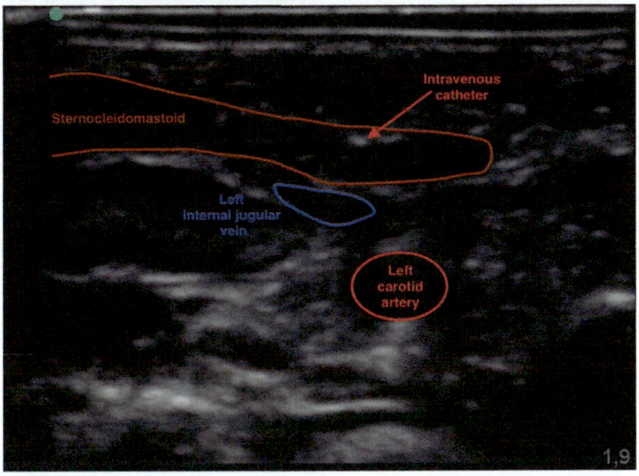

Fig. 1.15 The DNTP technique is performed in SAX view; the tip of the needle is identified as entering the sternocleidomastoid muscle

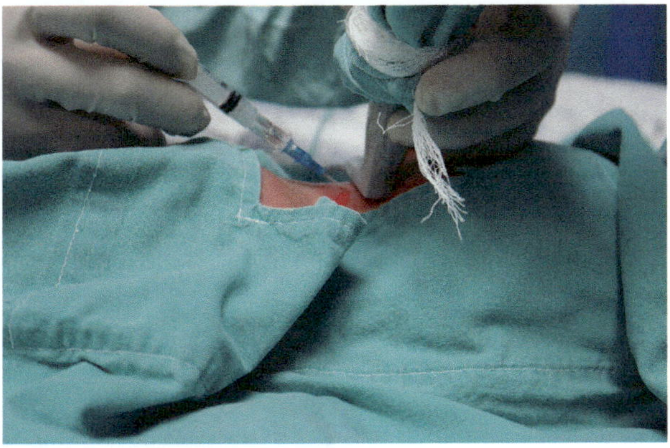

Fig. 1.16 As the intravenous catheter progresses, the transducer sweeps proximally. In this figure, the hockey stick transducer moves away from the puncture start site

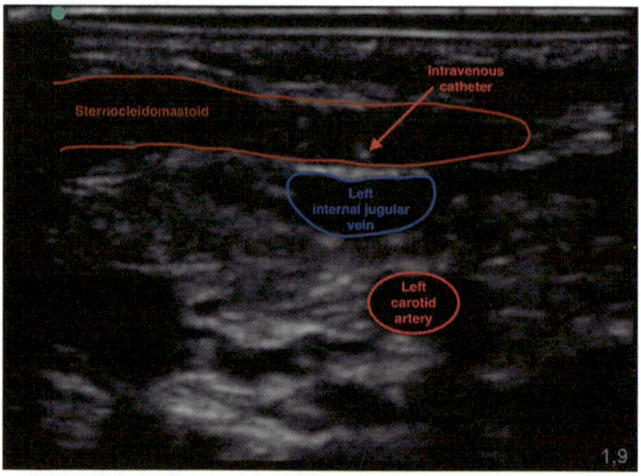

Fig. 1.17 SAX view, the tip of the intravenous catheter is passing through the sternocleidomastoid muscle

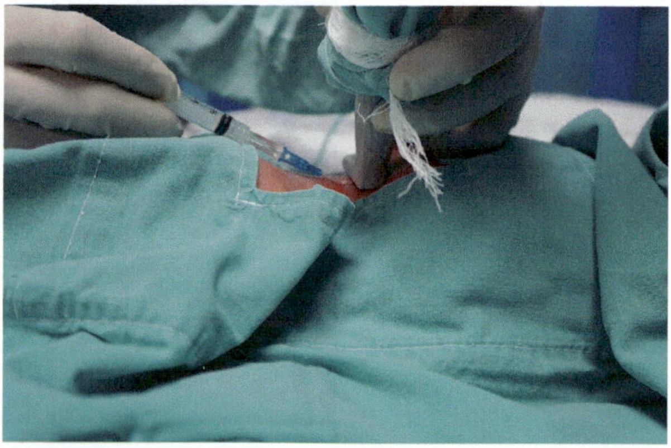

Fig. 1.18 The transducer has been moved more proximally, and the puncture angle has changed to target the selected vein

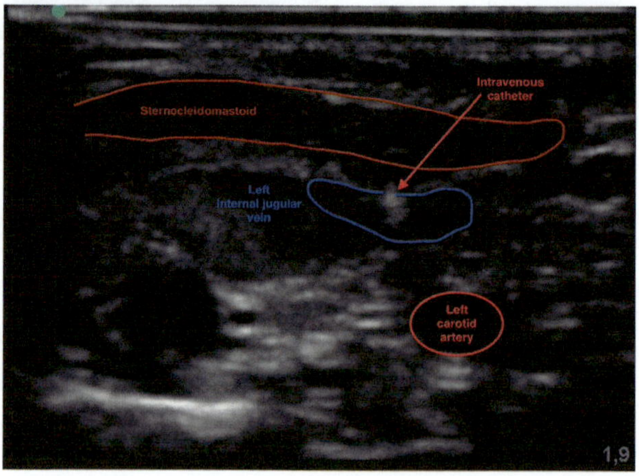

Fig. 1.19 SAX view. The tip of the intravenous catheter is penetrating the anterior wall of the vein

- In some cases of very deep vessels, both techniques can be used, starting in SAX view to find if the puncture follows the proper trajectory of the vessel and then continuing the puncture in LAX view to not puncture the posterior wall.

1.10 Catheter Fixation

- In our protocol, we fix the catheter to the skin with a 4–0 nonabsorbable monofilament suture in neonates and 3–0 in other age groups.
- Then we cover it with a sterile dressing.
- In the case of PICC, we use the fixation equipment that the catheter comes with.

Chapter 2
Right Internal Jugular Vein in Pediatrics

2.1 Patient Positioning

- The patient is a 1-year-old weighing 10 kg.
- Position the patient supine close to the head of the bed.
- Position the patient's head slightly to the left.
- Place a roll under the shoulders to increase the length of the cervical region and create a wider space between the clavicle and the jaw (Fig. 2.1).
- Gently hold the upper extremities with the arms caudal.

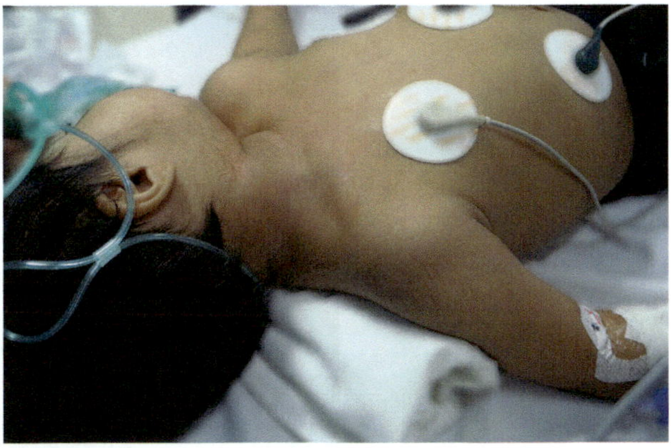

Fig. 2.1 Patient positioning

F. Montes-Tapia, *Atlas of Ultrasound-Guided Central Venous Catheter Placement*, https://doi.org/10.1007/978-3-031-61887-1_2

2.2 Scanning Technique

- Do a preliminary vascular assessment (non-sterile), known as rapid central vein assessment (RaCeVA).
- The operator stands at the patient's head.
- Position the ultrasound on the patient's right or left side or foot level.
- A high-frequency linear transducer (13–6 MHz), with a hockey stick-type probe or a probe as long as 5 cm, can be used.
- Hold the transducer with your left hand and with the transducer transverse to the neck and the tip of the hockey stick transducer to the patient's left side (Fig. 2.2).
- Begin the scan of the vessels in a short-axis (SAX) view in the middle of the neck and sweep down.
- Scan Sedillot's triangle (two borders of the sternocleidomastoid and the clavicle as the base).
- Visualization of the right internal jugular vein (RIJV) and right carotid artery (RCA) (Figs. 2.3 and 2.4).

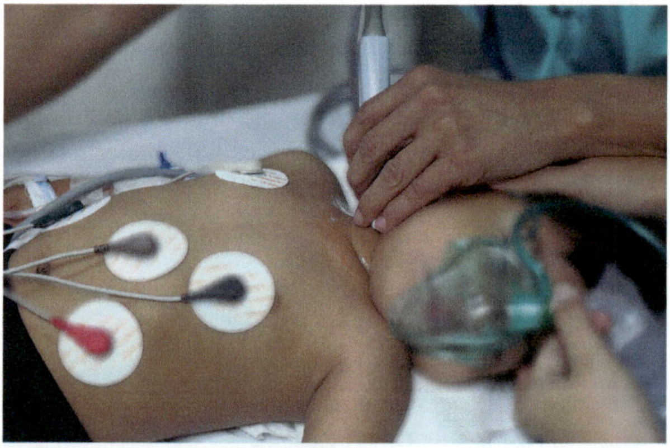

Fig. 2.2 Preliminary vascular assessment

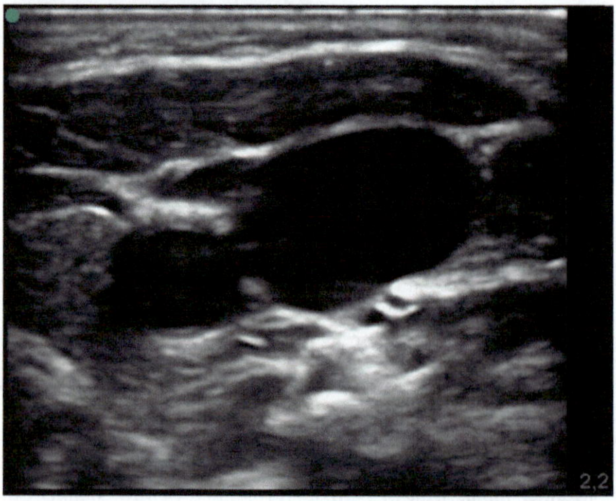

Fig. 2.3 Visualization of the RIJV and RCA
- The depth of the scan is 2,2 cm

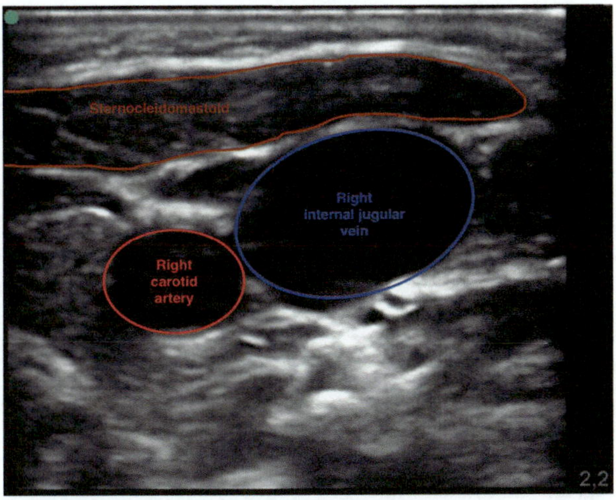

Fig. 2.4 Identifying structures
- The RIJV is in the most common position, lateral to the RCA
- Both structures are under the sternocleidomastoid muscle
- The diameter of the RIJV is 0.99 cm

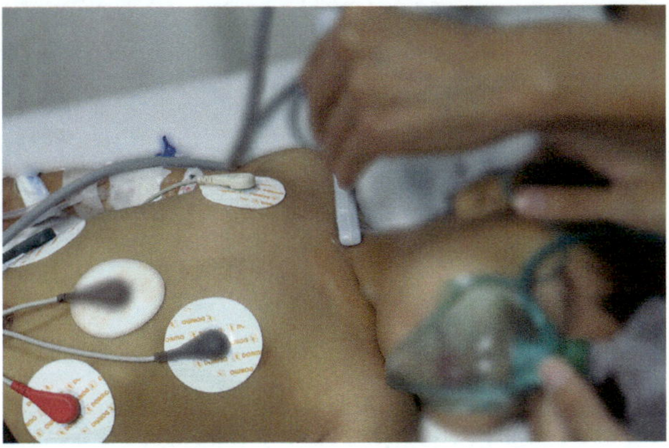

Fig. 2.5 Finishing the RIJV scan above the clavicle

- Sweep down the transducer and finish the scan of the right internal jugular vein (RIJV) just above the clavicle (Fig. 2.5).

2.3 Local Anesthesia Application

- Operator's view.
- Operator stands at the patient's head (Fig. 2.6).
- Patient with the head to the left.
- For infiltration, use a small needle 25–27 G (Fig. 2.7).
- Use lidocaine 1%.
- Infiltrate 1–1,5 cm before the chosen venipuncture site to anesthetize the oblique puncture path as well as the fixation site of the catheter holder.

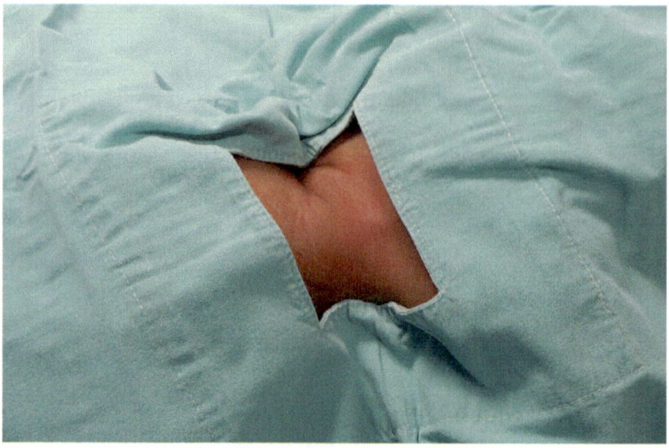

Fig. 2.6 Operator's view

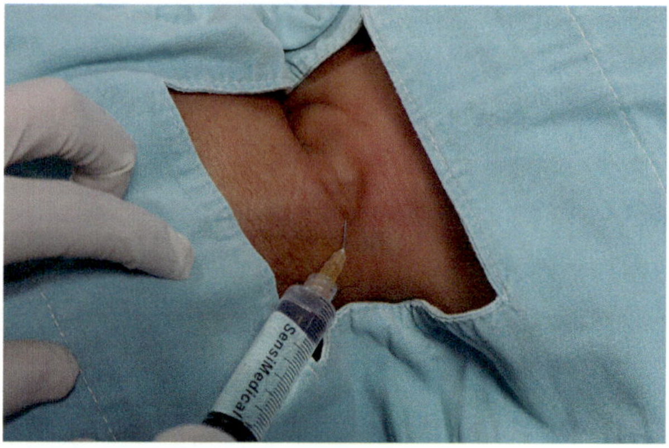

Fig. 2.7 Infiltration with lidocaine

2.4 Steps for Real-Time Ultrasound-Guided Access to the Right Internal Jugular Vein in Pediatrics

2.4.1 *Step 01*

- A 13-cm, 4 Fr, double-lumen catheter will be placed.
- Operator's view.
- Hold the transducer in your left hand.
- Locate the RIJV in SAX view and position the vein in the center of the screen (Figs. 2.8 and 2.9).
- Perform the puncture in the central part of the footprint length as long as the image of the RIJV is in the center of the screen, as seen in Fig. 2.8.
- Perform the puncture with a 21-G introducer needle with the right hand (Fig. 2.10).
- Start the puncture at an angle of 20–30° in relation to the skin.

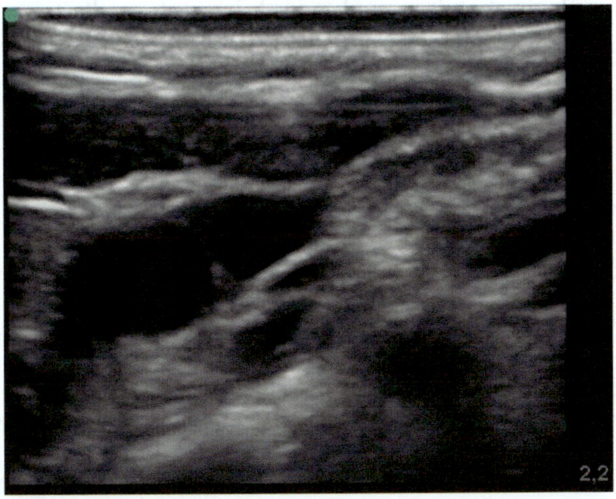

Fig. 2.8 Identifying structures
- The tip of the introducer needle is identified as a bright hyperechoic (white) dot
- The introducer needle passes the skin; however, the path defined by the dotted line is not in relation to the RIJV. The puncture is lateral to the vein
- The RIJV is deformed by compression of the tissues caused by the puncture

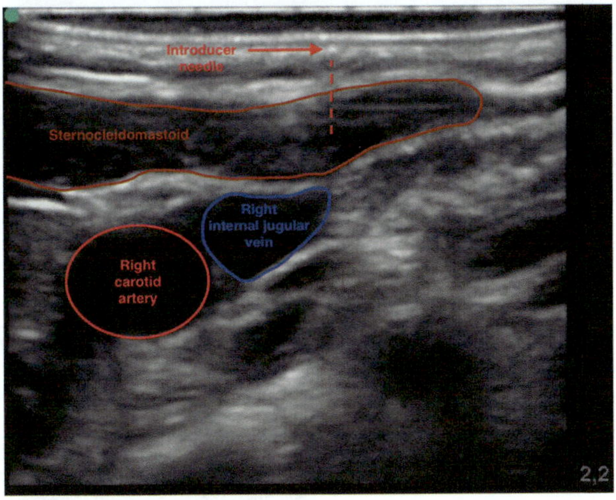

Fig. 2.9 Puncture at an angle of 20–30° in relation to the skin and in the central part of the length of the footprint

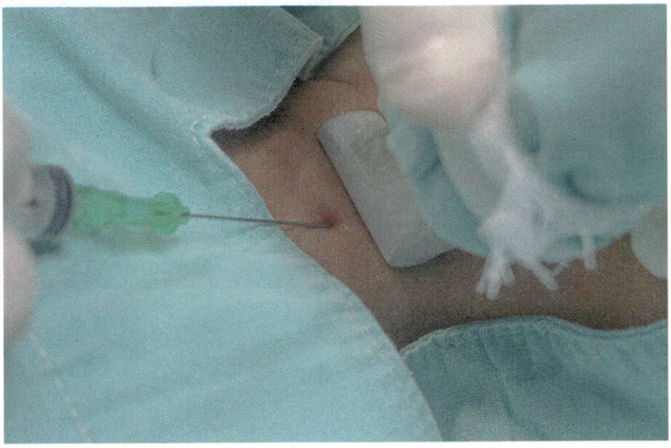

Fig. 2.10 SAX view of the start of the RIJV puncture

- Begin the ultrasound-guided dynamic needle tip positioning (DNTP) to guide the puncture in real time.

2.4.2 *Step 02*

- Operator's view.
- Correct the puncture by real-time ultrasound-guided DNTP toward medial to continue the trajectory to the RIJV (Fig. 2.11).
- SAX view of the puncture progression (Figs. 2.12 and 2.13).

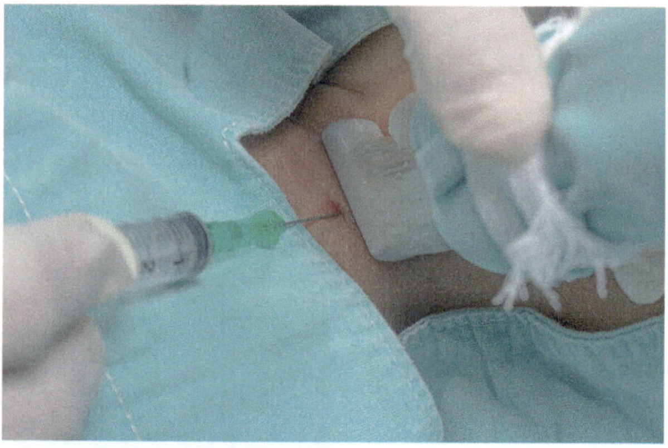

Fig. 2.11 Progression of the puncture

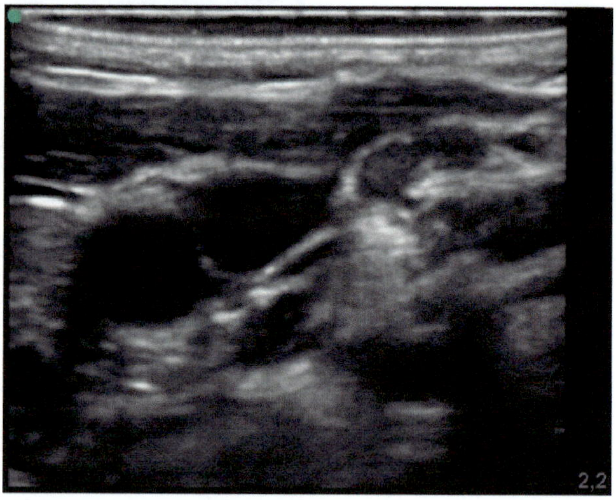

Fig. 2.12 SAX view of the puncture progression

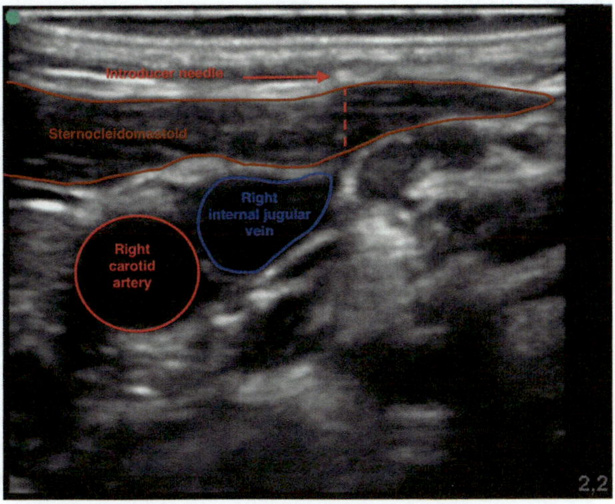

Fig. 2.13 Identifying structures
- A bright hyperechoic (white) dot identifies the tip of the introducer needle
- Progress has been made with deep insertion of the introducer needle; however, the puncture is still lateral. It needs to be done more medially
- The red dotted line indicates the direction of the puncture

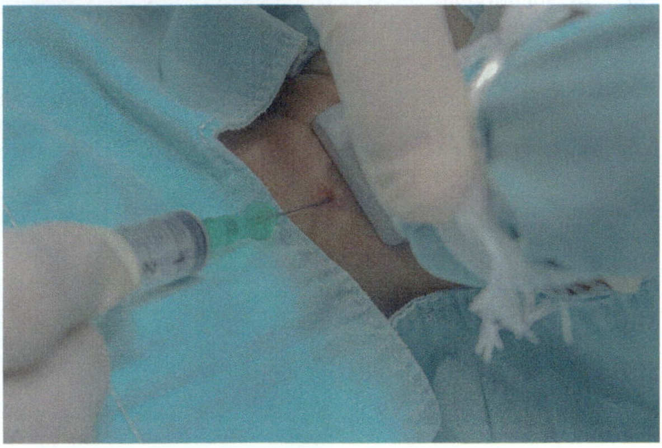

Fig. 2.14 Medial modification of the puncture

2.4.3 Step 03

- Change the direction of the puncture in real time, guided by ultrasound, while inserting the introducer needle (Fig. 2.14).
- Ultrasonographic image of the correction of the direction of the puncture (Figs. 2.15 and 2.16).

2.4.4 Step 04

- Extract and reintroduce the introducer needle a few millimeters to better change the puncture trajectory. Sweep up and then down the transducer to follow the needle tip (Fig. 2.17).

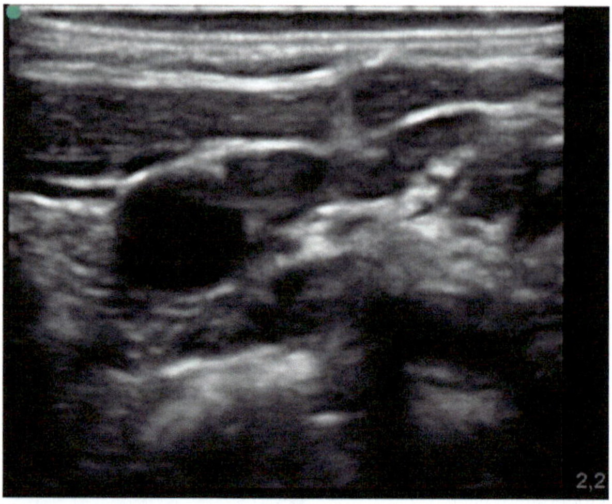

Fig. 2.15 SAX view of the change of direction and insertion of the introducer needle

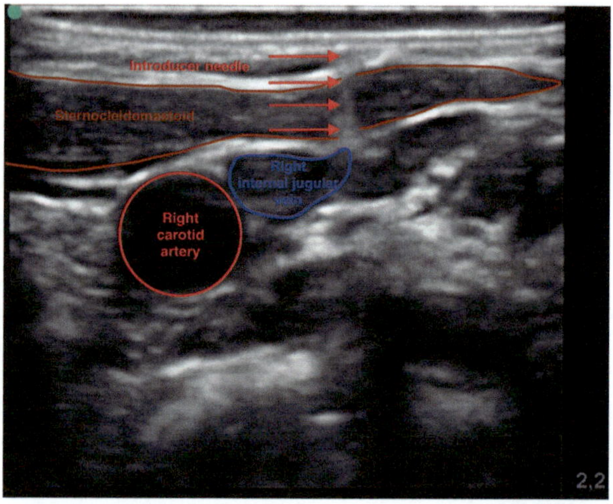

Fig. 2.16 Identifying structures

- The introducer needle has already penetrated the sternocleidomastoid, and the trajectory has not been completely modified. The puncture is still lateral

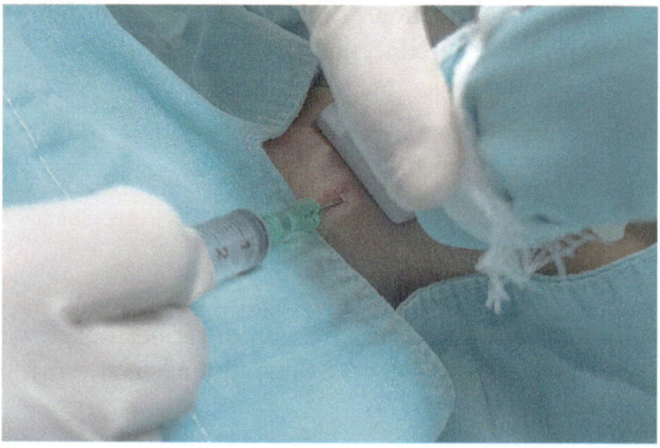

Fig. 2.17 Modification of the direction of the puncture through the extraction and reintroduction of the introducer needle

- Ultrasound view of the extraction of the introducer needle to the sternocleidomastoid muscle (Figs. 2.18 and 2.19).
- Ultrasound view of the reintroduction of the introducer needle (Figs. 2.20 and 2.21).
- Ultrasound view of the correct progression of the puncture to the direction of the RIJV (Figs. 2.22 and 2.23).

2.4.5 Step 05

- Sweep down the transducer to perform DNTP (Fig. 2.24).

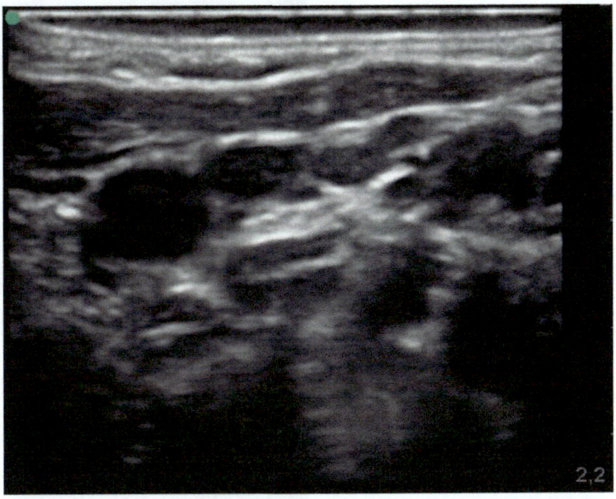

Fig. 2.18 SAX view of the extraction of the introducer needle

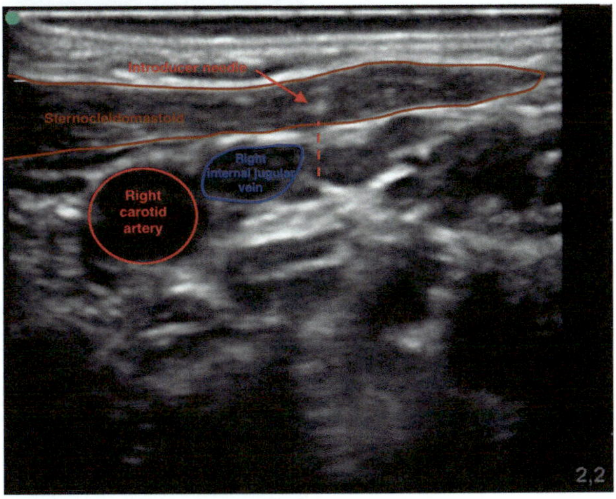

Fig. 2.19 Identifying structures
- The introducer needle has been moved back into the sternocleidomastoid muscle

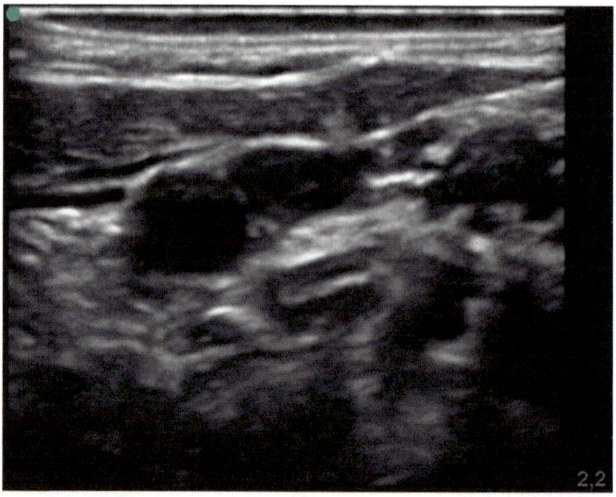

Fig. 2.20 SAX view of the redirection of the introducer needle

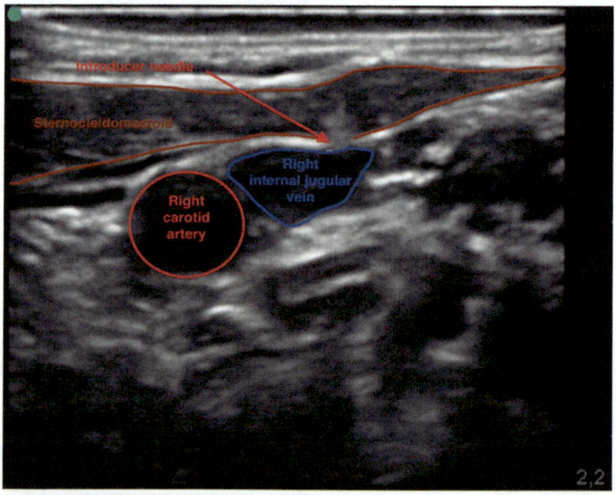

Fig. 2.21 Identifying structures

- The puncture is resumed now in a better trajectory directed toward the anterior wall of the RIJV
- The introducer needle again penetrates the sternocleidomastoid muscle

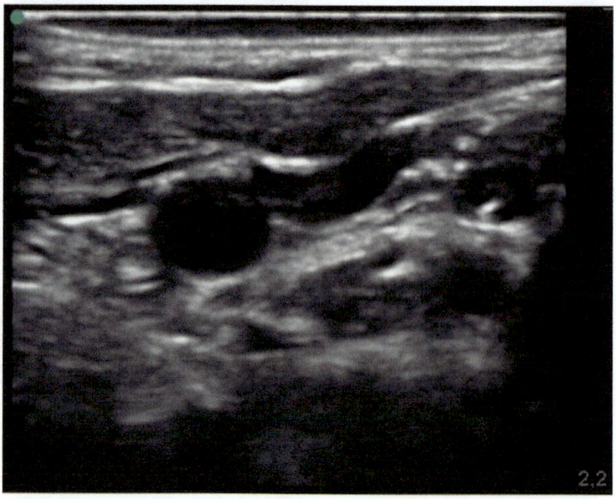

Fig. 2.22 SAX view of the puncture progression

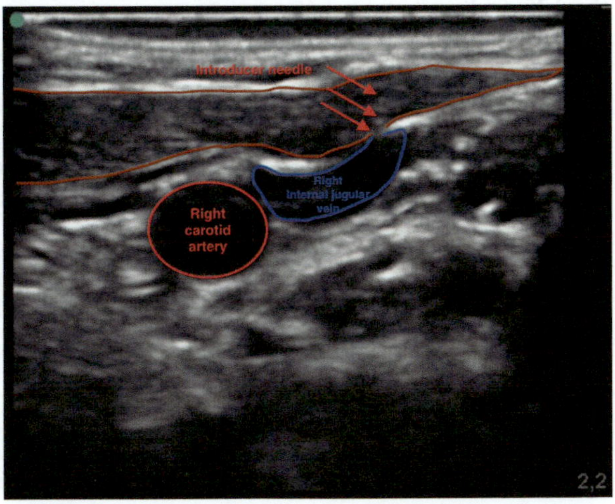

Fig. 2.23 Identifying structures
- The introducer needle reaches the anterior wall of the RIJV

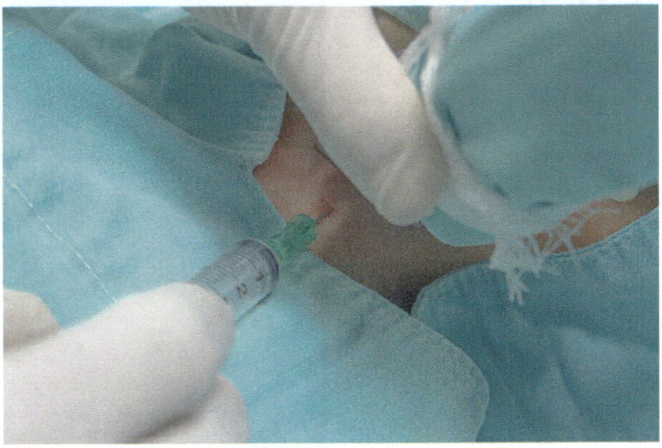

Fig. 2.24 Operator's view. Sweep down the transducer to DNTP

- Once you have identified that the introducer needle is over the anterior wall of the RIJV in the screen, cannulate the vein.
- Ultrasound view of the cannulation of the RIJV (Figs. 2.25 and 2.26).

2.4.6 Step 06

- Once you have identified on the screen the cannulation of the RIJV, set the transducer aside and maintain gentle negative pressure on the syringe plunger.
- Stop advancing when a flash of blood appears in the barrel of the syringe (Fig. 2.27).
- Hold the needle hub with your left hand and remove the syringe (Fig. 2.28).

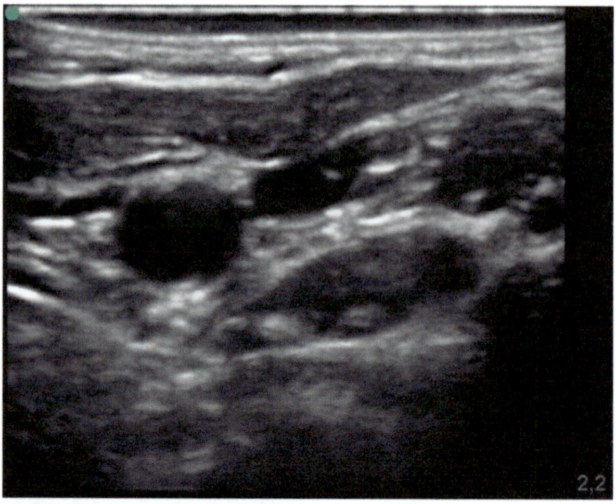

Fig. 2.25 SAX view of the cannulation of the RIJV

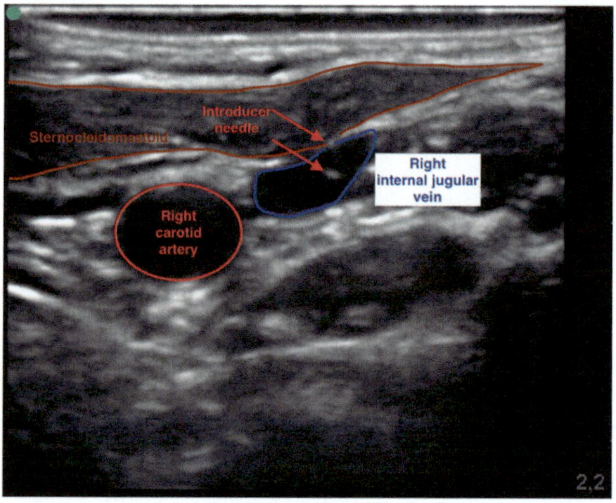

Fig. 2.26 Identifying structures

- The bright hyperechoic (white) dot, which is the tip of the introducer needle, is intravascular
- When this intravascular location is identified, the puncture is no longer continued

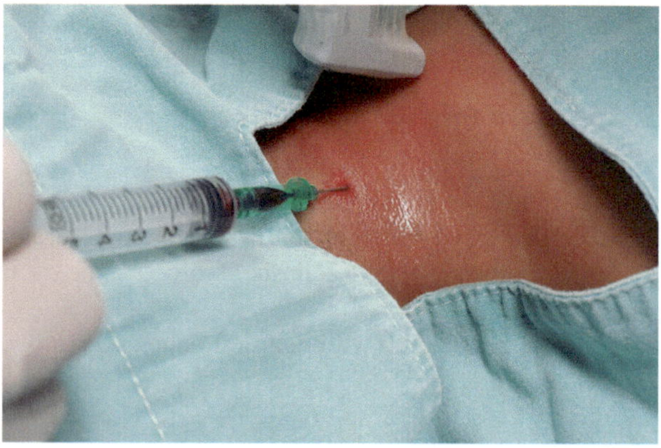

Fig. 2.27 Maintain a gentle negative pressure on the syringe plunger until a flash of blood appears in the barrel of the syringe

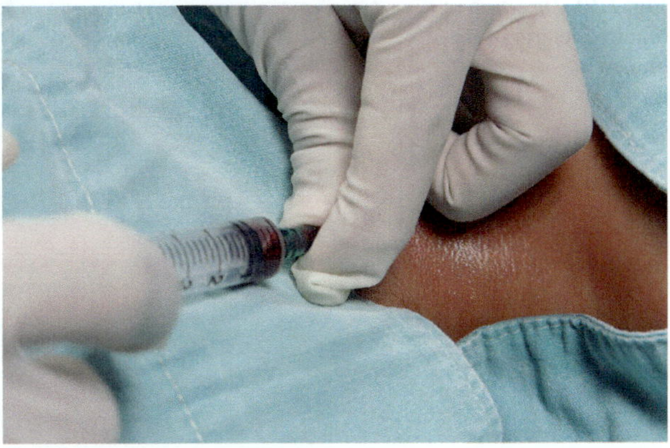

Fig. 2.28 Remove the syringe

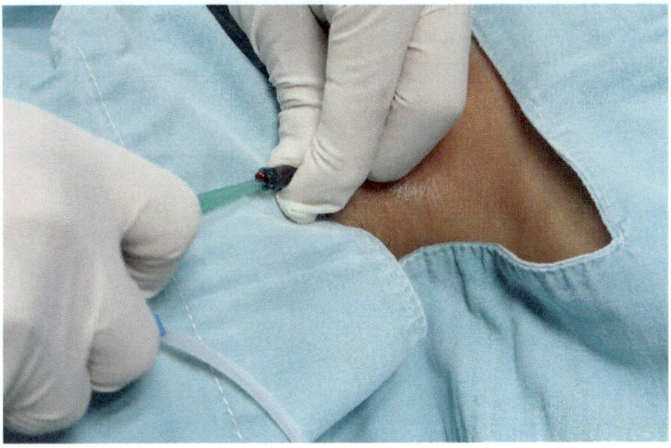

Fig. 2.29 Introduction of the guidewire through the introducer needle

2.4.7 Step 07

- Proceed to introduce the guide to place the CVC using Seldinger's technique.
- Introduce the 0.018". guidewire through the introducer needle. The J-tip can be passed (Fig. 2.29).
- Only insert the required guidewire length into the vein, always holding the needle hub so the needle does not move (Fig. 2.30).
- Scan to confirm the intravenous location of the guidewire. Place the transducer transverse on the neck (Fig. 2.31).
- Ultrasound view of the guidewire in SAX view (Figs. 2.32 and 2.33).
- You can also scan the guidewire in the LAX view. This scan is not necessary if you already identified the guidewire in SAX view (Fig. 2.34).
- Ultrasound view of the guidewire in LAX view (Figs. 2.35 and 2.36).

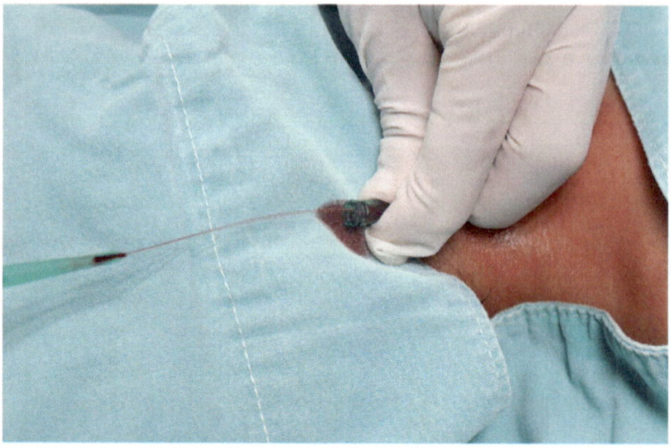

Fig. 2.30 Insertion of the required length of the guidewire

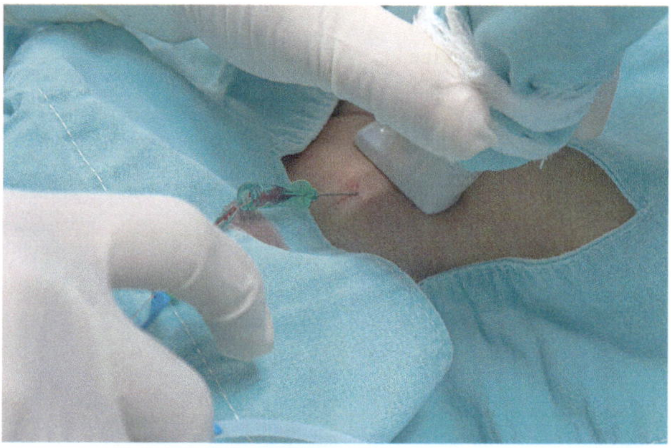

Fig. 2.31 Scanning in SAX view, hockey stick transducer transverse on the neck

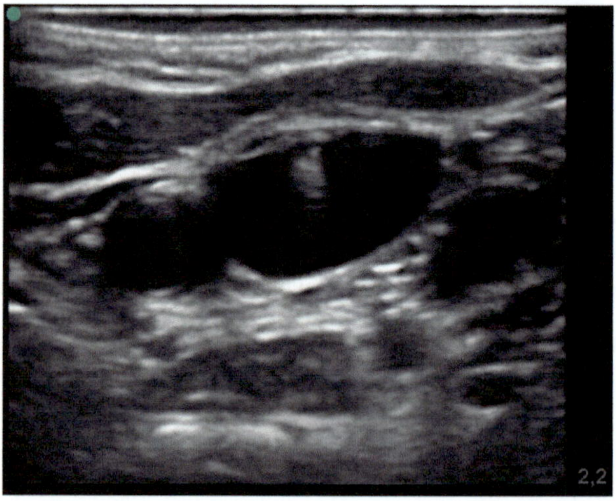

Fig. 2.32 SAX view of the intravascular guidewire

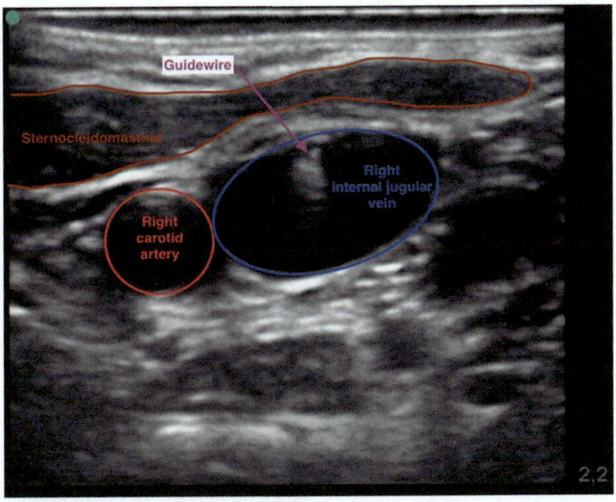

Fig. 2.33 Identifying structures

- The guidewire is intravascular. It is identified as a more hyperechoic dot with the comet tail sign

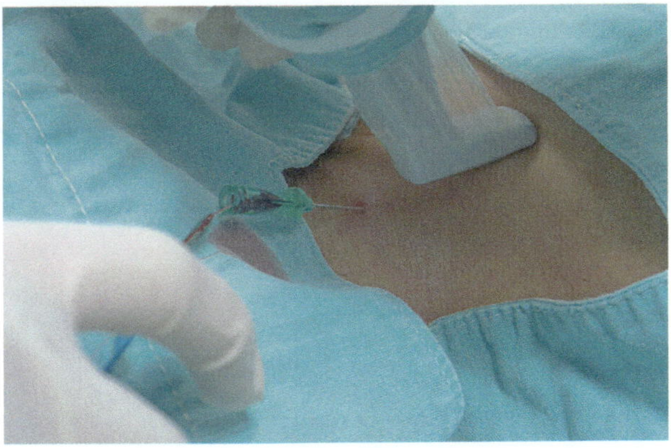

Fig. 2.34 Guidewire scan in LAX view

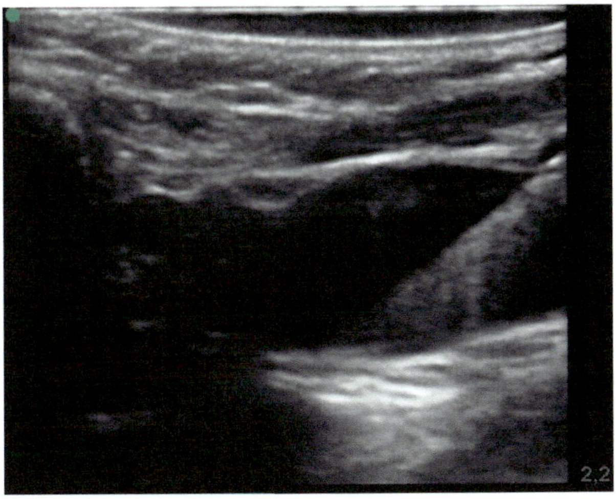

Fig. 2.35 LAX view of the guidewire in the RIJV

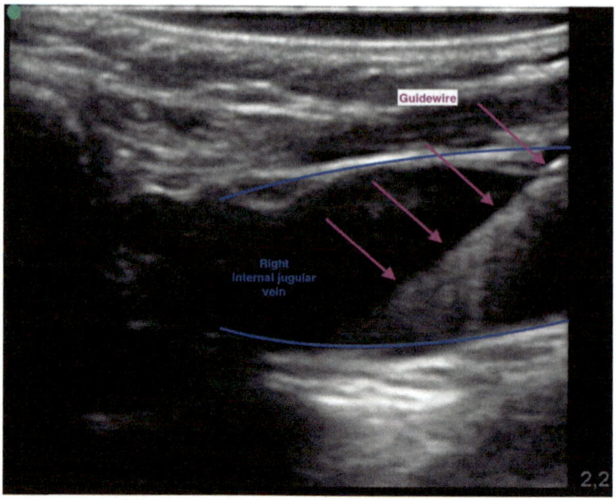

Fig. 2.36 Identifying structures

- The guidewire within the RIJV. Subsequent reverberation of the guidewire is seen

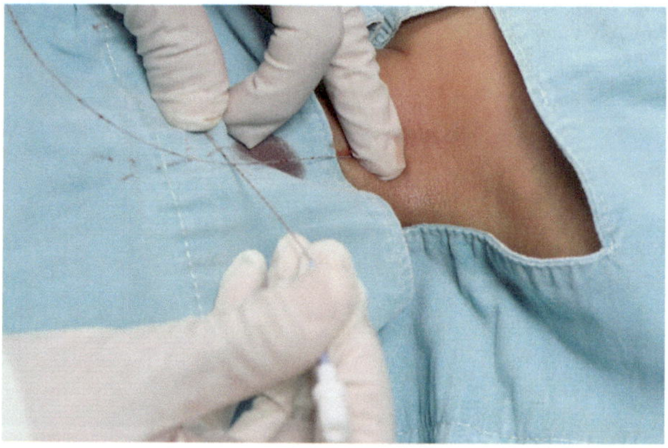

Fig. 2.37 Introduction of the dilator over the guidewire

2.4.8 Step 08

- With the middle finger of the left hand, occlude the entrance of the guidewire to the skin to avoid bleeding from the puncture.
- Grasp the guidewire with the same hand to help pass the dilator with the right hand (Fig. 2.37).
- Contract the skin with the left hand and begin introducing the dilator with the right hand (Fig. 2.38).
- Use a corkscrew motion as needed to insert the dilator gradually.
- The introduction of the dilator should be gentle so that the guidewire will not be bent.

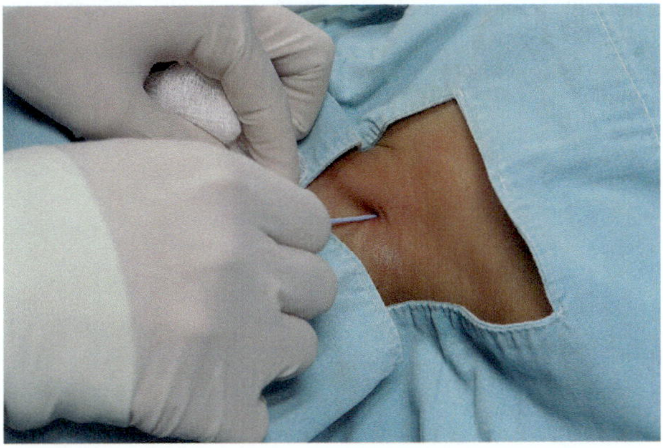

Fig. 2.38 Perform dilation of the path of the skin at the entrance of the RIJV

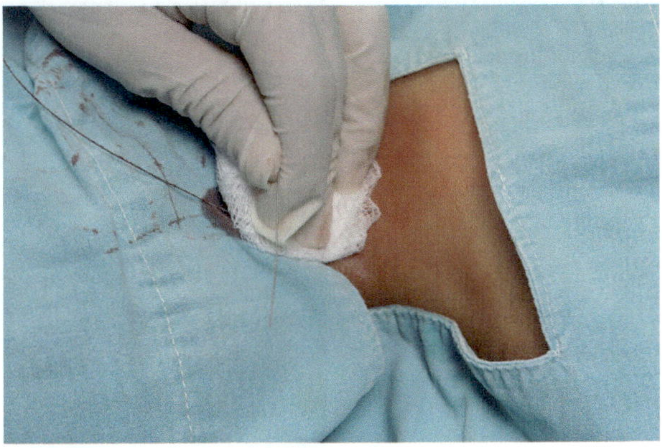

Fig. 2.39 Preparing to introduce the catheter by Seldinger's technique

2.4.9 Step 09

- When finished dilating, occlude the already dilated puncture entry site with gauze in your left hand to prevent bleeding.
- With the same hand, hold the wire to prepare to insert the catheter (Fig. 2.39).
- Advance the catheter over the guidewire (Seldinger's technique) (Fig. 2.40).
- When you have the required intravascular catheter length, remove the guidewire.
- Scan to confirm the intravenous location of the catheter.
- Scan the catheter in SAX view (Figs. 2.41 and 2.42) or LAX view; this scan is not necessary if you already identified the catheter in SAX view (Figs. 2.43 and 2.44).
- Check the venous return of the lines and clean them with a saline solution (Fig. 2.45).

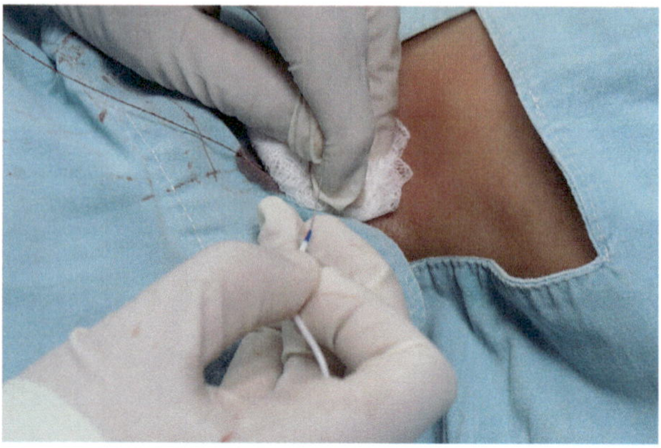

Fig. 2.40 Introduction of the catheter over the guidewire (Seldinger's technique)

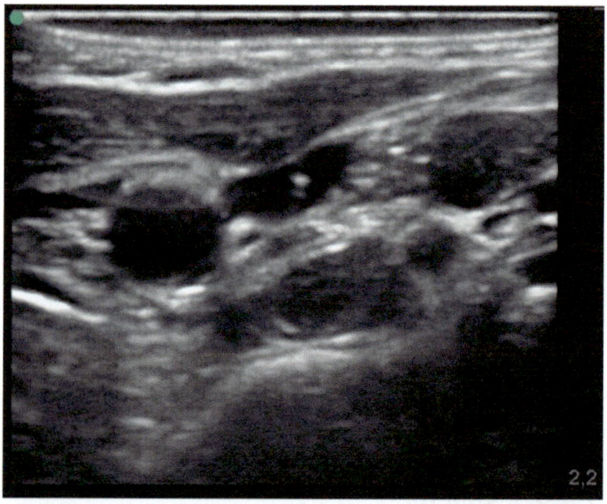

Fig. 2.41 Identifying structures

- Catheter inside the RIJV; two hyperechoic points can be seen

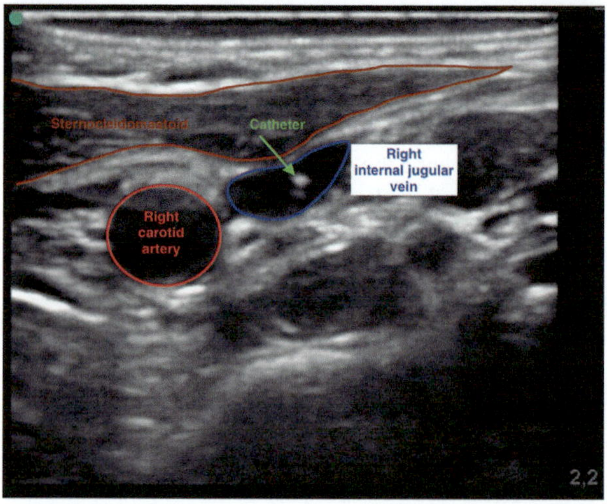

Fig. 2.42 LAX view of the catheter within the RIJV

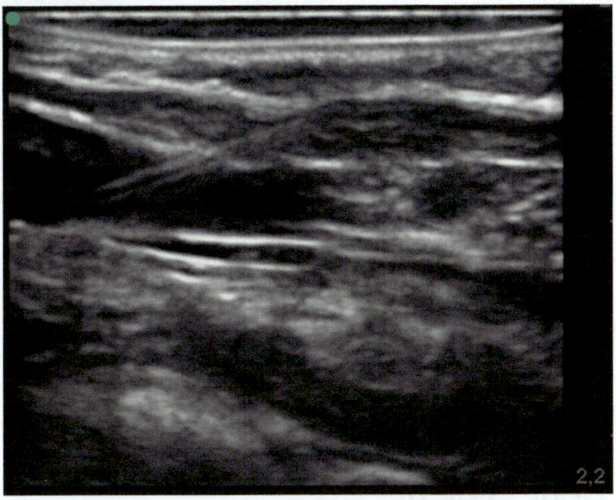

Fig. 2.43 Identifying structures

- This scan in LAX is not necessary if you have already identified the catheter in SAX
- Do the one you feel most comfortable with

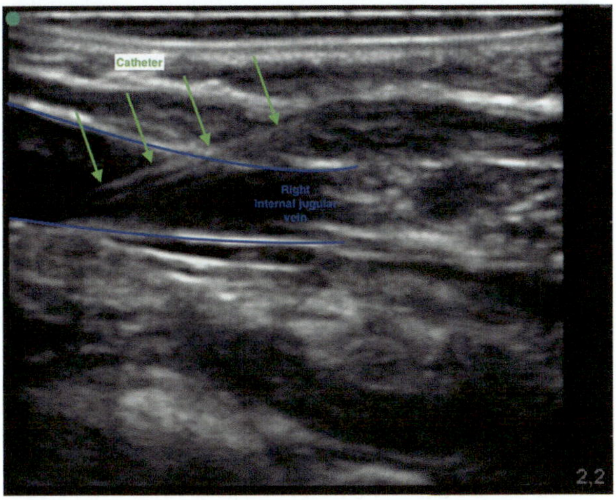

Fig. 2.44 Clean the lines with saline solution

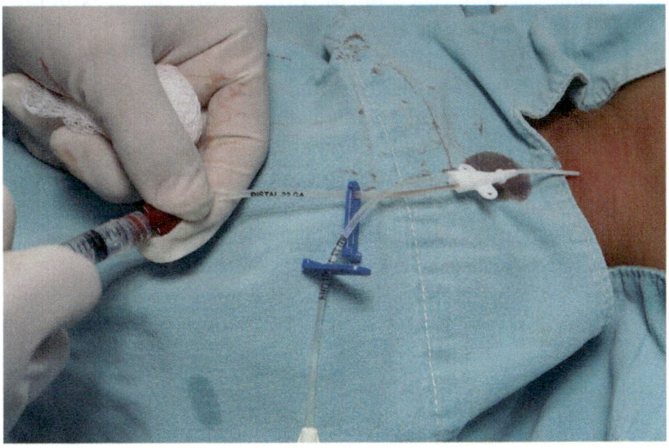

Fig. 2.45 SAX view of the intravascular catheter

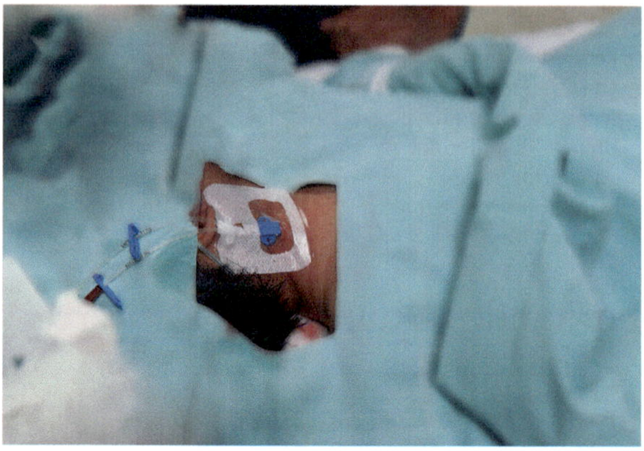

Fig. 2.46 Catheter with a sterile occlusive dressing

2.4.10 Step 10

- Secure the catheter and place a sterile occlusive dressing according to the institutional protocol (Fig. 2.46).

Sources

1. Spencer TR, Pittiruti M. Rapid central vein assessment (RaCeVA): a systematic, standardized approach for ultrasound assessment before central venous catheterization. J Vasc Access. 2019;20(3):239–49. https://doi.org/10.1177/1129729818804718. Epub 2018 Oct 4. PMID: 30286688.
2. Maddali MM, Al-Shamsi F, Arora NR, Panchatcharam SM. The optimal length of insertion for central venous catheters via the right internal jugular vein in pediatric cardiac surgical patients. J Cardiothorac Vasc Anesth. 2020;34(9):2386–91. https://doi.org/10.1053/j.jvca.2020.03.007.
3. Montes-Tapia F, Hernández-Trejo K, García-Rodríguez F, et al. Predicting the optimal depth of ultrasound-guided right internal jugular vein central venous catheters in neonates. J Pediatr Surg. 2020;55(9):1920–4. https://doi.org/10.1016/j.jpedsurg.2019.12.004.
4. Zanolla GR, Baldisserotto M, Piva J. How useful is ultrasound guidance for internal jugular venous access in children? J Pediatr Surg. 2018;53(4):789–93. https://doi.org/10.1016/j.jpedsurg.2017.08.010.
5. Montes-Tapia F, Rodríguez-Taméz A, Cura-Esquivel I, et al. Efficacy and safety of ultrasound-guided internal jugular vein catheterization in low-birth-weight newborn. J Pediatr Surg. 2016;51(10):1700–3. https://doi.org/10.1016/j.jpedsurg.2016.05.014.
6. Turker G, Kaya FN, Gurbet A, Aksu H, Erdogan C, Atlas A. Internal jugular vein cannulation: an ultrasound-guided technique versus a landmark-guided technique. Clinics (Sao Paulo). 2009;64(10):989–92. https://doi.org/10.1590/S1807-59322009001000009.
7. Morita M, Sasano H, Azami T, Sasano N, Katsuya H. The skin-traction method increases the cross-sectional area of the internal jugular vein by increasing its anteroposterior diameter. J Anesth. 2007;21(4):467–71. https://doi.org/10.1007/s00540-007-0562-6.

Chapter 3
Right Internal Jugular Vein in Neonates

3.1 Patient Positioning

- The patient is a newborn weighing 1190 g.
- Place the patient supine with the head near the edge of the crib where the procedure will be performed.
- Place a roll under the shoulders. Care must be taken to avoid hyperextending the neck, which can cause airway obstruction (Fig. 3.1).
- Turn the head to the left, not exceeding 60–70 degrees, since this maneuver can compromise venous return on the left side, decrease the caliber of the contralateral jugular vein, or change the relationship of the right internal jugular vein (RIJV) with the carotid.
- The objective of positioning the patient for this procedure is to increase the cervical area between the jaw and the clavicle since a newborn has a short neck, unlike other groups of pediatric age.

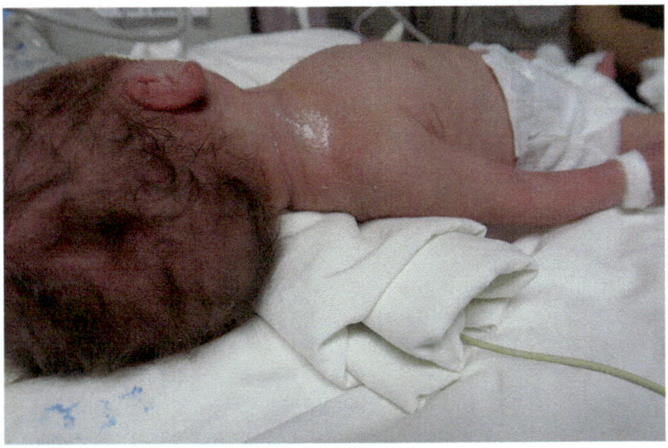

Fig. 3.1 Patient positioning

F. Montes-Tapia, *Atlas of Ultrasound-Guided Central Venous Catheter Placement*, https://doi.org/10.1007/978-3-031-61887-1_3

- Gently hold the arms, especially when the patient is not intubated, and place the arms in a lower direction close to the body. This maneuver helps pull the shoulder and clavicle downward, increasing the distance between the jaw and the clavicle.

3.2 Scanning Technique

- Do a preliminary vascular assessment (non-sterile), known as rapid central vein assessment (RaCeVA).
- The operator stands at the patient's head.
- Position the ultrasound on the patient's right or left side or foot level.
- Due to the patient's size, the use of a high-frequency linear transducer (13–6 MHz) with a hockey stick-type probe is recommended.
- Use your left hand to grasp the transducer.
- The smaller the newborn, the less compression the right internal jugular vein (RIJV) can withstand, and it may collapse. Therefore, holding the transducer with as little cervical compression as possible is recommended.
- Due to the normally short neck of the newborn, begin the scan of the vessels in short-axis (SAX) view in the middle of the neck and sweep down to the base of the neck (Fig. 3.2).
- Visualization of the right internal jugular vein (RIJV) and right carotid artery (RCA) (Figs. 3.3 and 3.4).
- In the initial scanning, we also measure the RIJV diameter and identify its relationship with adjacent structures (Figs. 3.5 and 3.6).
- Since Sedillot's triangle (composed of the edges of the sternocleidomastoid and the clavicle as its base) in children under 1500 g is very small, the puncture is made higher because the diameter of the transducer occupies most of this triangle, as seen in Fig. 3.2.

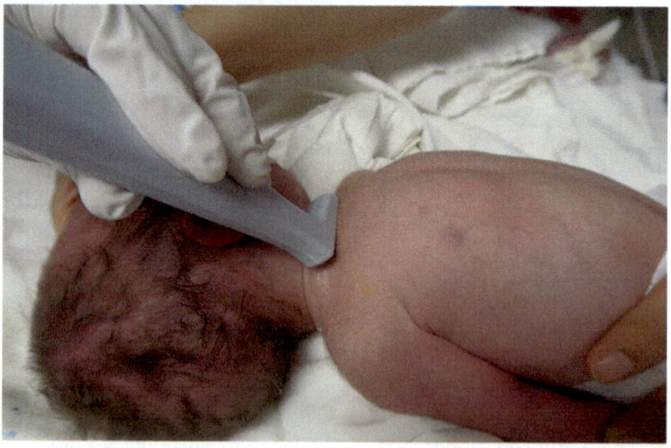

Fig. 3.2 Preliminary vascular assessment

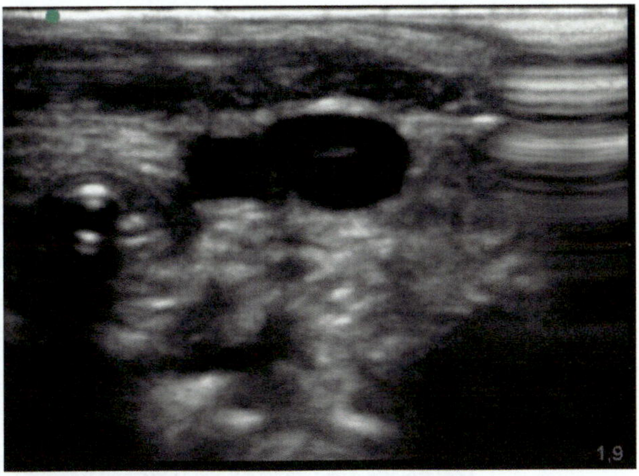

Fig. 3.3 SAX view of cervical vessels
- The scan depth is 1.9 cm
- Visualization of the RIJV and the right carotid artery (RCA)
- The mark on the side of the probe corresponds to the tip of the hockey stick transducer, which is identified on the screen as the aqua dot at the top left of the image. In this case, you are pointing to the patient's left side

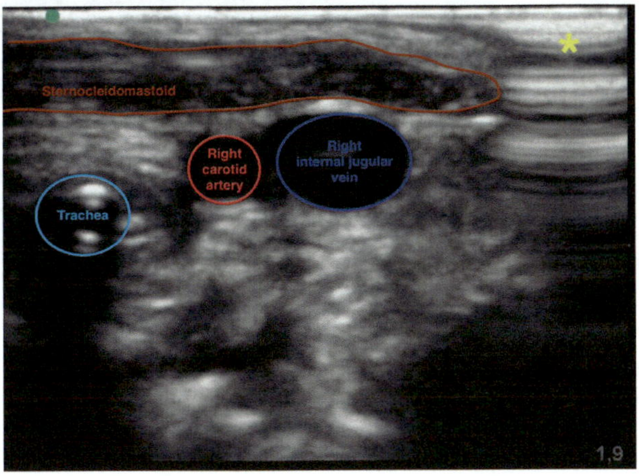

Fig. 3.4 Identifying structures
- In the uppermost part of the sternocleidomastoid muscle (SCM), the approximation of the two components, sternal and clavicular, can be seen
- The RIJV differs from the artery on compression since the vein will change to oval but not the artery
- The trachea is identified with an endotracheal tube
- * Indicates the lack of contact of the transducer on the patient's skin – In Fig. 3.2, the transducer's lateral part (right of the patient) is not in contact with the patient. This view is translated in this ultrasonographic image by transverse lines as barcodes that indicate this lack of contact of the transducer

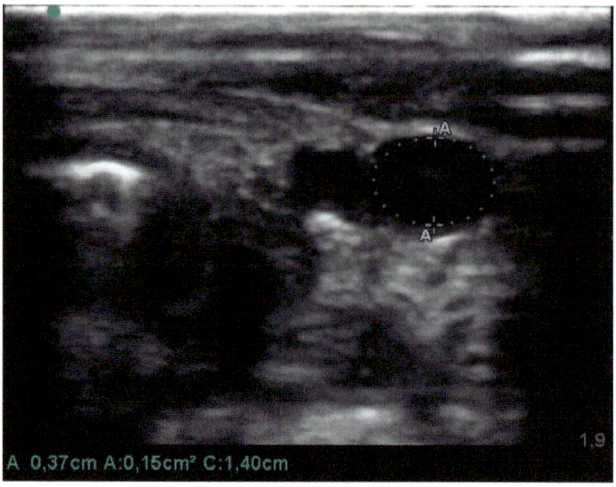

Fig. 3.5 We can measure the diameter of the RIJV 0,37 cm and an area of 0,15 cm²

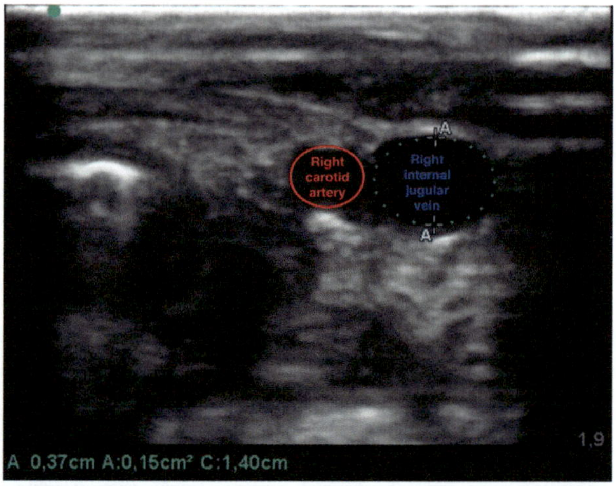

Fig. 3.6 Identifying structures
- The most common position of the RIJV is lateral to the carotid artery, as in this patient
- One of the reasons why the RIJV is positioned anterior to the carotid artery is when the patient is not well sedated. Once the patient is well sedated, the RIJV will be positioned mostly lateral to the RCA
- Turning the head to the contralateral side beyond 70° is another way to change the usual position of the RIJV

3.3 Local Anesthesia Application

- Operator's view: Stand at the patient's head.
- The head is at the bottom of the stretcher and turned to the left side (Fig. 3.7).
- Ultrasound-guided lidocaine infiltration in SAX at the angle of Sedillot's triangle (Fig. 3.8).

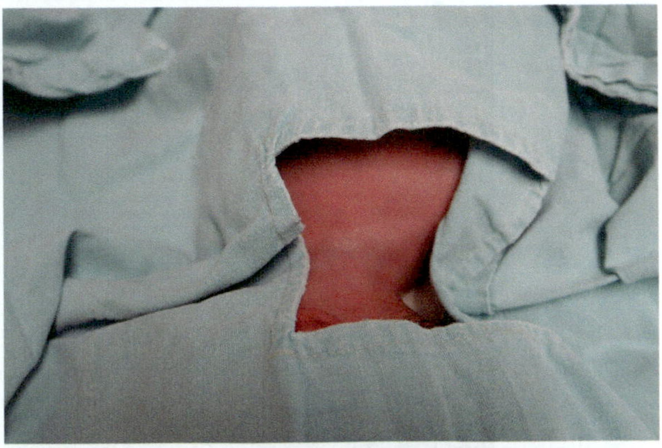

Fig. 3.7 Operator's view

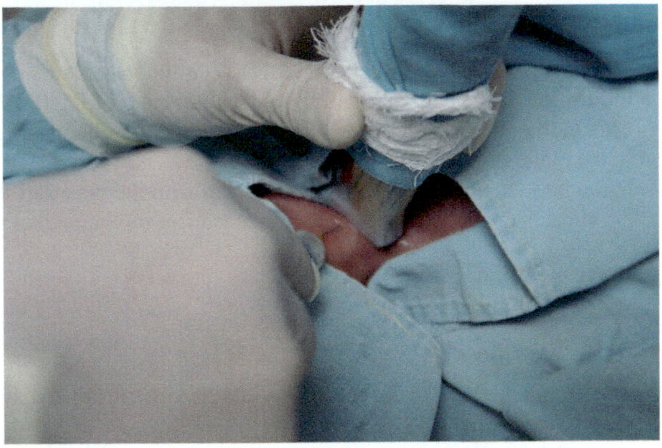

Fig. 3.8 Ultrasound-guided lidocaine infiltration in SAX

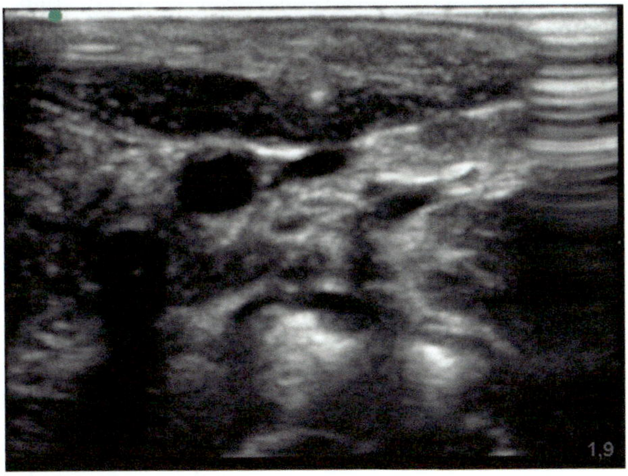

Fig. 3.9 SAX view of lidocaine infiltration

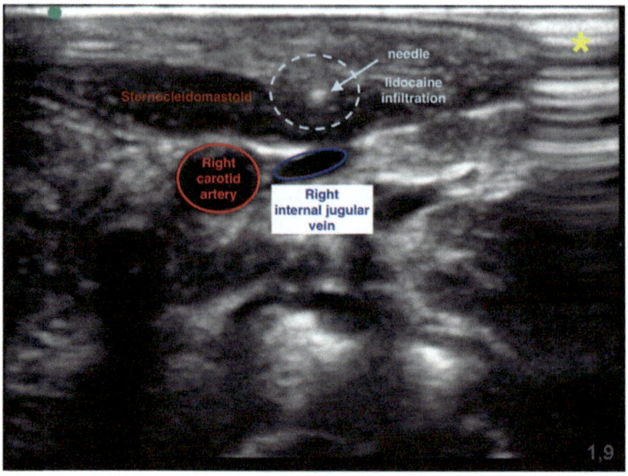

Fig. 3.10 Identifying structures
- The infiltration needle is identified between the subcutaneous tissue and the SCM muscle for infiltration of the path that will follow the puncture of the RIJV
- This moment of the procedure can be used to determine if the site of choice for the puncture is in the plane of the RIJV, as in this case
- It can be seen how the RIJV is compressed with the penetration of the infiltration needle
- * Indicates the lack of contact of the transducer on the patient's skin

- For infiltration, use a small needle 25–27 G.
- Use lidocaine 1%.
- Infiltrate 1–1,5 cm before the chosen venipuncture site to anesthetize the oblique puncture path as well as the fixation site of the catheter holder.
- Visualization of lidocaine infiltration (Figs. 3.9 and 3.10).

3.4 Steps for Real-Time Ultrasound-Guided Access to the Right Internal Jugular Vein in Neonates

3.4.1 Step 01

- A 13-cm, 4 Fr, double-lumen catheter will be placed.
- Operator's view.
- Hold the transducer in your left hand.
- Locate the RIJV in SAX and position the vein in the center of the screen (Figs. 3.11 and 3.12).
- Perform the puncture in the central part of the footprint length (Fig. 3.13) as long as the image of the chosen vessel is also in the center of the screen, as seen in Fig. 3.11.

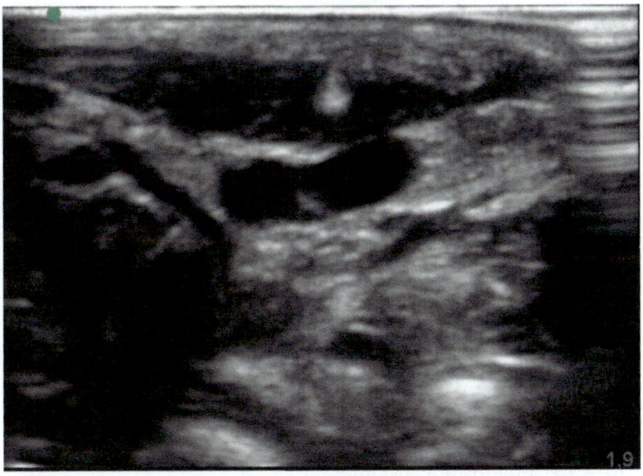

Fig. 3.11 Puncture in the central part of the length of the footprint

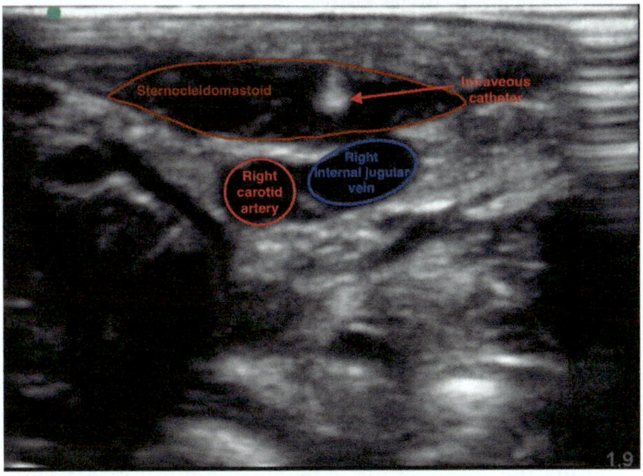

Fig. 3.12 Puncture at a 30–40° degree angle to the skin

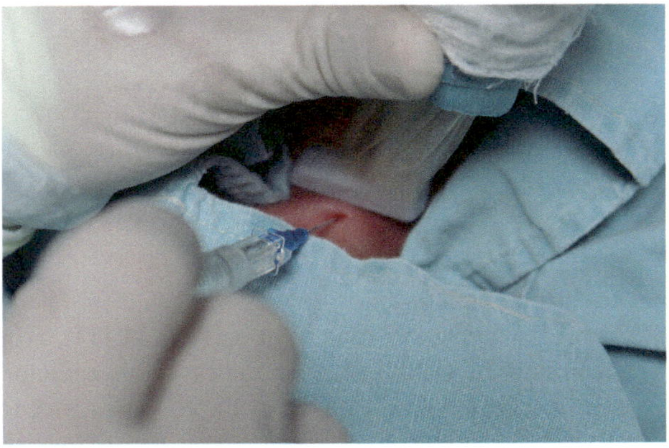

Fig. 3.13 SAX view of the start of the RIJV puncture with the intravenous catheter

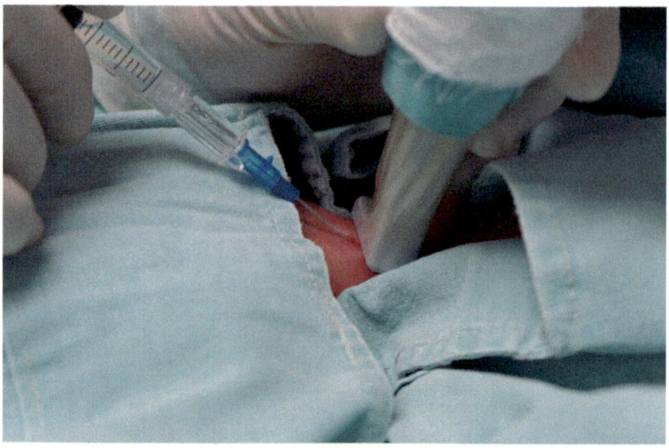

Fig. 3.14 Identifying structures
- In patients weighing less than 1500 g, the angle of the skin puncture allows the needle to pass the subcutaneous tissue easily
- The intravenous catheter can already be seen in the SCM. The intravenous catheter may only be seen in the subcutaneous tissue in children with a more prominent fat pad
- The RIJV is deformed by compression that begins in the anteroposterior direction; from there, its circular shape changes to oval

- Utilize the right hand to perform the puncture with a 22-G intravenous catheter (Fig. 3.13).
- Cannulate the vein with the intravenous catheter (I prefer this method in newborns, even more in premature ones).
- In infants less than 1000 g or with a vein diameter less than 1,4 mm, a 24-G intravenous catheter is preferable for a puncture with a 0.014" micro-guide.
- Start the puncture at a 30–40° degree angle to the skin (Fig. 3.14).
- Then begin the ultrasound-guided dynamic needle tip positioning (DNTP) to guide the intravenous catheter puncture; in other words, sweep down the transducer as you progress with the puncture (Figs. 3.11 and 3.12).

3.4.2 *Step 02*

- Modify the puncture angle to 20–30° (Fig. 3.15).
  - The puncture angle is modified so the vein is not crossed but cannulated.
- Restart the puncture.
- Sweep down the transductor to perform DNTP.
- It can now be visualized as the intravenous catheter has traversed the ECM and is located in the anterior wall of the RIJV (Figs. 3.16 and 3.17).

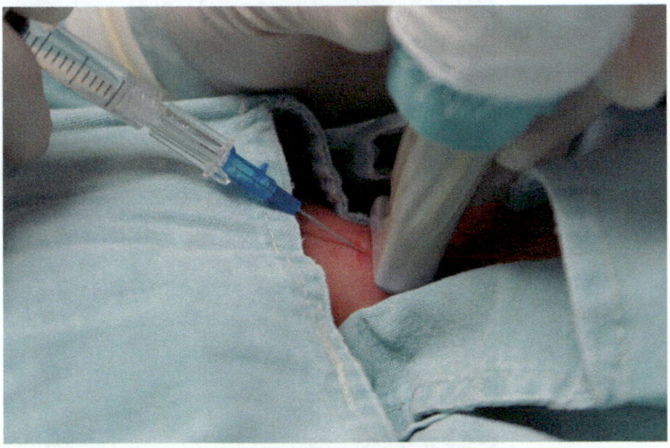

Fig. 3.15 Modify the puncture angle to 20–30°

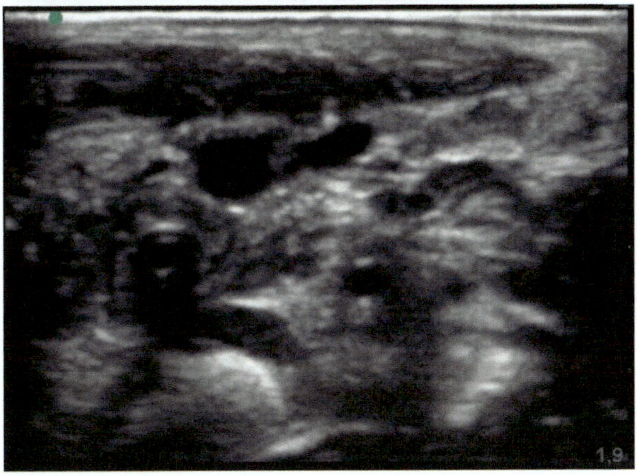

Fig. 3.16 SAX view of the intravenous catheter reaching the anterior wall of the RIJV, right in the middle of the vein

3.4.3 Step 03

- Continuing with the puncture (Fig. 3.18), once you identify that the vein will be penetrated on the ultrasound screen (Figs. 3.19 and 3.20), start with negative pressure on the syringe plunger.
- As experience is gained, a loss of resistance in the puncture may be felt when entering the lumen of the vein. That will be the moment to stop the puncture and start aspiration.

3.4.4 Step 04

- When positioning the intravascular intravenous catheter, apply gentle negative pressure on the syringe plunger as you advance the needle (Fig. 3.21).
- Ultrasound view of the RIJV cannulation (Figs. 3.22 and 3.23).

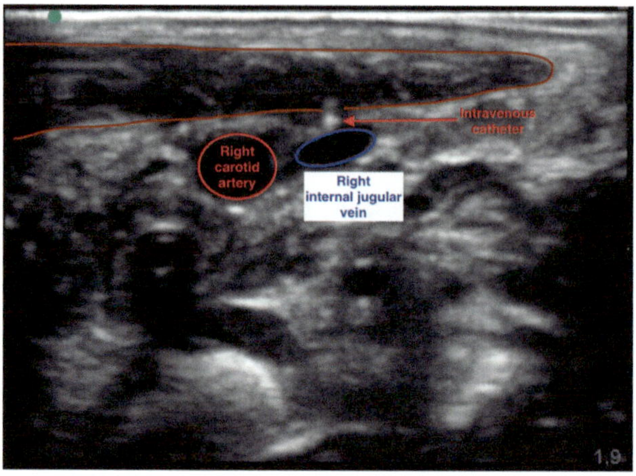

Fig. 3.17 Identifying structures

- A bright hyperechoic (white) dot identifies the tip of the intravenous catheter
- The intravenous catheter has crossed the SCM and is in the anterior wall of the RIJV
- The RIJV is more deformed in its anteroposterior direction due to compression by the intravenous catheter puncture
- The RCA is not deformed since no compression is exerted in its direction

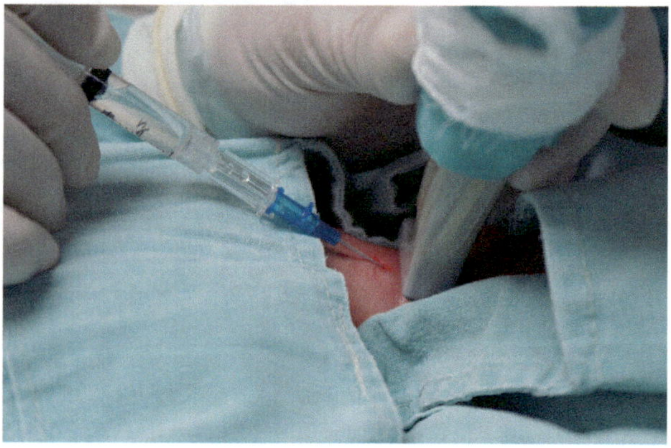

Fig. 3.18 Continue with the puncture and sweep down the transducer to DNTP

3.4.5 Step 05

- Once you have identified the cannulation of the RIJV, set the transducer aside and maintain gentle negative pressure on the syringe plunger.
- Stop advancing when a flash of blood appears in the barrel of the syringe.
- The catheter hub is held firmly so that the catheter tube does not move outward with the suction maneuver (Fig. 3.24).
- Remove the puncture needle and move the catheter tube inside the RIJV to cannulate the vein (Fig. 3.25).

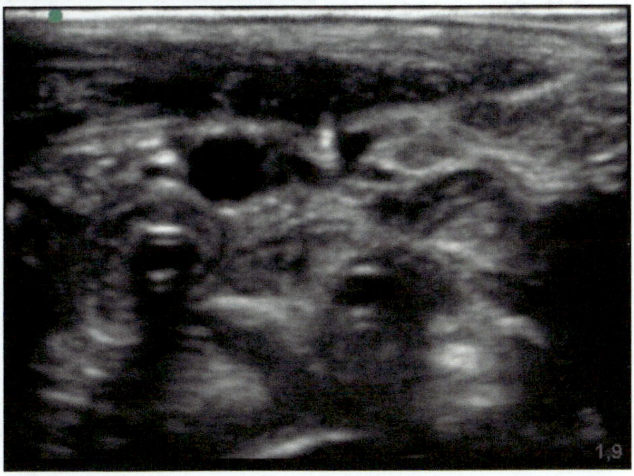

Fig. 3.19 SAX view of the cannulation of the RIJV with the intravenous catheter

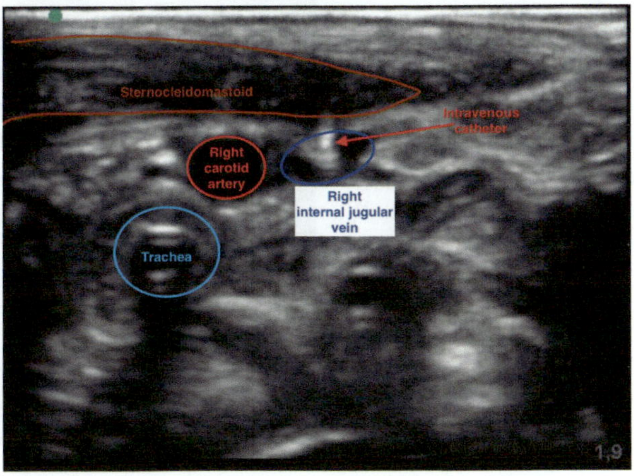

Fig. 3.20 Identifying structures
- The intravenous catheter is located inside the RIJV
- The RIJV is recovering its volume because the intravenous catheter no longer compresses the structures anterior to the vein

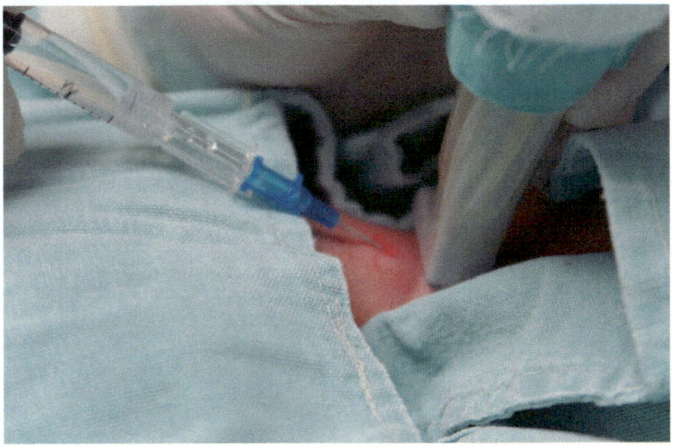

Fig. 3.21 Canalizing the RIJV

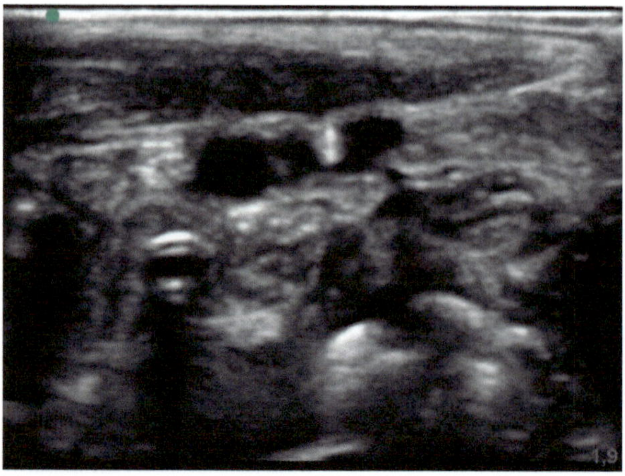

Fig. 3.22 SAX view of the cannulation of the RIJV, right in the central part of the vein

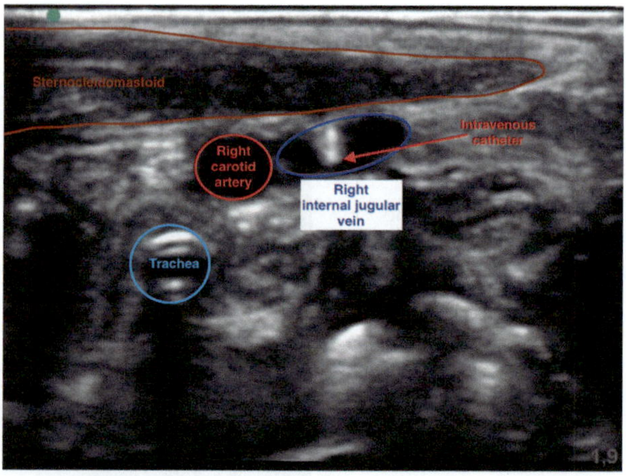

Fig. 3.23 Identifying structures

- Once the RIJV is cannulated, the intravenous catheter is introduced further without puncturing the posterior wall
- Once again, the RIJV has decreased in the anteroposterior caliber but with a smaller decrease than when the procedure began since we are only cannulating the vein

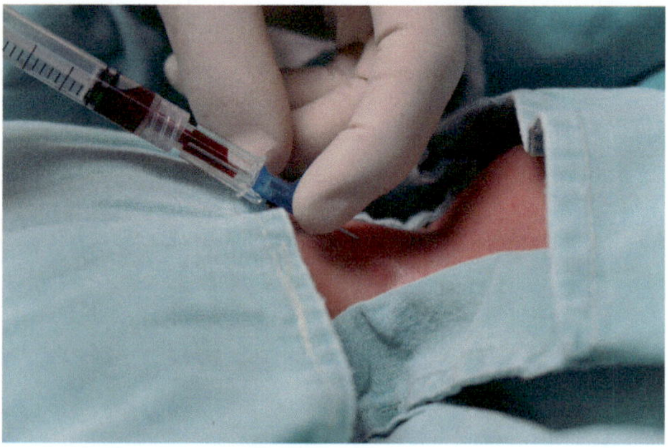

Fig. 3.24 Corroborating the return of blood

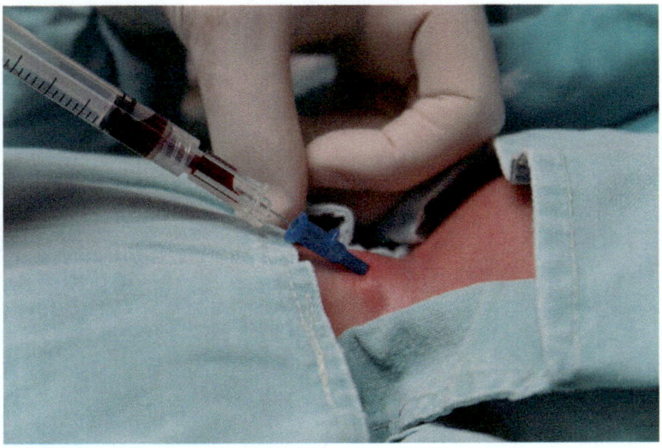

Fig. 3.25 Cannulation of the RIJV

- Once the catheter tube is inserted, the needle is removed. This skill must be practiced to not accidentally remove the catheter.
- Another technique to cannulate the vein is:
  - Once the intravascular location is confirmed by ultrasound, change the puncture angle to 10–20°, and under ultrasonographic view, the intravascular catheter is advanced without puncturing the posterior wall. Then, the puncture needle is withdrawn, and the entire length of the cannula is left in the vessel.

3.4.6 Step 06

- Before you pass the guidewire, check for free blood flow through the catheter tube cannulating the RIJV (Fig. 3.26).
- If there is no blood flow, one of the causes is that the catheter tube was bent intravascularly, so you will need to extract it gently with an aspiration maneuver until blood flows. Then, we will proceed to pass the guidewire.
- Another cause of a lack of blood flow in patients with prominent fat pads is a catheter tube bent by the subcutaneous tissue. Also, the SCM can occlude the catheter tube due to compression in inadequately sedated patients. In this case, performing the puncture with an introducer needle and not an intravenous catheter is preferable.
- Separate the syringe from the catheter hub; to do this, hold the catheter hub firmly so that the catheter tube does not move out of the vein. It must be remembered that the vascular diameters of newborns are millimeters and even more so in premature babies (Fig. 3.27).

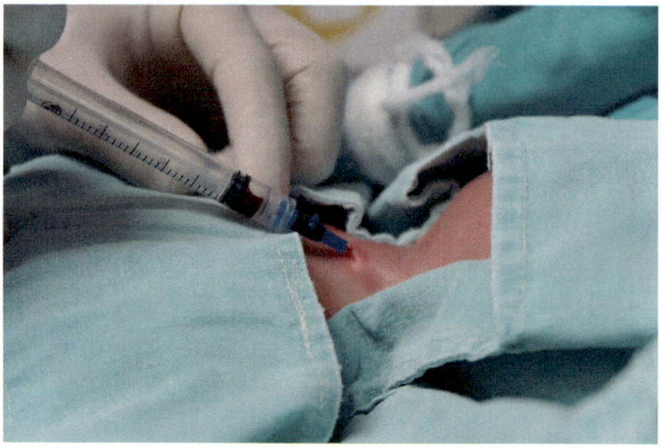

Fig. 3.26 Corroborating cannulation of the RIJV

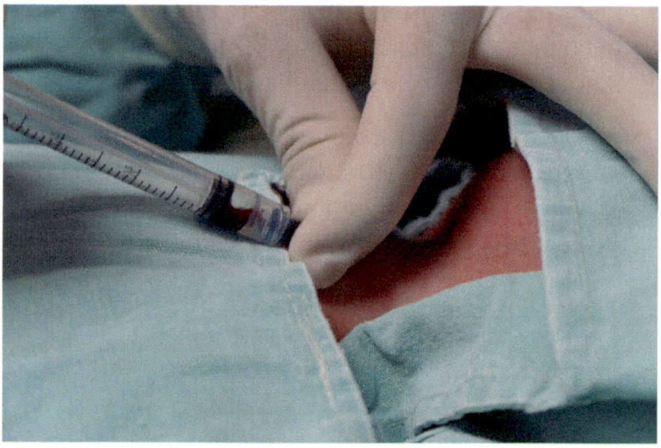

Fig. 3.27 Remove the syringe

3.4.7 Step 07

- Firmly hold the catheter hub. In some patients, it will give a blood return. In extremely premature babies, on occasions, the blood return is not demonstrated (Fig. 3.28).
- Introduce the guide through the catheter hub (Fig. 3.29). If you used the 22-G intravenous catheter (or the 21-G puncture needle), the 0.018" guidewire is correct.
  - If you cannot pass the guidewire and prove that the catheter tube or needle is in the RIJV lumen, try passing the straight part of the guidewire, not the J curved.
- If you performed the puncture with a 24-G intravenous catheter in prematurely less than 1000 g, use a 0.014" guidewire.
- Be sure to pass only enough to be intravascular and not reach the heart.

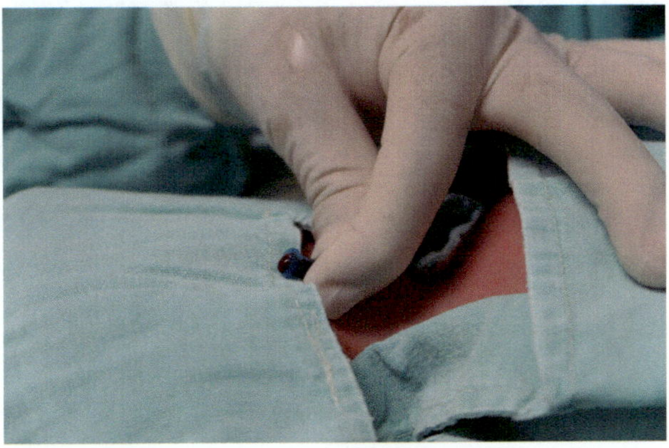

Fig. 3.28 Manual fixation of the intravenous catheter

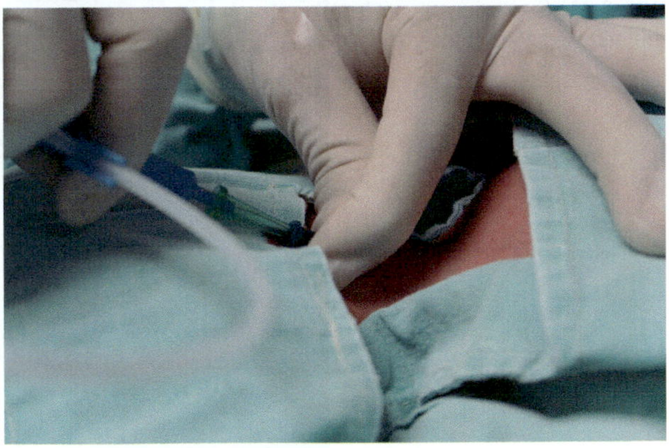

Fig. 3.29 Introduction of the guidewire through the intravenous cannula

- Scan to confirm the intravenous location of the guidewire. Place the transducer transverse on the neck (Fig. 3.30).
- Ultrasound view of the guidewire in SAX view (Figs. 3.31 and 3.32).

3.4.8 Step 08

- With the middle finger of the left hand, occlude the entry of the guide into the skin and expose the distal tip of the guide to pass the dilator (Fig. 3.33).
- Perform dilation with the right hand and countertraction of the skin with the left hand, and with a "screw" maneuver, the path of the skin and subcutaneous cell tissue is dilated up to the entrance of the RIJV (Fig. 3.34).
- Carefully perform this procedure at this age; it will not require a skin incision.
- If a lot of subcutaneous pressure is exerted without countertraction, the guidewire can be bent, hindering dilation and passage of the central venous catheter.

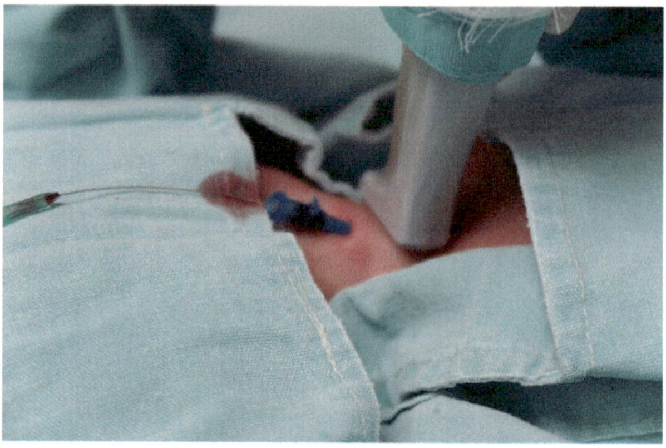

Fig. 3.30 Scanning in SAX view, hockey stick transducer, transverse on the neck

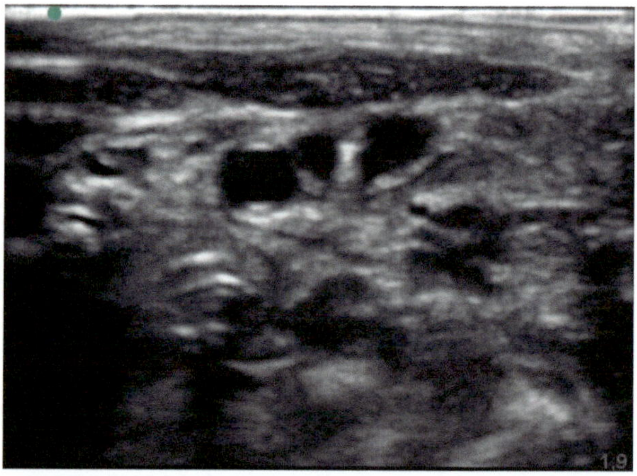

Fig. 3.31 SAX view of the intravascular guidewire

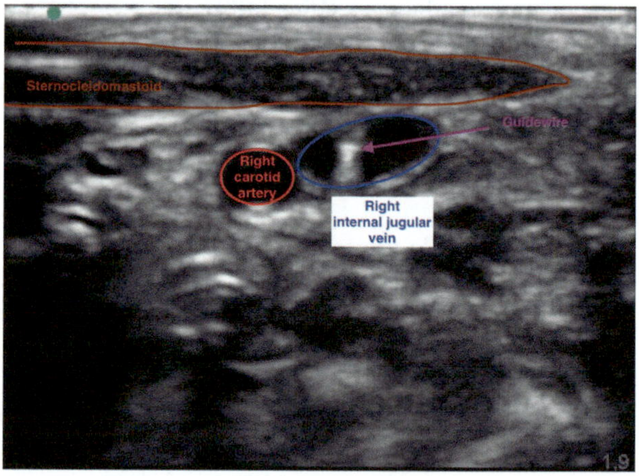

Fig. 3.32 Identifying structures

- The guidewire in the RIJV appears more echogenic with the comet tail sign and can be followed by sliding the transducer to the clavicle

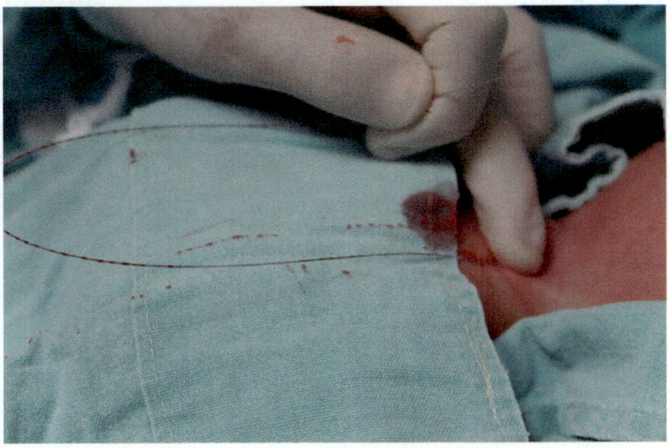

Fig. 3.33 Exposition of the distal tip of the guidewire to pass the dilator

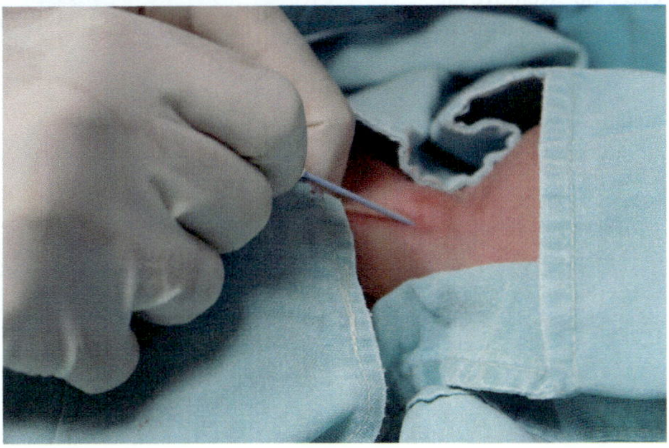

Fig. 3.34 Perform dilation of the path of the skin at the entrance of the RIJV

- Extract the dilator and, with the index finger of the left hand, occlude the exit in the skin so the patient does not bleed (Fig. 3.35).

3.4.9 Step 09

- Advance the catheter over the guidewire (Seldinger's technique) (Fig. 3.36).
- When you have the required intravascular catheter length, remove the guidewire.
- Scan the RIJV in SAX view to corroborate the intravascular CVC (Figs. 3.37 and 3.38).

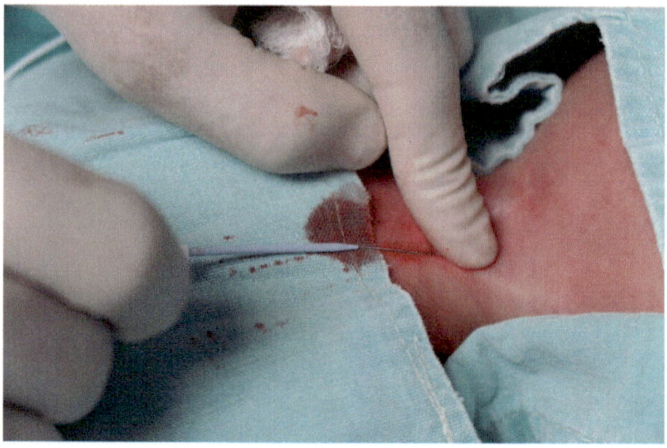

Fig. 3.35 Extract the dilator

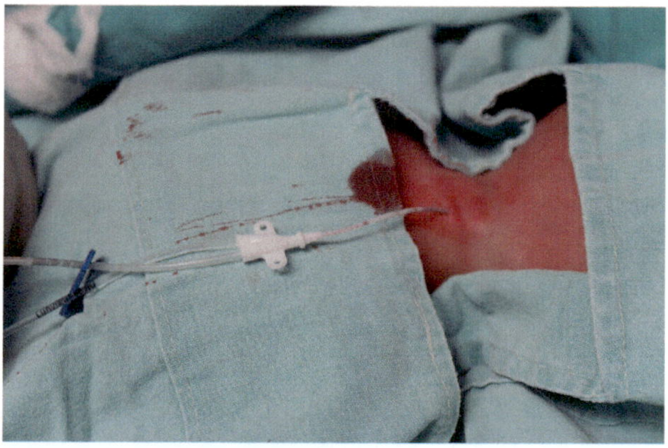

Fig. 3.36 Remove the guidewire and leave the intravascular CVC

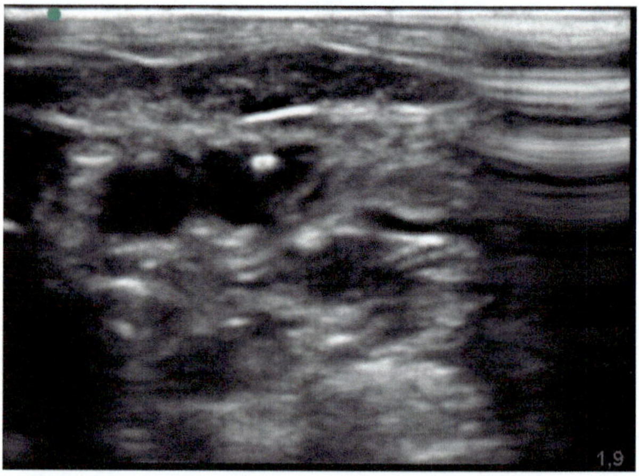

Fig. 3.37 SAX view of the catheter

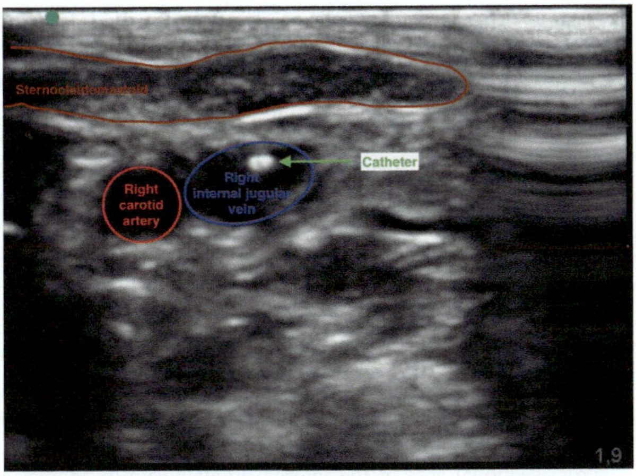

Fig. 3.38 Identifying structures
- The RIJV has been restored almost completely in its diameter
- The catheter inside the RIJV; the two lumens can be identified
- No residual perivascular hematoma is seen

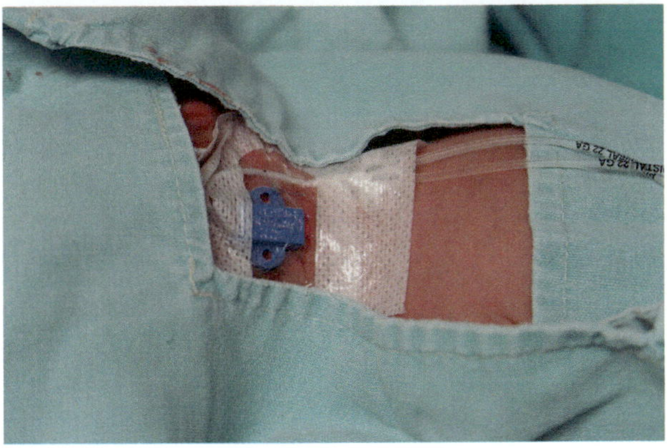

Fig. 3.39 Catheter with a sterile occlusive dressing

3.4.10 Step 10

- Secure the catheter and place a sterile occlusive dressing according to the institutional protocol (Fig. 3.39).

Sources

1. Spencer TR, Pittiruti M. Rapid central vein assessment (RaCeVA): a systematic, standardized approach for ultrasound assessment before central venous catheterization. J Vasc Access. 2019;20(3):239–49. https://doi.org/10.1177/1129729818804718. Epub 2018 Oct 4. PMID: 30286688.

2. Maddali MM, Al-Shamsi F, Arora NR, Panchatcharam SM. The optimal length of insertion for central venous catheters via the right internal jugular vein in pediatric cardiac surgical patients. J Cardiothorac Vasc Anesth. 2020;34(9):2386–91. https://doi.org/10.1053/j.jvca.2020.03.007.
3. Montes-Tapia F, Hernández-Trejo K, García-Rodríguez F, et al. Predicting the optimal depth of ultrasound-guided right internal jugular vein central venous catheters in neonates. J Pediatr Surg. 2020;55(9):1920–4. https://doi.org/10.1016/j.jpedsurg.2019.12.004.
4. Zanolla GR, Baldisserotto M, Piva J. How useful is ultrasound guidance for internal jugular venous access in children? J Pediatr Surg. 2018;53(4):789–93. https://doi.org/10.1016/j.jpedsurg.2017.08.010.
5. Montes-Tapia F, Rodríguez-Taméz A, Cura-Esquivel I, et al. Efficacy and safety of ultrasound-guided internal jugular vein catheterization in low-birth-weight newborn. J Pediatr Surg. 2016;51(10):1700–3. https://doi.org/10.1016/j.jpedsurg.2016.05.014.
6. Turker G, Kaya FN, Gurbet A, Aksu H, Erdogan C, Atlas A. Internal jugular vein cannulation: an ultrasound-guided technique versus a landmark-guided technique. Clinics (Sao Paulo). 2009;64(10):989–92. https://doi.org/10.1590/S1807-59322009001000009.
7. Morita M, Sasano H, Azami T, Sasano N, Katsuya H. The skin-traction method increases the cross-sectional area of the internal jugular vein by increasing its anteroposterior diameter. J Anesth. 2007;21(4):467–71. https://doi.org/10.1007/s00540-007-0562-6.

Chapter 4
Left Internal Jugular Vein in Pediatrics

4.1 Patient Positioning

- The patient is a 6-month-old patient weighing 3.8 kg.
- Position the patient supine near the head of the bed.
- Position the patient's head slightly to the right (Fig. 4.1).
- Place a roll under the shoulders to increase the length of the cervical region and create a wider space between the clavicle and jaw.
- Gently hold the upper extremities with the arms caudal.
- Due to the malnutrition of this patient, Sedillot's triangle can be seen very clearly due to the prominence of the two heads (clavicular and sternal) of the sternocleidomastoid muscle (SCM) (Fig. 4.2).

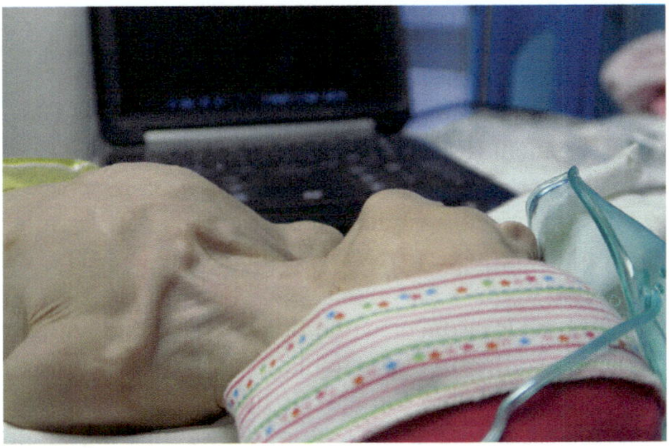

Fig. 4.1 Patient positioning

F. Montes-Tapia, *Atlas of Ultrasound-Guided Central Venous Catheter Placement*, https://doi.org/10.1007/978-3-031-61887-1_4

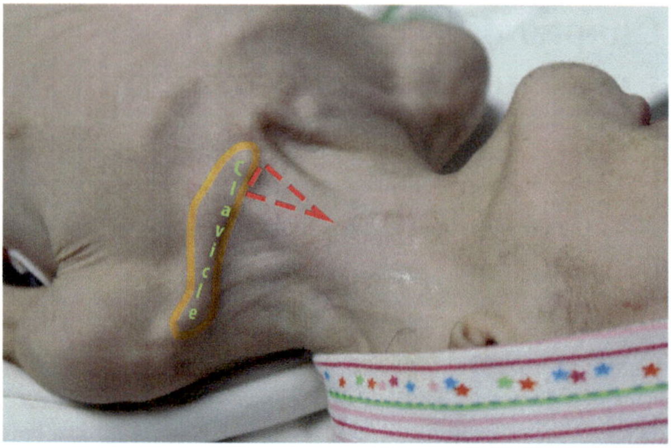

Fig. 4.2 Sedillot's triangle

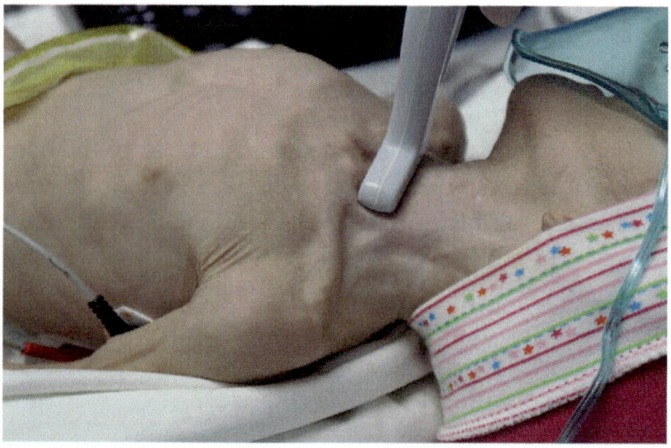

Fig. 4.3 Place the transducer transversely in the Sedillot's triangle for SAX view

4.2 Scanning Technique

- Do a preliminary vascular assessment (non-sterile), known as rapid central vein assessment (RaCeVA).
- The operator stands at the patient's head.
- Position the ultrasound on the patient's left or right side or foot level.
- A high-frequency linear transducer (13–6 MHz) with a hockey stick-type probe can be used.
- Hold the transducer with your left hand and with the transducer transverse to the neck and the tip of the hockey stick transducer to the patient's left side.
- Begin the scan of the vessels in the middle of the neck and sweep down.
- Finish scanning at the base of the Sedillot's triangle (Fig. 4.3).
- View of the left carotid artery (LCA) and left internal jugular vein (LIJV) in short-axis (SAX) view (Figs. 4.4 and 4.5).

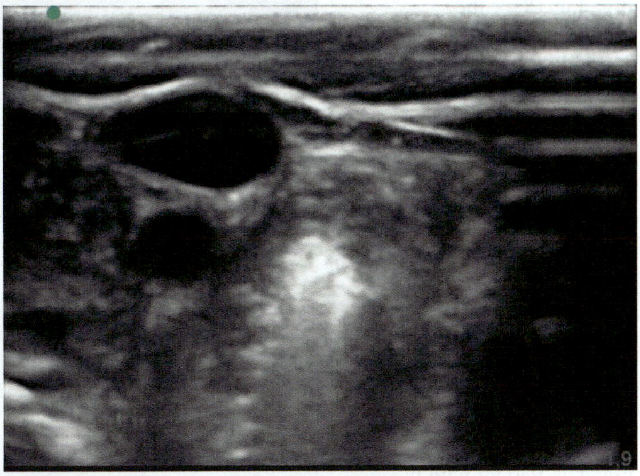

Fig. 4.4 SAX view of cervical vessels
- The depth of the scan is 1,9 cm
- The diameter of the RIJV is 0,55 cm

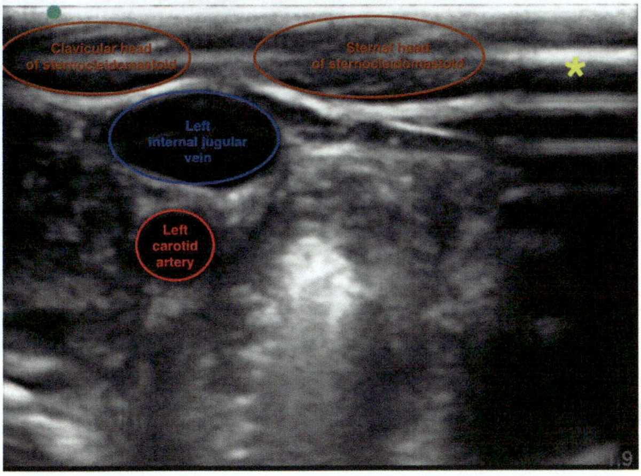

Fig. 4.5 Identifying structures
- The LIJV is anterior to the LCA
- You can see the two separate heads of the SCM in relation to Sedillot's triangle
- * Indicates the lack of contact of the transducer on the patient's skin
  – In Fig. 4.3, the transducer's medial part (right of the patient) is not in contact with the patient. This view is translated in this ultrasonographic image by transverse lines as barcodes that indicate this lack of contact of the transducer

- Scan the vessels in the long-axis (LAX) view; however, you can see that it practically involves the entire neck length, and there would be no space to perform the puncture (Fig. 4.6).

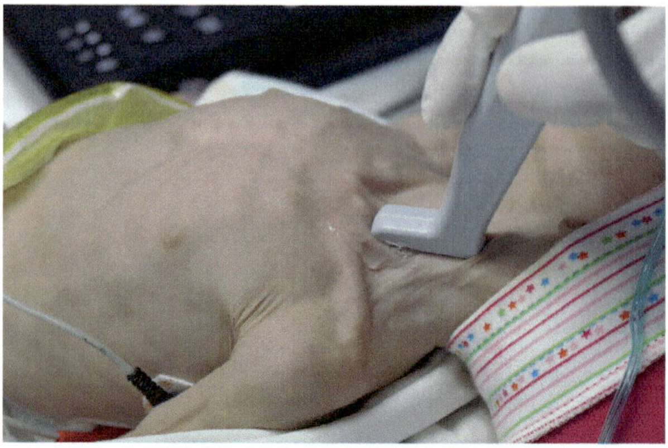

Fig. 4.6 Place the transducer longitudinally in Sedillot's triangle for LAX view

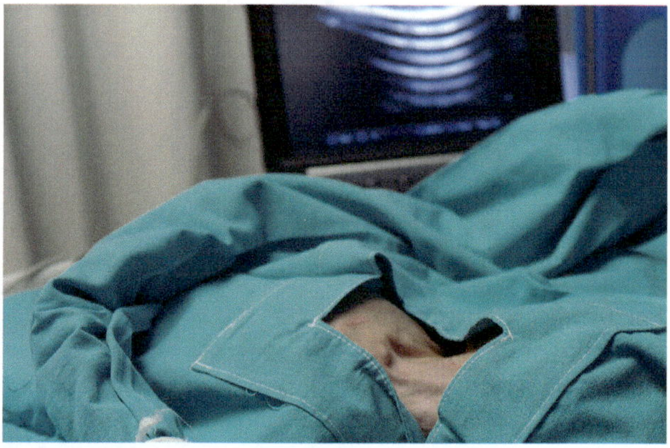

Fig. 4.7 Patient with the head to the right

4.3 Local Anesthesia Application

- Patient with the head to the right (Fig. 4.7).
- The sterile field only leaves the cervical, upper pectoral, and left shoulder regions uncovered.
- Real-time ultrasound-guided lidocaine infiltration (Fig. 4.8).
- For infiltration, use a small needle 25–27 G.
- Use lidocaine 1%.
- Ultrasound-guided infiltration is 1–1,5 cm before the chosen venipuncture site to anesthetize the oblique puncture path as well as the fixation site of the catheter holder.

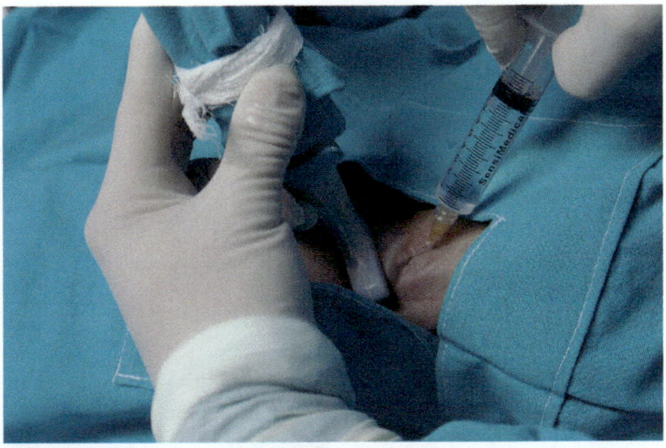

Fig. 4.8 Ultrasound-guided infiltration of lidocaine

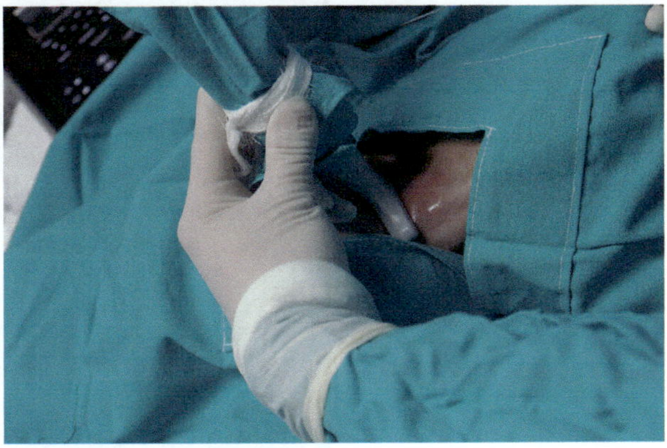

Fig. 4.9 Place the transducer transversely in Sedillot's triangle for SAX view

4.4 Steps for Real-Time Ultrasound-Guided Access to the Left Internal Jugular Vein in Pediatrics

4.4.1 Step 01

- A 13-cm, 4 Fr, double-lumen catheter will be placed.
- Hold the transducer in your left hand (Fig. 4.9).
- Locate the LIJV in SAX view and position the vein in the center of the monitor.
- SAX view of the cervical veins (Figs. 4.10 and 4.11).

4.4.2 Step 02

- Perform the puncture with a 22-G intravenous catheter or use a 21-G introducer needle.

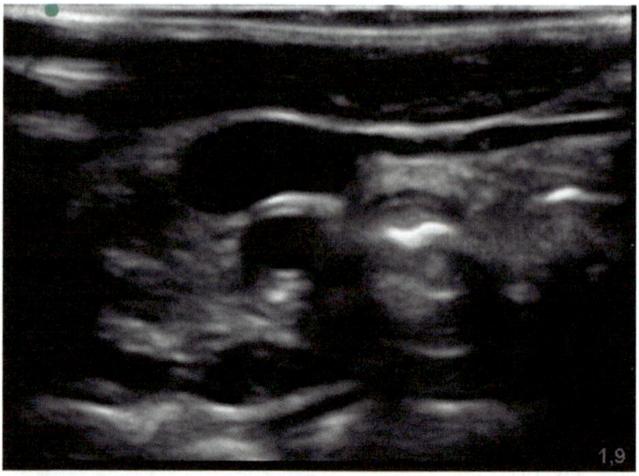

Fig. 4.10 SAX view of cervical vessels

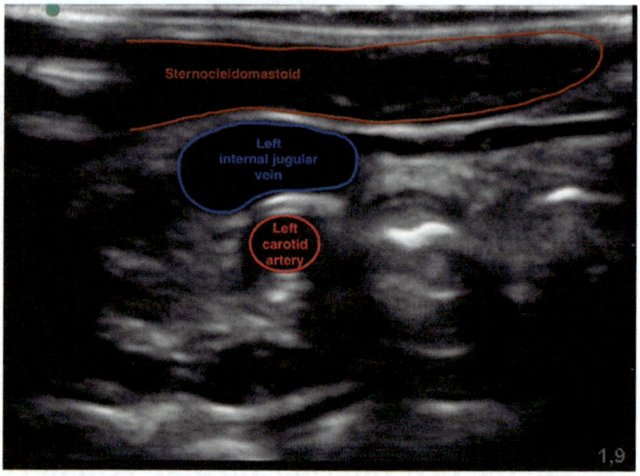

Fig. 4.11 Identifying structures
- The compression exerted by the transducer slightly deforms the vein
- The LIJV over the LCA

- Perform the puncture in the central part of the footprint length as long as the image of the LIJV is in the center of the screen, as seen in Fig. 4.12. This maneuver will make it easier for the puncture to be carried out (Fig. 4.13).
- Start the puncture with an angle of 40–50° in relation to the skin.
- Begin the ultrasound-guided dynamic needle tip positioning (DNTP) to guide the puncture in real time.
- The intravascular catheter has penetrated the skin and is passing the sternocleidomastoid muscle (SCM) (Figs. 4.12 and 4.14).

4.4.3 Step 03

- Continue the puncture with DTNP of the intravenous catheter (Fig. 4.15).
- As you advance with a real-time ultrasound-guided puncture, there is sweep down displacement of the transducer (Fig. 4.16).

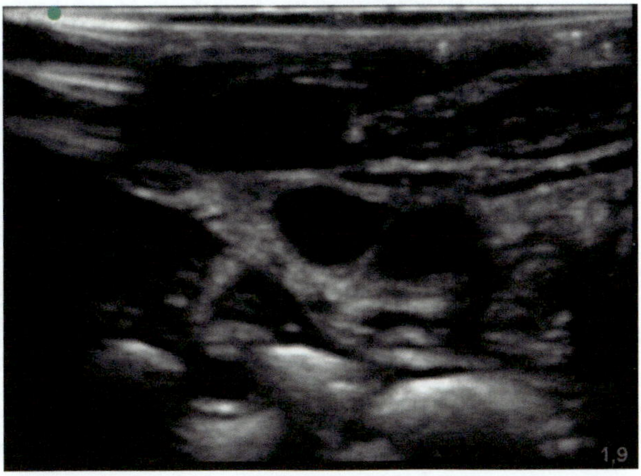

Fig. 4.12 Puncture at a 40–50° angle in relation to the skin and the central part of the footprint length

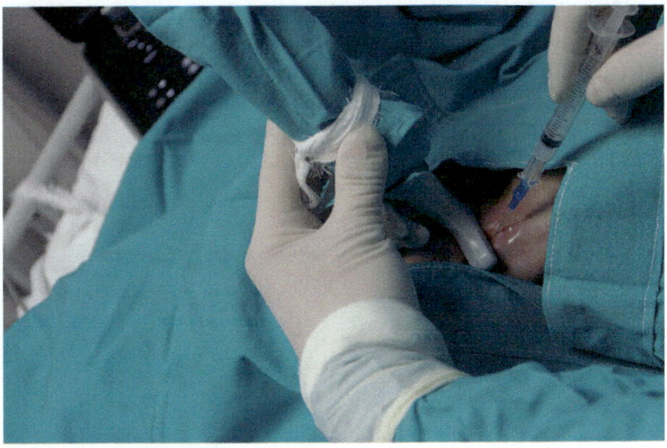

Fig. 4.13 SAX view of the start of the LIJV puncture with the intravenous catheter

- Always keep the puncture in the middle of the transducer.
- Progression of the puncture, the intravenous catheter is in the SCM (Figs. 4.17 and 4.18).

4.4.4 Step 04

- Operator view.
- Operator stands at the patient's head.
- Continue the puncture in the central part of the length of the hockey stick transducer (Fig. 4.19).
- Once you have identified on the screen that the intravenous catheter is at the anterior wall of the LIJV (Figs. 4.20 and 4.21), the vein will be cannulated and advance the puncture.
- Stop the puncture (Fig. 4.22) when it is seen on the screen (Figs. 4.23 and 4.24) that the intravenous catheter has cannulated the LIJV.

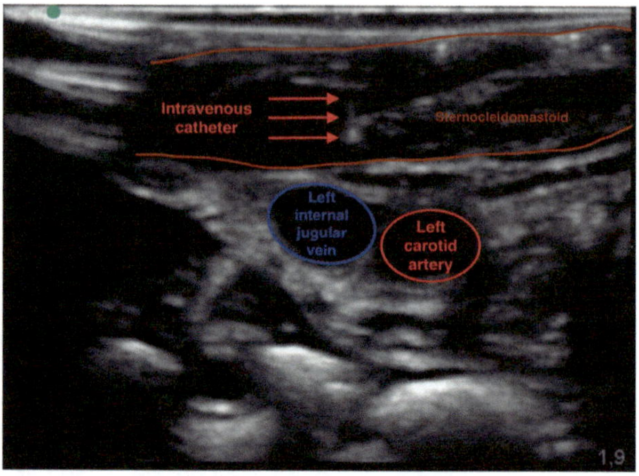

Fig. 4.14 Identifying structures
- Now, the LIJV has been mobilized, maintaining a lateral position to the LCA
- The intravenous catheter tip is identified as a bright hyperechoic (white) dot
- The intravascular catheter has penetrated the skin and is passing the SCM
- This rapid penetration of the puncture is due to the angle with which we are starting the puncture and because of the little subcutaneous tissue
- The trajectory of the intravascular catheter is in the direction of the LIJV

Fig. 4.15 Begin with DNTP (sweep down the transductor) of the intravenous catheter puncture

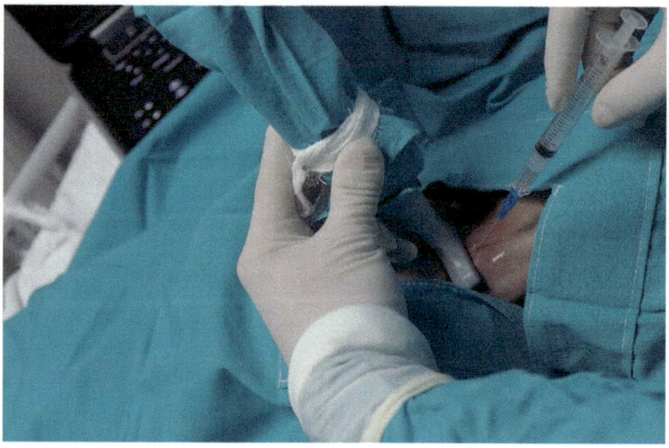

4.4.5 Step 05

- Once you have identified on the screen the intravascular intravenous catheter, set the transducer aside.
- Hold the flange of the intravenous catheter hub with your left hand.

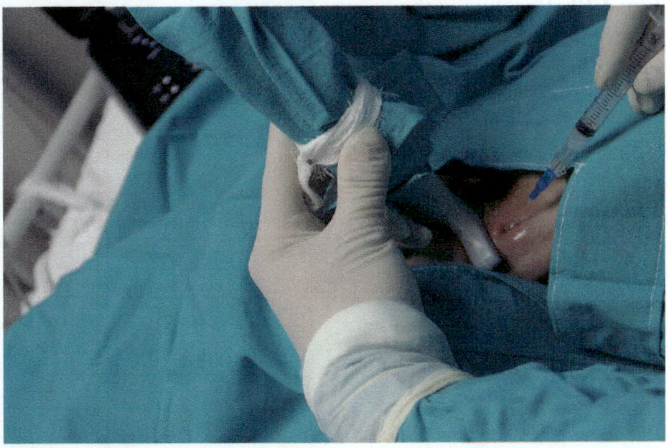

Fig. 4.16 Sweep down the transducer to follow the intravenous catheter tip on the screen (Figs. 4.17 and 4.18)

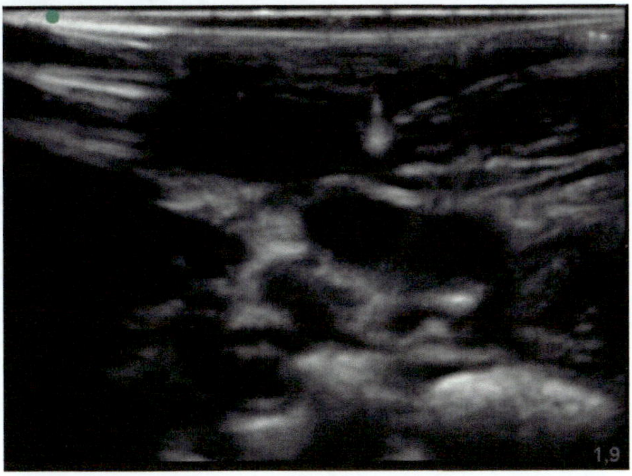

Fig. 4.17 SAX view of the progress of the puncture by the intravascular catheter

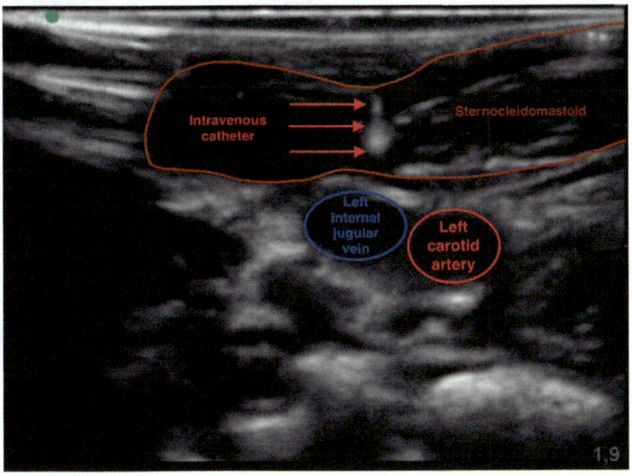

Fig. 4.18 Identifying structures

- The tip of the intravenous catheter is identified as a bright hyperechoic (white) dot
- The puncture is developing in the direction of the center of the LIJV

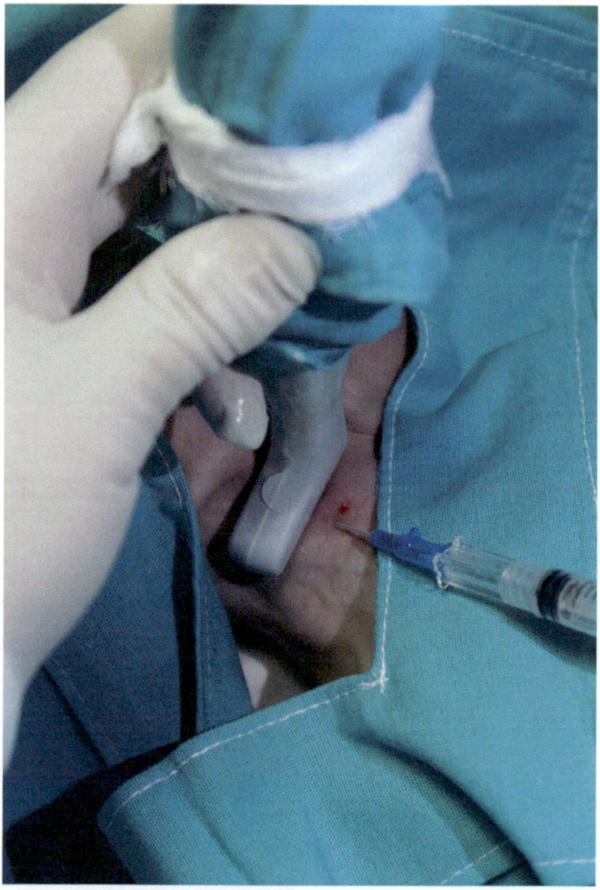

Fig. 4.19 Puncture in the central part of the length of the hockey stick transducer

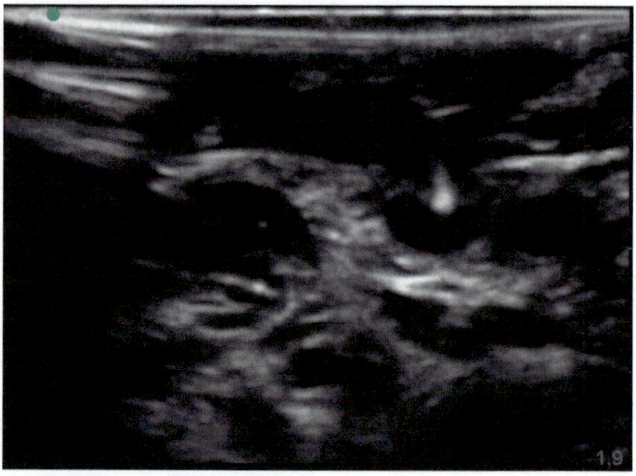

Fig. 4.20 SAX view of the intravenous catheter reaching the LIJV

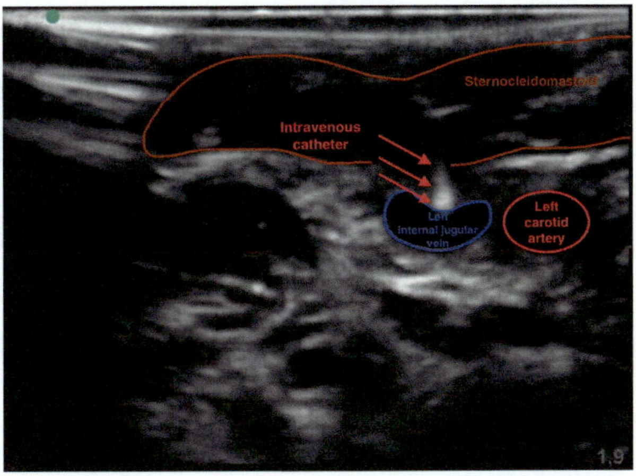

Fig. 4.21 Identifying structures

- The intravenous catheter has reached the anterior wall of the LIJV, right in the middle of the vein
- The LIJV is deformed by compression of the puncture

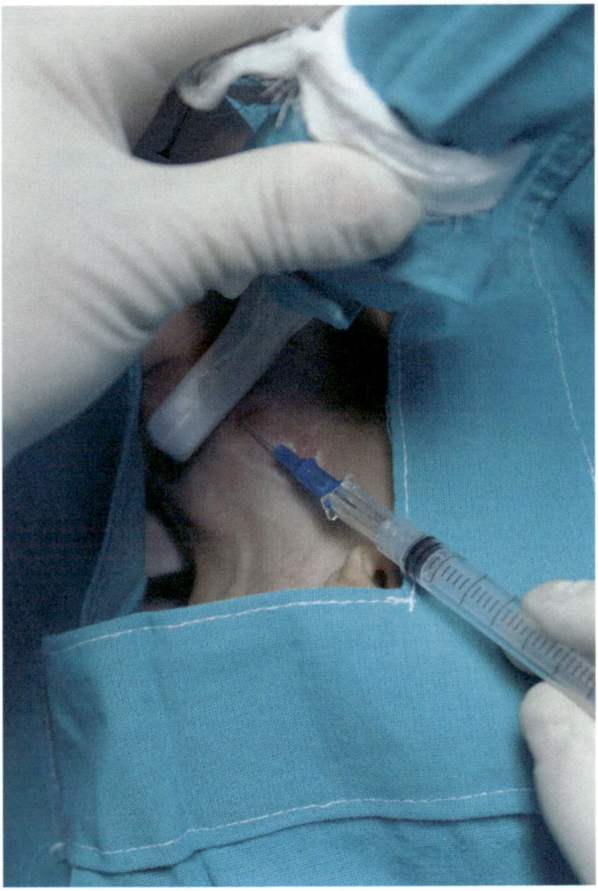

Fig. 4.22 Stop the puncture when it is seen that the intravenous catheter has cannulated the LIJV

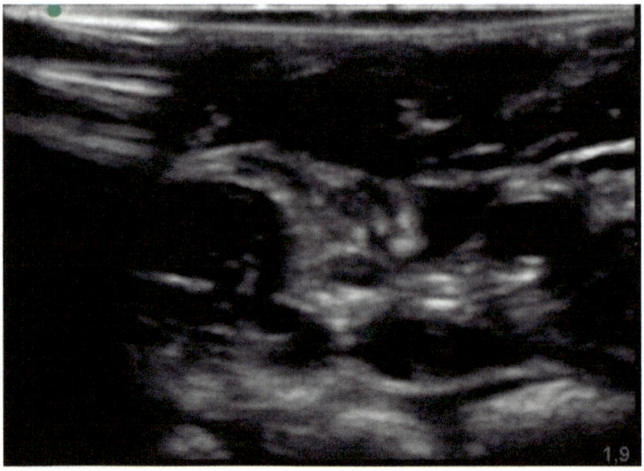

Fig. 4.23 SAX view of the puncture of the LIJV

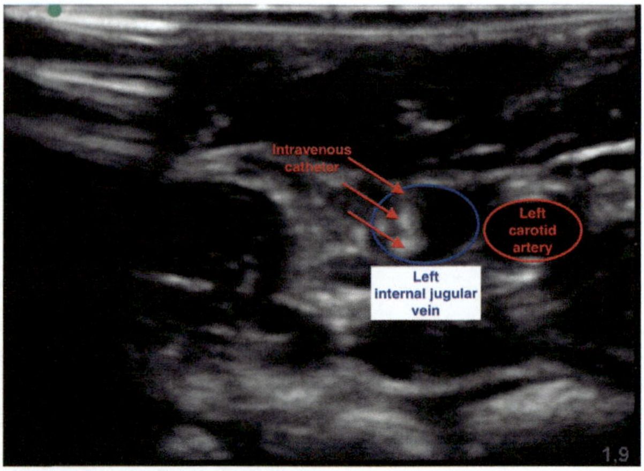

Fig. 4.24 Identifying structures
- The intravenous catheter is located inside the LIJV
- Since there is no further compression with the puncture, the vein recovers its shape

- Apply gentle negative pressure on the syringe plunger (Fig. 4.25).
- If the vein is well cannulated, the aspiration will rapidly extract blood (Fig. 4.26).

4.4.6 Step 06

- Hold the flange of the intravenous catheter hub and insert it, displacing it from the puncture needle to cannulate the vein (Fig. 4.27).
- Remove the puncture needle and move the catheter tube inside the LIJV to cannulate the vein (Fig. 4.28).
- Once the catheter tube is inserted, the needle is removed. This skill must be practiced to not accidentally remove the catheter.
- Another technique to cannulate the vein is:

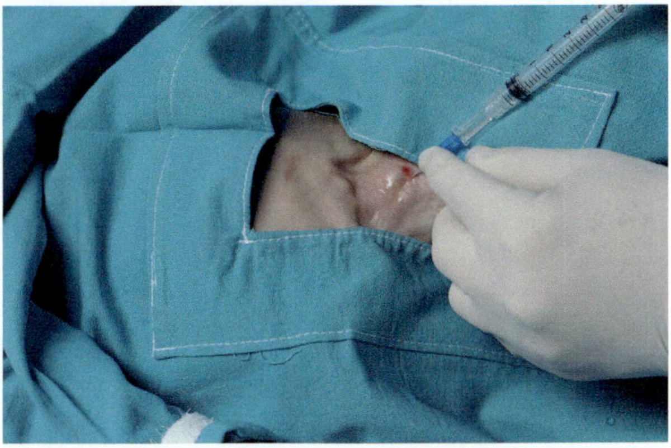

Fig. 4.25 Maintain gentle negative pressure on the syringe plunger

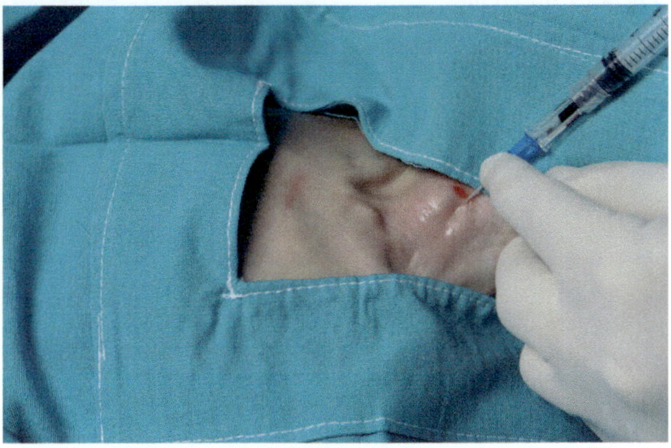

Fig. 4.26 Return of blood in the syringe

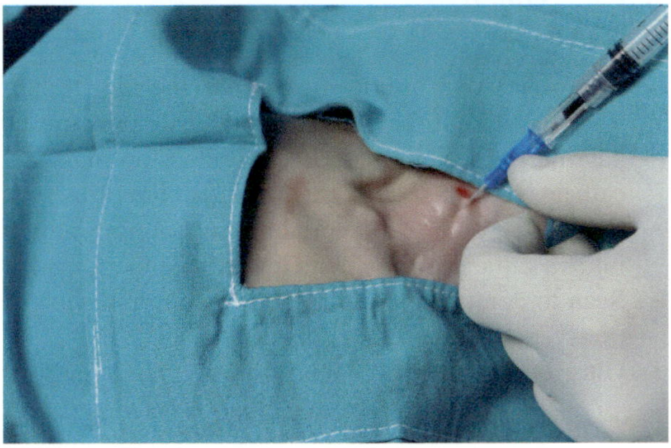

Fig. 4.27 Hold the flange of the intravenous catheter hub and insert it

o Once the intravascular location is confirmed by ultrasound, change the puncture angle to 10–20°, and under ultrasonographic guide, the intravenous catheter is advanced without puncturing the posterior wall. Then, the puncture needle is withdrawn, and the entire length of the cannula is left in the vessel.

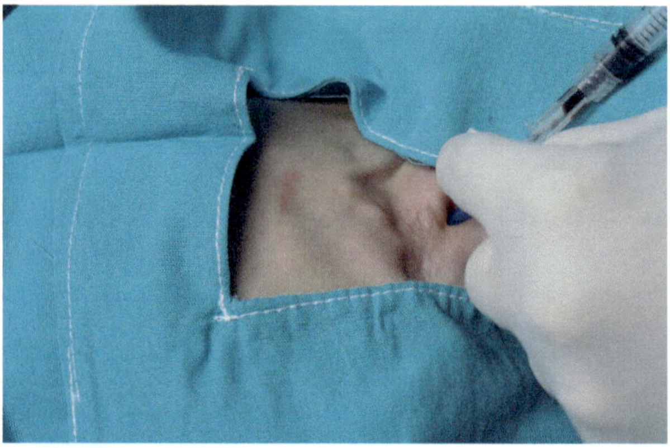

Fig. 4.28 Remove the puncture needle and move the catheter tube inside the LIJV

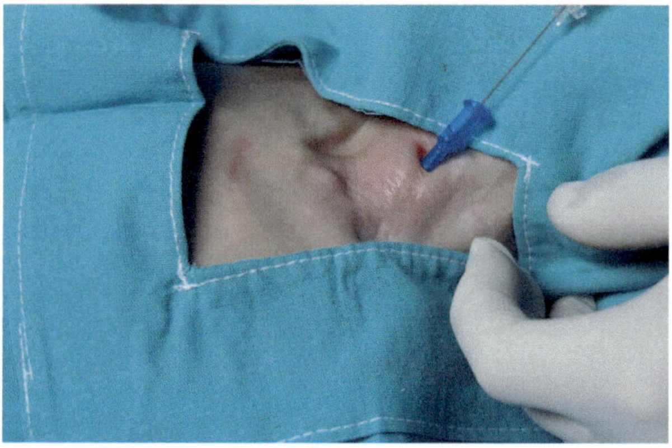

Fig. 4.29 Insert the guidewire

4.4.7 Step 07

- Insert the 0.018" guidewire through the catheter hub (Fig. 4.29).
- The J-tip end of the guide should easily pass through. If it does not, you can try passing the straight end. If it still does not pass, there may be a chance that the catheter tube has accidentally slipped out of the vein.
- On the left side, it is preferable to pass the J-tip, as this will help navigate the intravascular pathway, which is very sinuous up to the superior cava vein.
- Scan to confirm the intravenous location of the guidewire. Place the transducer transverse on the neck (Fig. 4.30).
- Ultrasound view of the guidewire in SAX view (Figs. 4.31 and 4.32).

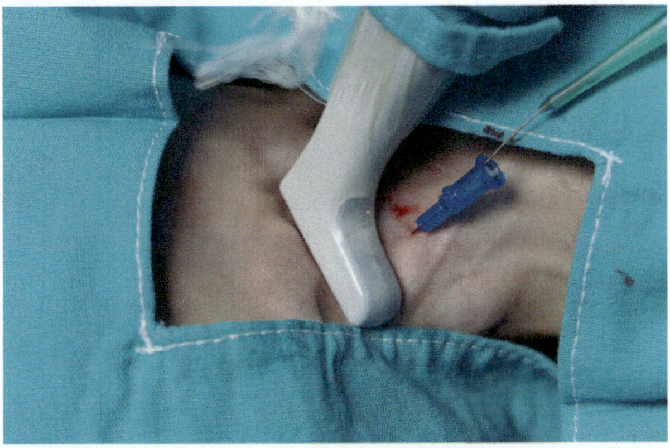

Fig. 4.30 Scanning in SAX view, hockey stick transducer, transverse on the neck

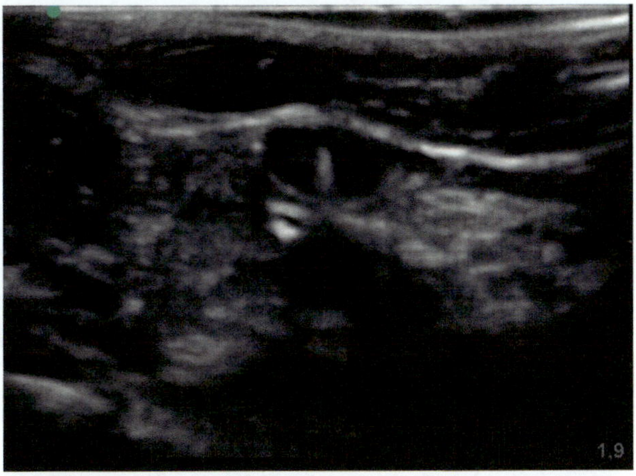

Fig. 4.31 SAX view of the intravascular guidewire

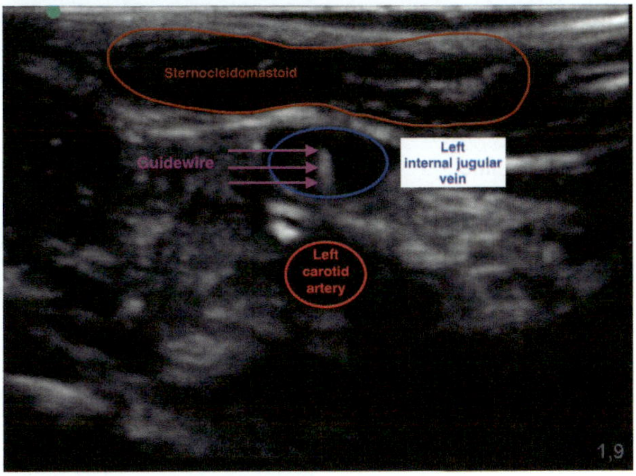

Fig. 4.32 Identifying structures

- The guidewire is found intravascularly. It is identified as a more hyperechoic dot point with the comet tail sign
- The LIJV has again been placed anterior to the LCA

4.4.8 *Step 08*

- Perform dilation with the right hand and countertraction of the skin with the left hand, and with a "screw" maneuver, the path of the skin and subcutaneous tissue is dilated up to the entrance of the LIJV (Fig. 4.33).
- Carefully perform this procedure at this age; it will not require a skin incision.
- The introduction of the dilator should be gentle so that the guide is not bent (Fig. 4.34).
- If a lot of subcutaneous pressure is exerted without countertraction, the guidewire can be bent, hindering dilation and passage of the central venous catheter.

4.4.9 *Step 09*

- Advance the catheter over the guidewire (Seldinger's technique).
- When you have the required intravascular catheter length, remove the guidewire (Fig. 4.35).

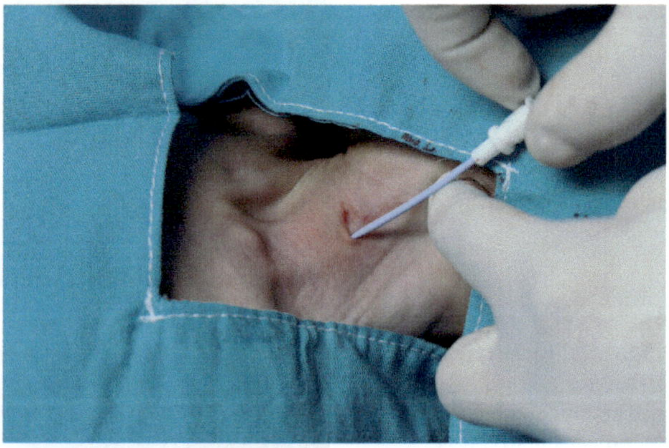

Fig. 4.33 Dilate the skin and subcutaneous tissue path to the LIJV

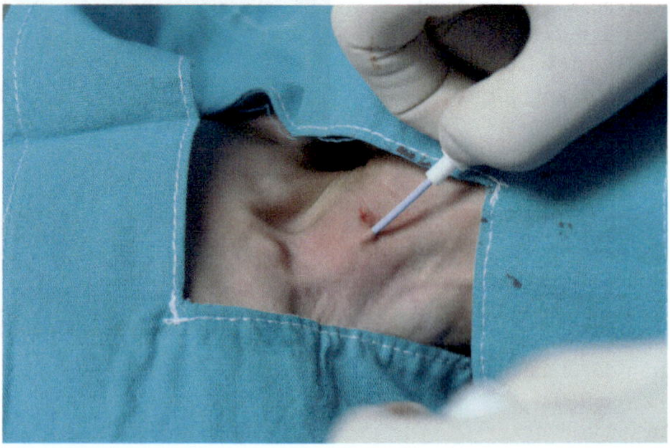

Fig. 4.34 Gentle introduction of the dilatator

- Scan to confirm the intravenous location of the catheter.
- Scan the catheter in LAX view at the level of the left supraclavicular fossae (Figs. 4.36 and 4.37).

4.4.10 Step 10

- Secure the catheter and apply a sterile dressing according to the institutional protocol (Fig. 4.38).

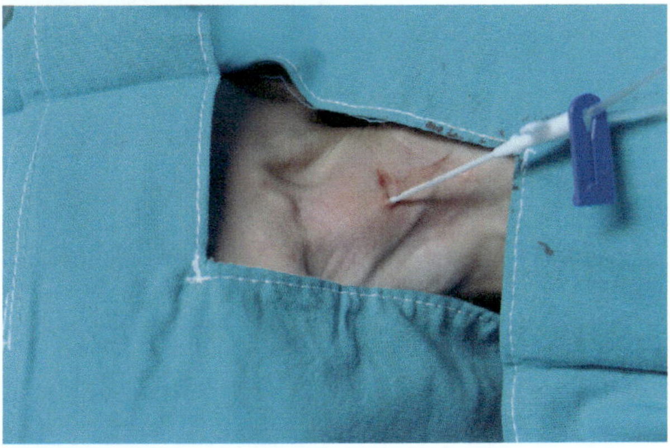

Fig. 4.35 Introduce the required catheter length

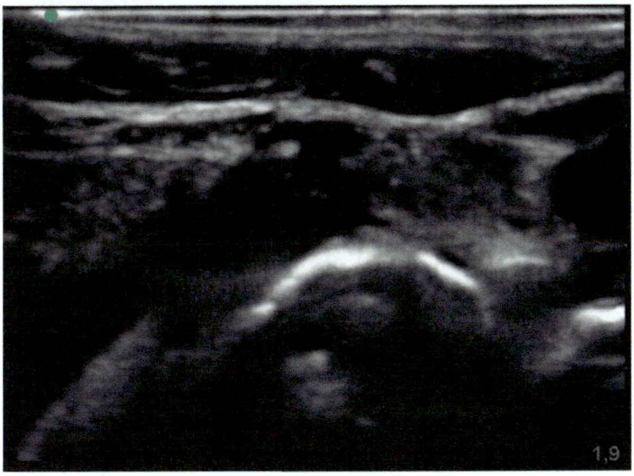

Fig. 4.36 LAX view of the intravascular catheter at the level of supraclavicular fossae

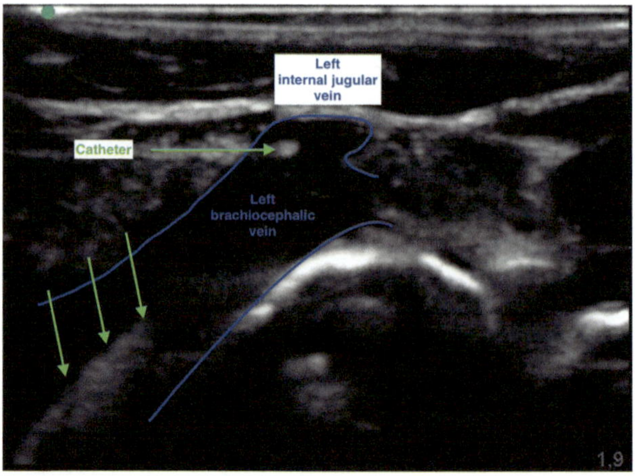

Fig. 4.37 Identifying structures

- With the transducer in the left supraclavicular fossae, the path of the catheter is evident
- In the LIJV that forms the LBCV, the catheter is identified as a hyperechoic dot
- In the LBCV, the catheter can be seen in the LAX view

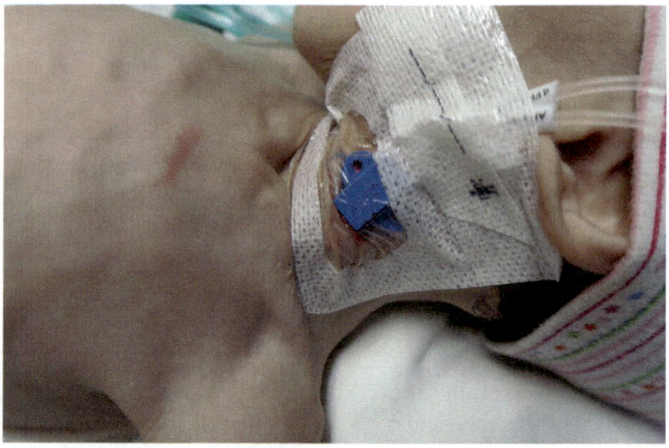

Fig. 4.38 Catheter with a sterile occlusive dressing

Sources

1. Spencer TR, Pittiruti M. Rapid central vein assessment (RaCeVA): a systematic, standardized approach for ultrasound assessment before central venous catheterization. J Vasc Access. 2019;20(3):239–49. https://doi.org/10.1177/1129729818804718. Epub 2018 Oct 4. PMID: 30286688.
2. Maddali MM, Al-Shamsi F, Arora NR, Panchatcharam SM. The optimal length of insertion for central venous catheters via the right internal jugular vein in pediatric cardiac surgical patients. J Cardiothorac Vasc Anesth. 2020;34(9):2386–91. https://doi.org/10.1053/j.jvca.2020.03.007.
3. Montes-Tapia F, Hernández-Trejo K, García-Rodríguez F, et al. Predicting the optimal depth of ultrasound-guided right internal jugular vein central venous catheters in neonates. J Pediatr Surg. 2020;55(9):1920–4. https://doi.org/10.1016/j.jpedsurg.2019.12.004.
4. Zanolla GR, Baldisserotto M, Piva J. How useful is ultrasound guidance for internal jugular venous access in children? J Pediatr Surg. 2018;53(4):789–93. https://doi.org/10.1016/j.jpedsurg.2017.08.010.

5. Montes-Tapia F, Rodríguez-Taméz A, Cura-Esquivel I, et al. Efficacy and safety of ultrasound-guided internal jugular vein catheterization in low-birth-weight newborn. J Pediatr Surg. 2016;51(10):1700–3. https://doi.org/10.1016/j.jpedsurg.2016.05.014.
6. Turker G, Kaya FN, Gurbet A, Aksu H, Erdogan C, Atlas A. Internal jugular vein cannulation: an ultrasound-guided technique versus a landmark-guided technique. Clinics (Sao Paulo). 2009;64(10):989–92. https://doi.org/10.1590/S1807-59322009001000009.
7. Morita M, Sasano H, Azami T, Sasano N, Katsuya H. The skin-traction method increases the cross-sectional area of the internal jugular vein by increasing its anteroposterior diameter. J Anesth. 2007;21(4):467–71. https://doi.org/10.1007/s00540-007-0562-6.

Chapter 5
Left Internal Jugular Vein in Neonates

5.1 Patient Positioning

- The patient is a newborn weighing 3500 g.
- Position the patient supine near the head of the crib.
- Position the patient's head slightly to the right.
- Place a roll under the shoulders to increase the length of the cervical region and create a wider space between the clavicle and jaw (Fig. 5.1).
- Gently hold the upper extremities with the arms caudal.

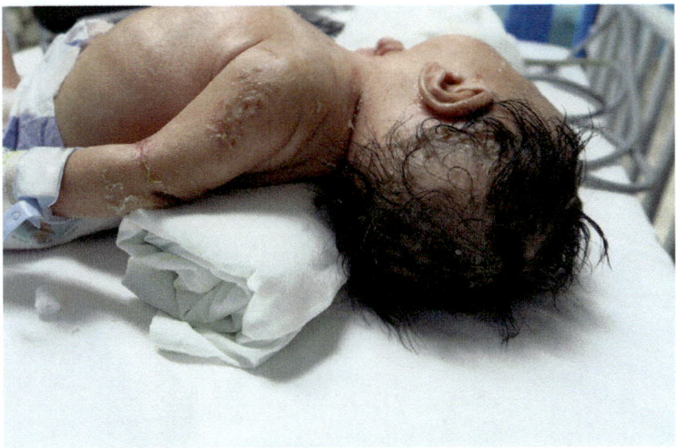

Fig. 5.1 Patient positioning

F. Montes-Tapia, *Atlas of Ultrasound-Guided Central Venous Catheter Placement*, https://doi.org/10.1007/978-3-031-61887-1_5

5.2 Scanning Technique

- Do a preliminary vascular assessment (non-sterile), known as rapid central vein assessment (RaCeVA).
- The operator stands at the patient's head.
- Position the ultrasound on the patient's right or left side or foot level.
- Due to the patient's size, a high-frequency linear transducer (13–6 MHz) with a hockey stick-type probe is recommended.
- Hold the transducer with your left hand and begin scanning with the transducer transverse to the neck and the tip of the hockey stick transducer to the patient's left side (Fig. 5.2).
- Begin the scan of the vessels in a short-axis (SAX) view in the middle of the neck and sweep down to the clavicle.
- Scan Sedillot's triangle (two borders of the sternocleidomastoid and the clavicle as the base).
- Visualize the arrangement of the left carotid artery (LCA) and left internal jugular vein (LIJV) and measure the diameter of the LIJV (Figs. 5.3 and 5.4).

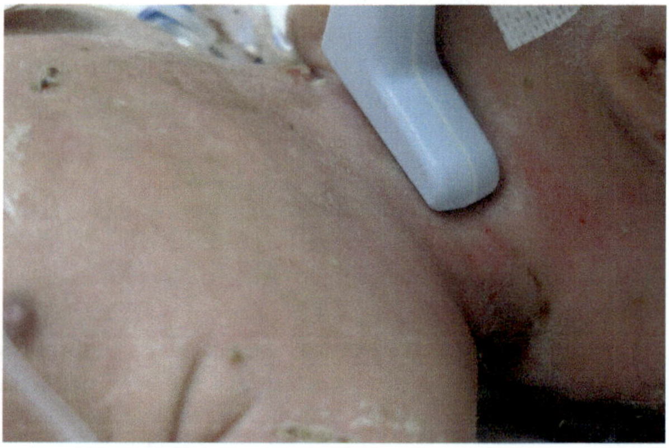

Fig. 5.2 Place the transducer transversely in Sedillot's triangle for SAX view

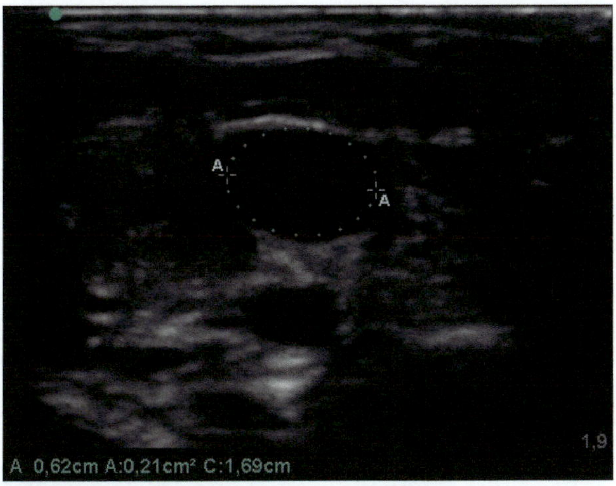

Fig. 5.3 SAX view of cervical vessels
- The depth of the scan is 1.9 cm
- Visualization of the LIJV and LCA
- The mark on the side of the probe corresponds to the tip of the hockey stick transducer, which is identified on the screen as the aqua dot at the top left of the image. In this case, you are pointing to the patient's left side
- The diameter of the LIJV is 0,62 cm with an area of 0,21 cm^2

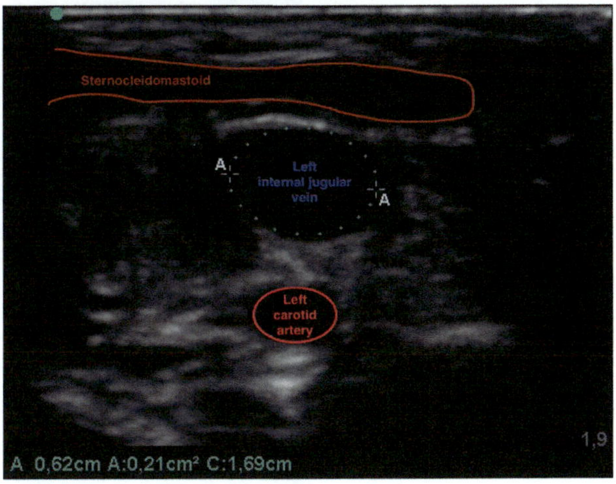

Fig. 5.4 Identifying structures
- In the uppermost part of the sternocleidomastoid muscle (SCM), the approximation of the two components, sternal and clavicular, can be seen
- The LIJV is located anterior to the LCA

5.3 Local Anesthesia Application

- The head is turned to the right side (Fig. 5.5).
- The sterile field only leaves the cervical, upper pectoral, and left shoulder regions uncovered.
- The operator stands at the patient's head (Fig. 5.6).

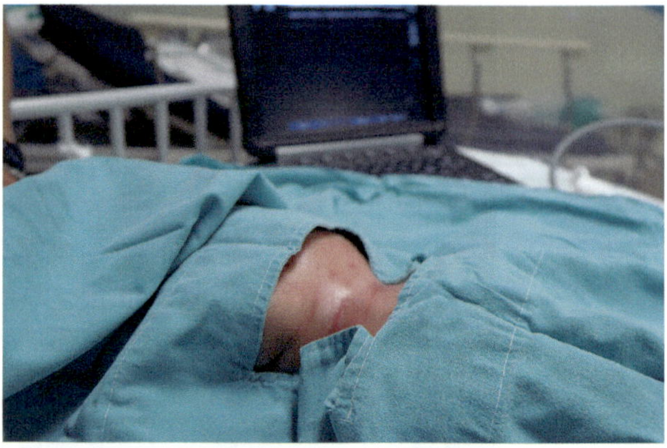

Fig. 5.5 The head is turned to the right side

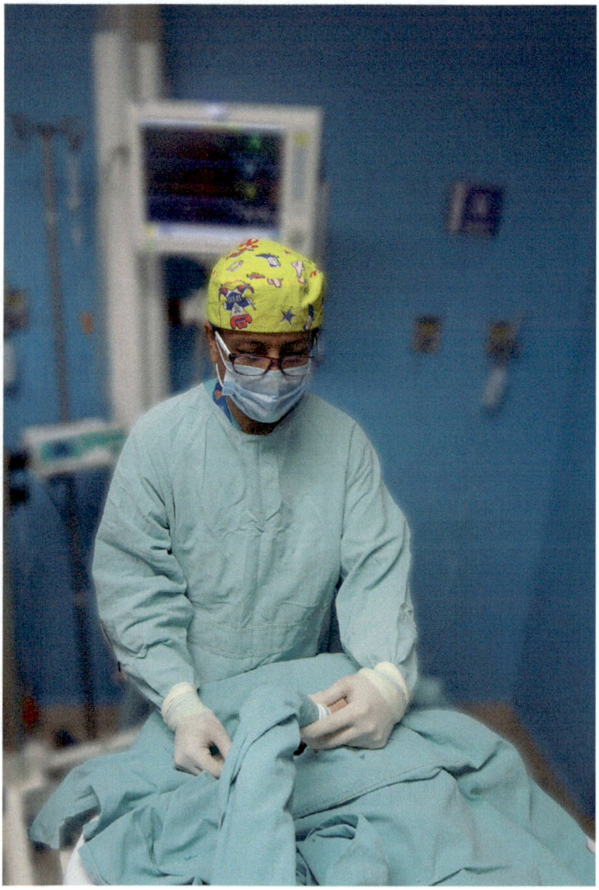

Fig. 5.6 The operator stands at the patient's head

- Use your left hand to grasp the transducer.
- Scan the LIJV and center it in the middle of the length of the transducer to visualize the vein in the central part of the screen (Fig. 5.7).
- SAX view of cervical vessels (Figs. 5.8 and 5.9).
- Real-time ultrasound-guided lidocaine infiltration (Fig. 5.10).
- For infiltration, use a small needle 25–27 G.
- Use lidocaine 1%.
- Infiltrate 1–1,5 cm before the chosen venipuncture site to anesthetize the oblique puncture path as well as the fixation site of the catheter holder.
- Ultrasound-guided lidocaine infiltration in SAX (Figs. 5.11 and 5.12).

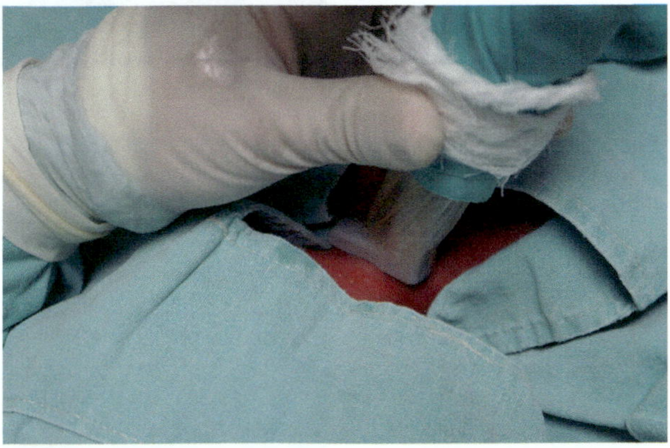

Fig. 5.7 Operator view. Scan the LIJV and center it in the middle of the transducer length

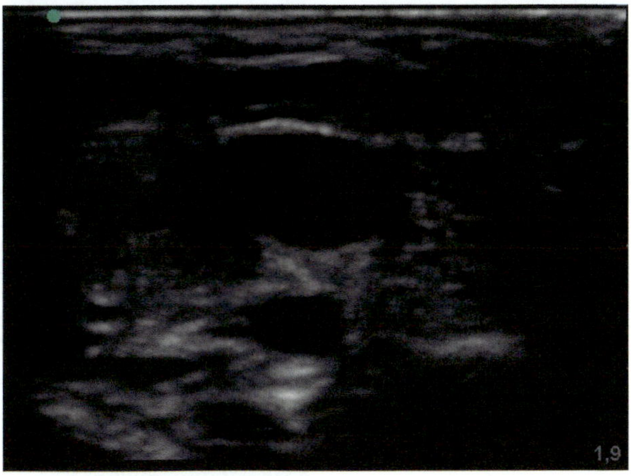

Fig. 5.8 SAX view of cervical vessels

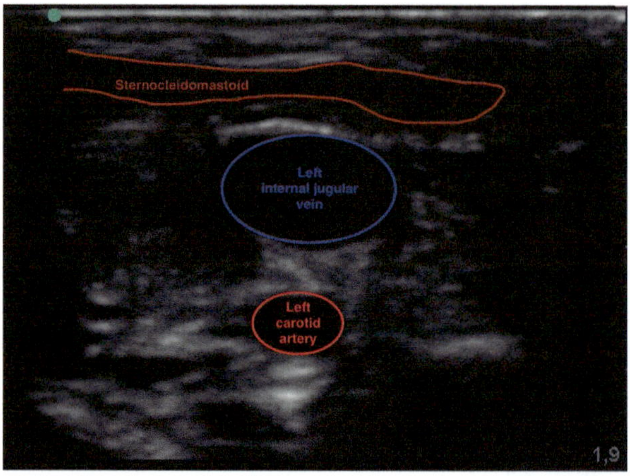

Fig. 5.9 Identifying structures

- The LIJV, scanned in the middle of the transducer length, shows the vein in the middle of the ultrasound screen and the LCA is below

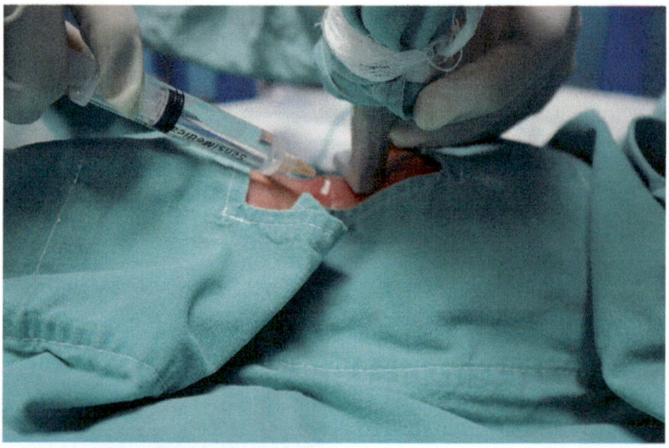

Fig. 5.10 Ultrasound-guided lidocaine infiltration in SAX

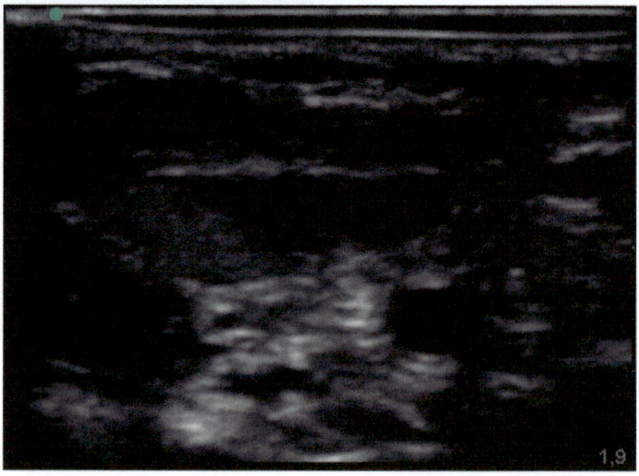

Fig. 5.11 SAX view of lidocaine infiltration

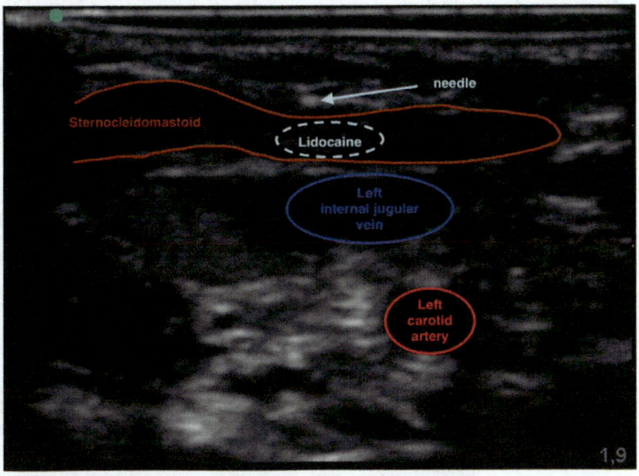

Fig. 5.12 Identifying structures
- The infiltration needle is identified between the subcutaneous tissue and the sternocleidomastoid muscle (SCM) for infiltration of the path that will follow the puncture of the LIJV
- This moment of the procedure can be used to determine if the site of choice for the puncture is in the plane of the LIJV, as in this case
- It can be seen how the LIJV is compressed with the penetration of the infiltration needle

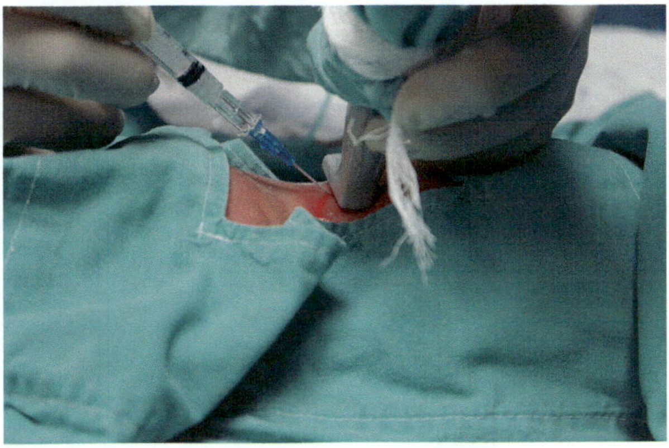

Fig. 5.13 Puncture in the central part of the length of the footprint

5.4 Steps for Real-Time Ultrasound-Guided Access to the Left Internal Jugular Vein in Neonates

5.4.1 Step 01

- A 13-cm, 4 Fr, double-lumen catheter will be placed.
- Hold the transducer in your left hand.
- Perform the puncture in the central part of the length of the footprint with a 22-G intravenous catheter with the right hand (Fig. 5.13).
- Start the puncture with a 40–50° angle in relation to the skin.

- Begin the ultrasound-guided dynamic needle tip positioning (DNTP) to guide the puncture in real time.
- Progression of the puncture; the intravenous catheter is in the SCM (Figs. 5.14, 5.15, 5.16 and 5.17).

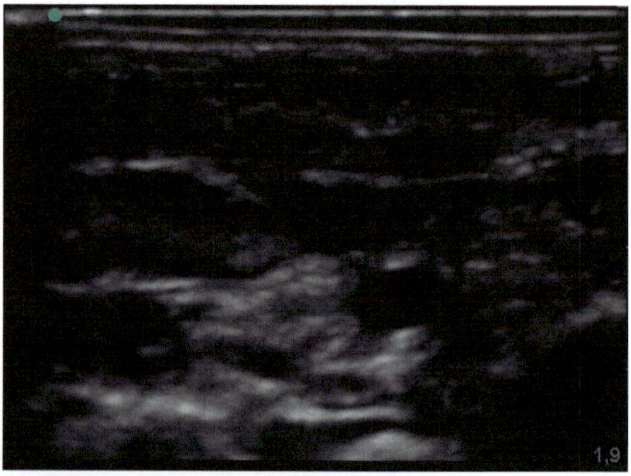

Fig. 5.14 SAX view of the start of the LIJV puncture with the intravenous catheter

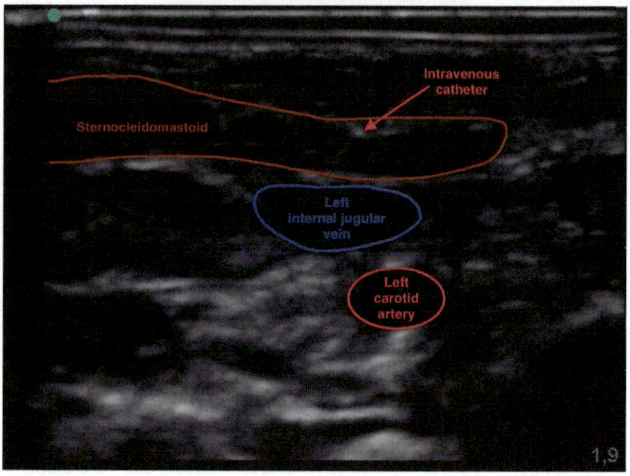

Fig. 5.15 Identifying structures
- The intravenous catheter tip is identified as a bright hyperechoic (white) dot
- The intravascular catheter has penetrated the skin and is in the SCM
- This rapid penetration of the puncture is due to the angle with which we are starting the puncture
- The trajectory of the intravascular catheter is in the direction of the LIJV

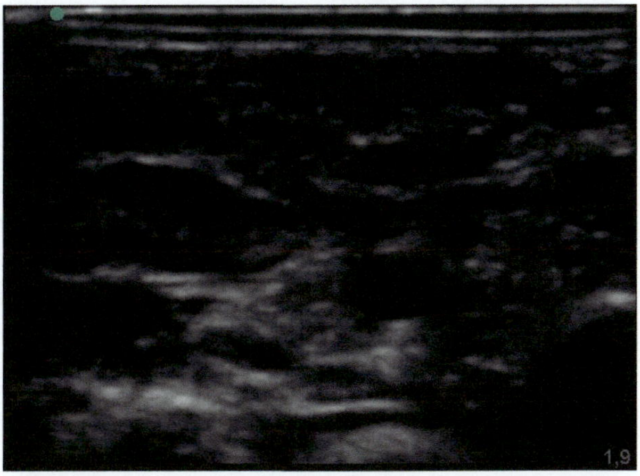

Fig. 5.16 SAX view of the progression of the puncture

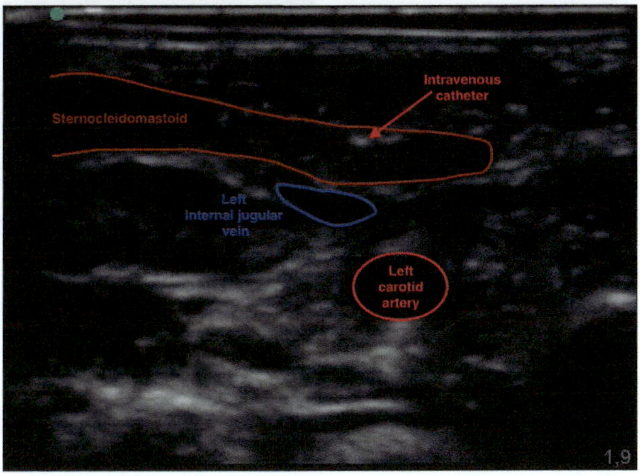

Fig. 5.17 Identifying structures
- The LIJV is more collapsed due to the compression performed with the intravenous catheter

5.4.2 Step 02

- Continue with DNTP to guide the puncture in real time; in other words, sweep down the transducer as the puncture progresses (Fig. 5.18).
- Always keep the puncture in the middle of the transducer.
- SAX view of the progression of the puncture (Figs. 5.19, 5.20, 5.21, 5.22).

5.4.3 Step 03

- Always keep the puncture in the central part of the length of the hockey stick transducer (Fig. 5.23).

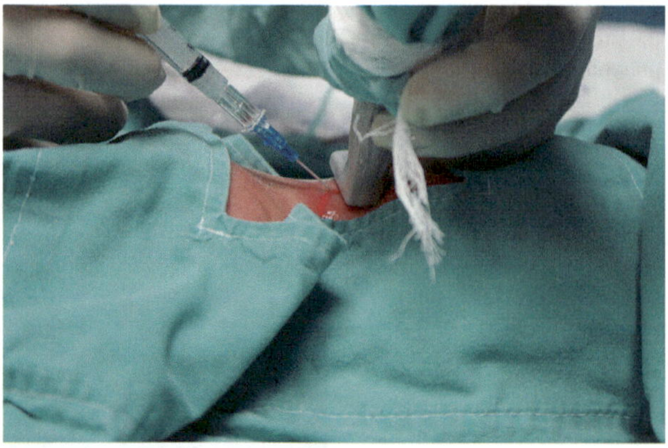

Fig. 5.18 Sweep down the transducer as you progress with the puncture

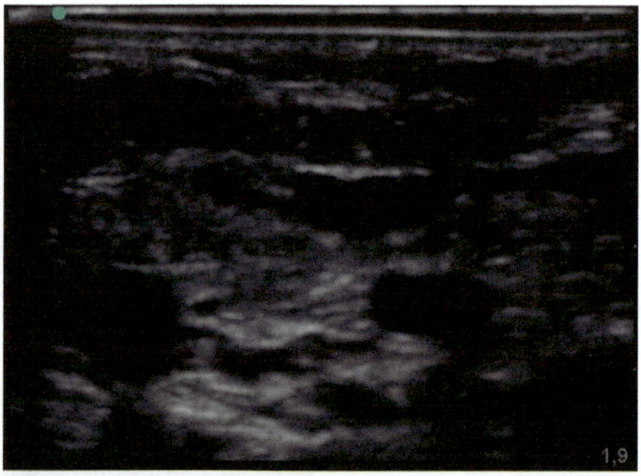

Fig. 5.19 SAX view of the progression of the puncture

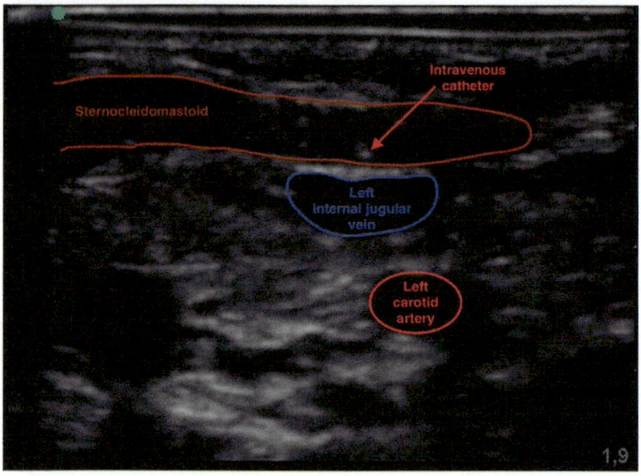

Fig. 5.20 Identifying structures

- The intravenous catheter tip is going through the SCM muscle
- The puncture is developing in the direction of the center of the LIJV

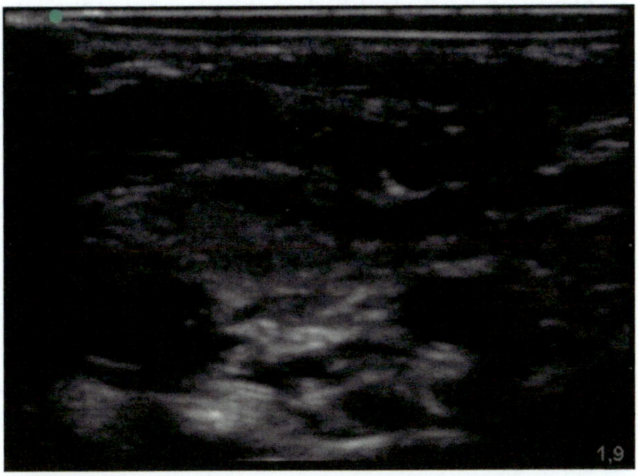

Fig. 5.21 SAX view of the progression of the puncture

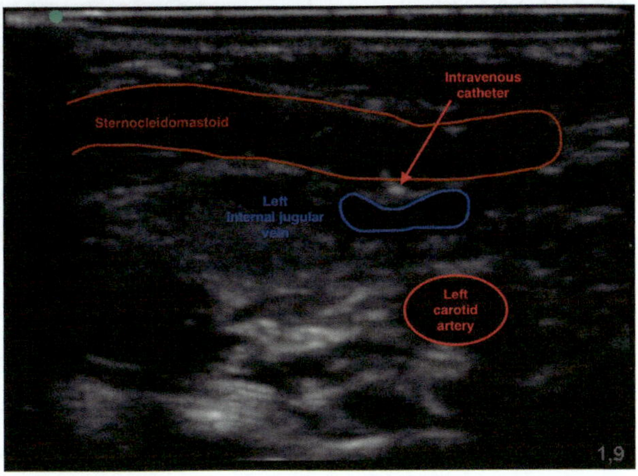

Fig. 5.22 Identifying structures

- The intravenous catheter has reached the anterior wall of the LIJV, right in the middle of the vein
- The LIJV is deformed by compression of the puncture

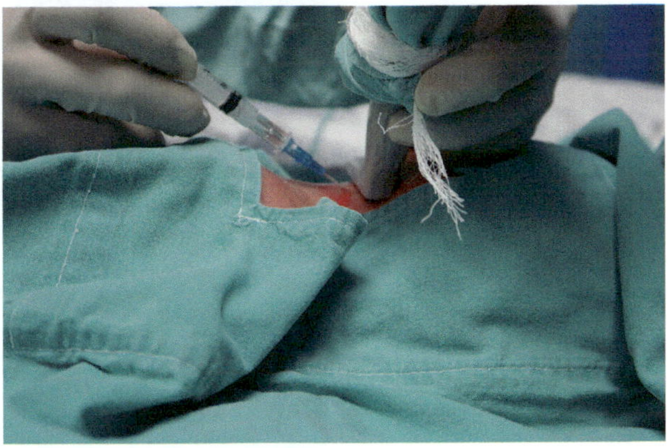

Fig. 5.23 Keep the puncture in the middle of the length of the transducer

- Once you have identified on the screen that the intravenous catheter is penetrating the anterior wall of the LIJV (Figs. 5.24 and 5.25), the vein will be cannulated and advance the puncture.

5.4.4 Step 04

- Once you have identified the cannulation of the LIJV, change the puncture angle to less than 10° to cannulate with a more intravenous catheter inside the vein lumen (Fig. 5.26).
- Perform the cannulation with DNTP of the intravenous catheter so as not to penetrate the posterior wall.

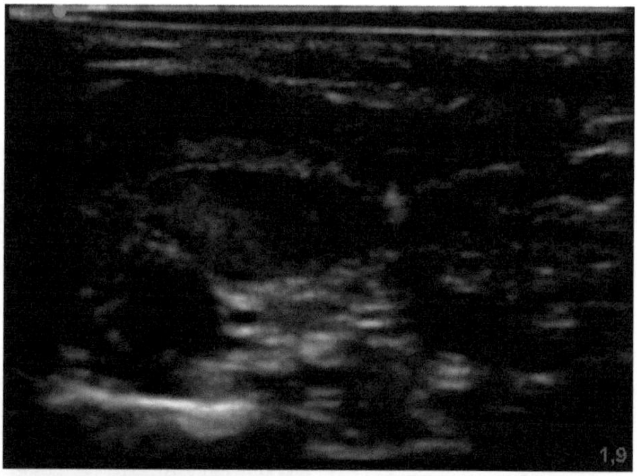

Fig. 5.24 SAX view of the intravenous catheter reaching the LIJV

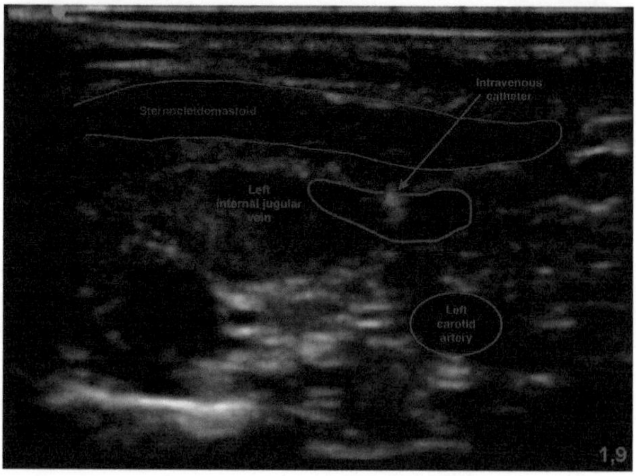

Fig. 5.25 Identifying structures
- The intravenous catheter tip is entering the LIJV

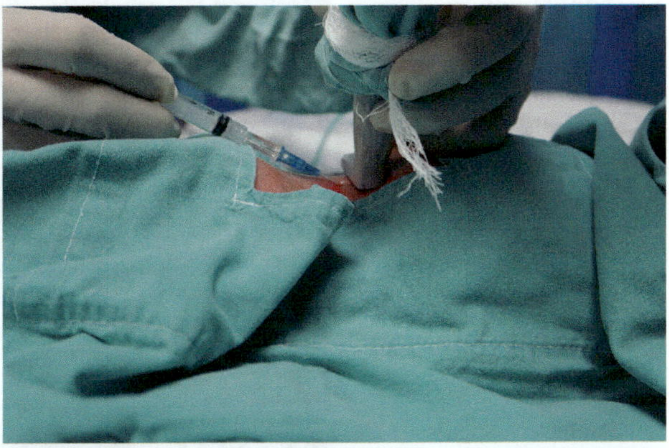

Fig. 5.26 Modify the puncture angle to less than 10°

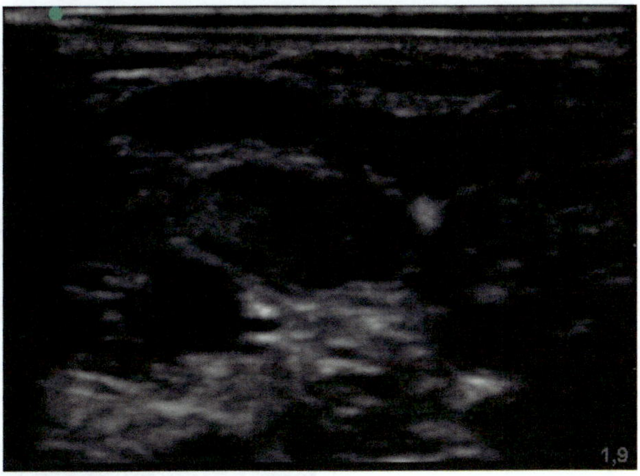

Fig. 5.27 SAX view of the cannulation with the intravenous catheter

- SAX view of the cannulation with the intravenous catheter (Figs. 5.27, 5.28, 5.29 and 5.30).

5.4.5 Step 05

- Apply gentle negative pressure on the syringe plunger when positioning the intravascular intravenous catheter.
- Set the transducer aside and aspirate the syringe.
- When a flash of blood appears in the barrel of the syringe, stop advancing (Fig. 5.31).
- The catheter hub is held firmly so that the catheter tube does not move outward with the suction maneuver.

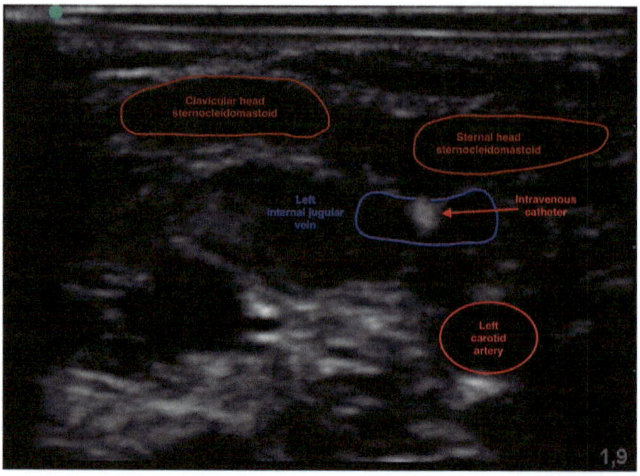

Fig. 5.28 Identifying structures
- The puncture angle has been modified to canalize the LIJV with a more intravenous catheter

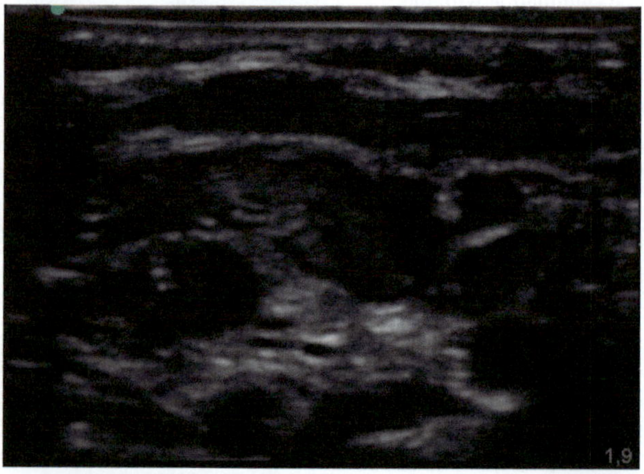

Fig. 5.29 SAX view of the cannulation progression

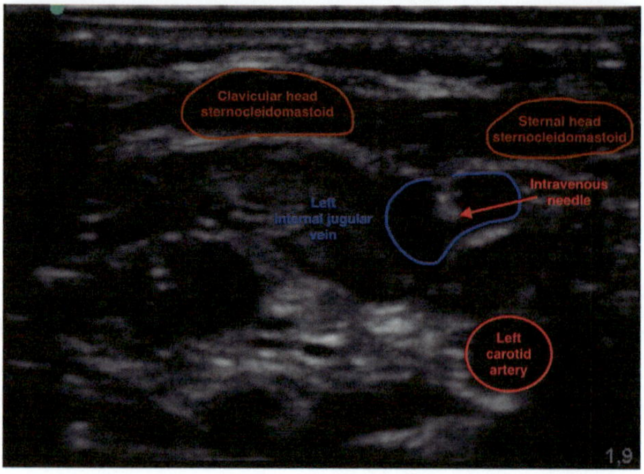

Fig. 5.30 Identifying structures
- Cannulation with the intravenous catheter has progressed without penetrating the posterior wall, and the LIJV is more medial in the direction of the LBCV
- The two heads of the SCM muscle are visualized, indicating the base of Sedillot's triangle

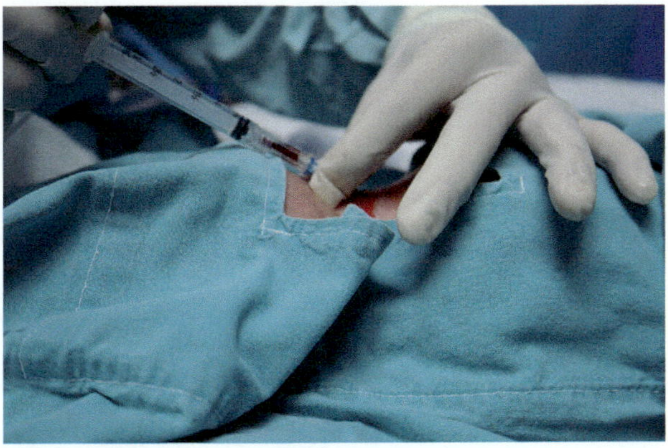

Fig. 5.31 Maintain gentle negative pressure on the syringe plunger

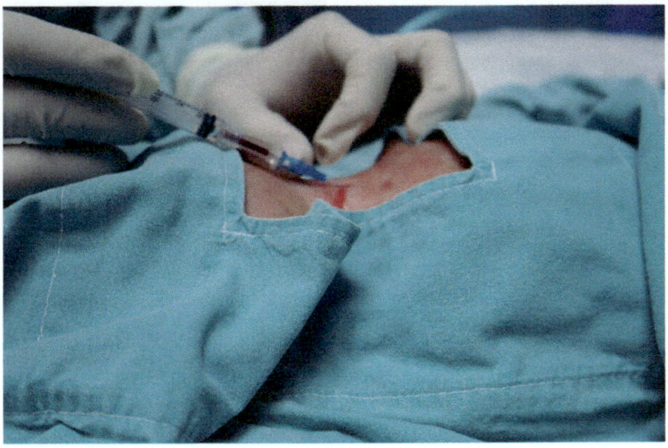

Fig. 5.32 Hold the flange of the intravenous catheter hub and insert it

5.4.6 Step 06

- Hold the flange of the intravenous catheter hub and insert it, displacing it from the puncture needle to cannulate the vein (Fig. 5.32).
- Continue introducing the catheter tube by pushing the flange of the intravenous catheter hub to cannulate the vein (Fig. 5.33).
- Once the entire catheter tube is inserted, remove the puncture needle (Fig. 5.34).
- Once the catheter tube is inserted, the needle is removed. This skill must be practiced to not remove the catheter accidentally (Fig. 5.35).
- Before you pass the guidewire, check for free blood flow through the catheter tube cannulating the LIJV (Fig. 5.36).
  - If there is no blood flow, one of the causes is that the catheter tube was bent intravascularly, so you will need to extract it gently with an aspiration maneuver until blood flows. Then, we will proceed to pass the guidewire.

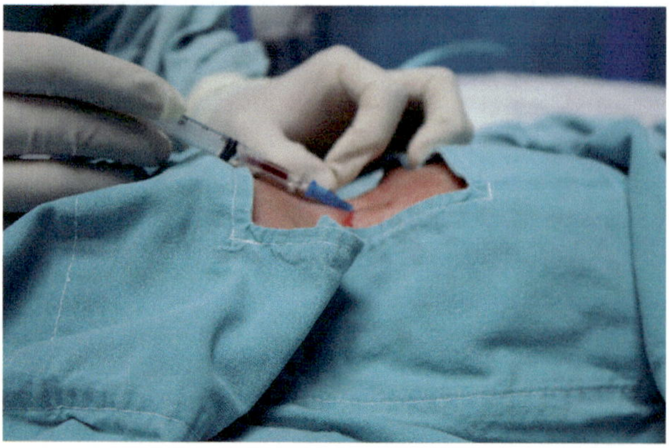

Fig. 5.33 Introducing the catheter tube

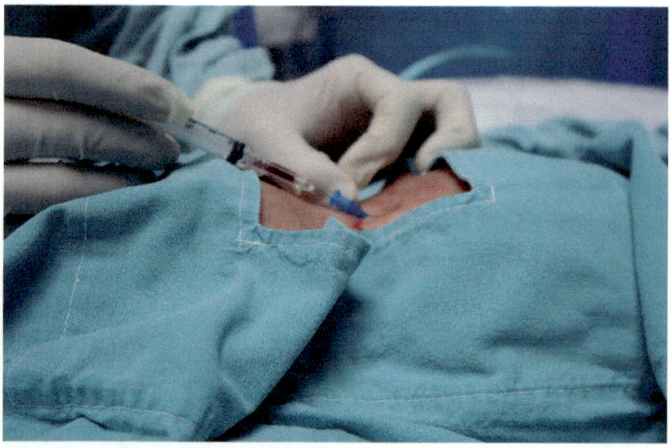

Fig. 5.34 Removal of the puncture needle

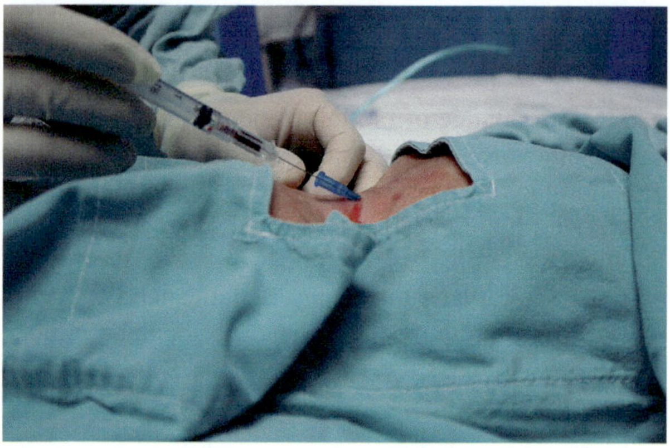

Fig. 5.35 Insert the catheter and remove the needle

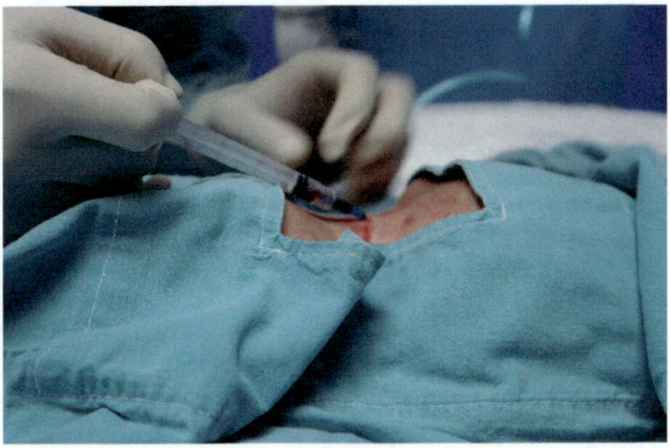

Fig. 5.36 Check for free blood flow through the catheter tube cannulating the LIJV

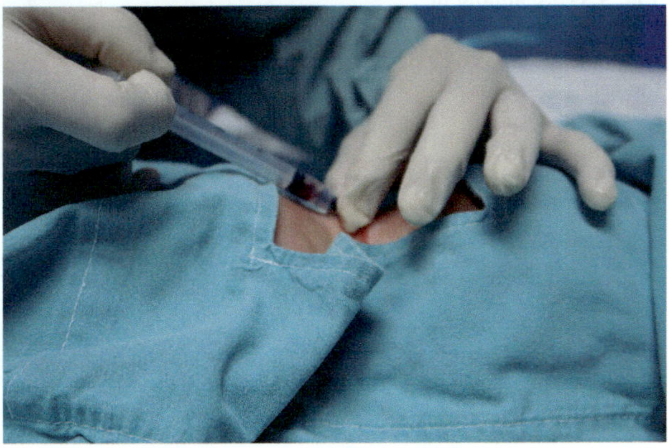

Fig. 5.37 Remove the syringe

   - A bent catheter tube is another cause of a lack of blood flow in patients with prominent fat pads. Also, the SCM can occlude the catheter tube due to compression in inadequately sedated patients. In this case, performing the puncture with an introducer needle is preferable.

- Firmly hold the catheter hub and remove the syringe (Fig. 5.37).

5.4.7 Step 07

- Insert the 0.018" guidewire through the catheter hub (Fig. 5.38).
- The J-tip end of the guide should easily pass through. If it does not, you can try passing the straight end. If it still does not pass, there may be a chance that the catheter tube has accidentally slipped out of the vein.

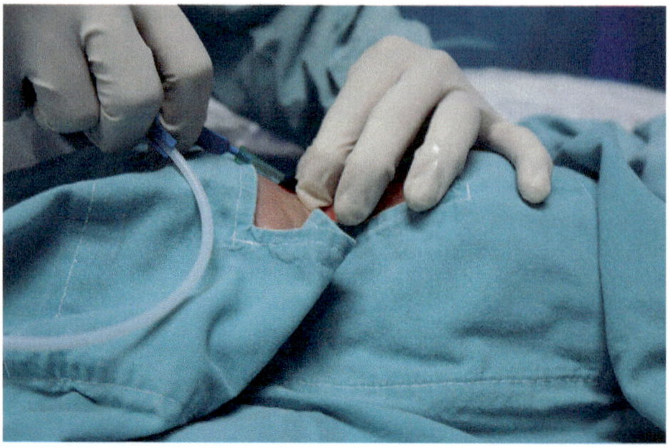

Fig. 5.38 Insert the guidewire

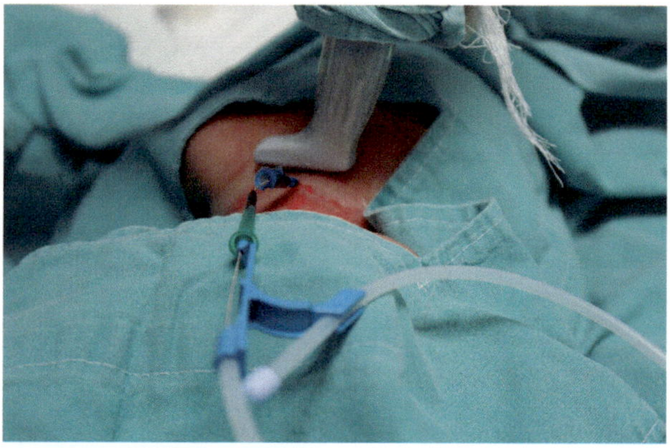

Fig. 5.39 Scanning in SAX view, hockey stick transducer, transverse on the neck

- On the left side, it is preferable to pass the J-tip, as this will help navigate the intravascular pathway, which is very sinuous up to the superior cava vein (SCV).
- If you performed the puncture with a 24-G intravenous catheter in prematurely less than 1000 g, use a 0.014" guidewire.
- Check the intravenous location of the guidewire in SAX (Fig. 5.39).
- Scan for the intravascular guidewire in SAX (Figs. 5.40 and 5.41).
- With the index finger of the left hand and a gauze, occlude the entry of the guide into the skin and remove the catheter tube (Fig. 5.42).

5.4.8 *Step 08*

- Grasp the guidewire with the left hand to introduce the dilator with the right hand (Fig. 5.43).
- Perform dilation with the right hand and countertraction of the skin with the left hand (Fig. 5.44).

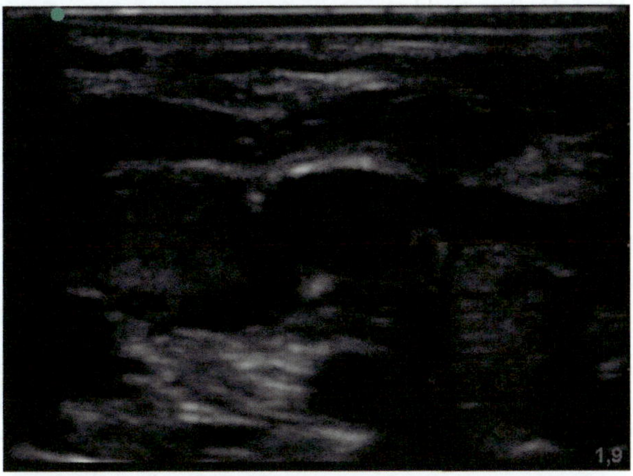

Fig. 5.40 SAX view of the intravascular guidewire

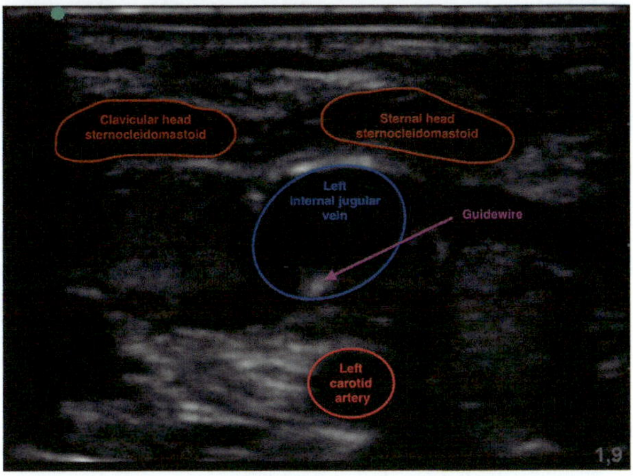

Fig. 5.41 Identifying structures

- The guidewire is found intravascularly. It is identified as a more hyperechoic dot

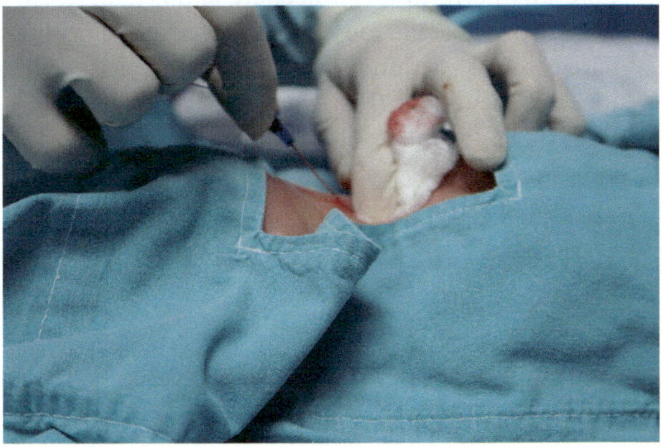

Fig. 5.42 Remove the catheter tube

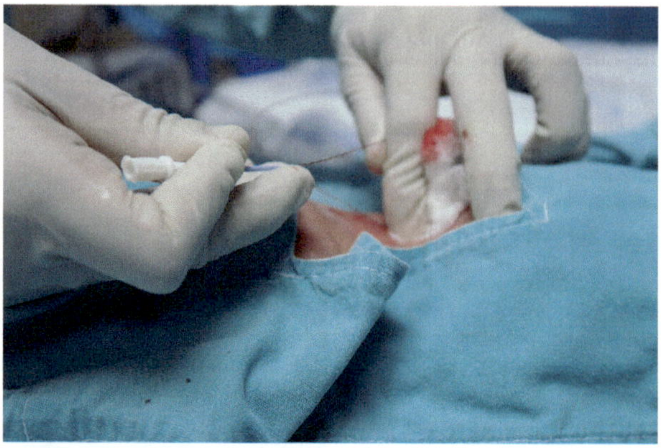

Fig. 5.43 Pass the dilator with the right hand

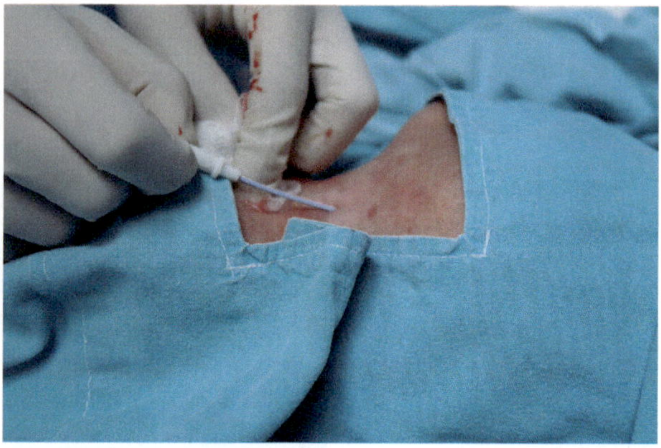

Fig. 5.44 Perform dilation

- Perform dilation with a "screw" maneuver. The skin path is dilated up to the entrance of the LIJV (Fig. 5.45).
- Carefully perform this procedure at this age; it will not require a skin incision.
- If a lot of subcutaneous pressure is exerted without countertraction, the guidewire can be bent, hindering dilation and passage of the central venous catheter.
- Remove the dilator (Fig. 5.46).
- With the index finger of the left hand and a gauze, occlude the entry of the guide into the skin (Fig. 5.47).

5.4.9 Step 09

- Grasp the guidewire with the left hand to introduce the catheter with the right hand. Advance the catheter over the guidewire (Seldinger's technique) (Fig. 5.48).

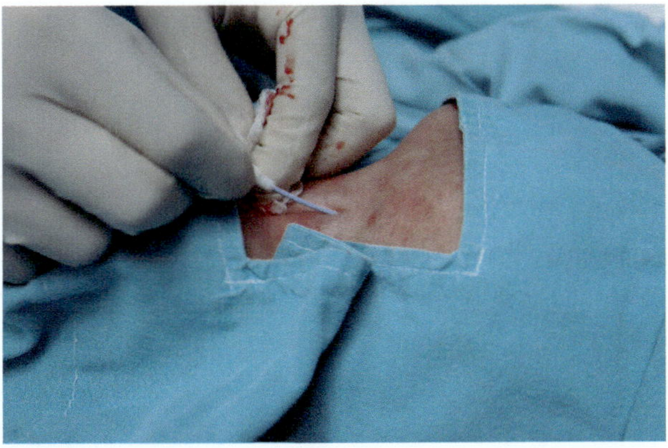

Fig. 5.45 Dilation with the right hand and a "screw" maneuver

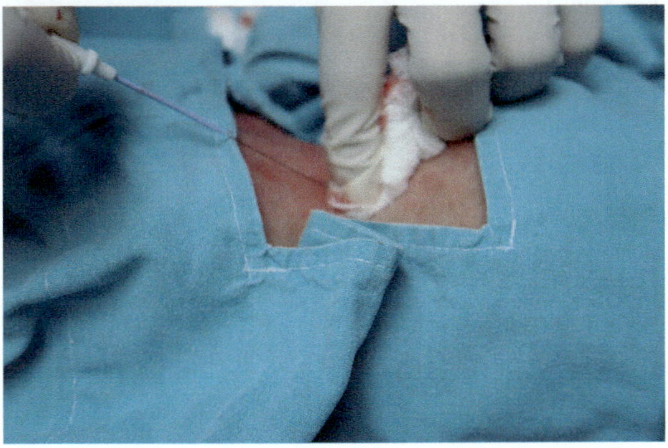

Fig. 5.46 Remove the dilator

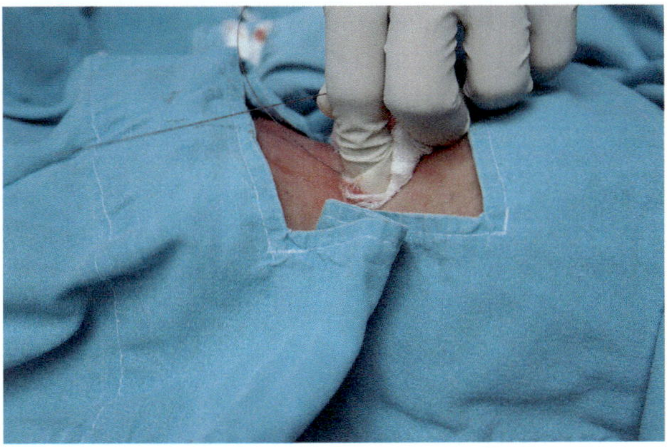

Fig. 5.47 Remove the dilator and block the entry of the guide into the skin

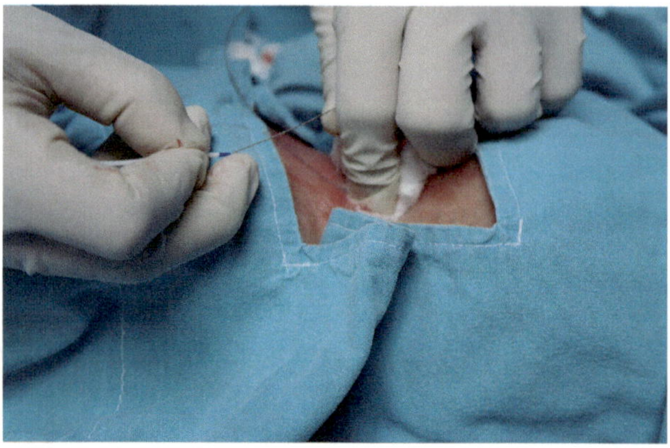

Fig. 5.48 Introduce the catheter over the guidewire (Seldinger's technique)

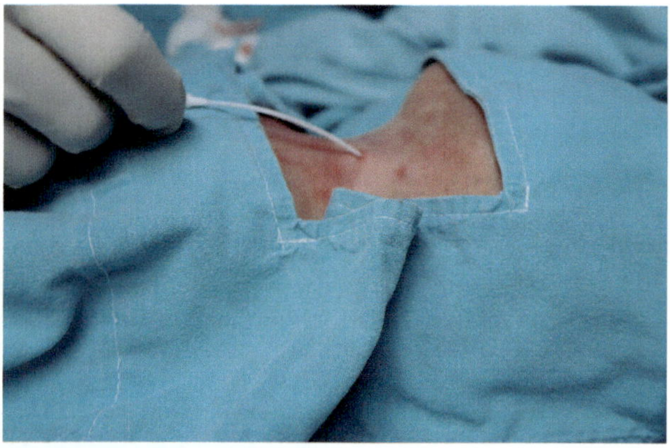

Fig. 5.49 Introduce the required intravascular catheter length

- When you have the required intravascular catheter length, remove the guidewire (Fig. 5.49).

5.4.10 Step 10

- Scan to confirm the intravenous location of the catheter (Fig. 5.50).
- SAX view of the intravascular catheter (Figs. 5.51 and 5.52).

5.4.11 Step 11

- Secure the catheter and apply a sterile dressing according to the institutional protocol (Fig. 5.53).

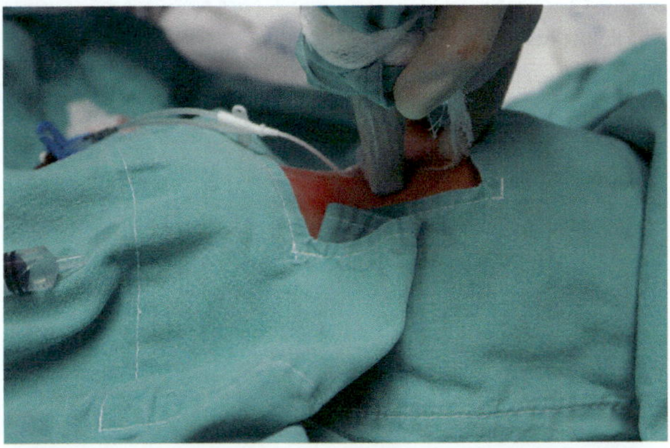

Fig. 5.50 Scan the catheter in the SAX view

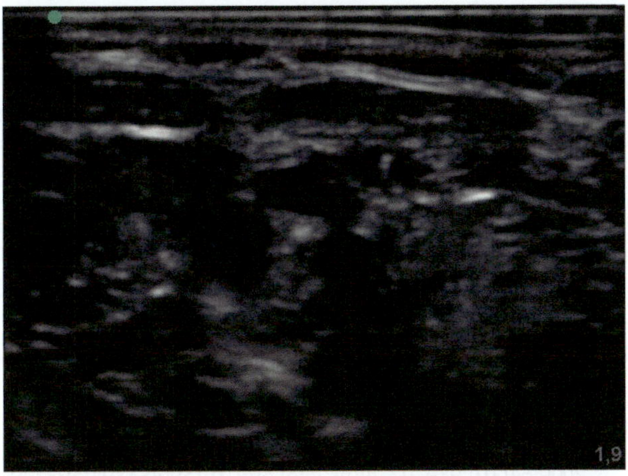

Fig. 5.51 SAX view of the intravascular catheter

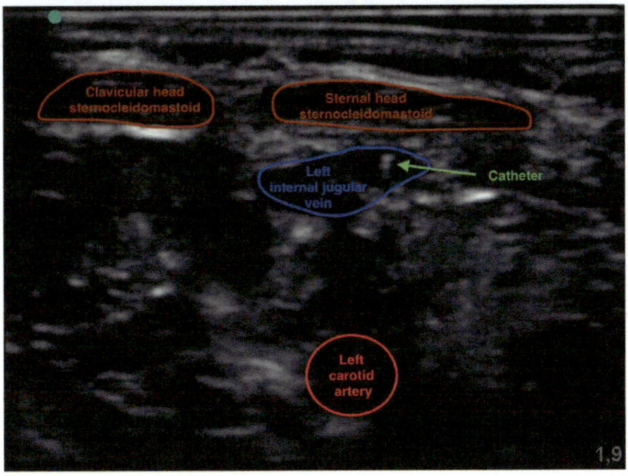

Fig. 5.52 Identifying structures

- Catheter inside the LIJV; the two lumens can be identified
- No residual perivascular hematoma is seen

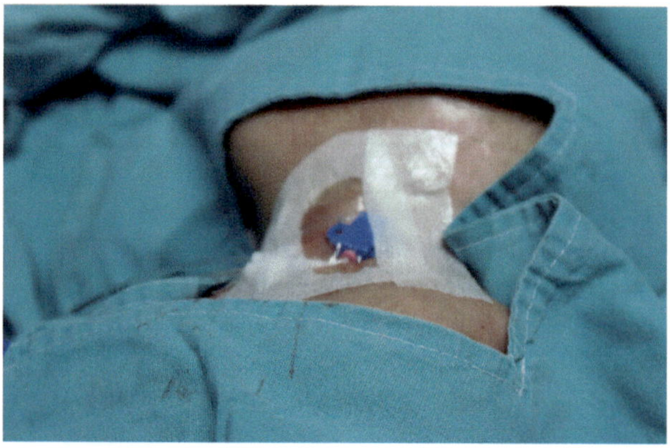

Fig. 5.53 Catheter with a sterile occlusive dressing

Sources

1. Spencer TR, Pittiruti M. Rapid central vein assessment (RaCeVA): a systematic, standardized approach for ultrasound assessment before central venous catheterization. J Vasc Access. 2019;20(3):239–49. https://doi.org/10.1177/1129729818804718. Epub 2018 Oct 4. PMID: 30286688.
2. Tan Y, Tu Z, Ye P, et al. Ultrasound guidance for internal jugular vein cannulation in neonates: modified dynamic needle tip positioning short-axis out-of-plane technique versus long-axis in-plane technique, a randomized controlled trial. J Vasc Access. 2022;23(6):922–9. https://doi.org/10.1177/11297298211015043.
3. Zanolla GR, Baldisserotto M, Piva J. How useful is ultrasound guidance for internal jugular venous access in children? J Pediatr Surg. 2018;53(4):789–93. https://doi.org/10.1016/j.jpedsurg.2017.08.010.
4. Turker G, Kaya FN, Gurbet A, Aksu H, Erdogan C, Atlas A. Internal jugular vein cannulation: an ultrasound-guided technique versus a landmark-guided technique. Clinics (Sao Paulo). 2009;64(10):989–92. https://doi.org/10.1590/S1807-59322009001000009.
5. Morita M, Sasano H, Azami T, Sasano N, Katsuya H. The skin-traction method increases the cross-sectional area of the internal jugular vein by increasing its anteroposterior diameter. J Anesth. 2007;21(4):467–71. https://doi.org/10.1007/s00540-007-0562-6.
6. Sigaut S, Skhiri A, Stany I, et al. Ultrasound guided internal jugular vein access in children and infant: a meta-analysis of published studies. Paediatr Anaesth. 2009;19(12):1199–206. https://doi.org/10.1111/j.1460-9592.2009.03171.x.

Chapter 6
Infraclavicular Right Subclavian Vein in Pediatrics

6.1 Patient Positioning

- The patient is a 7-year-old patient weighing 21.9 kg.
- Position the patient in supine near the right side of the bed or stretcher (Fig. 6.1).
- Place the patient's head centered or slightly to the left.
- Place a roll under the shoulders to create a wide space between the clavicle and the first rib (Fig. 6.2).
- Gently restraint the upper extremities with the arms caudal.

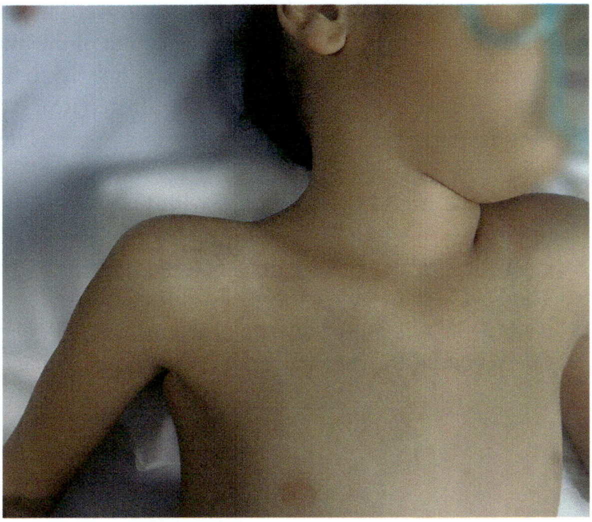

Fig. 6.1 Patient positioning

F. Montes-Tapia, *Atlas of Ultrasound-Guided Central Venous Catheter Placement*, https://doi.org/10.1007/978-3-031-61887-1_6

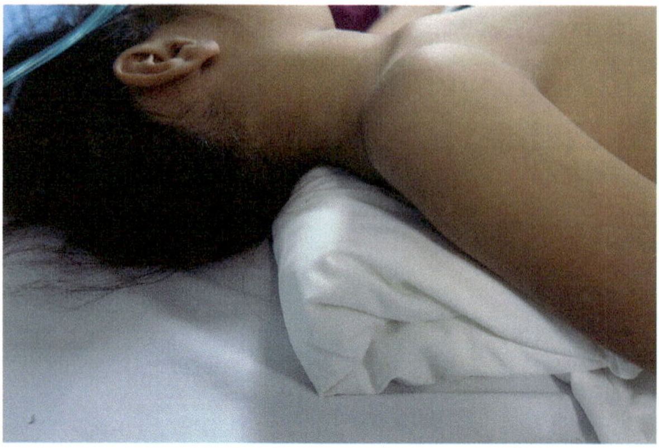

Fig. 6.2 A roll under the shoulders

6.2 Scanning Technique

- The operator stands on the right side of the patient (Fig. 6.3).
- Place the ultrasound in any of these three positions: next to the left shoulder, the right shoulder, or above the head.
- A high-frequency linear transducer (13–6 MHz) with a probe of less than 5 cm footprint can be used.
- Hold the transducer with your left hand and scan the subclavian vessels in a long-axis (LAX) view placing the transducer obliquely in the external third of the clavicle and with the position indicator toward the neck (Fig. 6.4).
- Place the image of the clavicle in the center of the ultrasound screen. The clavicle produces an inferior acoustic shadow (Figs. 6.5, 6.6, 6.7 and 6.8).
- First, visualize the right subclavian artery (RSCA) (Figs. 6.5 and 6.6), which runs deeper in relation to the clavicle and is more lateral than the right subclavian vein (RSCV).
- Sweep the transducer medially, with the transducer obliquely over the clavicle toward the junction of the middle and inner thirds, to locate the RSCV.
- LAX view of the RSCV (Figs. 6.7 and 6.8).
- The RSCV has two anatomical differences from the RSCA. The first difference is the RSCV is more superficial than the RSCA and runs closer to the clavicle. The second difference is the RSCV is more medial than the artery.

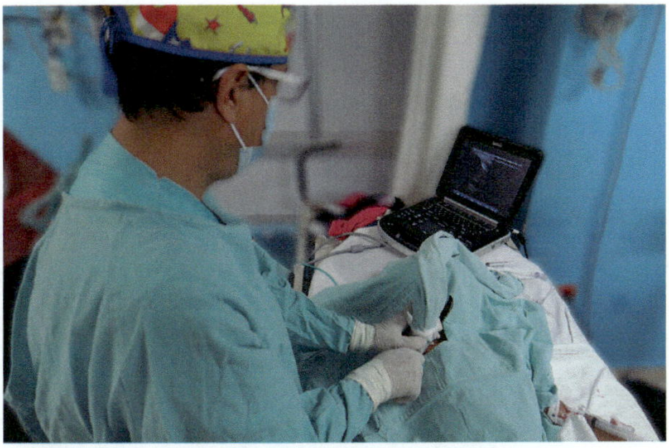

Fig. 6.3 Position of the operator and the ultrasound

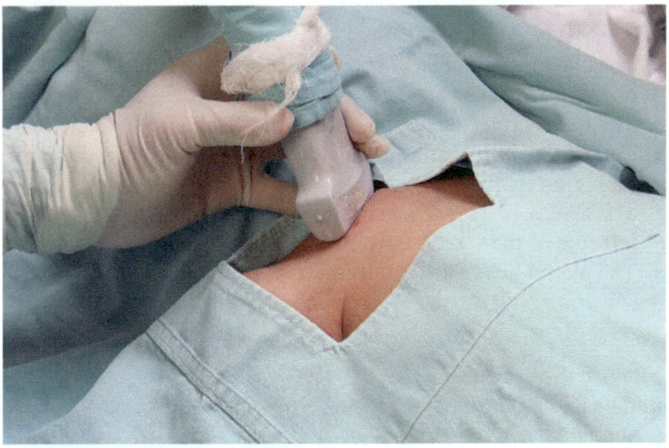

Fig. 6.4 Hold the transducer with the left hand and place it oblique to the clavicle, in the external third of the clavicle

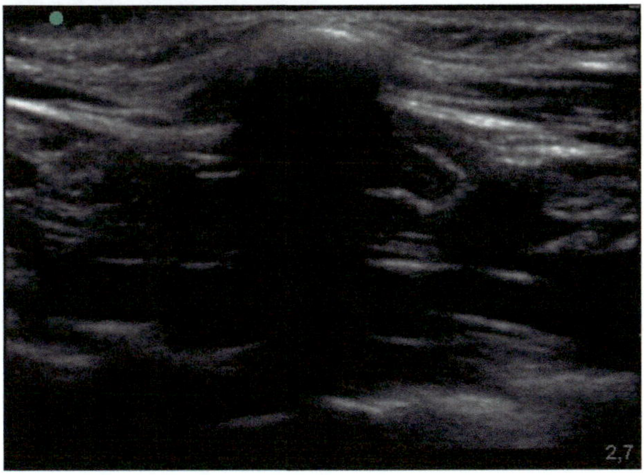

Fig. 6.5 Scan of the external third of the clavicle. LAX view of the RSCA

- The position indicator directed toward the neck
- The scan depth is 2,7 cm

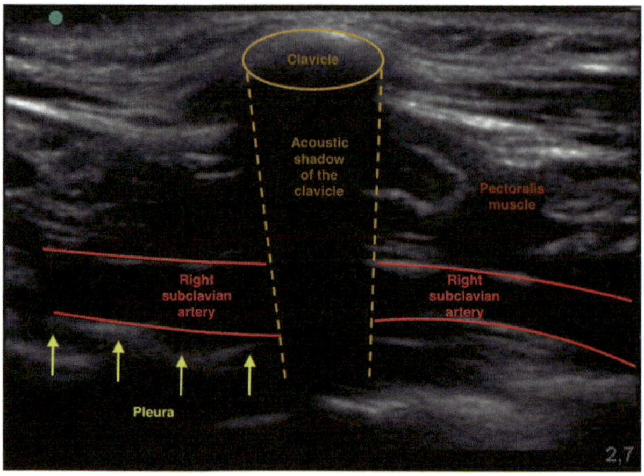

Fig. 6.6 Identifying structures

- The clavicle is in the center of the transducer (Fig. 6.4), and it is seen in the center of the image on the screen. The acoustic shadow causes the structures below it not to be visualized
- The RSCA runs deeper in relation to the clavicle and lateral to the vein
- The RSCA in its extrathoracic portion on the right side of the screen corresponds to the pectoral region
- The RSCA in its thoracic portion is identified toward the cervical region, in other words, on the left side of the screen (toward the probe mark)
- The pleura lies below the inferior wall of the thoracic portion of the RSCA

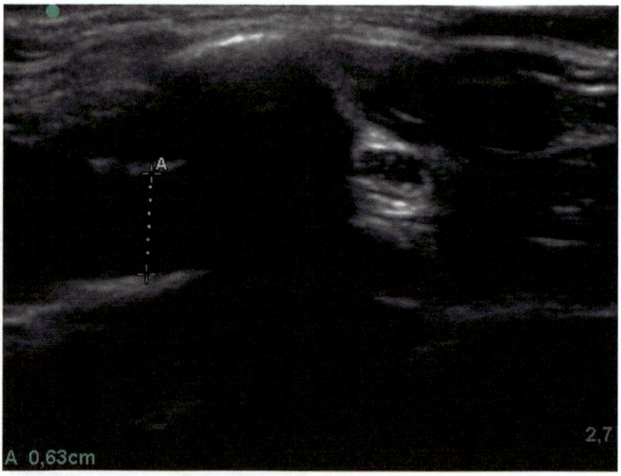

Fig. 6.7 Scan between the middle and inner thirds of the clavicle. LAX view of the RSCV

- The diameter of the RSCV is 0,63 cm

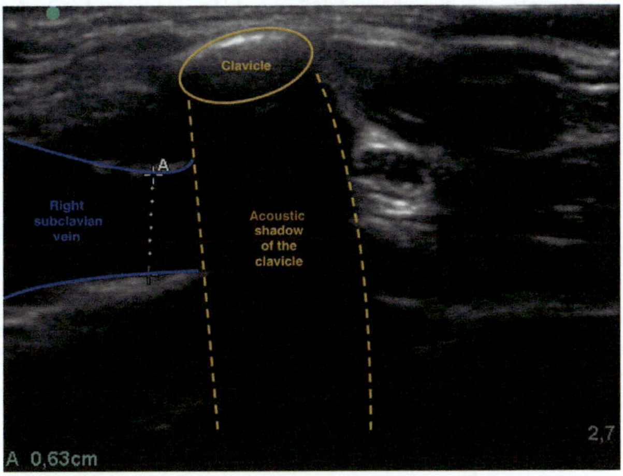

Fig. 6.8 Identifying structures
- The thoracic RSCV is identified on the left side of the screen (toward the mark of the probe), which is toward the cervical region
- The extrathoracic portion of the RSCV is not seen with the position of the transducer in this image
- The RSCV is more superficial than the RSCA and runs closer to the clavicle

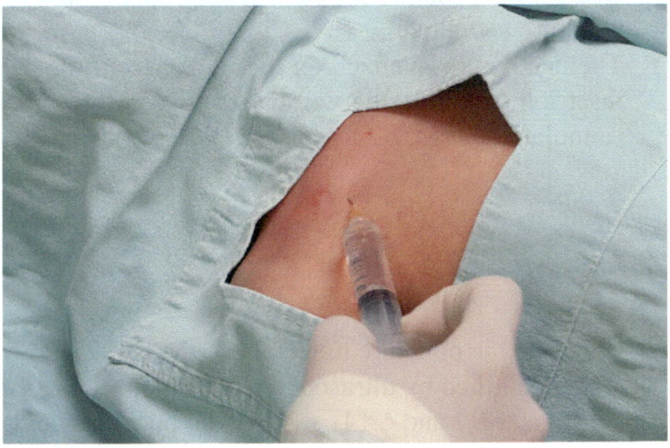

Fig. 6.9 Lidocaine infiltration

6.3 Local Anesthesia Application

- The sterile field only leaves the cervical, upper pectoral, and right shoulder regions uncovered.
- For infiltration, use a small needle 25–27 G.
- Use lidocaine 1%.
- After ultrasound localization of the area to be punctured, infiltration of the marked site is performed.
- Infiltrate 1–1,5 cm before the chosen venipuncture site to anesthetize the oblique puncture path as well as the fixation site of the catheter holder (Fig. 6.9).

6.4 Steps for Real-Time Ultrasound-Guided Access to Infraclavicular Right Subclavian Vein in Pediatric

6.4.1 Step 01

- We will use an Arrow® 4 Fr, 13-cm, double-lumen catheter.
- The operator stands on the right side of the patient (Fig. 6.3).
- Hold the transducer with your left hand and scan the RSCV in the LAX view in the junction of the middle and inner thirds of the left clavicle.
- Use the 21-G introducer needle that comes with the catheter kit.
- Once you identify the RSCV at the LAX view on the screen, the introducer needle is aligned following the direction of the transducer and the central part of the thickness of the transducer (Fig. 6.10).
- Start the puncture at an angle of 20–30° degrees to penetrate the skin and enter the subcutaneous tissue.
- Begin with dynamic needle tracking (DNT), the basis of the ultrasound-guided puncture technique.
- The needle is visualized on the screen from the beginning of the puncture. The insertion of the needle will be monitored throughout the puncture until venous cannulation (Figs. 6.11 and 6.12).

6.4.2 Step 02

- Continue the puncture trajectory to the subclavian vein seen on the screen.
- Once identified by ultrasound that you have reached the lower edge of the clavicle (Figs. 6.13 and 6.14), modify the puncture angle.

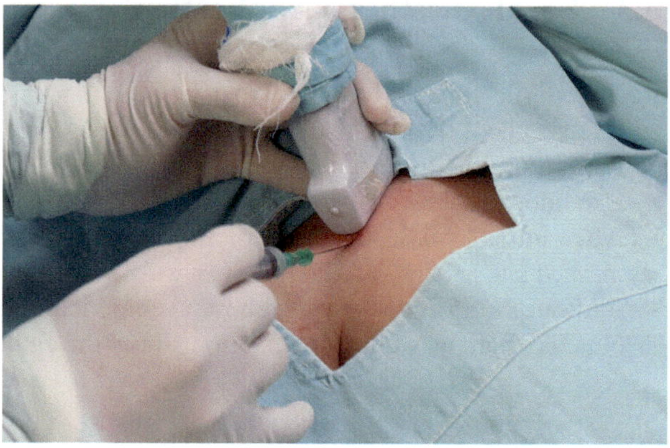

Fig. 6.10 The introducer needle follows the direction of the transducer and the central part of the thickness of the transducer, at an angle of 20 to 30°

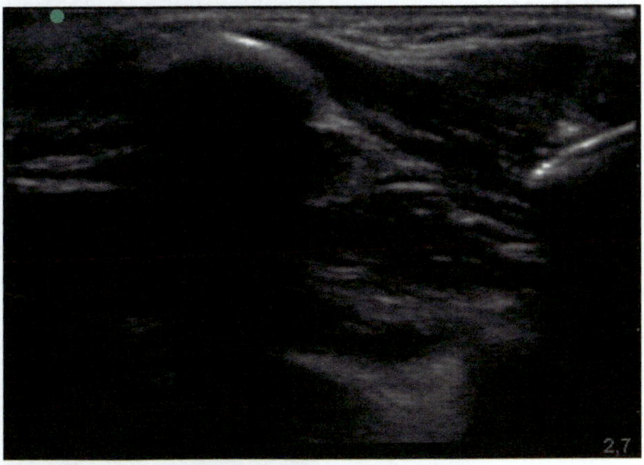

Fig. 6.11 Scan between the middle and inner thirds of the clavicle. LAX view of the start of the puncture of the RSCV
- The scan depth is 2,7 cm

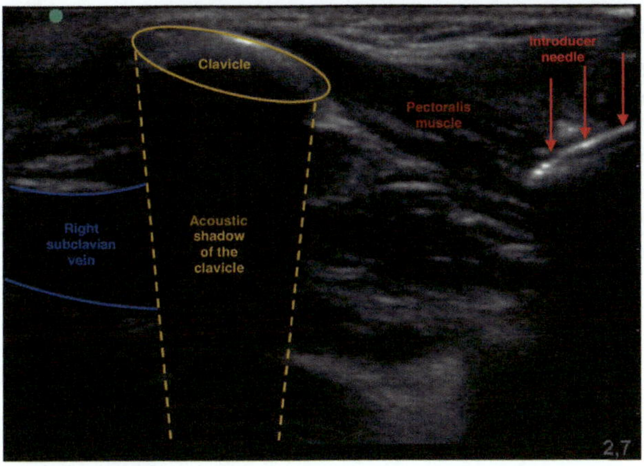

Fig. 6.12 Identifying structures
- Position the right clavicle in the center of the screen; to do this, place the clavicle in the middle of the probe and oblique to this
- The acoustic shadow of the clavicle hides the course at this level of the RSCV
- The trajectory of the introducer needle is not yet aligned with the disposition of the thoracic RSCV

- Modify the puncture angle to less than 10° or almost parallel to the thoracic wall to pass the introducer needle under the clavicle (Fig. 6.15).
- With this puncture modification, you will notice that the clavicle does not interfere with the advancement of the introducer needle, and thus it will pass easily (Figs. 6.16 and 6.17).
- The angle of puncture will depend on the age of the patient. A more acute inclination will be used with more weight and age.

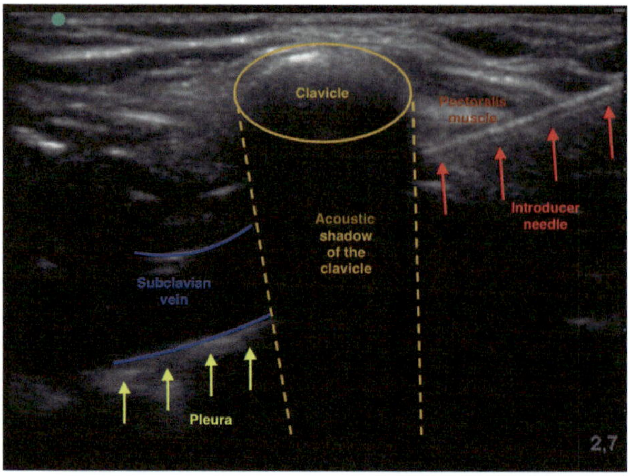

Fig. 6.13 Modify the puncture angle to less than 10 °

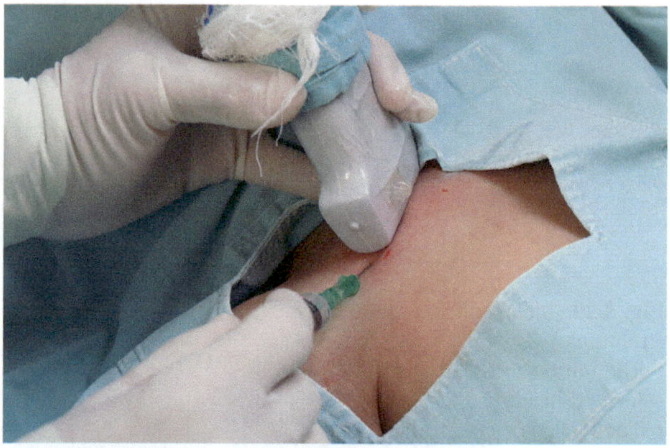

Fig. 6.14 LAX view of the progress of the puncture and arrival of the introducer needle at the lower edge of the clavicle

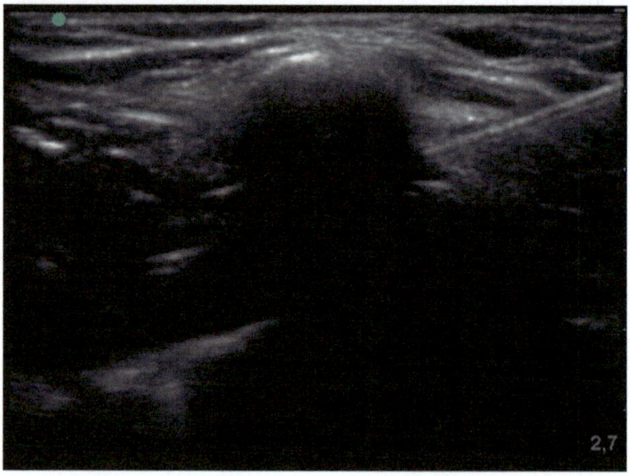

Fig. 6.15 Identifying structures

- The introducer needle has advanced through the pectoralis muscle reaching the lower border of the clavicle

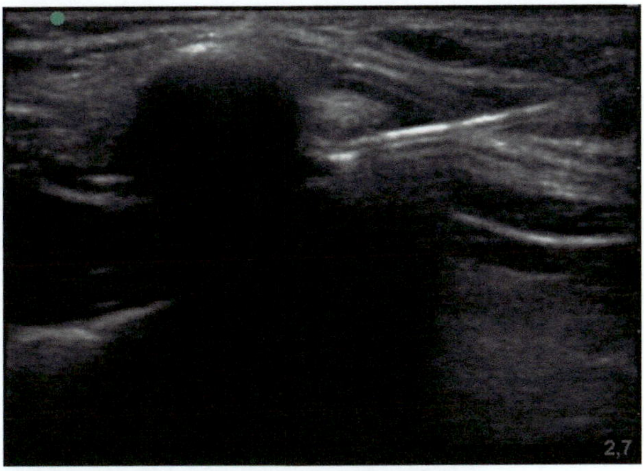

Fig. 6.16 LAX view of the puncture angle modification to less than 10° (see Fig. 6.15) in relation to the anterior thoracic wall so the introducer needle passes under the clavicle

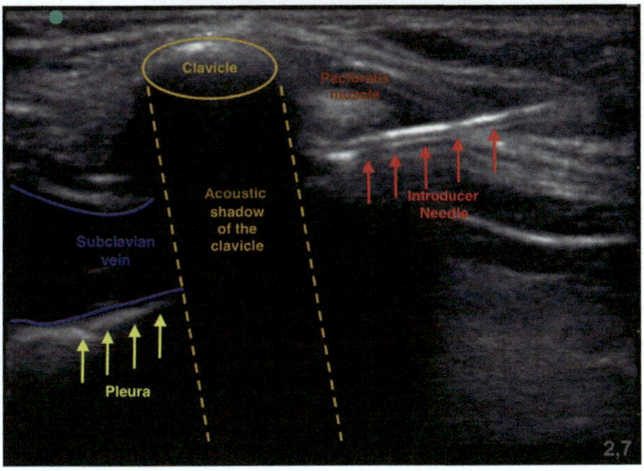

Fig. 6.17 Identifying structures
- Start of the infraclavicular puncture trajectory. You will not see a segment of the puncture needle below the clavicle due to the acoustic shadow of the clavicle
- Therefore, the puncture is advanced following the trajectory toward the RSCV
- The direction of the introducer needle runs parallel to the pleura, making it impossible to puncture it and cause a pneumothorax
- Maintain gentle negative pressure on the syringe plunger as you advance the needle

6.4.3 Step 03

- Stop advancing the puncture when a flash of blood appears in the barrel of the syringe (Fig. 6.18).
- When you cannulate the RSCV, you will feel a loss of resistance and the return of blood in the barrel of the syringe.
- LAX view of the cannulation of the RSCV (Figs. 6.19 and 6.20).
- Once you have identified cannulation of the RSCV, set the transducer aside.

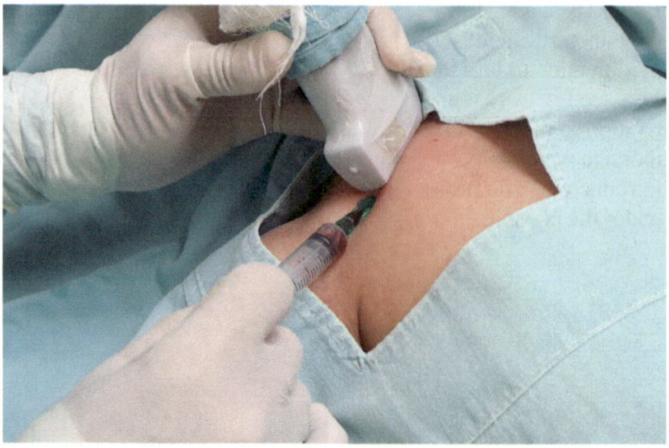

Fig. 6.18 A flash of blood appears in the barrel of the syringe

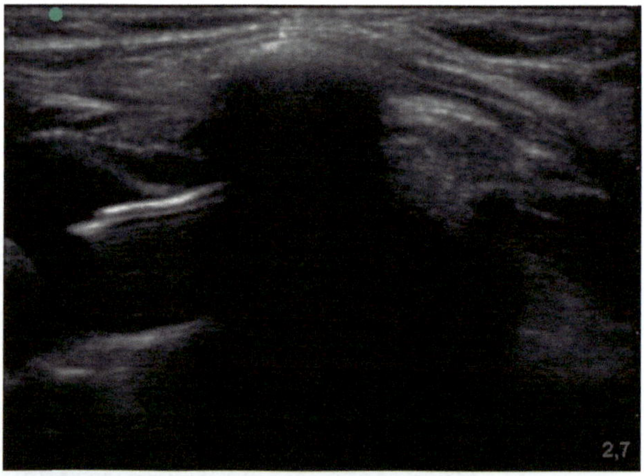

Fig. 6.19 LAX view of the cannulation of the RSCV

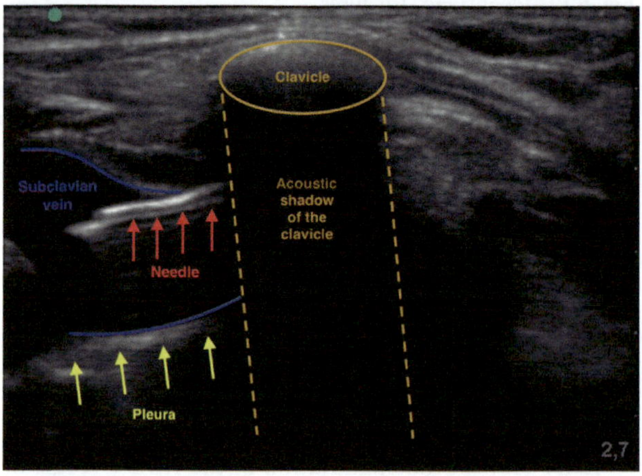

Fig. 6.20 Identifying structures

- Infraclavicular cannulation of the RSCV
- The puncture is performed with two safety elements:
- Visualization of the needle tip so as not to puncture other structures than the RSCV
- Keep the trajectory of the puncture parallel to the pleura and thus prevent puncturing it

6.4.4 Step 04

- Hold the needle hub firmly so the needle is not displaced (Fig. 6.21).
- Insert the 0.018" guidewire, which should go through easily (Fig. 6.22).
- The J-tip end of the guide should easily pass through. If it does not, you can try passing the straight end. If it still does not pass, there may be a chance that the introducer needle has accidentally slipped out of the vein.
- After introducing enough guidewire, remove the introducer needle.
- Place the transducer obliquely over the clavicle toward the junction of the middle and inner thirds, to locate the right subclavian vein.
- Verify the intravascular location of the guidewire by ultrasound (Fig. 6.23).
- LAX view of the intravascular guidewire (Figs. 6.24 and 6.25).
- Scan the right cervical area in SAX view (Fig. 6.26).
- Check that the guidewire is not lodged in the ipsilateral RIJV, which would have to be modified toward the superior cava vein before dilating the trajectory (Figs. 6.27 and 6.28).

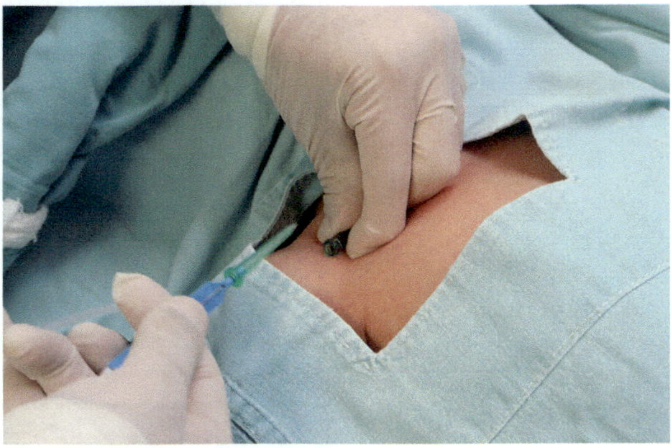

Fig. 6.21 Hold the needle hub

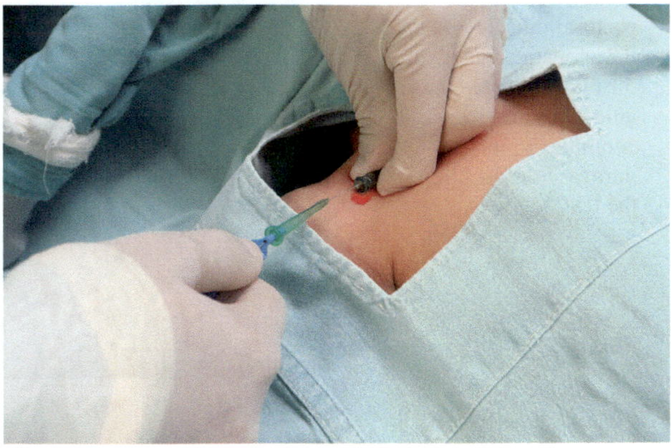

Fig. 6.22 Introduce the guidewire

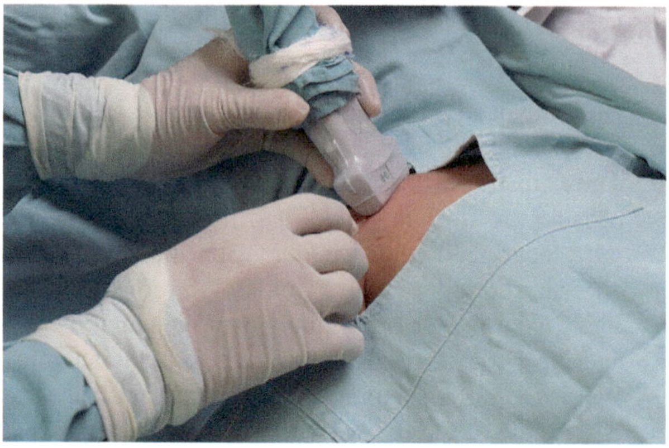

Fig. 6.23 Scan the intravascular location of the guidewire in LAX

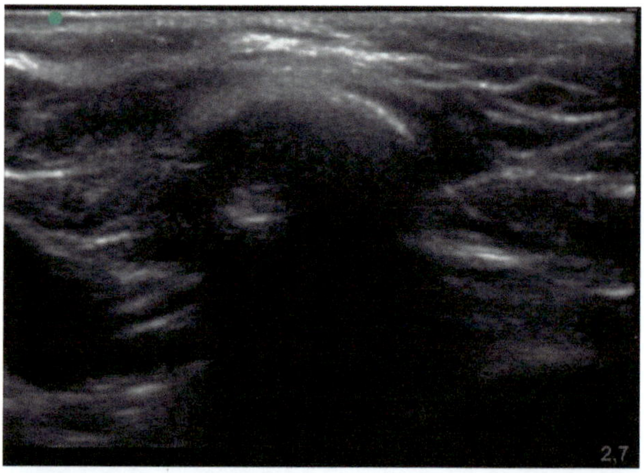

Fig. 6.24 LAX view of the intravascular guidewire

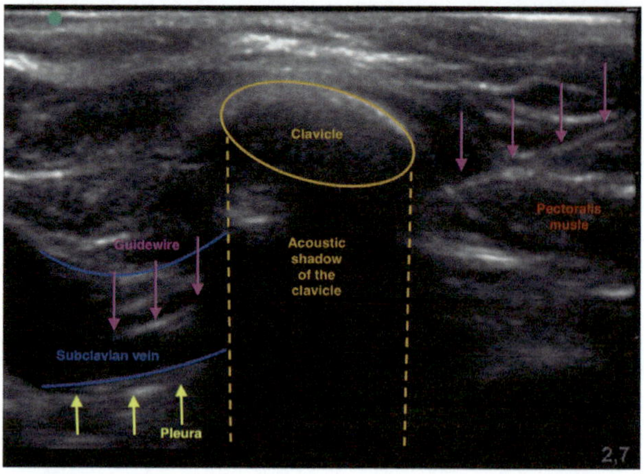

Fig. 6.25 Identifying structures

- The course of the guidewire through the pectoral muscle and then the acoustic shadow of the clavicle hides the guidewire and then continues to its intravascular location in the RSCV

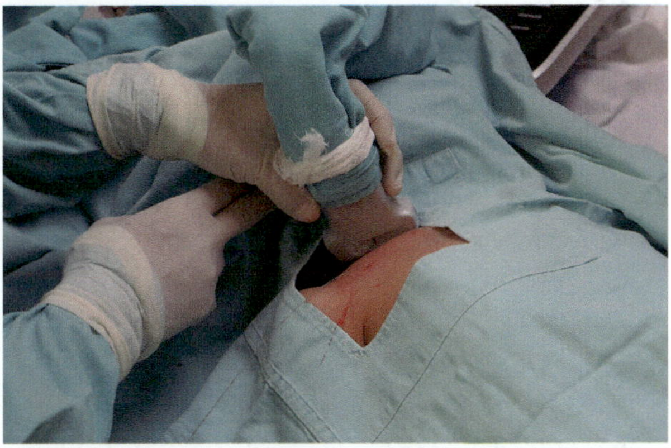

Fig. 6.26 Scan the cervical vessels (RIJV and RCA)

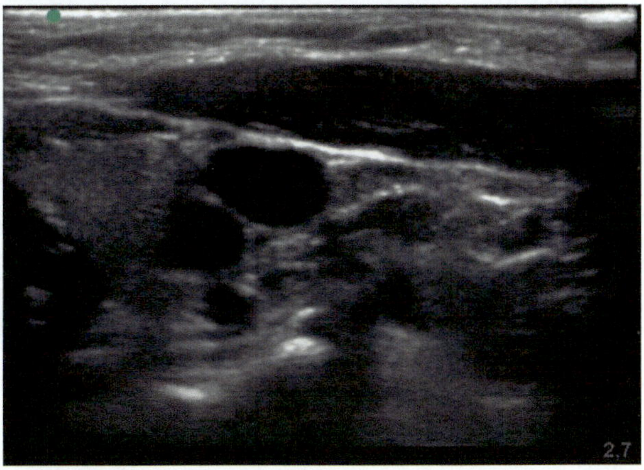

Fig. 6.27 SAX view of cervical vessels

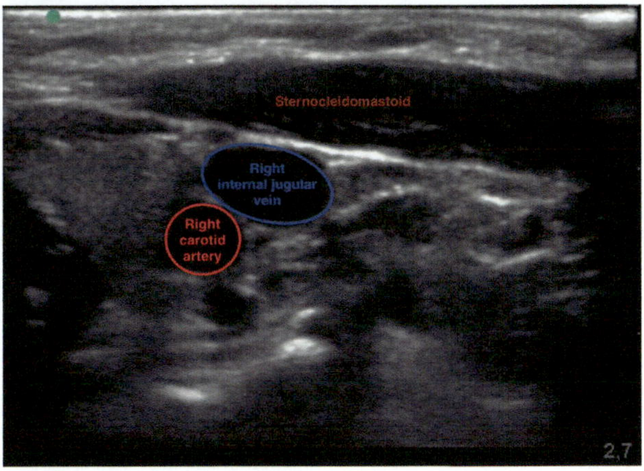

Fig. 6.28 Identifying structures

- The RIJV and the RCA without guidewire

6.4.5 *Step 05*

- Perform dilation with the right hand, and retract the skin with the left hand and with a "screw" maneuver.
- Dilate the path of the skin up to the entrance of the RIJV (Fig. 6.29).
- If a lot of subcutaneous pressure is exerted without countertraction, the guidewire can be bent, hindering dilation and passage of the catheter.

6.4.6 *Step 05*

- Introduce the central venous catheter using Seldinger's technique and remove the guidewire.
- Check the venous return of the lines and clean them with a solution (Fig. 6.30).

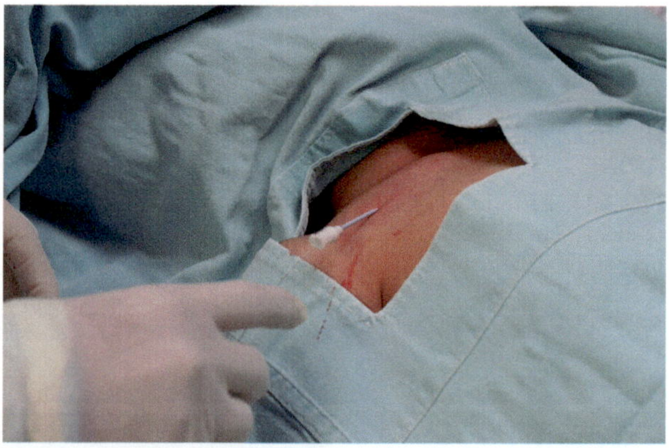

Fig. 6.29 Dilation of the skin path at the entrance to the RSCV

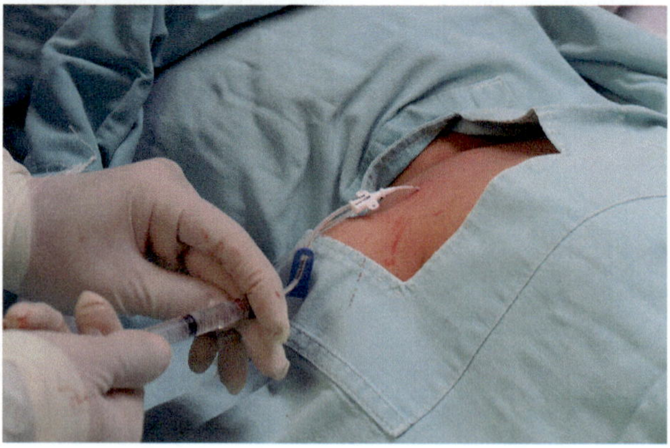

Fig. 6.30 Introduce the required intravascular catheter length

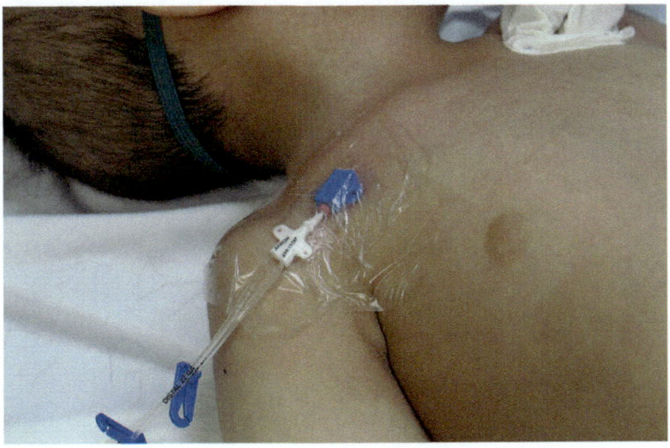

Fig. 6.31 Dressing according to the institutional protocol

6.4.7 *Step 06*

- Secure the catheter and place a sterile occlusive dressing according to the institutional protocol (Fig. 6.31).

Sources

1. Pirotte T, Veyckemans F. Ultrasound-guided subclavian vein cannulation in infants and children: a novel approach. Br J Anaesth. 2007;98(4):509–14. https://doi.org/10.1093/bja/aem041. Epub 2007 Mar 1.
2. Park SI, Kim YH, So SY, Kim MJ, Kim HJ, Kim JK. Ultrasound-guided subclavian catheterization in pediatric patients with a linear probe: a case series. Korean J Anesthesiol. 2013;64(6):541–4. https://doi.org/10.4097/kjae.2013.64.6.541. Epub 2013 Jun 24. PMID: 23814657.
3. Byon HJ, Lee GW, Lee JH, Park YH, Kim HS, Kim CS, Kim JT. Comparison between ultrasound-guided supraclavicular and infraclavicular approaches for subclavian venous catheterization in children—a randomized trial. Br J Anaesth. 2013;111(5):788–92. https://doi.org/10.1093/bja/aet202. Epub 2013 Jun 10.
4. Nardi N, Wodey E, Laviolle B, De La Brière F, Delahaye S, Engrand C, Gauvrit C, Dessard S, Defontaine A, Ecoffey C. Effectiveness and complications of ultrasound-guided subclavian vein cannulation in children and neonates. Anaesth Crit Care Pain Med. 2016;35(3):209–13. https://doi.org/10.1016/j.accpm.2015.09.007. Epub 2016 Feb 26.
5. Rezayat T, Stowell JR, Kendall JL, Turner E, Fox JC, Barjaktarevic I. Ultrasound-guided cannulation: time to bring subclavian central lines Back. West J Emerg Med. 2016;17(2):216–21. https://doi.org/10.5811/westjem.2016.1.29462. Epub 2016 Mar 2.

Chapter 7
Infraclavicular Right Subclavian Vein in Neonates

7.1 Patient Positioning

- The patient is a newborn weighing 3270 g.
- Position the newborn in supine close to the right side of the thermal crib.
- Place the patient's head centered or slightly to the left.
- Place a roll under the shoulders to create a wide space between the clavicle and the first rib (Fig. 7.1).
- Gently restrain the upper extremities with the arm caudal.
- Place the ultrasound device in any of these three positions: above the left shoulder, above the head, or next to the right shoulder.
- Due to the patient's size, a high-frequency linear transducer (13–6 MHz) with a hockey stick-type probe can be used.

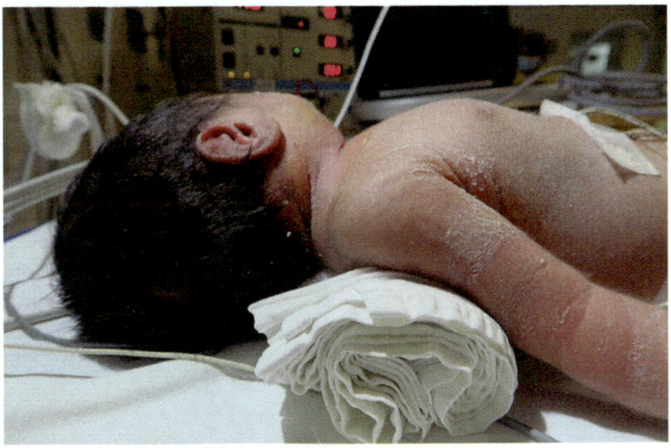

Fig. 7.1 Patient positioning

F. Montes-Tapia, *Atlas of Ultrasound-Guided Central Venous Catheter Placement*, https://doi.org/10.1007/978-3-031-61887-1_7

7.2 Scanning Technique

- Do a preliminary vascular assessment (non-sterile), known as rapid central vein assessment (RaCeVA).
- The operator stands on the right side of the patient.
- Hold the transducer with your left hand and scan the subclavian vessels in long-axis (LAX) placing the transducer obliquely in the external third of the clavicle and with the tip of the hockey stick transducer toward the neck (Fig. 7.2).
- Start the search of the subclavian vessels in the external third of the clavicle, placing the transducer obliquely over the clavicle.
- Place the image of the clavicle in the center of the ultrasound screen. The clavicle produces an inferior acoustic shadow (Fig. 7.3).
- First, visualize the right subclavian artery (RSCA) (Figs. 7.3 and 7.4), which runs deeper in relation to the clavicle and is lateral than the right subclavian vein (RSCV).

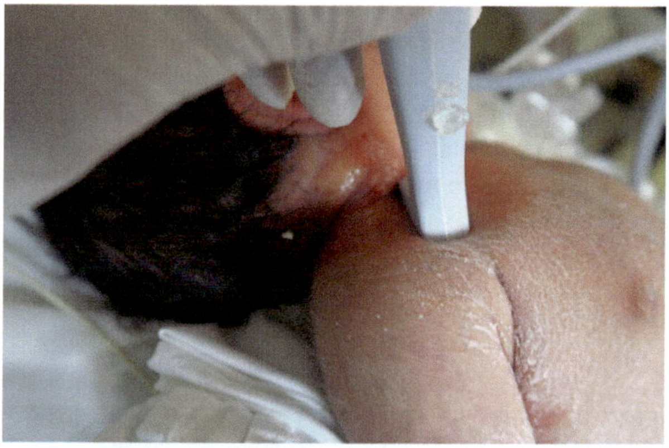

Fig. 7.2 Hold the transducer with the left hand and place it obliquely to the clavicle, in the external third of the clavicle

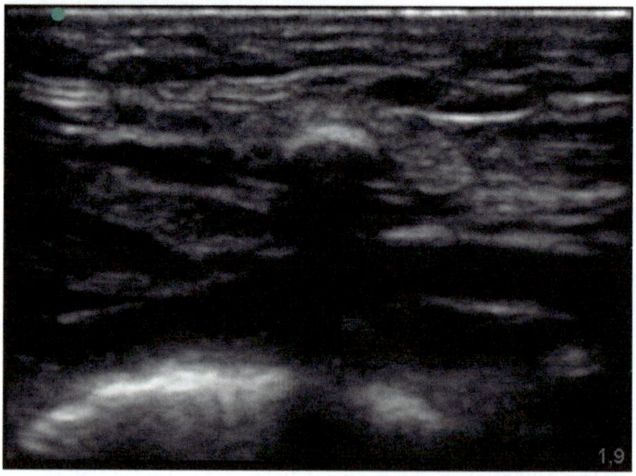

Fig. 7.3 Scan of the external third of the clavicle. LAX view of the RSCA

- The position indicator corresponds to the tip of the hockey stick transductor, directed toward the neck (Fig. 7.2).
- The scan depth of 1,9 cm

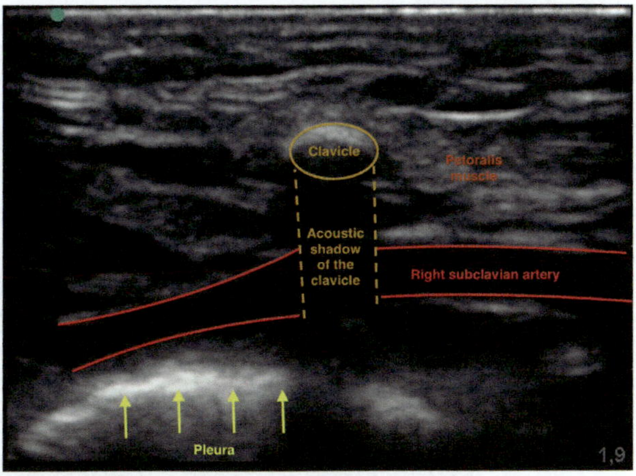

Fig. 7.4 Identifying structures

- The clavicle is in the center of the transducer (Fig. 7.2), and it is seen in the center of the image on the screen. The acoustic shadow causes that the structures below it cannot be visualized
- The RSCA runs deeper in relation to the clavicle and lateral to the vein
- The RSCA in its extrathoracic portion on the right side of the screen corresponds to the pectoral region
- The RSCA in its thoracic portion is identified toward the cervical region, in other words, on the left side of the screen (toward the probe mark or the tip of the hockey stick transductor)
- The pleura lies below the inferior wall of the thoracic portion of the RSCA

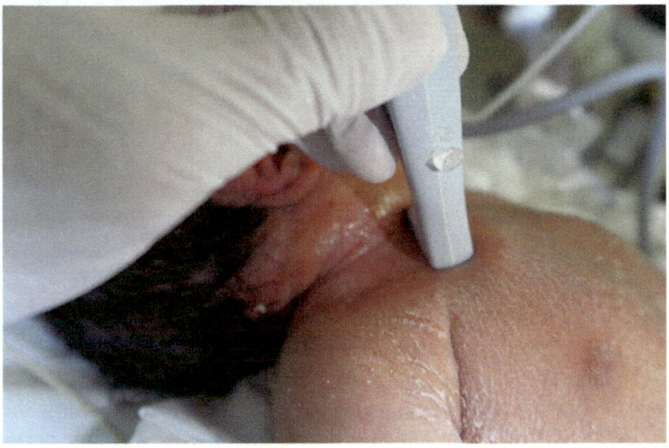

Fig. 7.5 Sweep the transductor from the external third of the clavicle (Fig. 7.2) to the junction of the middle and inner third

- Sweep the transductor across the external third of the clavicle to the junction of the middle and inner third to locate RSCV (Fig. 7.5).
- LAX view of RSCV (Figs. 7.6 and 7.7).
- The RSCV has two anatomical differences from the RSCA. The first difference is the RSCV is more superficial than the RSCA and runs closer to the clavicle. The second difference is the RSCV is more medial than the RSCA.

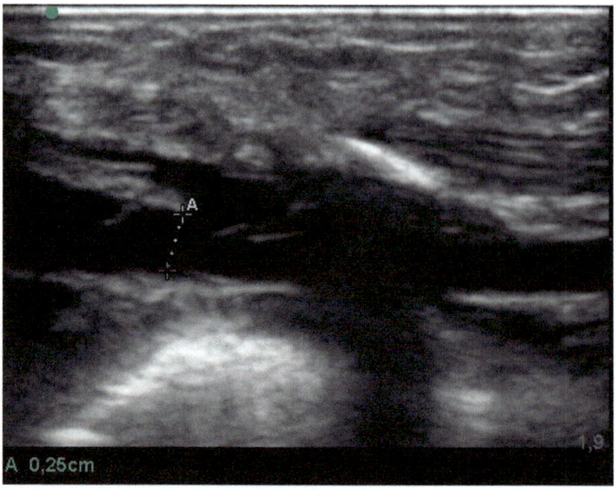

Fig. 7.6 Scan between the middle and inner thirds of the clavicle. LAX view of the RSCV

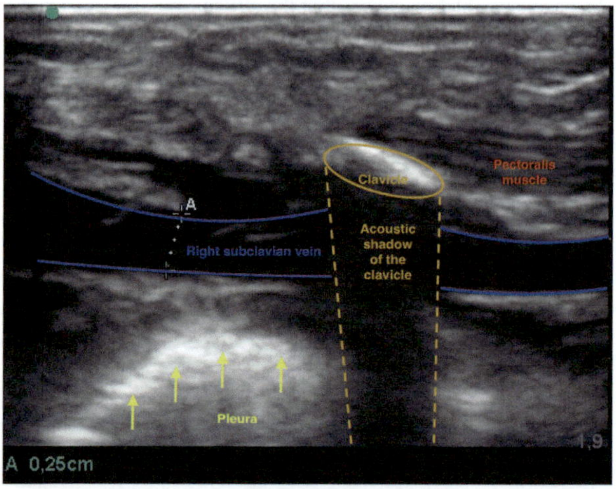

Fig. 7.7 Identifying structures
- The RSCV in its extrathoracic portion on the right side of the screen corresponds to the pectoral region
- The clavicle that causes an acoustic shadow does not allow the visualization of structures
- The RSCV in its thoracic portion is identified toward the cervical region, in other words, on the left side of the screen (toward the tip of the hockey stick transductor)
- The diameter of the RSCV is 0,25 cm

7.3 Local Anesthesia Application

- The patient is on high-frequency oscillatory ventilation.
- The sterile field only leaves the cervical, upper pectoral, and right shoulder regions uncovered (Fig. 7.8).
- Real-time ultrasound-guided lidocaine infiltration.
- For infiltration, use a small needle 25–27 G.
- Use lidocaine 1%.
- Subcutaneous infiltration with lidocaine in the puncture tract 1,5–2 cm before the chosen venipuncture site to anesthetize the oblique puncture path as well as the fixation site of the catheter holder (Fig. 7.9).
- LAX view of lidocaine infiltration (Figs. 7.10 and 7.11).

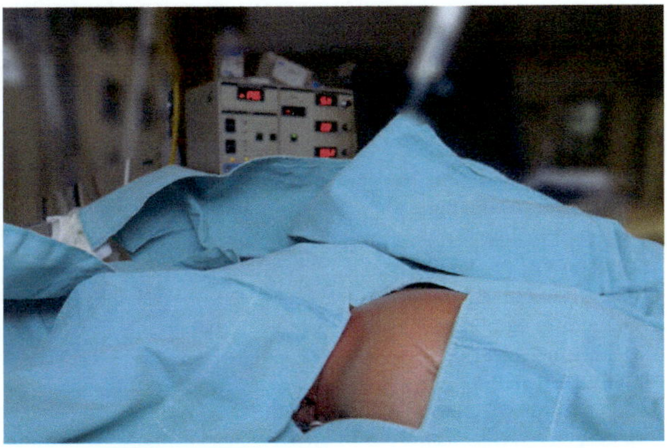

Fig. 7.8 The sterile field only leaves the cervical, upper pectoral, and right shoulder regions uncovered

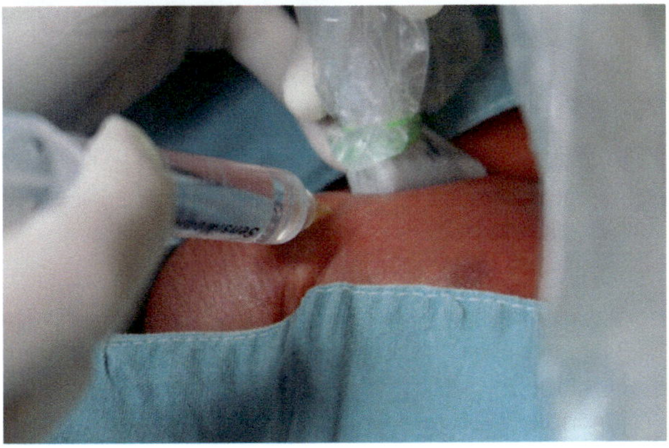

Fig. 7.9 Real-time ultrasound-guided lidocaine infiltration

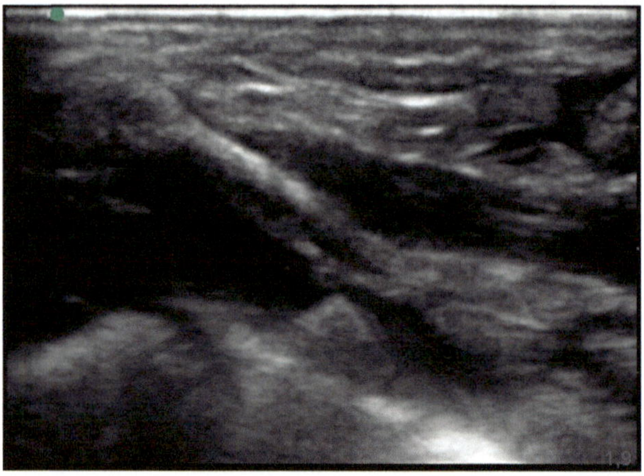

Fig. 7.10 LAX view of lidocaine infiltration

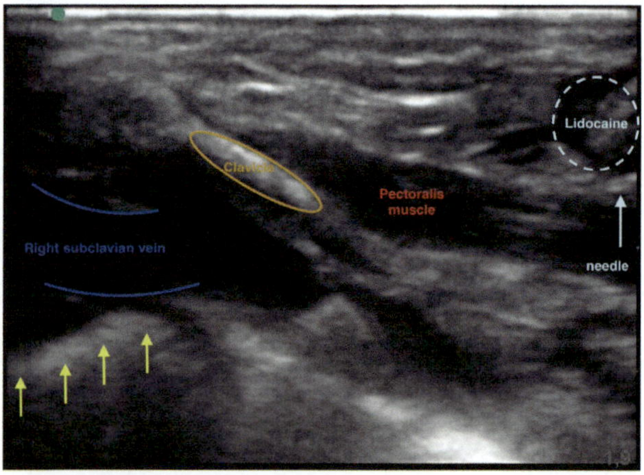

Fig. 7.11 Identifying structures
- The infiltration needle is identified between the subcutaneous tissues for infiltration of the path that will follow the puncture of the RSCV
- This moment of the procedure can be used to determine if the site of choice for the puncture is in the plane of the RSCV, as in this case

7.4 Steps for Real-Time Ultrasound-Guided Access to Infraclavicular Right Subclavian Vein in Neonates

7.4.1 Step 01

- We will use a Vygon® 3 Fr, 10-cm, double-lumen catheter.
- The operator stands on the right side of the newborn.
- Hold the transducer with your left hand and scan the RSCV in LAX view, in the junction of the middle and inner thirds of the right clavicle.
- The catheter 3 Fr. Vygon® has a 21-G introducer needle that is echogenic, which substantially improves visualization.

- Once you identify the RSCV at the LAX view on the screen, the introducer needle is aligned following the direction of the tip of the hockey stick transducer and the central part of the thickness of the transducer (Fig. 7.12).
- Start the puncture at an angle of 30° to 45° degrees to penetrate the skin and enter the subcutaneous tissue.
- Begin with dynamic needle tracking (DNT), the basis of the ultrasound-guided puncture technique.
- The needle is visualized on the screen from the beginning of the puncture. The introducer needle is monitored throughout the procedure until venous cannulation.
- LAX view of the start of the puncture (Figs. 7.13 and 7.14).

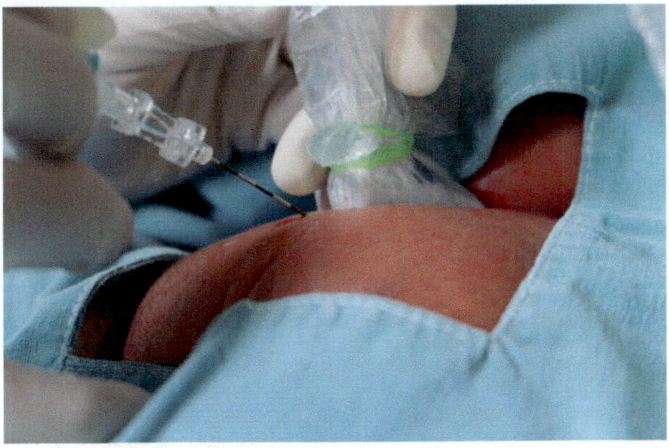

Fig. 7.12 The introducer needle is aligned to the central part of the thickness of the transducer and following the direction of the tip of the hockey stick transducer, at an angle of 30–45°

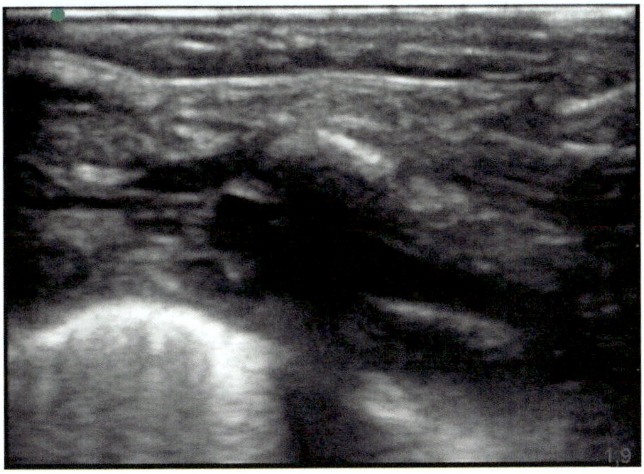

Fig. 7.13 Scan between the middle and inner thirds of the clavicle. LAX view of the start of the puncture of the RSCV
- The scan depth is 1,9 cm

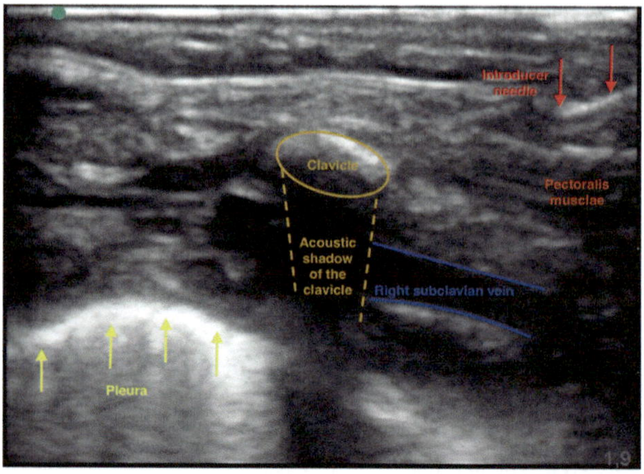

Fig. 7.14 Identifying structures

- Position the right clavicle in the center of the screen; to do this, place the clavicle in the middle of the probe and oblique to this. The acoustic shadow of the clavicle hides the course at this level of the RSCV
- The trajectory of the introducer needle is not yet aligned with the disposition of the thoracic RSCV

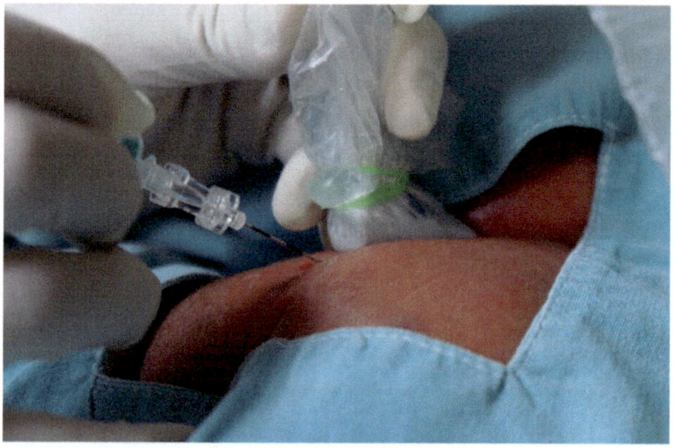

Fig. 7.15 Sweep the transductor medially over the clavicle and modify the puncture medially

7.4.2 Step 02

- Modify the scan, sweep medially the transductor over the clavicle to identify the thoracic portion of the RSCV, and then modify the direction of the puncture to follow the course of the vein (Fig. 7.15).
- With this modification of the scan and following the course of the thoracic portion of the RSCV, continue the puncture (Figs. 7.16 and 7.17).

7.4.3 Step 03

- Once identified by ultrasound that you have reached the lower edge of the clavicle (Figs. 7.18 and 7.19), modify the puncture angle.
- Modify the puncture angle to less than 10° or almost parallel to the chest wall to pass the introducer needle under the clavicle (Fig. 7.20).

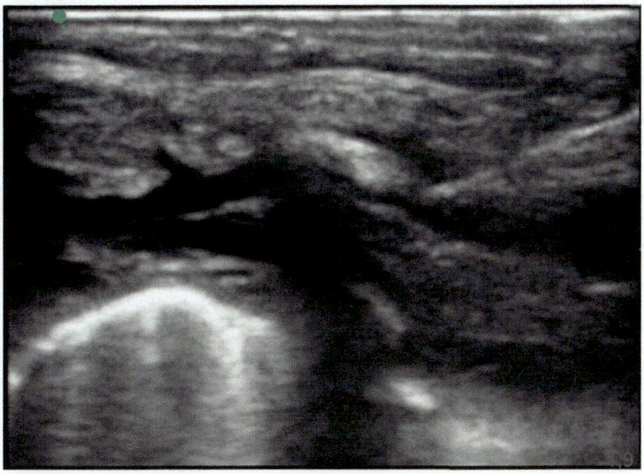

Fig. 7.16 LAX view of the advancement of the puncture
- Now with the modification of the more medial scan, the thoracic portion of the RSCV is visualized

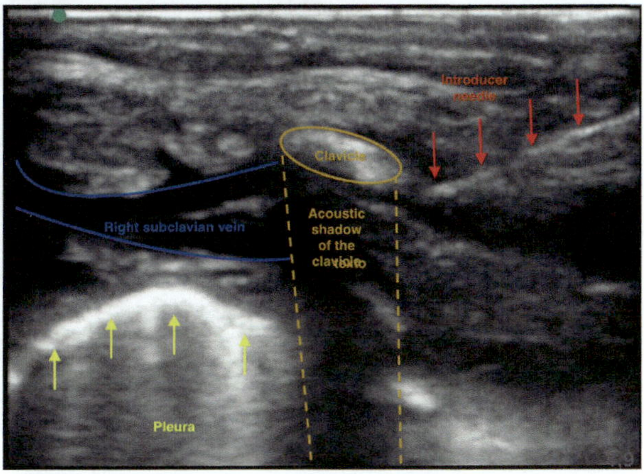

Fig. 7.17 Identifying structures
- The thoracic portion of the RSCV can now be seen
- The introducer needle has advanced through the pectoral muscles reaching the lower border of the clavicle

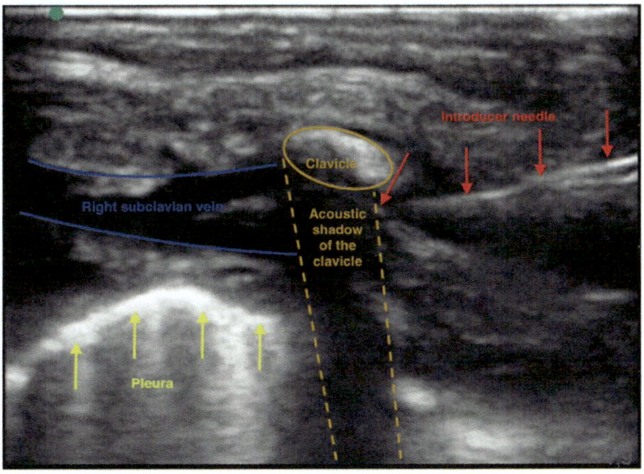

Fig. 7.18 Modification of the puncture angle to less than 10°

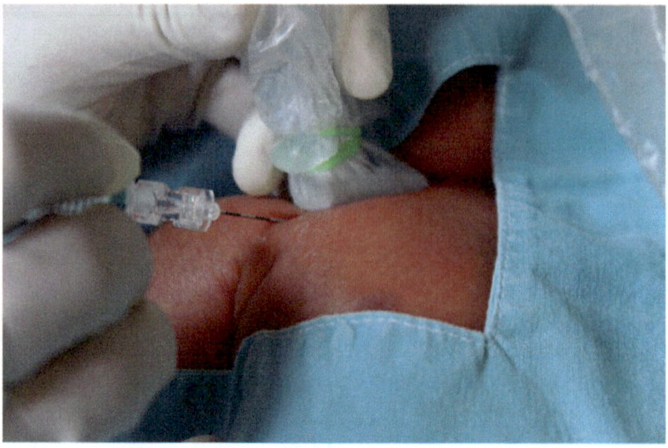

Fig. 7.19 LAX view of the advancement of the puncture with modification of the angle of puncture

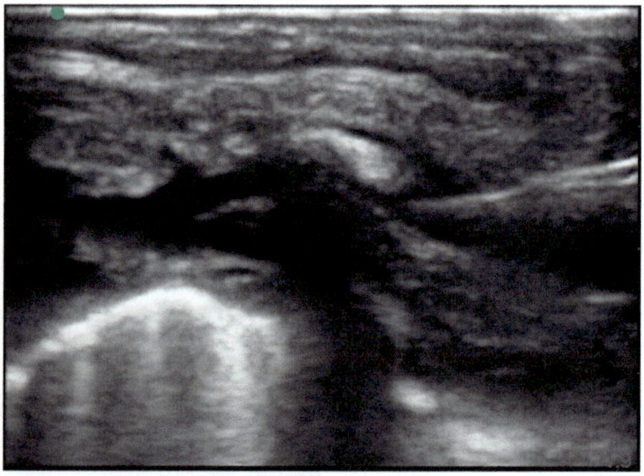

Fig. 7.20 Identifying structures

- Puncture angle modification to less than 10° in relation to the anterior chest wall (Fig. 7.18) so the introducer needle will pass under the clavicle

- With this puncture modification, you will notice that the clavicle does not interfere with the advancement of the introducer needle, and thus it will pass easily.
- Continue the puncture trajectory to the subclavian vein seen on the screen.
- The clavicle is not an impassable obstacle at this age as long as the roll has been properly positioned under the shoulders.

7.4.4 Step 04

- Continue advancing the introducer needle under DNT. This maneuver will guide you to change direction in real time if the puncture is going in an inappropriate direction (Fig. 7.21).

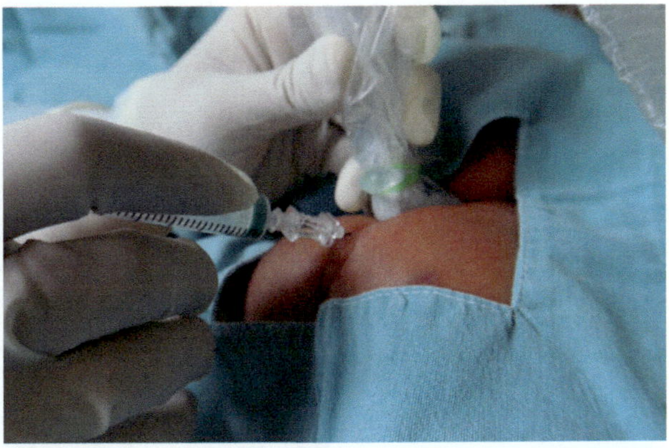

Fig. 7.21 Slide the transducer to cephalic area and continue the puncture following the trajectory of the RSCV under DNT

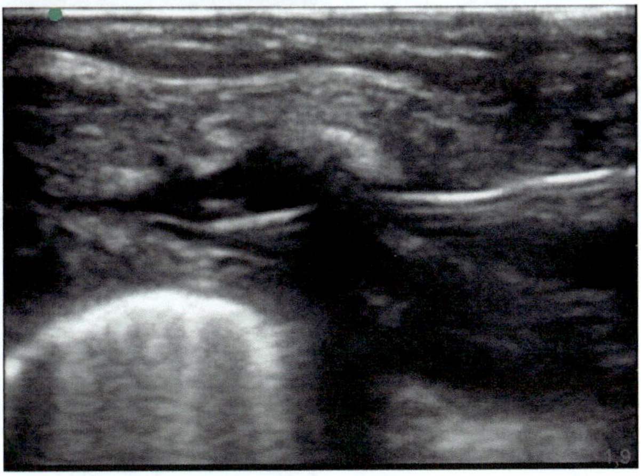

Fig. 7.22 LAX view of the cannulation of the RSCV by the introducer needle

- When you pass under the clavicle, you will not see the tip of the needle. If it is in the correct path of the footprint, the tip of the needle will be seen after the clavicle.
- In this patient, to perform DNT of the introducer needle, slide the transducer toward the head and maintain the transducer oblique to the clavicle.
- In this case, it is identified that the introducer needle is cannulating the RSCV but in the direction of the posterior wall (Figs. 7.22 and 7.23).
- Maintain gentle negative pressure on the syringe plunger as you advance the needle.
- Change the trajectory of the puncture under ultrasonographic guidance to make it more horizontal and that the tip of the introducer needle is not in the direction of the posterior wall of the RSCV (Fig. 7.24).
- Therefore, the puncture is advanced following the trajectory toward the RSCV (Figs. 7.25 and 7.26).

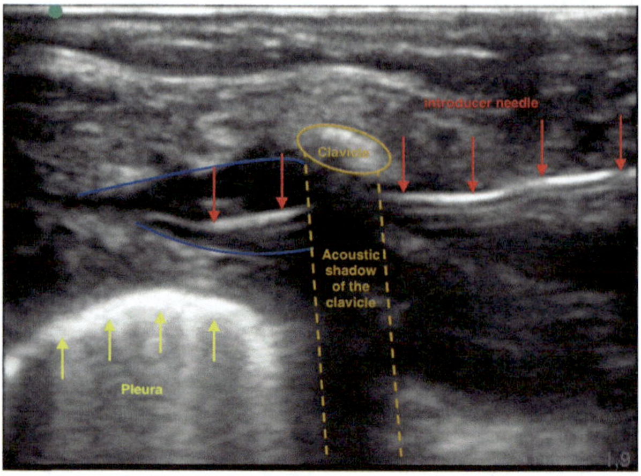

Fig. 7.23 Identifying structures
- Start of the infraclavicular puncture trajectory. You will not see a segment of the introducer needle below the clavicle due to the acoustic shadow of the clavicle
- At this level, the puncture has a trajectory toward the posterior wall

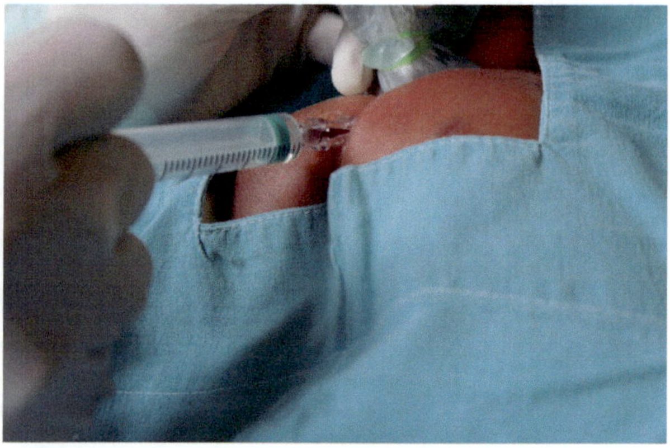

Fig. 7.24 Change the trajectory of the puncture under ultrasonographic guidance to make it more horizontal. A flash of blood appears in the barrel of the syringe

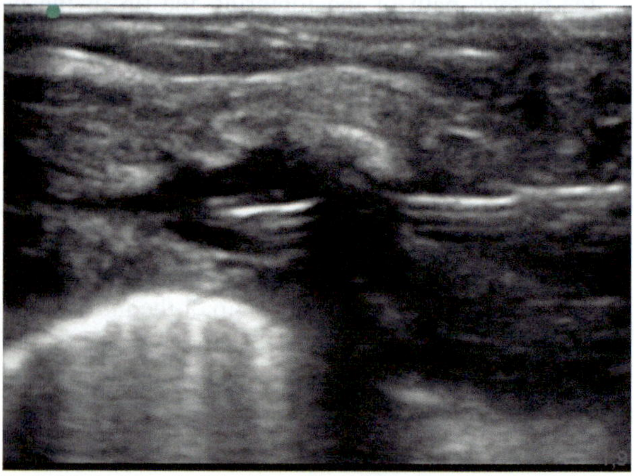

Fig. 7.25 LAX view of the horizontal trajectory change of the introducer needle

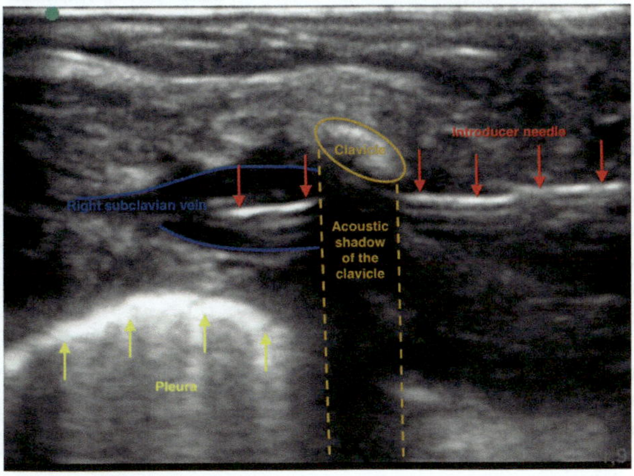

Fig. 7.26 Identifying structures
- Infraclavicular cannulation of the thoracic portion of the RSCV
- Now the tip of the introducer needle is not in the direction of the posterior wall but with the lumen of the vein and parallel to the pleura
- The thoracic portion of the RSCV is still not completely visualized, so slide the transducer toward cephalic and obliquely to the clavicle

Fig. 7.27 Scanning by sliding the transducer toward the head, to follow the trajectory of the puncture with DNT. LAX view

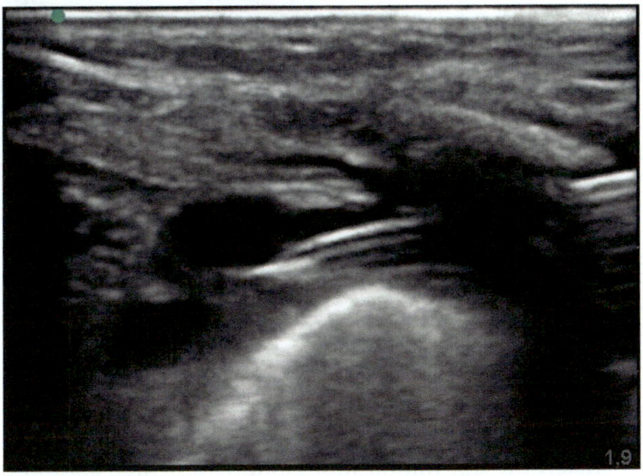

- With this change of trajectory, the direction of the introducer needle runs parallel to the pleura, making it impossible to puncture it and cause a pneumothorax (Figs. 7.27 and 7.28).
- When you cannulate the RSCV, you will feel a loss of resistance and the return of blood in the barrel of the syringe. Then stop advancing with the puncture.

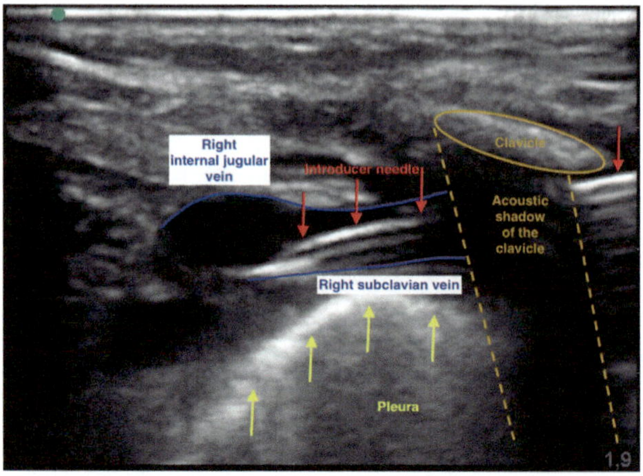

Fig. 7.28 Identifying structures
- Visualization of the RSCV cannulation
- The puncture is performed with two safety elements
  - Visualization of the needle tip so as not to puncture other structures than the RSCV
  - Keep the trajectory of the puncture parallel to the pleura and thus prevent puncturing it

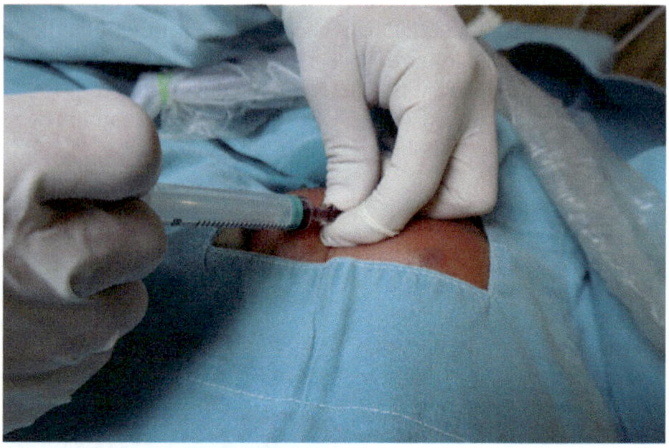

Fig. 7.29 Hold the needle hub

7.4.5 Step 05

- Hold the needle hub firmly with your left hand, so the needle is not displaced (Fig. 7.29).
- Insert the 0,3-mm nitinol guidewire, which should pass easily (Fig. 7.30).
- This type of guidewire is marked every 10 cm, so the guidewire should not go beyond the first 5 cm.
- After introducing enough guidewire, remove the introducer needle.
- Place the transducer obliquely over the clavicle toward the junction of the middle and inner thirds, to locate the right subclavian vein (Fig. 7.31).
- Verify the intravascular location of the guidewire by ultrasound (Figs. 7.32 and 7.33).

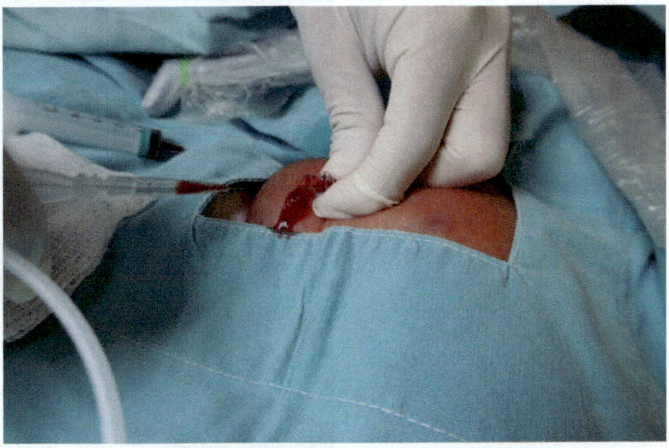

Fig. 7.30 Introducing the guidewire

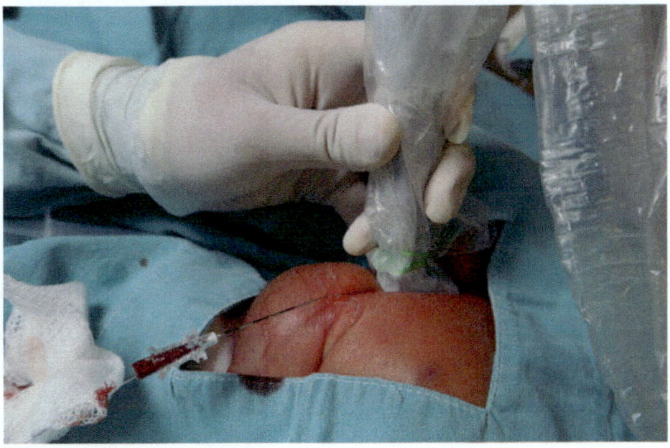

Fig. 7.31 Scan the intravascular location of the guidewire in LAX

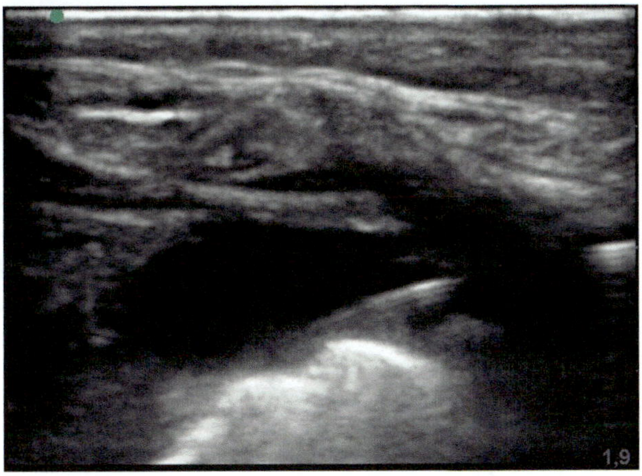

Fig. 7.32 LAX view of the intravascular guidewire

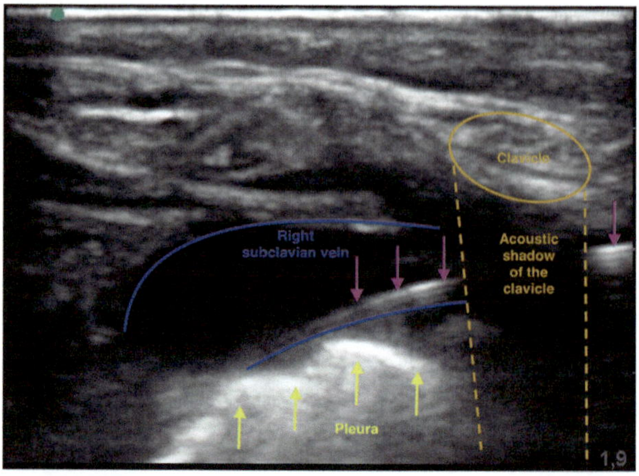

Fig. 7.33 Identifying structures
- The course of the guidewire through the pectoral muscle and then the acoustic shadow of the clavicle hides the guidewire and then continues to its intravascular location of the thoracic RSCV, with direction curving inferiorly toward the right brachiocephalic vein

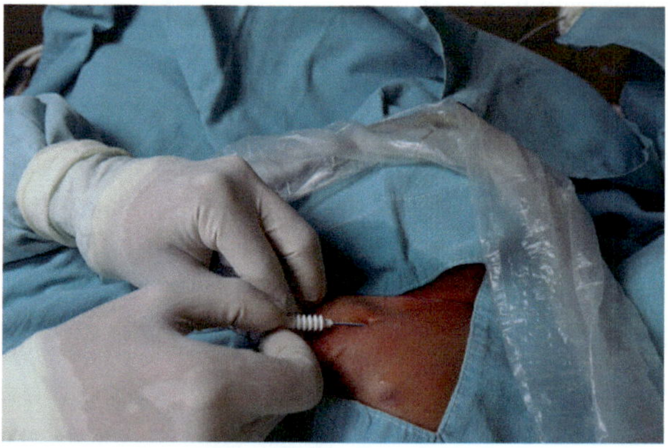

Fig. 7.34 Dilation of the skin path at the entrance to the RSCV

7.4.6 Step 06

- Perform dilation with the right hand and countertraction of the skin with the left hand and with a "screw" maneuver.
- Dilate the path of the skin up to the entrance of the RIJV (Fig. 7.34).
- If a lot of subcutaneous pressure is exerted without countertraction, the guidewire can be bent, hindering dilation and passage of the central venous catheter.
- Extract the dilator and, with the index finger of the left hand, occlude the exit in the skin so the patient does not bleed (Fig. 7.35).

7.4.7 Step 07

- When you finish dilating, occlude the already dilated puncture entry site with gauze and your left hand so it does not bleed.
- With the same hand, hold the wire to prepare to insert the catheter (Fig. 7.36).

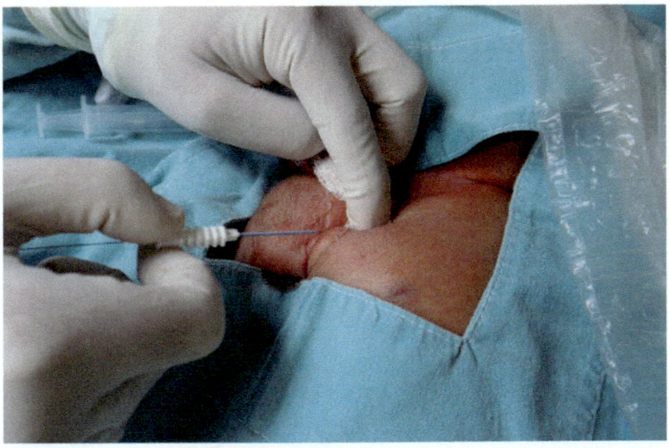

Fig. 7.35 Remove the dilator, applying compression to the skin entrance so that it does not bleed

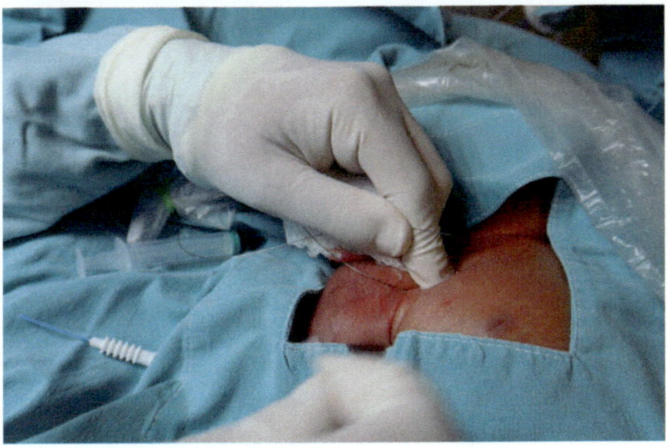

Fig. 7.36 Preparation to introduce the catheter over the guidewire (Seldinger's technique)

- Once you have inserted the catheter using Seldinger's technique, remove the guidewire, and check the venous return of the lines and clean them with a solution (Fig. 7.37).
- Place the transducer obliquely over the clavicle toward the junction of the middle and inner thirds, to locate the right subclavian vein.
- Scan to confirm the intravascular location of the catheter (Fig. 7.38).
- LAX view of the central venous catheter inside the RSCV (Figs. 7.39 and 7.40).
- Check the venous return of the lines and clean them with a solution.
- Another way to check the intravascular location of the CVC is to scan the supraclavicular fossae (Fig. 7.41).
- LAX view of the supraclavicular fossae with the catheter within the RSCV (Figs. 7.42 and 7.43).

7.4.8 Step 08

- Secure the catheter and place a sterile occlusive dressing according to the institutional protocol (Fig. 7.44).

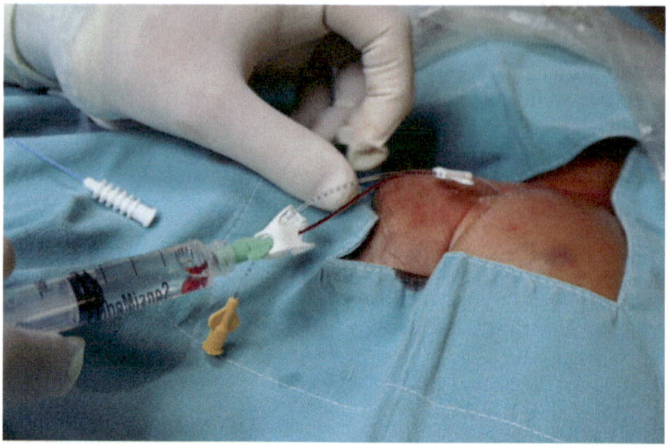

Fig. 7.37 Introduce the required intravascular catheter length

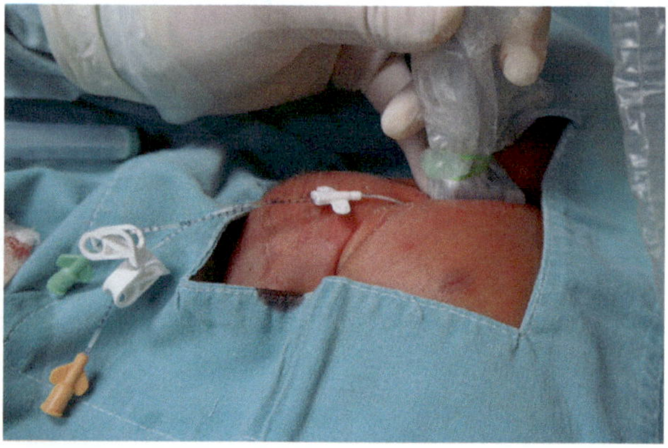

Fig. 7.38 Scan the intravascular location of the catheter in the RSCV

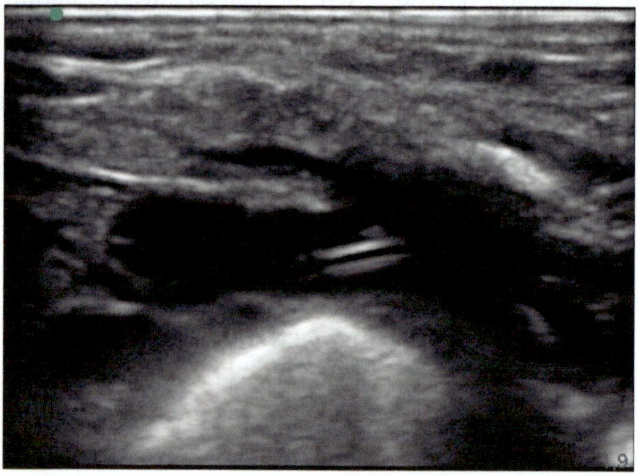

Fig. 7.39 LAX view of the central venous catheter inside the RSCV

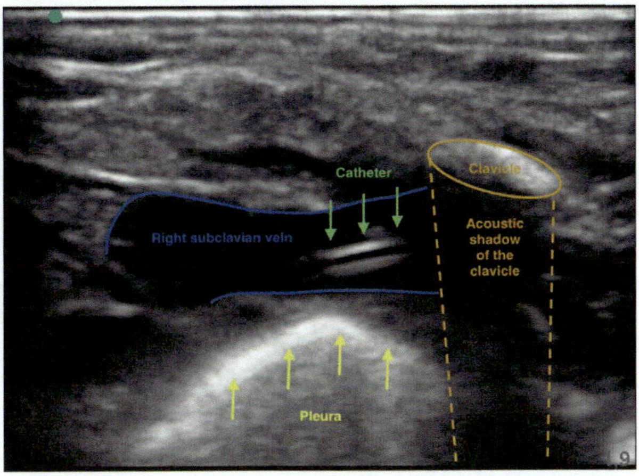

Fig. 7.40 Identifying structures
- Catheter inside the RSCV

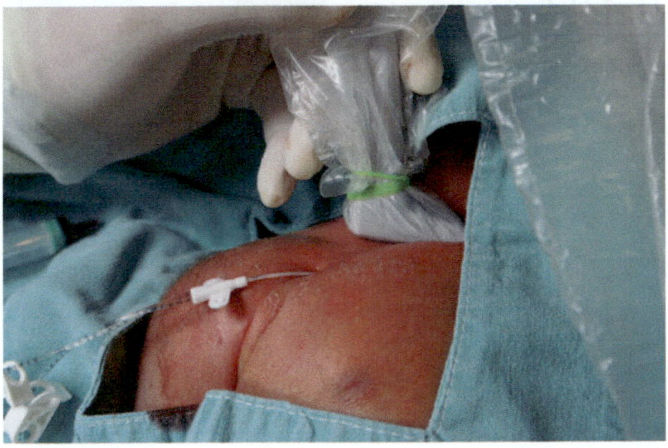

Fig. 7.41 Scan the supraclavicular fossae

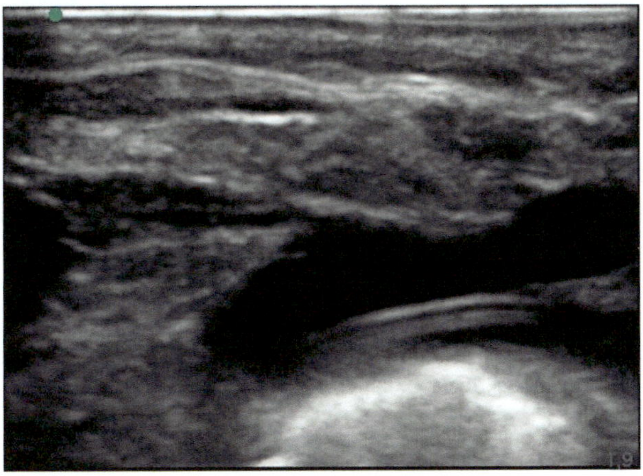

Fig. 7.42 LAX view of the right supraclavicular fossae

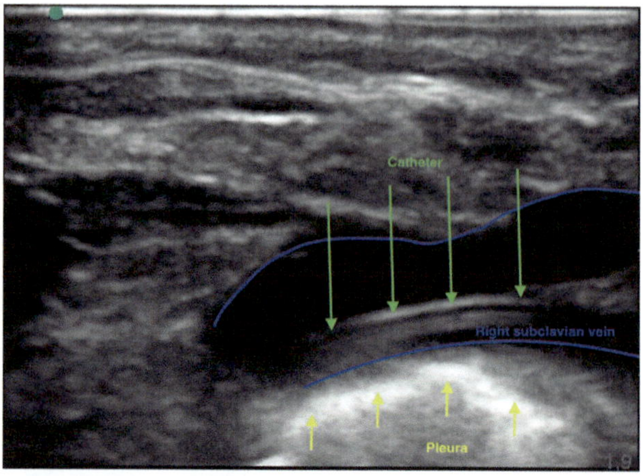

Fig. 7.43 Identifying structures

- The catheter is in the RSCV in a downward course toward the right brachiocephalic vein

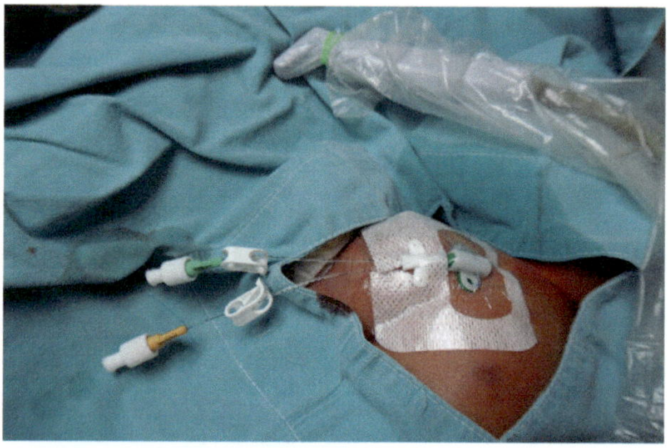

Fig. 7.44 Dressing according to the institutional protocol

Sources

1. Pirotte T, Veyckemans F. Ultrasound-guided subclavian vein cannulation in infants and children: a novel approach. Br J Anaesth. 2007;98(4):509–14. https://doi.org/10.1093/bja/aem041. Epub 2007 Mar 1.
2. Park SI, Kim YH, So SY, Kim MJ, Kim HJ, Kim JK. Ultrasound-guided subclavian catheterization in pediatric patients with a linear probe: a case series. Korean J Anesthesiol. 2013;64(6):541–4. https://doi.org/10.4097/kjae.2013.64.6.541. Epub 2013 Jun 24. PMID: 23814657.
3. Byon HJ, Lee GW, Lee JH, Park YH, Kim HS, Kim CS, Kim JT. Comparison between ultrasound-guided supraclavicular and infraclavicular approaches for subclavian venous catheterization in children—a randomized trial. Br J Anaesth. 2013;111(5):788–92. https://doi.org/10.1093/bja/aet202. Epub 2013 Jun 10.

4. Nardi N, Wodey E, Laviolle B, De La Brière F, Delahaye S, Engrand C, Gauvrit C, Dessard S, Defontaine A, Ecoffey C. Effectiveness and complications of ultrasound-guided subclavian vein cannulation in children and neonates. Anaesth Crit Care Pain Med. 2016;35(3):209–13. https://doi.org/10.1016/j.accpm.2015.09.007. Epub 2016 Feb 26.
5. Rezayat T, Stowell JR, Kendall JL, Turner E, Fox JC, Barjaktarevic I. Ultrasound-guided cannulation: time to bring subclavian central lines Back. West J Emerg Med. 2016;17(2):216–21. https://doi.org/10.5811/westjem.2016.1.29462. Epub 2016 Mar 2.

Chapter 8
Infraclavicular Left Subclavian Vein in Pediatrics

8.1 Patient Positioning

- The patient is an 8-month-old infant weighing 7 kg.
- Position the patient in dorsal decubitus close to the left side of the bed or stretcher.
- Place a roll under the shoulders to create a wide space between the clavicle and the first rib (Fig. 8.1).
- Place the patient's head centered or slightly to the right.
- Gently restrain the upper extremities with the arms caudal.
- Place the ultrasound in any of these positions: next to the left shoulder, above the head, or the right shoulder.
- A high-frequency linear transducer (13–6 MHz) with a hockey stick-type probe or a probe as long as 5 cm can be used.

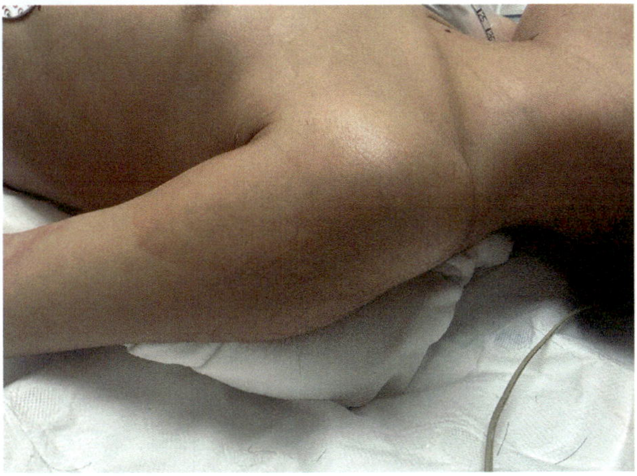

Fig. 8.1 Patient positioning

F. Montes-Tapia, *Atlas of Ultrasound-Guided Central Venous Catheter Placement*, https://doi.org/10.1007/978-3-031-61887-1_8

8.2 Scanning Technique

- Do a preliminary vascular assessment (non-sterile), known as rapid central vein assessment (RaCeVA).
- Hold the transducer with your left hand and scan the subclavian vessels in long axis (LAX), placing the transducer obliquely to the clavicle and with the position indicator toward the neck (Fig. 8.2).
- Start the search of the subclavian vessels in the external third of the clavicle, placing the transducer obliquely over the clavicle.
- Place the image of the clavicle in the center of the ultrasound screen. The clavicle produces an inferior acoustic shadow.
- First, visualize the left subclavian artery (LSCA) (Figs. 8.3 and 8.4), which runs deeper in relation to the clavicle and is more lateral than the left subclavian vein (LSCV).
- Sweep the transductor medially, with the transducer obliquely over the clavicle toward the junction of the middle and inner thirds, to locate the LSCV.
- LAX view of the LSCV (Figs. 8.5 and 8.6).
- The LSCV has two anatomical differences from the LSCA. The first difference is the LSCV is more superficial than the LSCA and runs closer to the clavicle. The second difference is the LSCV is more medial than the artery.

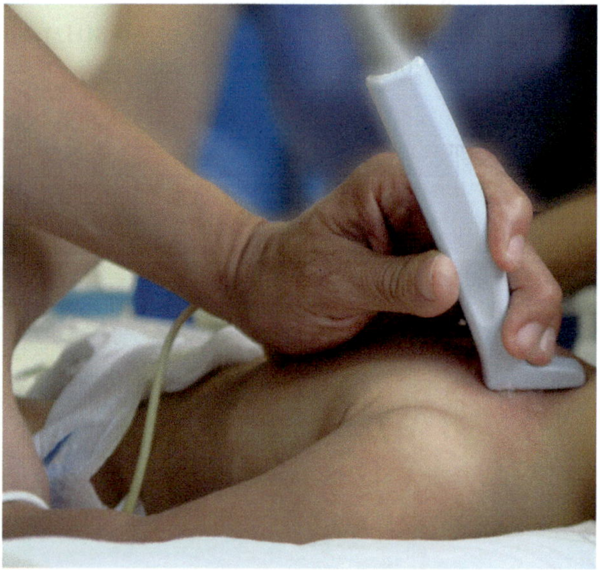

Fig. 8.2 Hold the transducer with the left hand and place it oblique to the clavicle, in the external third of the clavicle

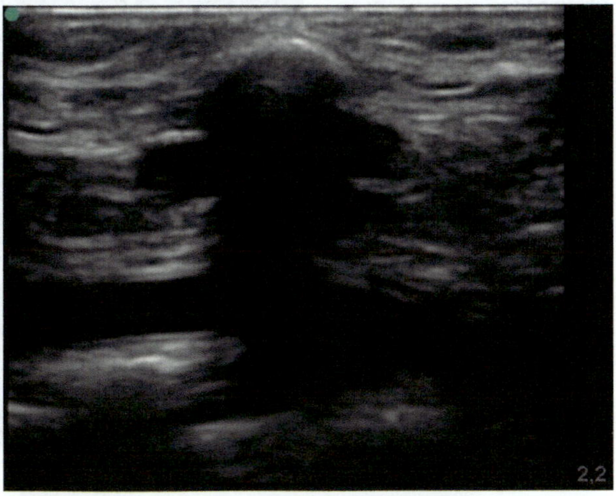

Fig. 8.3 Scan of the external third of the clavicle. LAX view of the LSCA
- The mark on the side of the probe corresponds to the tip of the hockey stick transducer, directed toward the neck
- The scan depth is 2,2 cm

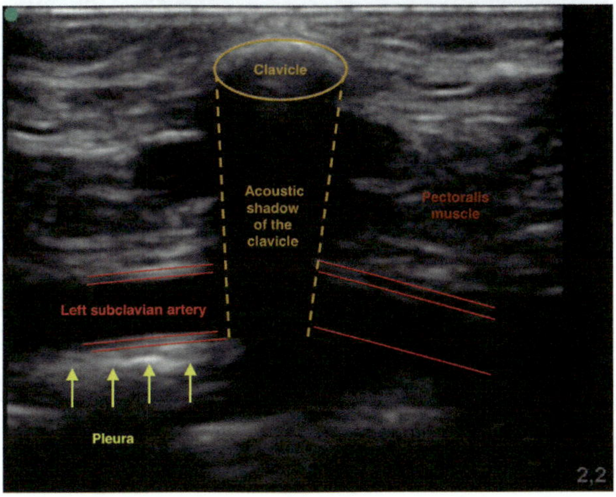

Fig. 8.4 Identifying structures
- The clavicle is in the center of the transducer (Fig. 8.2) and is seen in the center of the image on the screen. The acoustic shadow causes the structures below it not to be visualized
- The LSCA, with two echogenic layers of its wall, typical of an artery, runs deeper in relation to the clavicle and lateral to the vein
- The LSCA, in its extrathoracic portion on the right side of the screen, corresponds to the pectoral region
- The LSCA in its thoracic portion is identified toward the cervical region, in other words, on the left side of the screen (toward the tip of the hockey stick transductor)
- The pleura lies below the inferior wall of the thoracic portion of the LSCA

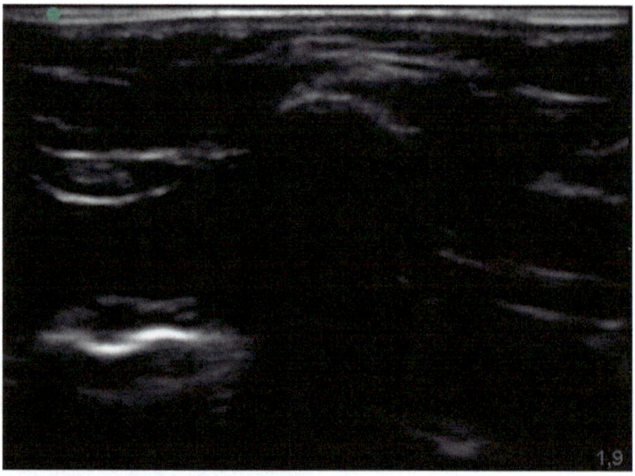

Fig. 8.5 Scan between the middle and inner third of the clavicle. LAX view of LSCV

- The scanning depth is changed to 1.9 cm because the LSCV is at a shallower depth and below the lower edge of the clavicle

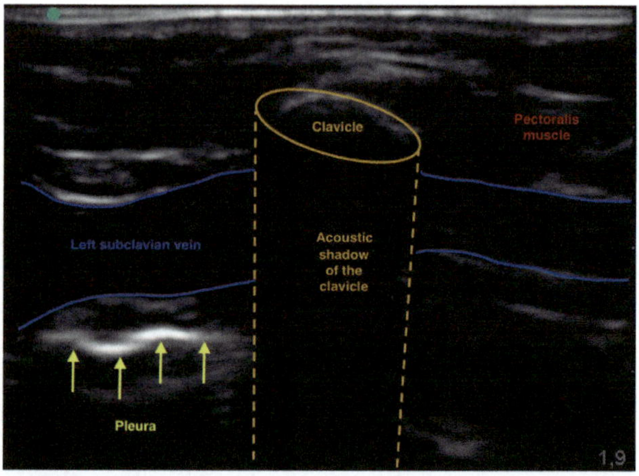

Fig. 8.6 Identifying structures

- The LSCV in its extrathoracic portion on the right side of the screen corresponds to the pectoral region
- Then, toward the cervical region, in other words, on the left side of the screen, the continuation of the thoracic LSCV is identified
- Just below the inferior wall of the LSCV, the pleura is identified

8.3 Local Anesthesia Application

- The sterile field only leaves the cervical, upper pectoral, and left shoulder regions uncovered.
- Real-time ultrasound-guided lidocaine infiltration.
- For infiltration, use a small needle 25–27 G.
- Use lidocaine 1%.
- Subcutaneous infiltration with lidocaine in the puncture tract 1,5–2 cm before the chosen venipuncture site to anesthetize the oblique puncture path as well as the fixation site of the catheter holder (Fig. 8.7).

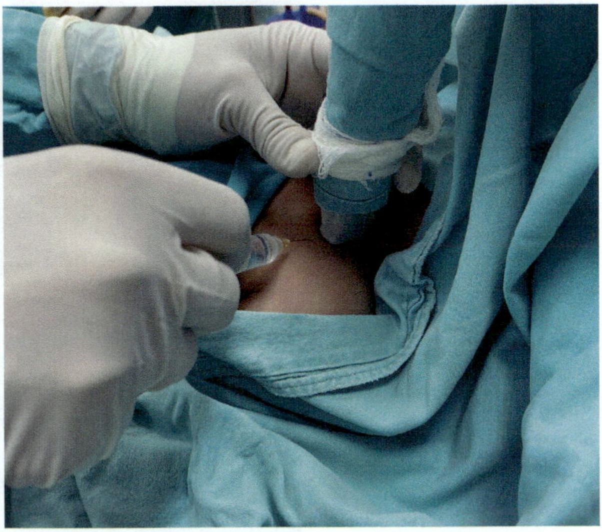

Fig. 8.7 Lidocaine infiltration

8.4 Steps for Real-Time Ultrasound-Guided Access to Infraclavicular Left Subclavian Vein in Pediatrics

8.4.1 Step 01

- We will use an Arrow® 4 Fr, 13-cm, double-lumen catheter.
- The operator stands on the patient's left side.
- The ultrasound is above the left shoulder.
- The sterile field only leaves the cervical, upper pectoral, and left shoulder regions uncovered (Fig. 8.8).
- Hold the transducer with your left hand and scan the LSCV in the LAX view in the junction of the middle and inner thirds of the left clavicle.
- Use the 21-G introducer needle that comes with the catheter kit.
- Once you identify the LSCV at the LAX view on the screen, the introducer needle is aligned following the direction of the tip of the hockey stick transducer and the central part of the thickness of the transducer (Fig. 8.9).
- Start the puncture at an angle of 30–45° degrees to penetrate the skin and enter the subcutaneous tissue.
- Begin with dynamic needle tracking (DNT), the basis of the ultrasound-guided puncture technique.
- The needle is visualized on the screen from the beginning of the puncture. The insertion of the needle will be monitored throughout the puncture until venous cannulation (Figs. 8.10 and 8.11).

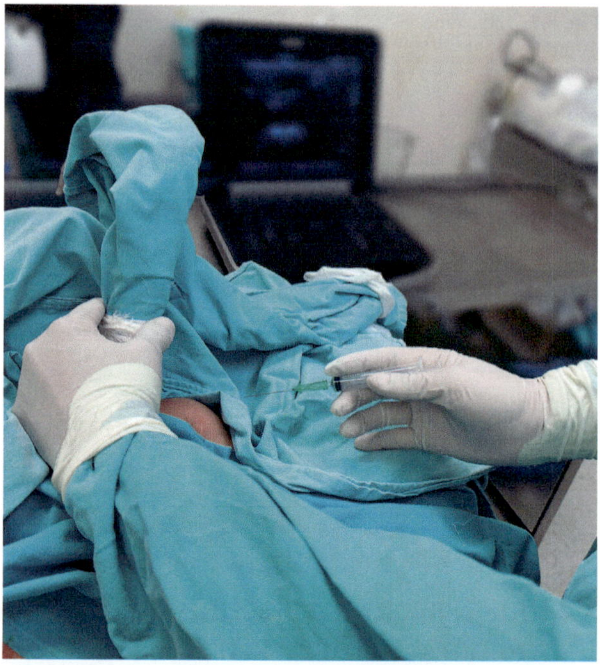

Fig. 8.8 The operator stands on the left side of the patient

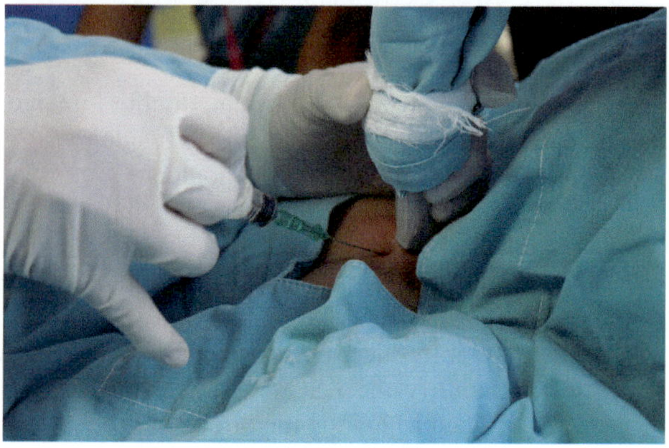

Fig. 8.9 The introducer needle is aligned to the central part of the thickness of the transducer and follows the direction of the tip of the hockey stick transducer at an angle of 30° to 45°

8.4.2 Step 02

- Once you identify on the ultrasound screen that you have reached the lower edge of the clavicle (Figs. 8.12 and 8.13), modify the puncture angle.
- Modify the puncture angle to less than 10° or almost parallel to the chest wall to pass the introducer needle below the clavicle (Fig. 8.14).
- Perform DNT; slide the transducer toward the head while advancing the puncture and maintaining the footprint oblique to the clavicle.

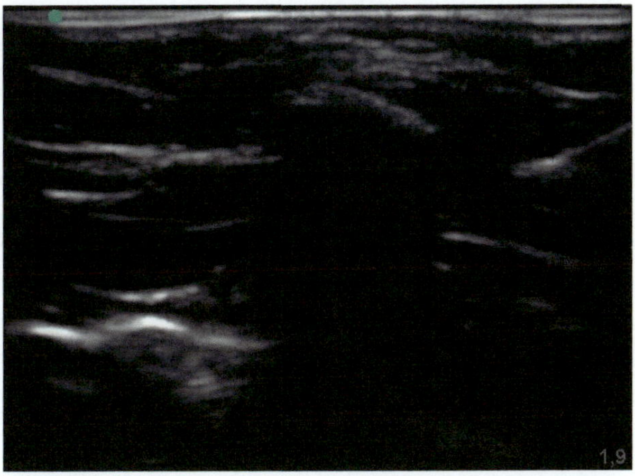

Fig. 8.10 Scan between the middle and inner thirds of the clavicle. LAX view of introducer needle entry into the subcutaneous tissue

- The scan depth is 1,9 cm

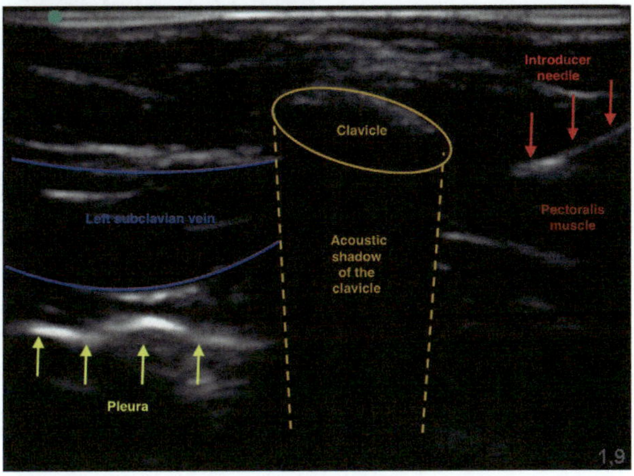

Fig. 8.11 Identifying structures

- Position the left clavicle in the center of the screen; to do this, place the clavicle in the middle of the probe and oblique to this
- The acoustic shadow of the clavicle hides the course at this level of the LSCV
- The introducer needle is not aligned with the disposition of the thoracic LSCV

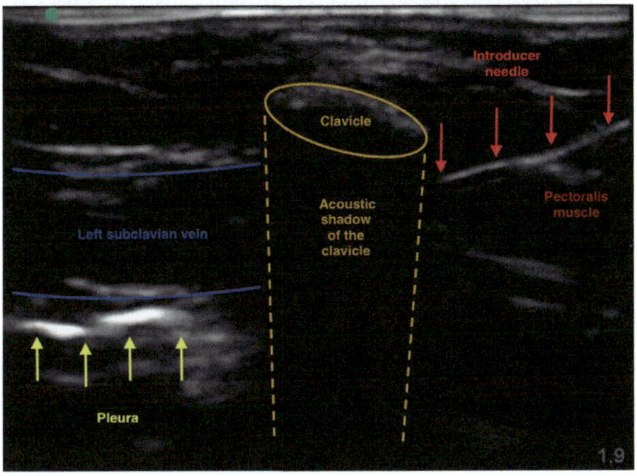

Fig. 8.12 Modification of the puncture angle

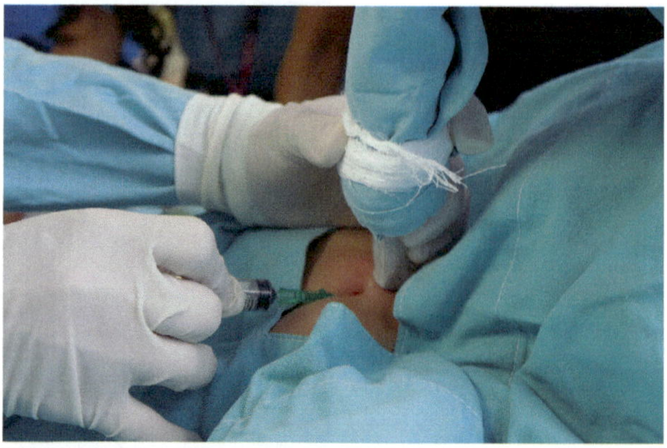

Fig. 8.13 LAX view of the progress of the puncture and arrival of the introducer needle at the lower edge of the clavicle

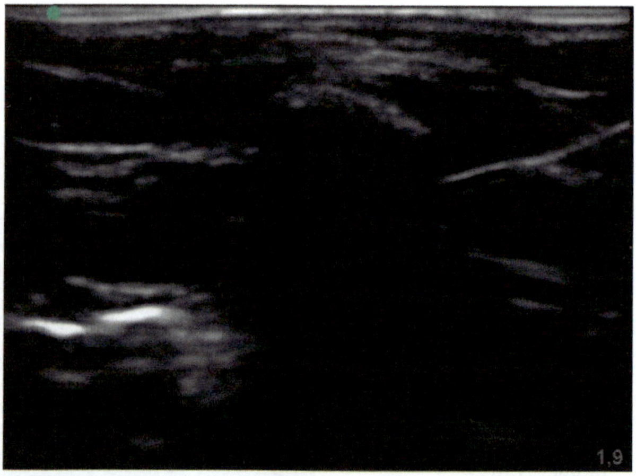

Fig. 8.14 Identifying structures
- The introducer needle has advanced through the pectoralis muscle, reaching the lower edge of the clavicle

- The puncture is advanced following the trajectory toward the LSCV, keeping the introducer needle parallel to the pleura (Figs. 8.15 and 8.16).
- With this modification of the puncture, you will notice that the clavicle does not get in the way of advancing the introducer needle, and thus it will easily pass.
- LAX view of initial canalization of the LSCV (Figs. 8.17 and 8.18).

8.4.3 Step 03

- Once you have identified canalization of the LSCV, set the transducer aside. Apply gentle negative pressure on the syringe plunger as you advance the needle (Fig. 8.19).
- LAX view of the LSCV cannulation (Figs. 8.20 and 8.21).

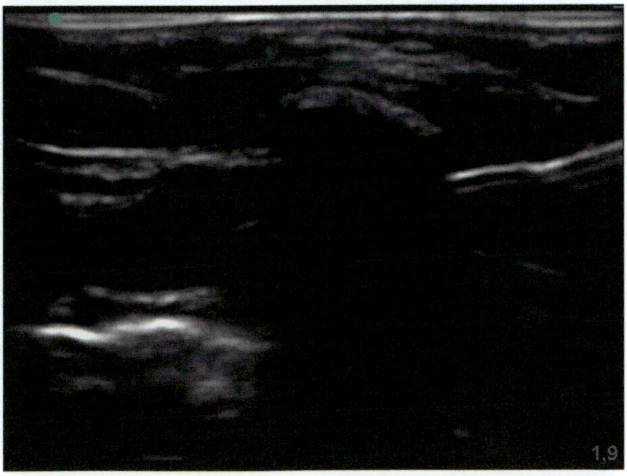

Fig. 8.15 LAX view of the puncture angle modification to less than 10° (see Fig. 8.14) in relation to the anterior chest wall so that the introducer needle passes below the clavicle

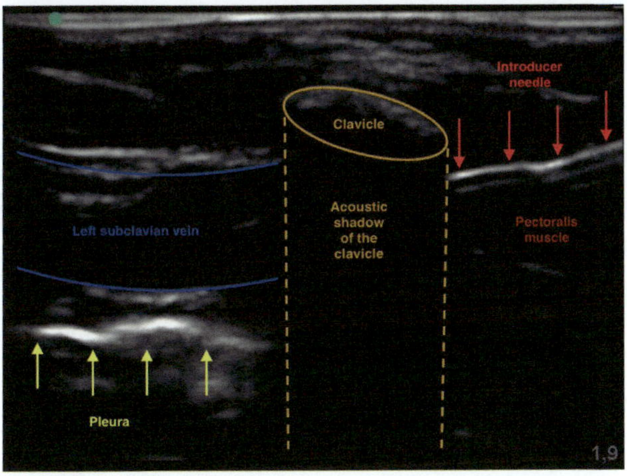

Fig. 8.16 Identifying structures

- At the beginning of the infraclavicular puncture trajectory, you will not visualize a segment of the introducer needle below the clavicle due to the acoustic shadow
- Therefore, the puncture is advanced following the trajectory toward the LSCV, keeping the introducer needle parallel to the pleura

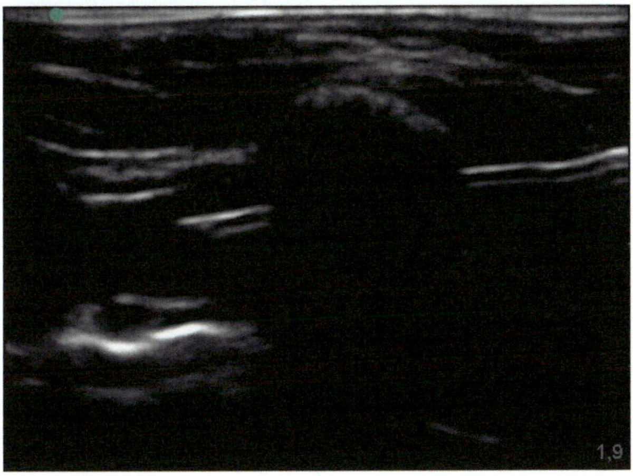

Fig. 8.17 LAX view of the LSCV infraclavicular puncture

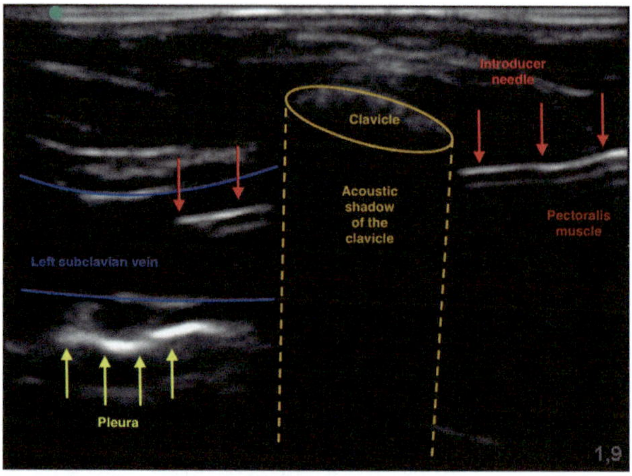

Fig. 8.18 Identifying structures
- Infraclavicular puncture enters the LSCV with the tip of the introducer needle.
- The puncture is performed with two security elements:
  - Complete visualization of the needle to prevent puncturing structures other than the LSCV
  - Keep the trajectory of the puncture parallel to the pleura and thus prevent puncturing it

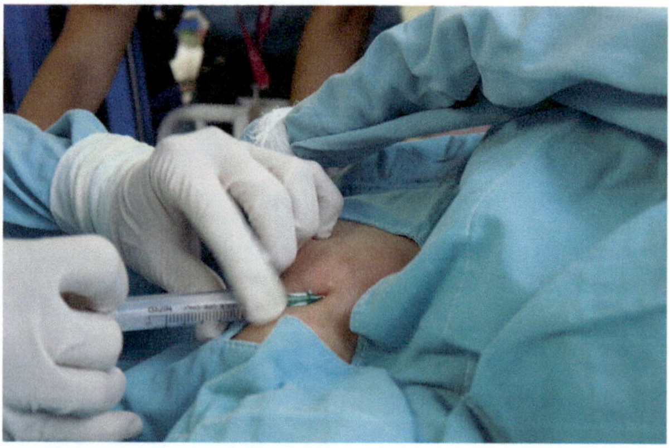

Fig. 8.19 Apply gentle negative pressure on the syringe plunger

- When you cannulate the vein, you will feel a loss of resistance and the return of blood in the barrel of the syringe (Fig. 8.22).
- Hold the needle hub firmly when checking for blood flow so the needle does not dislodge.

8.4.4 Step 04

- Insert the 0.18" guidewire, which should go through easily (Fig. 8.23).

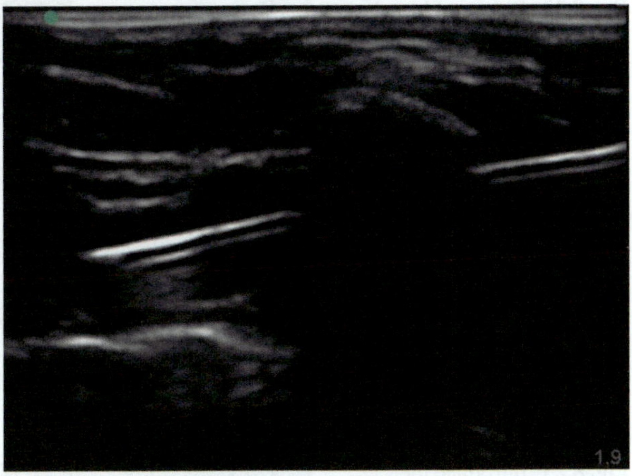

Fig. 8.20 LAX view of the LSCV cannulation

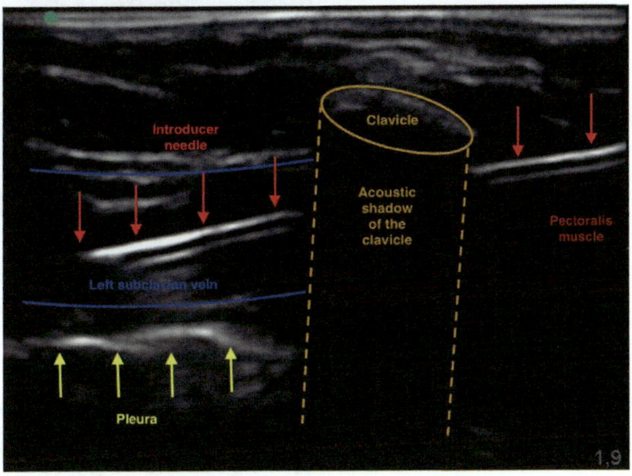

Fig. 8.21 Identifying structures

- Cannulation of the LSCV by the 21-G introducer needle

- When you have inserted enough guidewire, withdraw the introducer needle (Fig. 8.24).
- Verify the intravascular location of the guidewire by placing the transducer over the supraclavicular fossa (Fig. 8.25).
- LAX view of the intravascular guidewire (Figs. 8.26 and 8.27).

8.4.5 Step 05

- Perform dilation with the right hand, and retract the skin with the left hand and a "screw" maneuver.
- Dilate the path of the skin up to the entrance of the LSCV (Fig. 8.28).

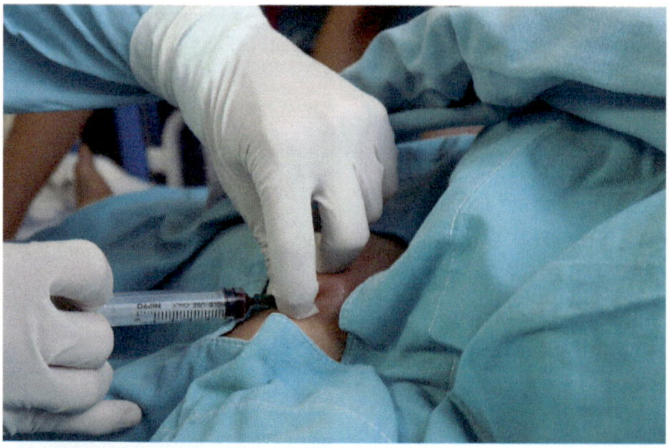

Fig. 8.22 Return of blood in the barrel of the syringe. Hold the needle hub

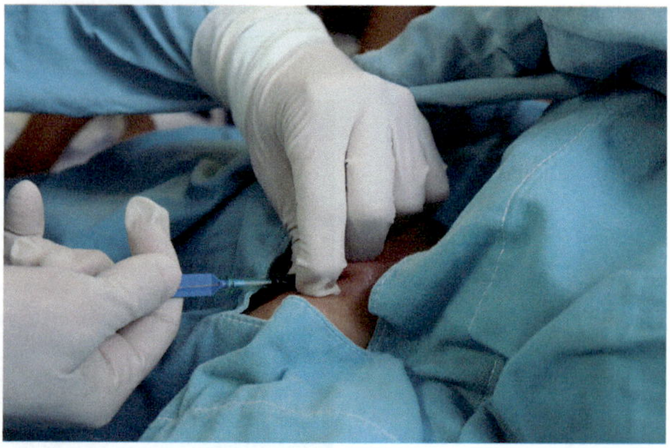

Fig. 8.23 Introduce the guidewire

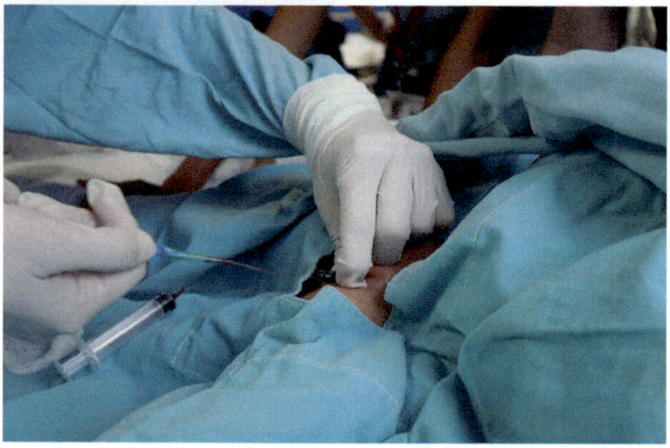

Fig. 8.24 Withdraw the introducer needle

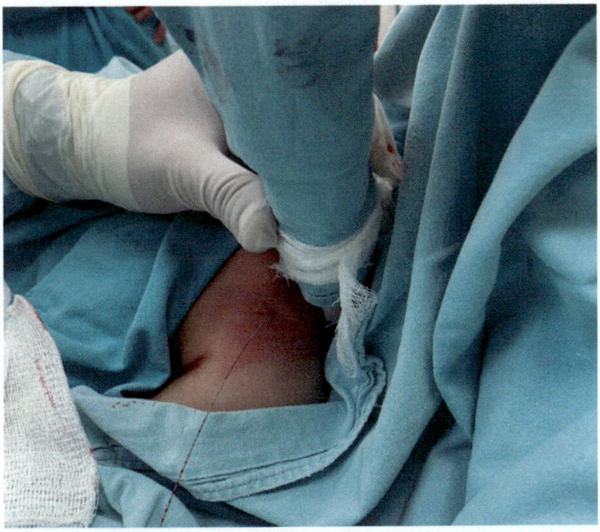

Fig. 8.25 Scan the intravascular location of the guidewire over the supraclavicular fossa

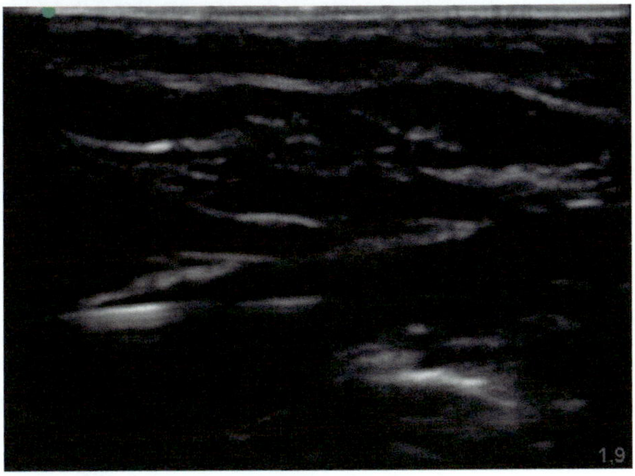

Fig. 8.26 LAX view of the intravascular guidewire

8.4.6 Step 06

- Introduce the central venous catheter using Seldinger's technique and remove the guidewire (Fig. 8.29).
- Place the transducer obliquely over the clavicle toward the junction of the middle and inner thirds, to locate the left subclavian vein.
- Scan the intravascular location of the catheter (Fig. 8.30).
- LAX view of the catheter in the LSCV (Figs. 8.31 and 8.32).
- Check the venous return of the lines and clean them with a solution.

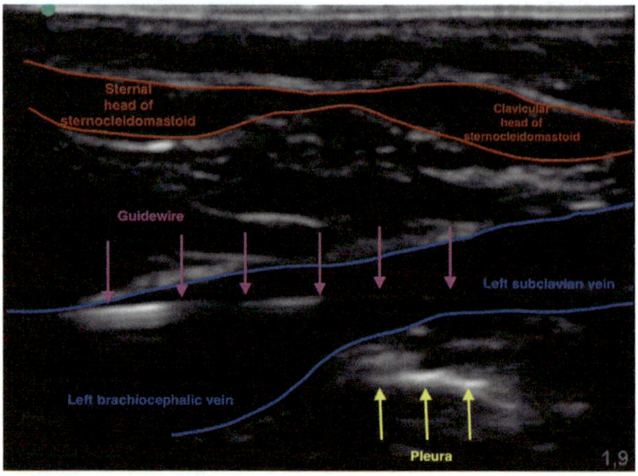

Fig. 8.27 Identifying structures

- The guidewire inside the LSCV and then LBCV

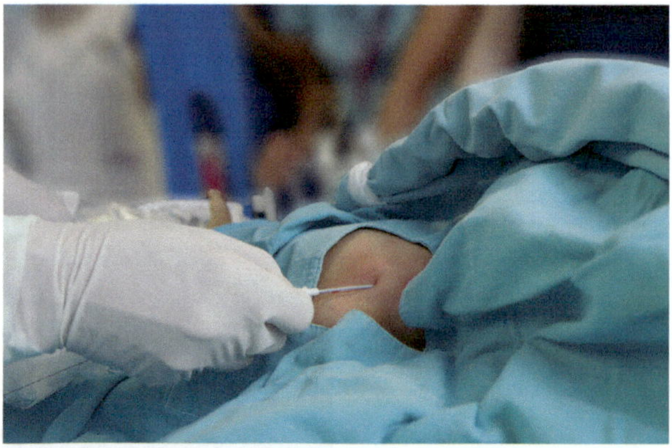

Fig. 8.28 Dilation of the skin path at the entrance to the LSCV

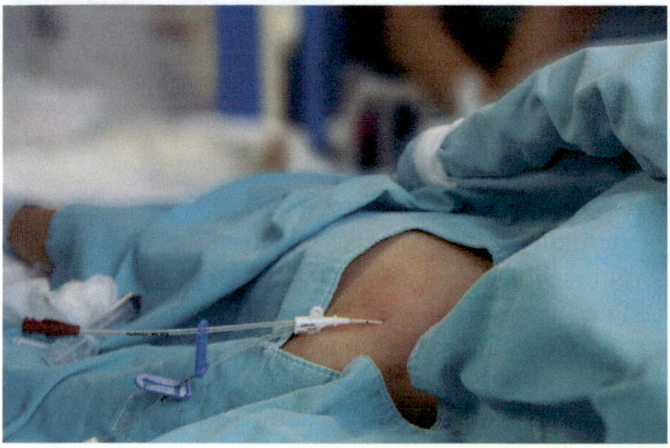

Fig. 8.29 Introduce the required intravascular catheter length

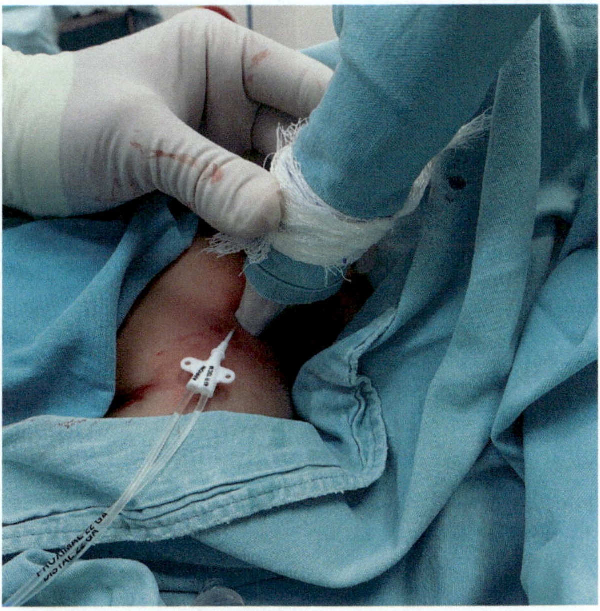

Fig. 8.30 Scan the intravascular location of the CVC in the LSCV

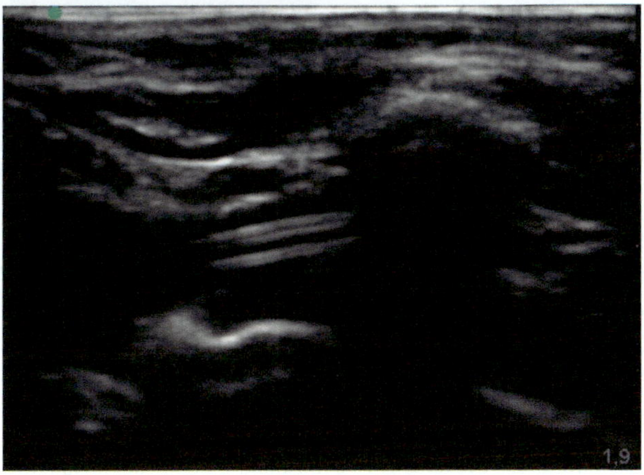

Fig. 8.31 LAX view of the catheter in the LSCV

8.4.7 Step 07

- Secure the catheter and place a sterile occlusive dressing according to the institutional protocol (Fig. 8.33).

Fig. 8.32 Identifying structures

- Central venous catheter inside the LSCV with visualization of the extrathoracic course toward the thoracic region only interrupted by the acoustic shadow of the clavicle

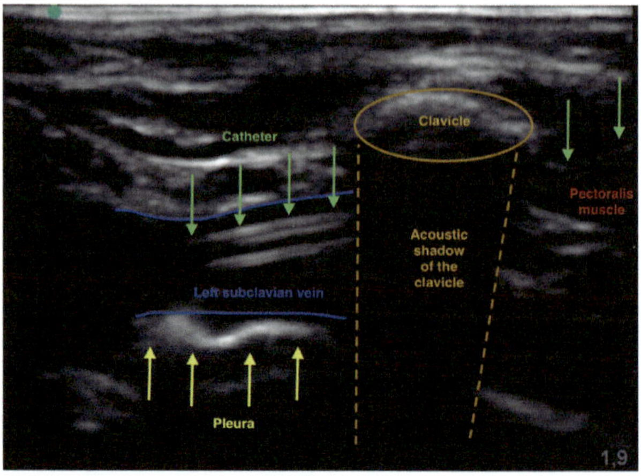

Fig. 8.33 Dressing according to the institutional protocol

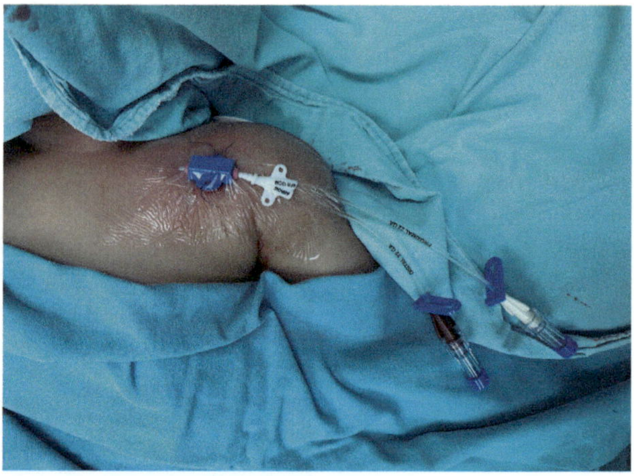

Sources

1. Pirotte T, Veyckemans F. Ultrasound-guided subclavian vein cannulation in infants and children: a novel approach. Br J Anaesth. 2007;98(4):509–14. https://doi.org/10.1093/bja/aem041. Epub 2007 Mar 1.
2. Park SI, Kim YH, So SY, Kim MJ, Kim HJ, Kim JK. Ultrasound-guided subclavian catheterization in pediatric patients with a linear probe: a case series. Korean J Anesthesiol. 2013;64(6):541–4. https://doi.org/10.4097/kjae.2013.64.6.541. Epub 2013 Jun 24. PMID: 23814657.
3. Byon HJ, Lee GW, Lee JH, Park YH, Kim HS, Kim CS, Kim JT. Comparison between ultrasound-guided supraclavicular and infraclavicular approaches for subclavian venous catheterization in children—a randomized trial. Br J Anaesth. 2013;111(5):788–92. https://doi.org/10.1093/bja/aet202. Epub 2013 Jun 10.

4. Nardi N, Wodey E, Laviolle B, De La Brière F, Delahaye S, Engrand C, Gauvrit C, Dessard S, Defontaine A, Ecoffey C. Effectiveness and complications of ultrasound-guided subclavian vein cannulation in children and neonates. Anaesth Crit Care Pain Med. 2016;35(3):209–13. https://doi.org/10.1016/j.accpm.2015.09.007. Epub 2016 Feb 26.
5. Rezayat T, Stowell JR, Kendall JL, Turner E, Fox JC, Barjaktarevic I. Ultrasound-guided cannulation: time to bring subclavian central lines Back. West J Emerg Med. 2016;17(2):216–21. https://doi.org/10.5811/westjem.2016.1.29462. Epub 2016 Mar 2.

Chapter 9
Infraclavicular Left Subclavian Vein in Neonates

9.1 Patient Positioning

- The patient is a 2880-g newborn.
- Position the newborn in supine close to the left side of the thermal crib (Fig. 9.1).
- Place the patient's head centered or slightly to the right.
- Gently restrain the upper extremities with the arm caudal.
- The operator stands on the left side of the patient.
- Place the ultrasound device in any of these three positions: above the right shoulder, above the head, or next to the left shoulder.
- Due to the patient's size, a high-frequency linear transducer (13–6 MHz) with a hockey stick-type probe can be used.

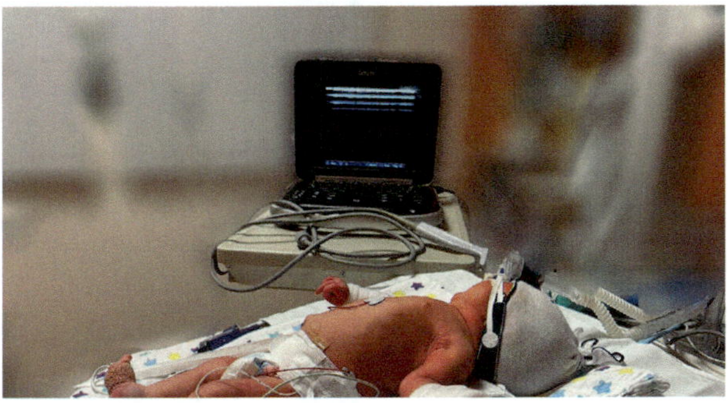

Fig. 9.1 Patient positioning

F. Montes-Tapia, *Atlas of Ultrasound-Guided Central Venous Catheter Placement*, https://doi.org/10.1007/978-3-031-61887-1_9

9.2 Scanning Technique

- Do a preliminary vascular assessment (non-sterile), known as rapid central vein assessment (RaCeVA).
- Hold the transducer with your left hand and scan the subclavian vessels in long axis (LAX), placing the transducer obliquely in the external third of the clavicle and with the tip of the hockey stick transducer toward the neck (Fig. 9.2).
- Start the search of the subclavian vessels in the external third of the clavicle, placing the transducer obliquely over the clavicle.
- Place the image of the clavicle in the center of the ultrasound screen. The clavicle produces an inferior acoustic shadow.
- First, visualize the left subclavian artery (LSCA) (Figs. 9.3 and 9.4), which runs deeper in relation to the clavicle and is more lateral than the left subclavian vein (LSCV).

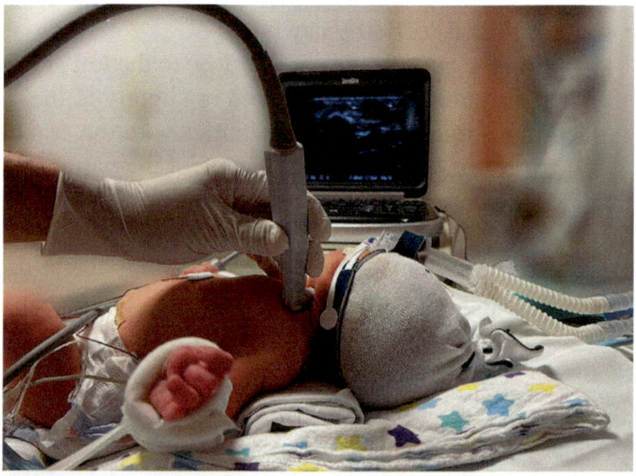

Fig. 9.2 Hold the transducer with the left hand and place it oblique to the clavicle, in the external third of the clavicle

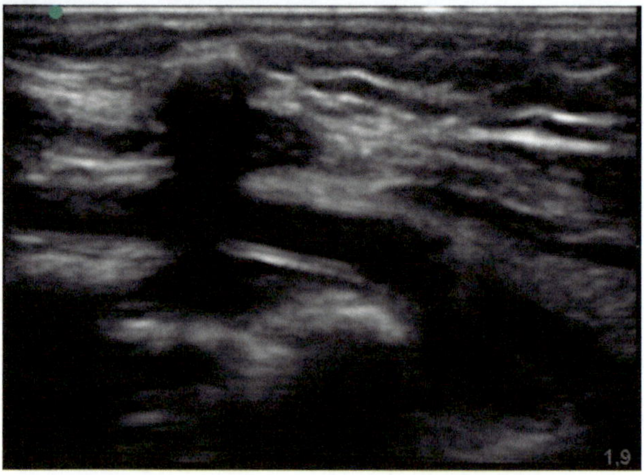

Fig. 9.3 Scan of the external third of the clavicle. LAX view of the LSCA

- The position indicator corresponds to the tip of the hockey stick transductor, directed toward the neck (Fig. 9.2)
- The scan depth is 1,9 cm

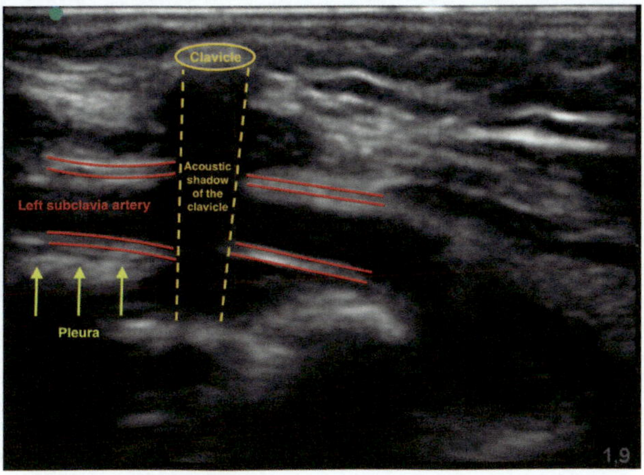

Fig. 9.4 Identifying structures

- The clavicle is not in the center of the transducer but in the upper half or closer to the tip; hence, the clavicle looks closer to the position indicator on the screen and closer to the left side of the screen
- The LSCA, with two echogenic layers of its wall, typical of an artery, runs deeper in relation to the clavicle and lateral to the vein
- The LSCA, in its extrathoracic portion on the right side of the screen, corresponds to the pectoral region
- The LSCA in its thoracic portion is identified toward the cervical region, in other words, on the left side of the screen (toward the probe mark or the tip of the hockey stick transductor)
- The pleura lies below the inferior wall of the thoracic portion of the LSCA

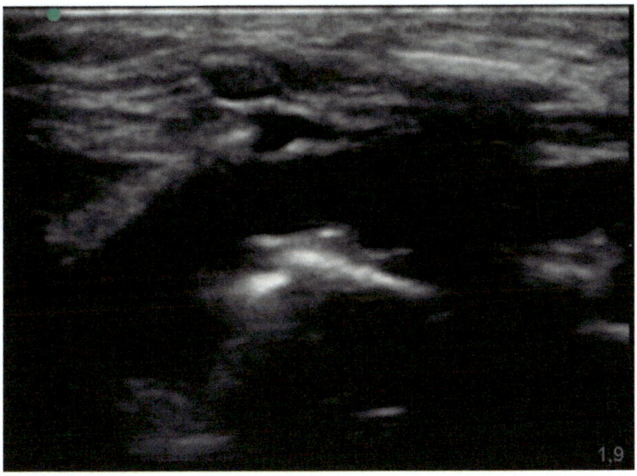

Fig. 9.5 Scan between the middle and inner thirds of the clavicle. LAX view of the LSCV

- Sweep the transductor across the external third of the clavicle to the junction of the middle and inner third to locate the LSCV.
- LAX view of the LSCV (Figs. 9.5 and 9.6).

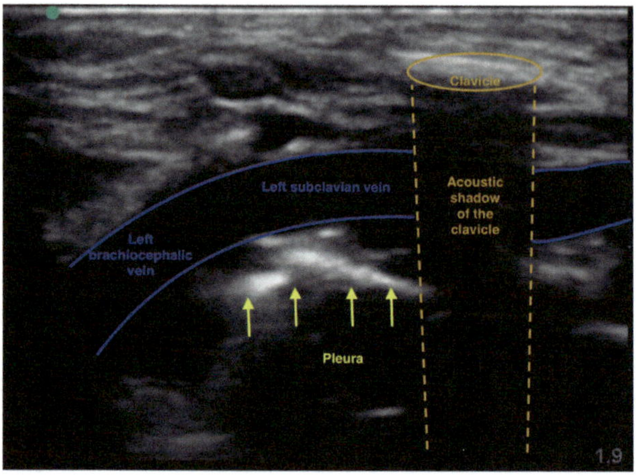

Fig. 9.6 Identifying structures

- The LSCV in its extrathoracic portion on the right side of the screen corresponds to the pectoral region
- The clavicle that causes an acoustic shadow does not allow the visualization of structures
- The LSCV in its thoracic portion is identified toward the cervical region, in other words, on the left side of the screen (toward the tip of the hockey stick transductor)
- The diameter of LSCV is 0,3 cm
- The LSCV continues with the LBCV, identified in a downward trajectory
- Just below the inferior wall of the LSCV, the pleura is identified

- The LSCV has two anatomical differences from the LSCA. The first difference is the LSCV is more superficial than the LSCA and runs closer to the clavicle. The second difference is the LSCV is more medial than the LSCA.

9.3 Local Anesthesia Application

- The sterile field only leaves the cervical, upper pectoral, and left shoulder regions uncovered.
- For infiltration, use a small needle 25–27 G.
- Use lidocaine 1%.
- After ultrasound localization of the area to be punctured, infiltration of the marked site is performed.
- Subcutaneous infiltration with lidocaine in the puncture tract 1,5–2 cm before the chosen venipuncture site to anesthetize the oblique puncture path as well as the fixation site of the catheter holder (Fig. 9.7).

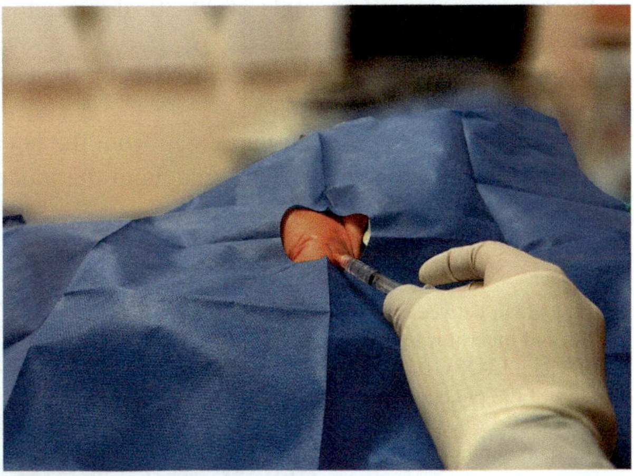

Fig. 9.7 Lidocaine infiltration

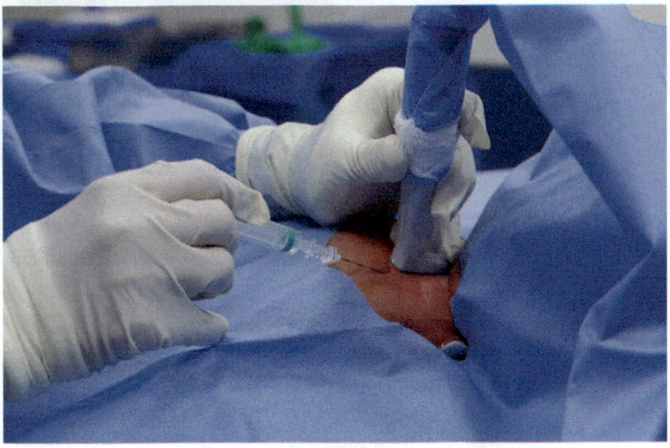

Fig. 9.8 The introducer needle is aligned to the central part of the thickness of the transducer following the direction of the tip of the hockey stick transducer at an angle of 20–30°

9.4 Steps for Real-Time Ultrasound-Guided Access to Infraclavicular Left Subclavian Vein in Neonates

9.4.1 Step 01

- We will use a Vygon® 3 Fr, 10-cm, double-lumen catheter.
- The operator stands on the left side of the newborn.
- Hold the transducer with your left hand and scan the LSCV in LAX view at the junction of the middle and inner thirds of the left clavicle.
- The catheter 3 Fr Vygon® has a 21-G introducer needle that is echogenic, which substantially improves visualization.
- Once you identify the LSCV at the LAX view on the screen, the introducer needle is aligned following the direction of the tip of the hockey stick transducer and the central part of the thickness of the transducer (Fig. 9.8).

- Start the puncture at an angle of 20–30° degrees to penetrate the skin and enter the subcutaneous tissue.
- Begin with dynamic needle tracking (DNT), the basis of the ultrasound-guided puncture technique.
- The needle is visualized on the screen from the beginning of the puncture. The introducer needle is monitored throughout the procedure until venous cannulation (Figs. 9.9 and 9.10).

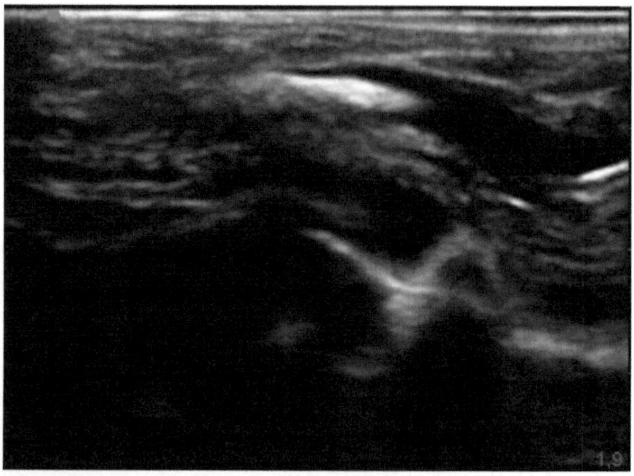

Fig. 9.9 Scan between the middle and inner thirds of the clavicle. LAX view of the start of the puncture of the LSCV
- The scan depth is 1,9 cm

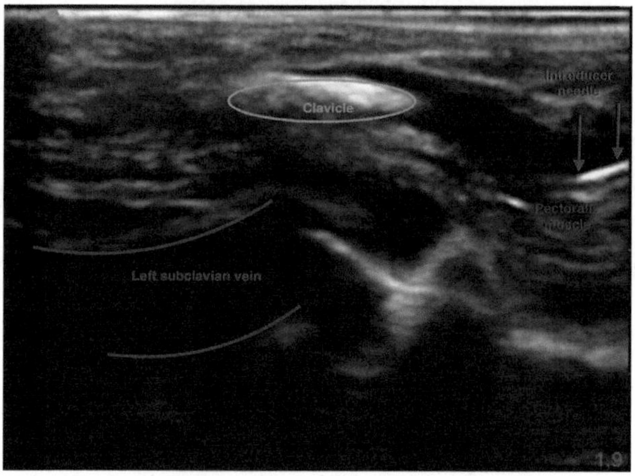

Fig. 9.10 Identifying structures
- Position the left clavicle in the center of the screen; to do this, place the clavicle in the middle of the probe and oblique to this (Fig. 9.8)
- The introducer needle can be seen penetrating the subcutaneous tissue of the anterior chest wall, corresponding to the right side of the image
- The LSCV is seen in line with the puncture needle

9.4.2 Step 02

- Once ultrasound identifies that you have reached the lower edge of the clavicle (Figs. 9.11 and 9.12), modify the puncture angle.
- Modify the puncture angle to less than 10 degrees or almost parallel to the chest wall to pass the needle below the clavicle (Fig. 9.13).
- The clavicle is not an impassable obstacle at this age as long as the roll has been properly positioned under the shoulders.

9.4.3 Step 03

- Continue advancing the introducer needle under DNT. This maneuver will guide you to change direction in real time if the puncture is going in an inappropriate direction (Fig. 9.14).

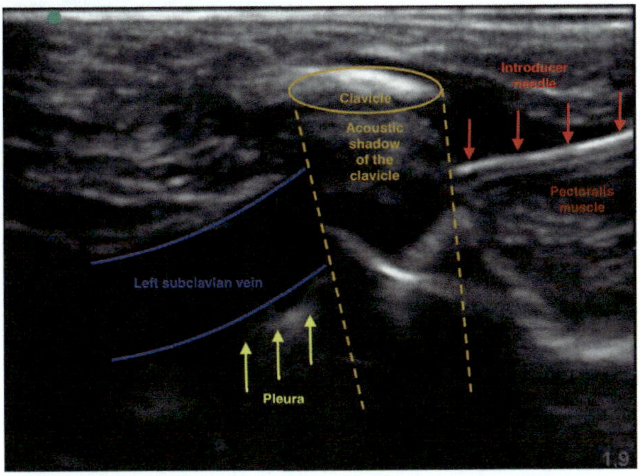

Fig. 9.11 Modification of the puncture angle to less than 10 degrees

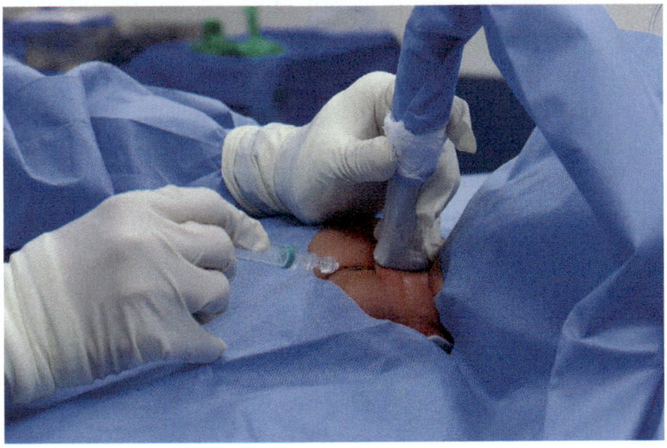

Fig. 9.12 LAX view of the progress of the puncture and arrival of the introducer needle at the lower edge of the clavicle

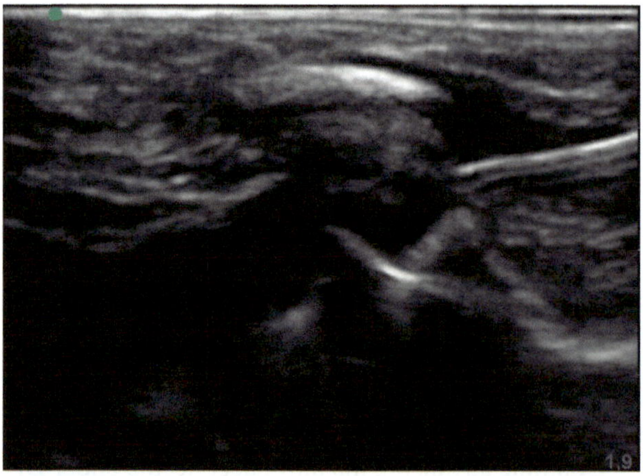

Fig. 9.13 Identifying structures
- The introducer needle has advanced through the pectoralis muscle, reaching the lower edge of the clavicle

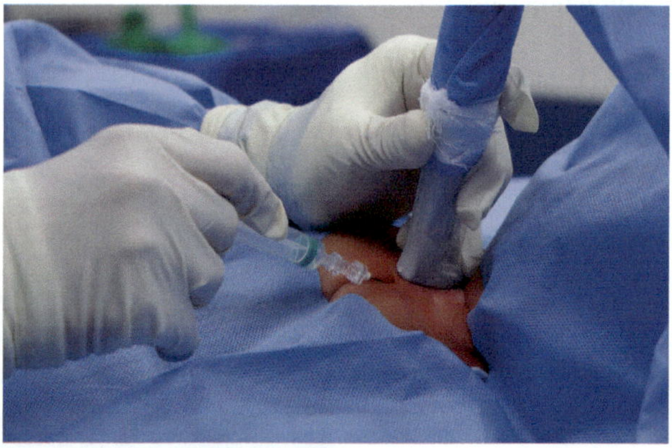

Fig. 9.14 Continue the puncture following the trajectory of the LSCV using dynamic needle tracking

- When you pass under the clavicle, you will not see the tip of the needle. If it is in the correct path of the footprint, the tip of the needle will be seen after the clavicle.
- In this patient, to perform DNT of the introducer needle, slide the transducer toward the head and maintain the transducer oblique to the clavicle.
- Advance the introducer needle, identifying that the needle passes below the clavicle, and maintain gentle negative pressure on the syringe plunger as you advance the needle.
- When you canalize the vein, you will feel a loss of resistance and the return of blood in the barrel of the syringe. Then stop advancing with the puncture (Fig. 9.15).
- LAX view of the canalization of the LSCV by the introducer needle (Figs. 9.16 and 9.17).

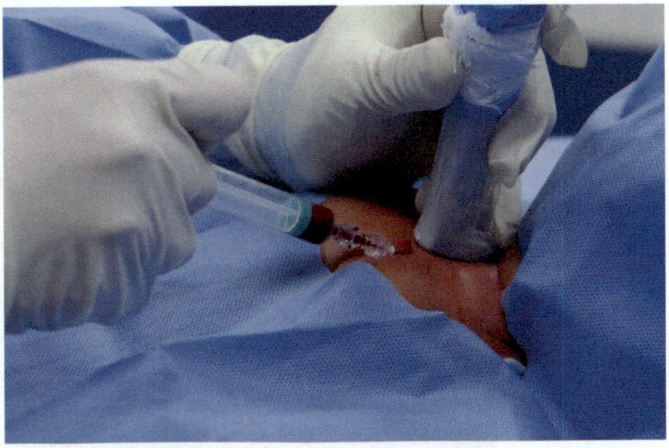

Fig. 9.15 A flash of blood appears in the barrel of the syringe

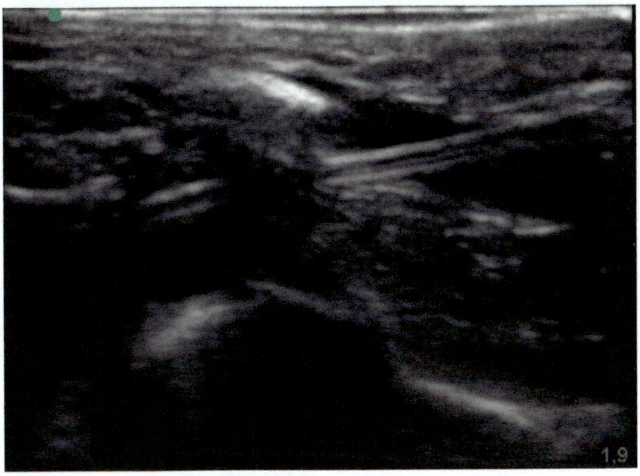

Fig. 9.16 LAX view of the canalization of the LSCV by the introducer needle

9.4.4 Step 04

- Firmly hold the needle hub with your left hand and remove the syringe.
- Insert the 0,3-mm nitinol guidewire, which should pass easily (Fig. 9.18).
- This type of guidewire is marked every 10 cm, so the guidewire should not go beyond the first 5 cm.
- After introducing enough guidewire, remove the introducer needle (Fig. 9.19).
- Scan the supraclavicular fossa to identify the intravascular guidewire (Fig. 9.20).
- LAX view of the intravascular guidewire within the LSCV (Fig. 9.21 and 9.22).

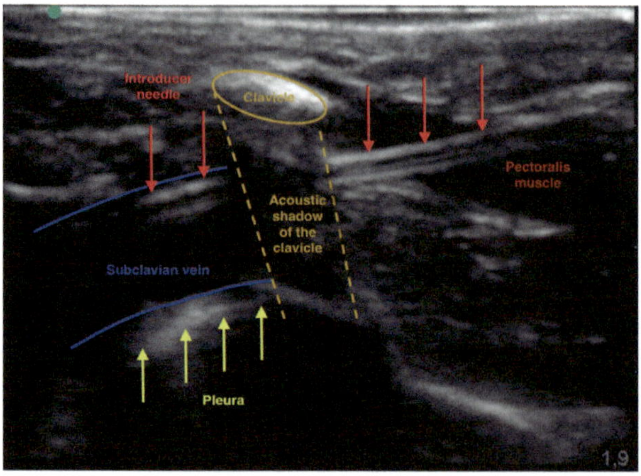

Fig. 9.17 Identifying structures

- Introducer needle canalizing the LSCV; at this moment, blood is returning in the puncture syringe, as shown in Fig. 9.15; therefore, needle progression stops
- The acoustic shadow of the clavicle does not allow seeing the infraclavicular section of the introducer needle
- The trajectory of the introducer needle is parallel to the pleura, making it almost impossible to puncture it. The entire length of the inserted introducer needle is identified

Fig. 9.18 Introduce the guidewire

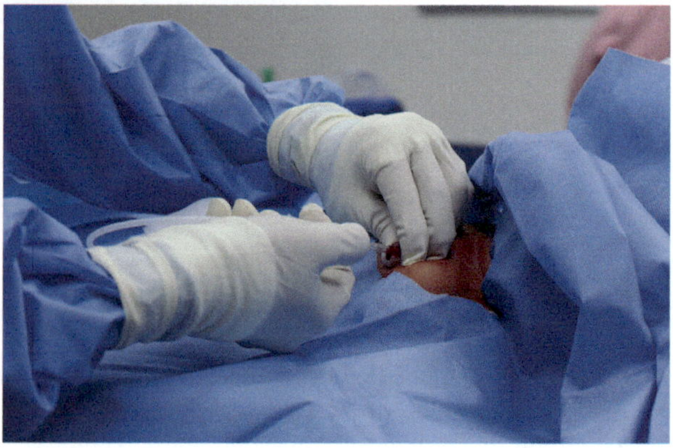

9.4.5 Step 05

- Perform dilation with the right hand and countertraction of the skin with the left hand and with a "screw" maneuver.
- Dilate the path of the skin up to the entrance of the LSCV (Fig. 9.23).
- If a lot of subcutaneous pressure is exerted without countertraction, the guidewire can be bent, hindering dilation and passage of the central venous catheter.

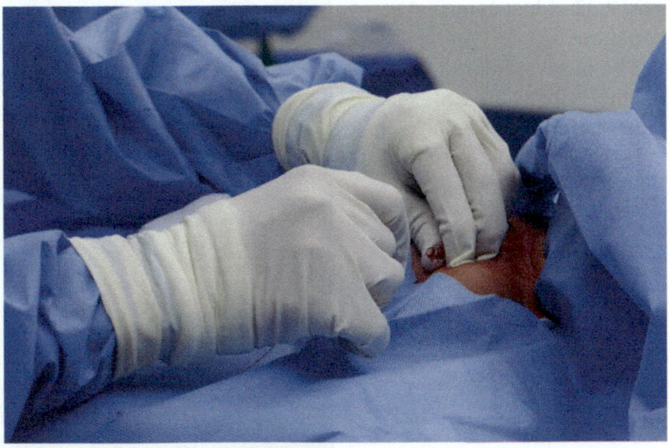

Fig. 9.19 Remove the introducer needle

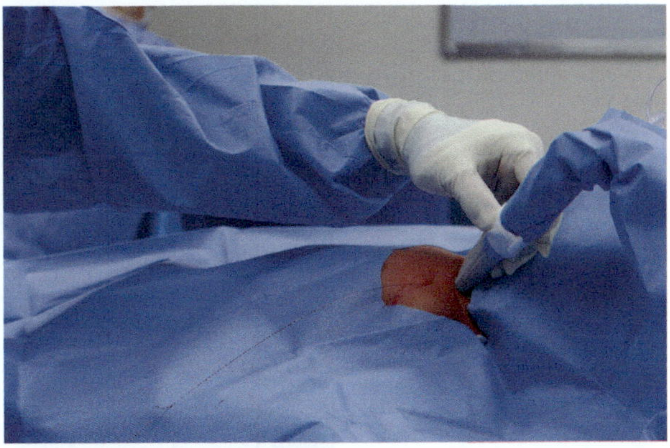

Fig. 9.20 Place the transducer in the supraclavicular fossa

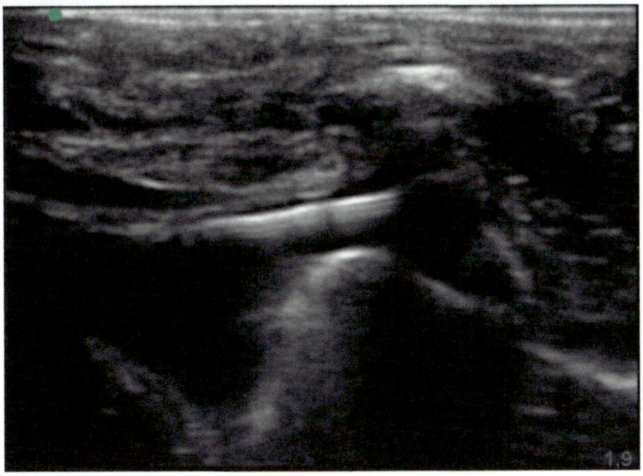

Fig. 9.21 LAX view of the intravascular guidewire within the LSCV

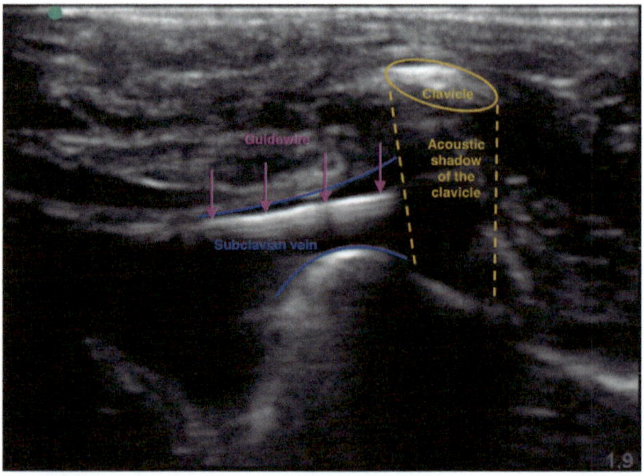

Fig. 9.22 Identifying structures

- The intravascular guidewire in the LSCV to the left brachiocephalic vein

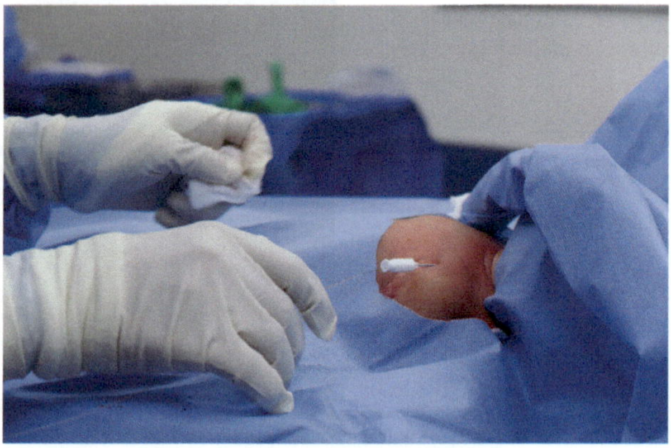

Fig. 9.23 Dilation of the skin path at the entrance to the LSCV

- After dilating, introduce the 3 Fr, 10-cm, double-lumen catheter with Seldinger's technique and remove the guidewire (Fig. 9.24).
- LAX view of the catheter inside the LSCV (Figs. 9.25 and 9.26).

9.4.6 Step 06

- Secure the catheter and place a sterile occlusive dressing according to the institutional protocol (Fig. 9.27).

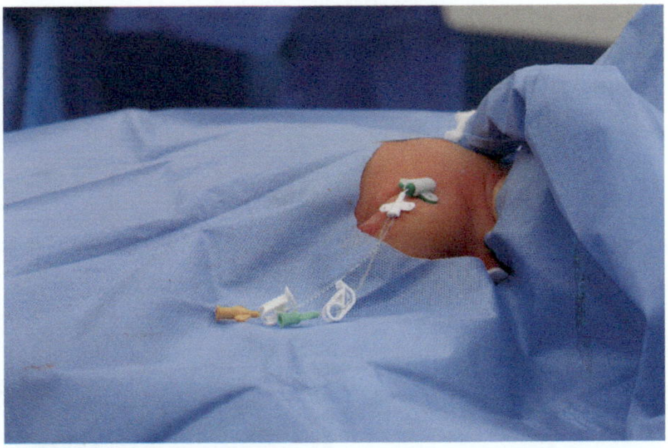

Fig. 9.24 Introduce the required intravascular catheter length

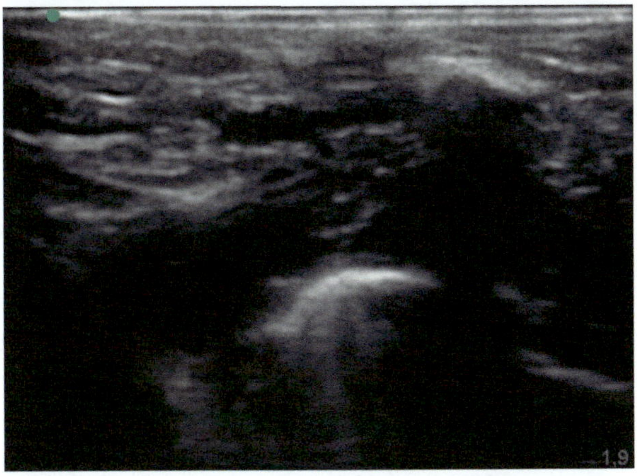

Fig. 9.25 LAX view of the catheter inside the LSCV

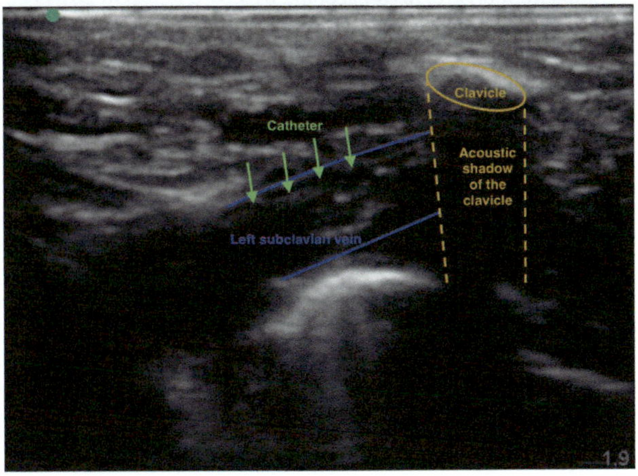

Fig. 9.26 Identifying structures

- Catheter inside the LSCV

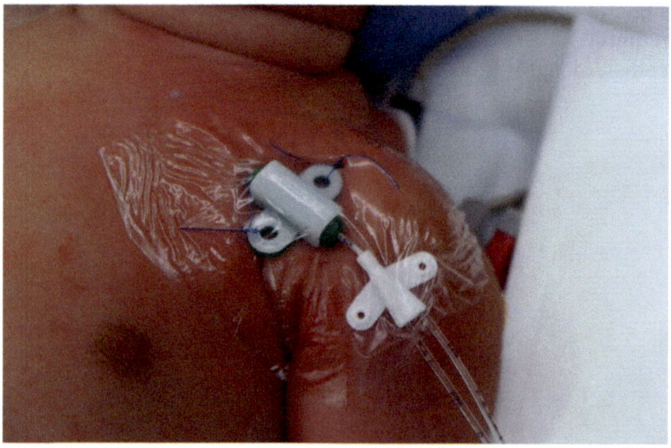

Fig. 9.27 Dressing according to the institutional protocol

Sources

1. Pirotte T, Veyckemans F. Ultrasound-guided subclavian vein cannulation in infants and children: a novel approach. Br J Anaesth. 2007;98(4):509–14. https://doi.org/10.1093/bja/aem041. Epub 2007 Mar 1.
2. Park SI, Kim YH, So SY, Kim MJ, Kim HJ, Kim JK. Ultrasound-guided subclavian catheterization in pediatric patients with a linear probe: a case series. Korean J Anesthesiol. 2013;64(6):541–4. https://doi.org/10.4097/kjae.2013.64.6.541. Epub 2013 Jun 24. PMID: 23814657.
3. Byon HJ, Lee GW, Lee JH, Park YH, Kim HS, Kim CS, Kim JT. Comparison between ultrasound-guided supraclavicular and infraclavicular approaches for subclavian venous catheterization in children—a randomized trial. Br J Anaesth. 2013;111(5):788–92. https://doi.org/10.1093/bja/aet202. Epub 2013 Jun 10.
4. Nardi N, Wodey E, Laviolle B, De La Brière F, Delahaye S, Engrand C, Gauvrit C, Dessard S, Defontaine A, Ecoffey C. Effectiveness and complications of ultrasound-guided subclavian vein cannulation in children and neonates. Anaesth Crit Care Pain Med. 2016;35(3):209–13. https://doi.org/10.1016/j.accpm.2015.09.007. Epub 2016 Feb 26.
5. Rezayat T, Stowell JR, Kendall JL, Turner E, Fox JC, Barjaktarevic I. Ultrasound-guided cannulation: time to bring subclavian central lines Back. West J Emerg Med. 2016;17(2):216–21. https://doi.org/10.5811/westjem.2016.1.29462. Epub 2016 Mar 2.

Chapter 10
Supraclavicular Right Subclavian Vein in Pediatrics

10.1 Patient Positioning

- The patient is a 1-year-old weighing 9,5 kg.
- Position the patient supine close to the head of the bed.
- Place the patient's head to the left (Fig. 10.1).
- Place a roll under the shoulders.
- Gently hold the upper extremities with the arms caudal.
- The objective of positioning the patient is to increase the length of the cervical region and create a wider space between the clavicle and the jaw to access the supraclavicular fossae.
- Place the ultrasound device next to the left or right shoulder or in front of the operator, that is, at the patient's feet (Fig. 10.2).

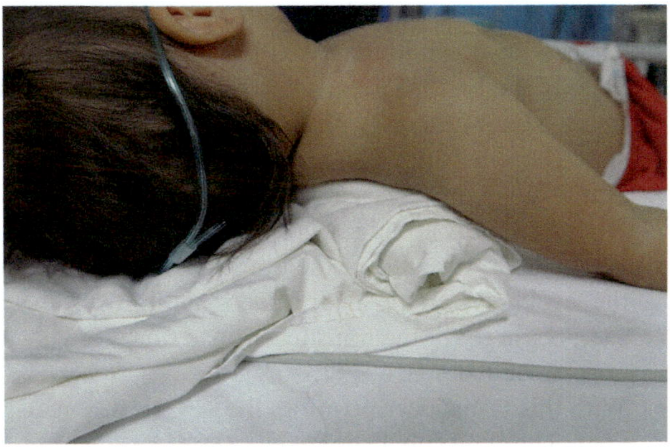

Fig. 10.1 Place a roll under the shoulders

F. Montes-Tapia, *Atlas of Ultrasound-Guided Central Venous Catheter Placement*, https://doi.org/10.1007/978-3-031-61887-1_10

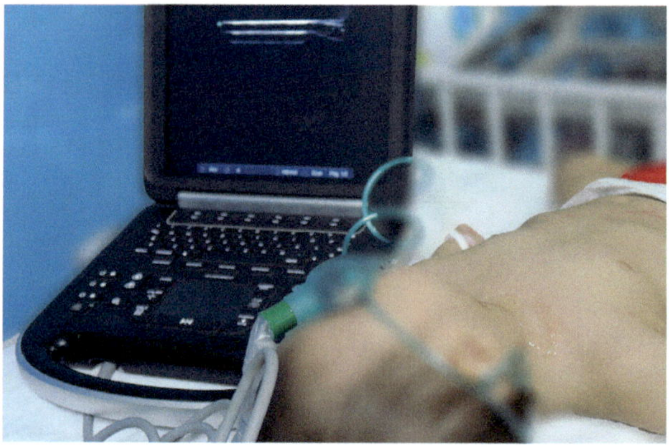

Fig. 10.2 Patient's head to the left and the ultrasound device next to the left shoulder

10.2 Scanning Technique

- Do a preliminary vascular assessment (non-sterile), known as rapid central vein assessment (RaCeVA).
- Stands at the patient's head, on the right side.
- Place the ultrasound device in front of the operator at the left or right shoulder.
- Because the supraclavicular fossa at this age is small, it is recommended to use a high-frequency linear transducer (13–6 MHz) with a hockey stick-type probe or for a patient of greater weight a larger probe.
- Hold the transducer with your left hand and begin the scanning with the transducer transverse to the middle of the neck and the tip of the hockey stick probe to the patient's left side (Fig. 10.3).
- At this level, visualize the right internal jugular vein (RIJV) and the right carotid artery (RCA) in short-axis (SAX) view (Figs. 10.4 and 10.5).
- Then, slide down to the base of the neck.
- Scan at the base of the neck, with the transducer transverse to the neck and the lower edge of the transducer in contact with the clavicle. This scan level corresponds to the base of Sedillot's triangle (Fig. 10.6).
- At this level, the cervical vessels are still visualized in SAX view. SAX view of RIJV and RCA at the base of the neck (Figs. 10.7 and 10.8).
- When the lower edge of the transducer contacts the upper edge of the clavicle at the level between the medial and inner thirds of the clavicle (supraclavicular fossae), begin to tilt the transducer posteriorly to view the subclavian vessels in the retroclavicular space (Fig. 10.9).
- With this transducer position, the vessels are visualized in the long-axis (LAX) view. The right subclavian artery (RSCA), the right carotid artery (RCA), and the brachiocephalic artery will be first visualized; the only vein visualized at this level is the RIJV (Figs. 10.10 and 10.11).

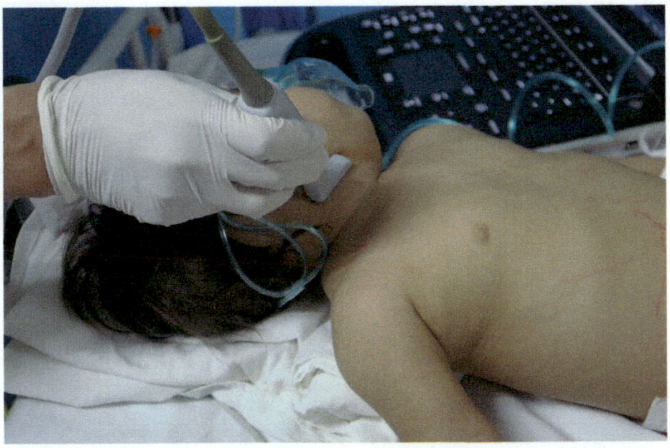

Fig. 10.3 Begin at the middle of the neck, and then sweep down to the base of the neck

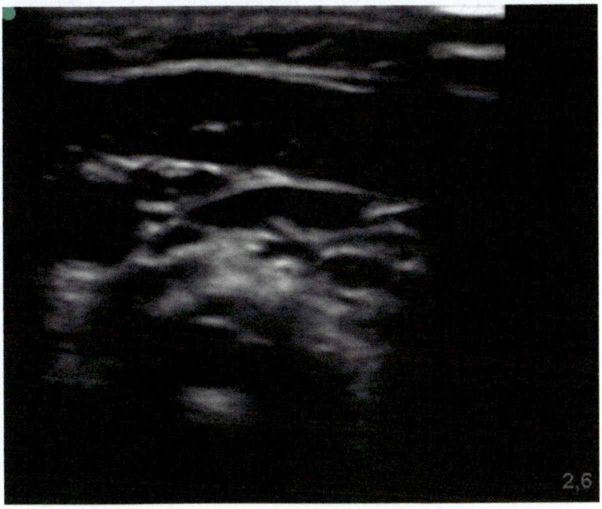

Fig. 10.4 SAX view of the cervical vessels

- The position indicator corresponds to the tip of the hockey stick transductor, directed toward the left side of the patient (Fig. 10.3)
- The scan depth is 2,6 cm

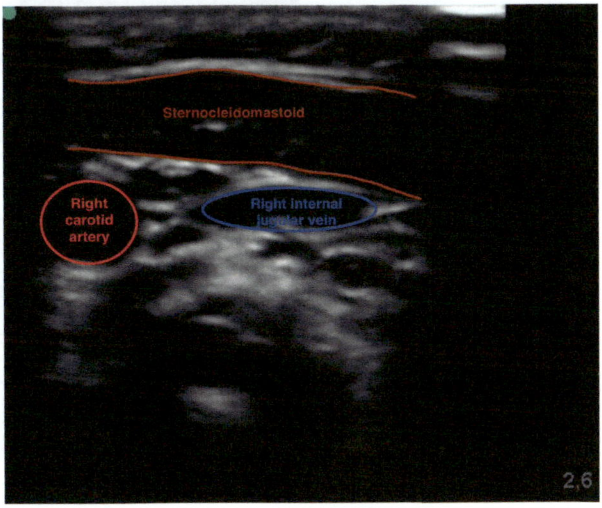

Fig. 10.5 Identifying structures

- RIJV and RCA under the sternocleidomastoid muscle

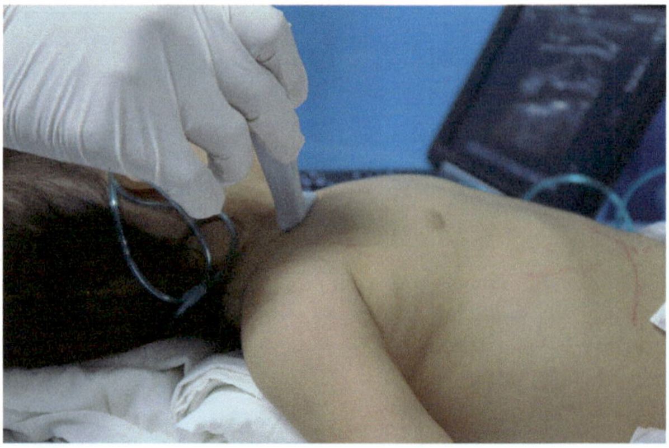

Fig. 10.6 Scan at the base of the neck

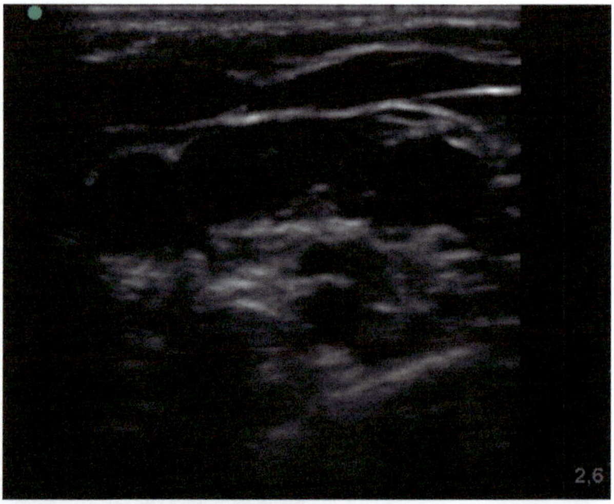

Fig. 10.7 SAX view of the RIJV and RCA at the base of the neck

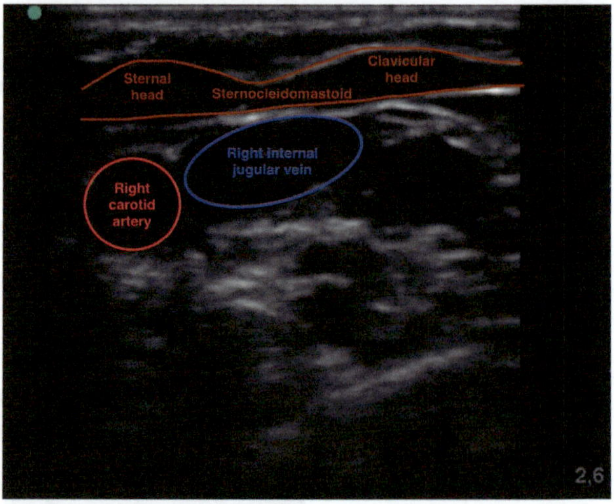

Fig. 10.8 Identifying structures

- The RIJV and RCA below the sternocleidomastoid muscle

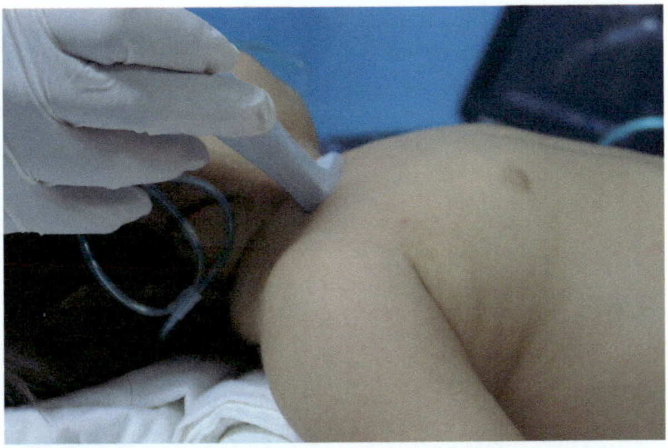

Fig. 10.9 Begin with a posterior tilt of the transducer, to begin with the visualization of the retroclavicular vessels

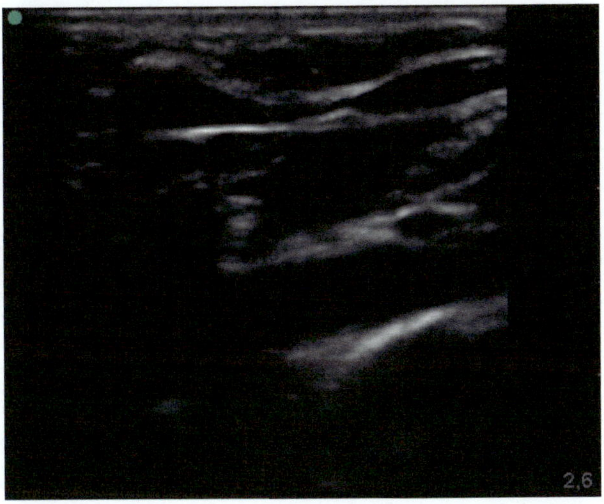

Fig. 10.10 LAX visualization of vessels in the right supraclavicular fossae

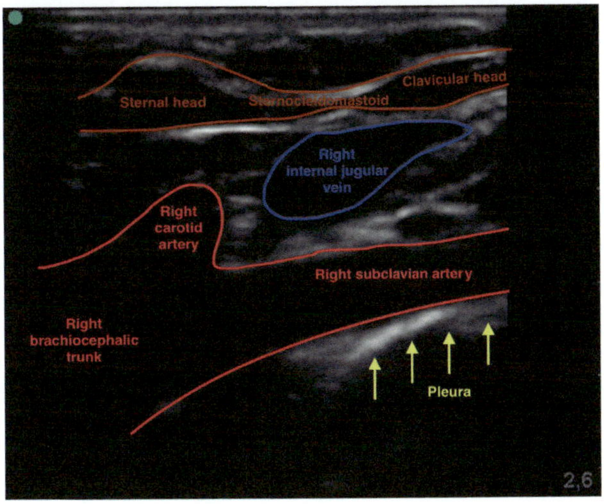

Fig. 10.11 Identifying structures

- The two heads of the sternocleidomastoid muscle are identified
- The RIJV close to joining the RSCV is appreciated
- The brachiocephalic artery originates the RCA and RSCA
- The pleura in contact with the lower border of the RSCA

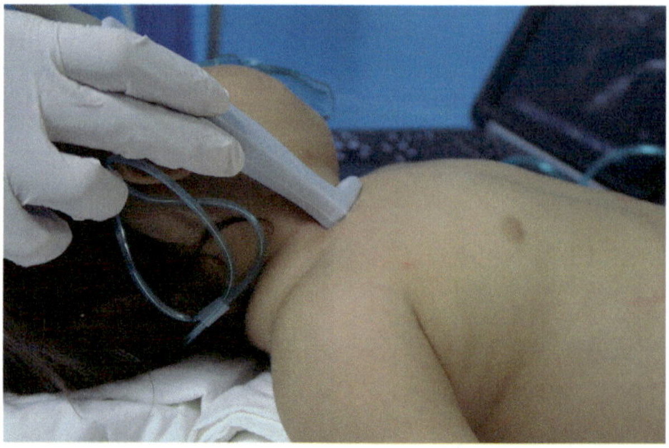

Fig. 10.12 Perform a more posterior tilt until the transducer shaft is almost in contact with the patient's jaw or until the retroclavicular venous vessels are visualized

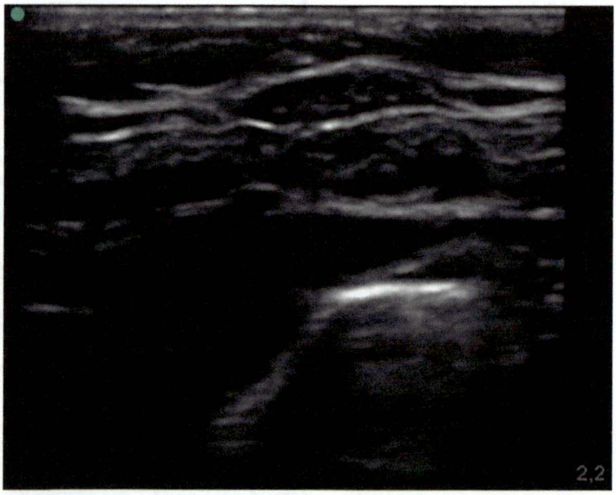

Fig. 10.13 LAX visualization of the retroclavicular veins
- Scan at a depth of 2,2 cm

- Tilt the transducer more posteriorly with the shaft of the transducer almost in contact with the patient's mandible (Fig. 10.12).
- The objective of more tilting is to visualize the retroclavicular vessels like the right subclavian vein (RSCV) and medially the right brachiocephalic vein (RBCV) because these are more anterior to the arteries (Figs. 10.13 and 10.14).

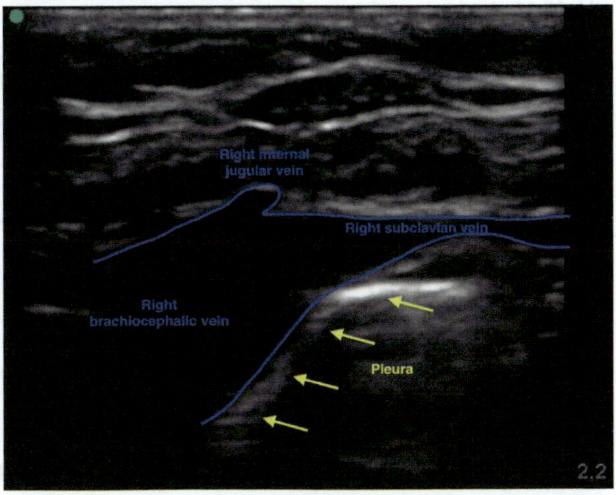

Fig. 10.14 Identifying structures
- The RSCV is at its junction with the RIJV draining into the RBCV
- The pleura is in close contact with the posterior wall of the RSCV and the RBCV

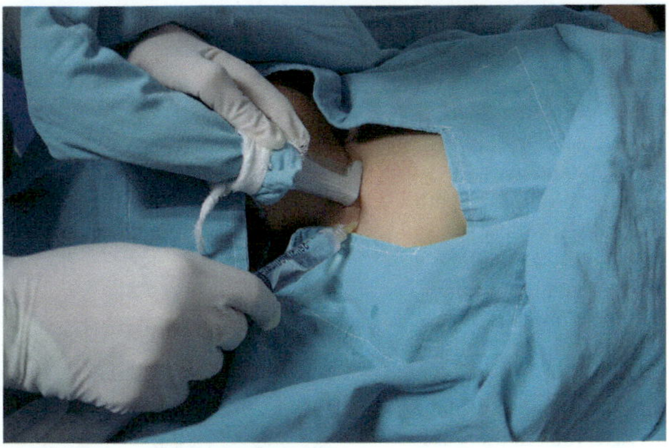

Fig. 10.15 Real-time ultrasound-guided lidocaine infiltration

10.3 Local Anesthesia Application

- The sterile field only leaves the cervical, upper pectoral, and right shoulder regions uncovered.
- Real-time ultrasound-guided lidocaine infiltration.
- For infiltration, use a small needle 25–27 G.
- Use lidocaine 1%.
- Subcutaneous infiltration with lidocaine in the puncture tract 1,5–2 cm before the chosen venipuncture site to anesthetize the oblique puncture path as well as the fixation site of the catheter holder (Fig. 10.15).
- LAX view of lidocaine infiltration (Figs. 10.16 and 10.17).

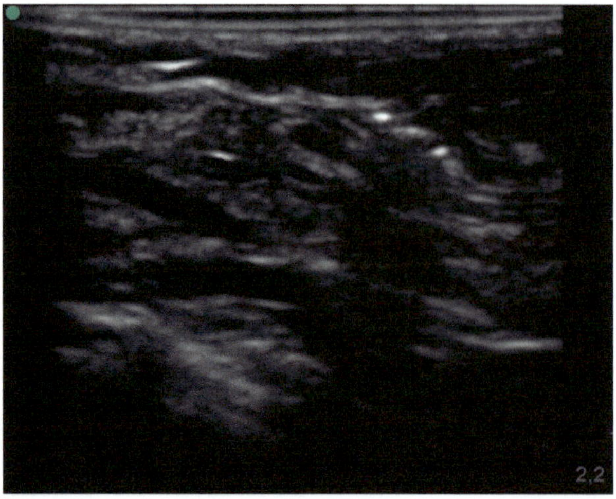

Fig. 10.16 LAX view of lidocaine infiltration

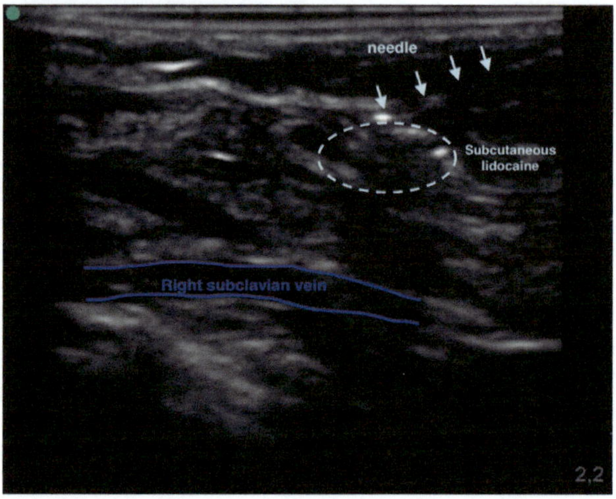

Fig. 10.17 Identifying structures
- The infiltration needle (25 G) is identified between the subcutaneous tissues for infiltration of the path that will follow the puncture of the RSCV
- This moment of the procedure can be used to determine if the site of choice for the puncture is in the plane of the RSCV, as in this case

10.4 Steps for Real-Time Ultrasound-Guided Access to Supraclavicular Right Subclavian Vein in Pediatrics

10.4.1 Step 01

- We will use an Arrow® 4 Fr, 13-cm, double-lumen catheter. This type of catheter has a 21-G introducer needle, or you can also use a 22-G intravenous catheter.
- Place the transducer at the level of the right supraclavicular fossa with the tip of the transducer to the left between the inner third of the clavicle and the sternal notch.

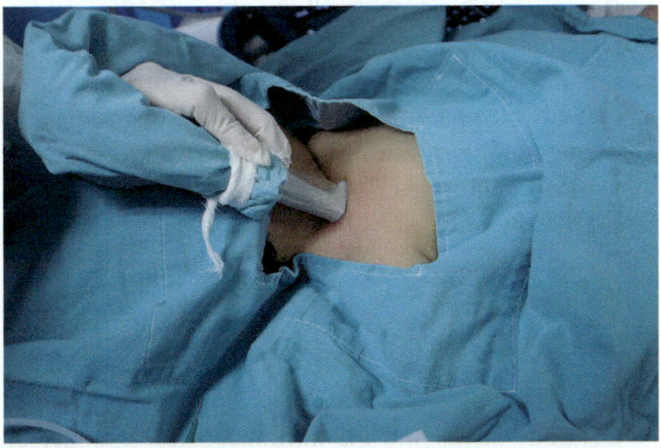

Fig. 10.18 Localization of the RSCV by placing the transducer in the right supraclavicular fossae with a posterior tilt

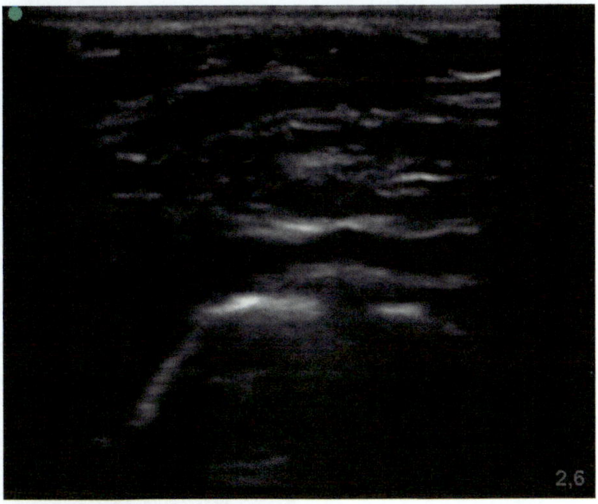

Fig. 10.19 Scan of the right supraclavicular fossae. LAX view of the RSCV

- Tilt the transducer posteriorly with the shaft almost in contact with the patient's mandible (Fig. 10.18).
- LAX view of the RSCV (Figs. 10.19 and 10.20).

10.4.2 Step 02

- Once you identify the RSCV at LAX view on the screen, perform the puncture with a 21-G introducer needle, which comes with the central venous catheter kit.
- Start the puncture at a 40–50-degree angle to the skin from lateral to medial.
- The introducer needle is aligned following the direction of the tip of the hockey stick transducer and the central part of the thickness of the transducer.

- Begin with dynamic needle tracking (DNT), the basis of the ultrasound-guided puncture technique.
- It is important to visualize the entire introducer needle at each moment of puncture advancement to avoid incidents. The needle is visualized on the screen from the beginning of the puncture and is monitored throughout the procedure until venous cannulation (Fig. 10.21).
- LAX view of the start of the puncture (Figs. 10.22 and 10.23).

10.4.3 *Step 03*

- Continue advancing the introducer needle under ultrasound guidance. Slide to medial the transductor to continue with real-time DNT (Fig. 10.24).

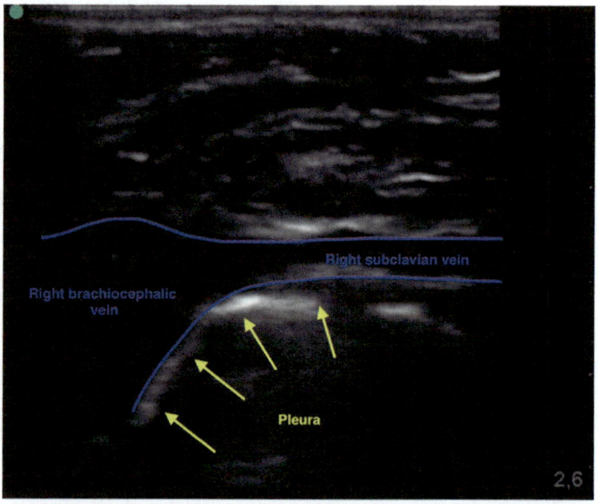

Fig. 10.20 Identifying structures
- The RSCV is anterior and more retroclavicular than the RSCA
- The pleura is in contact with the posterior wall of the RSCV and the lateral wall of the RBCV

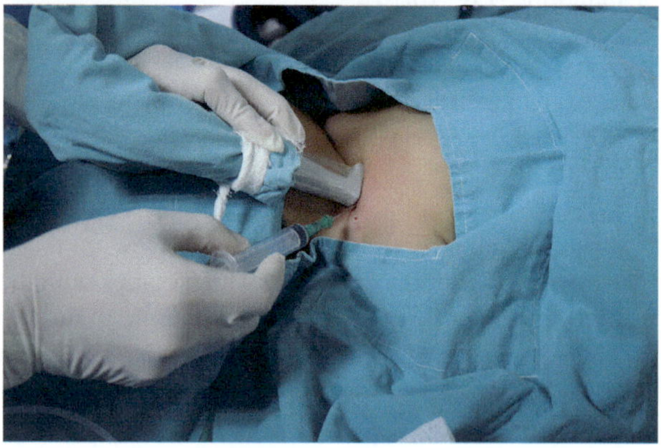

Fig. 10.21 The introducer needle is aligned to the central part of the thickness of the transducer and follows the direction of the tip of the hockey stick transducer at an angle of 40–50°

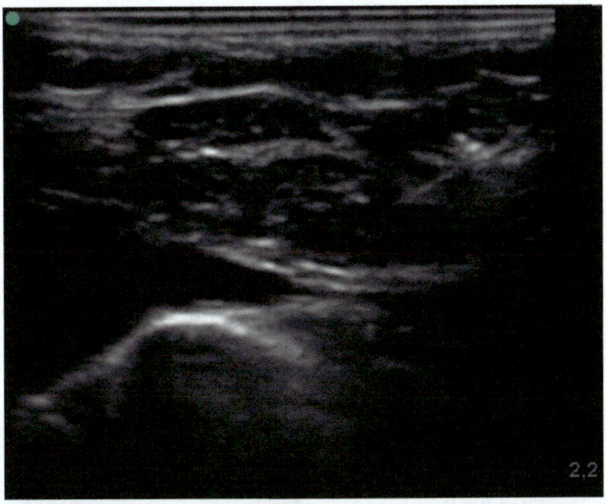

Fig. 10.22 Scan of the right supraclavicular fossae. LAX view of the start of the puncture

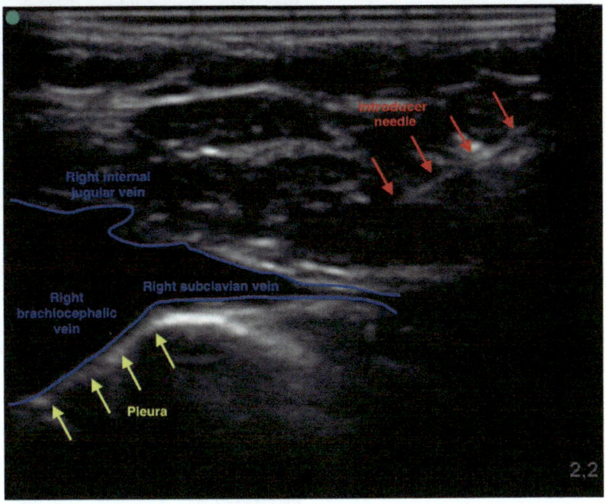

Fig. 10.23 Identifying structures

- The puncture has started, and the introducer needle is inserted in the direction of the RSCV
- The RSCV is compressed by the pressure applied to the penetration of the introducer needle

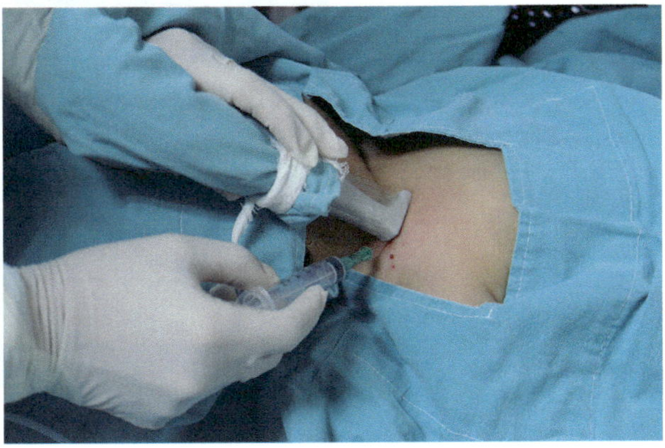

Fig. 10.24 Real-time dynamic needle tracking. During puncture advancement, the transducer slides from lateral to medial

- LAX view of the progression of the puncture in the appropriate direction of the RSCV (Figs. 10.25 and 10.26).

10.4.4 Step 04

- When you identify on the ultrasound screen that you are penetrating the RSCV, apply gentle negative pressure on the syringe plunger (Fig. 10.27).
- LAX view of the cannulation of the RSCV (Figs. 10.28 and 10.29).

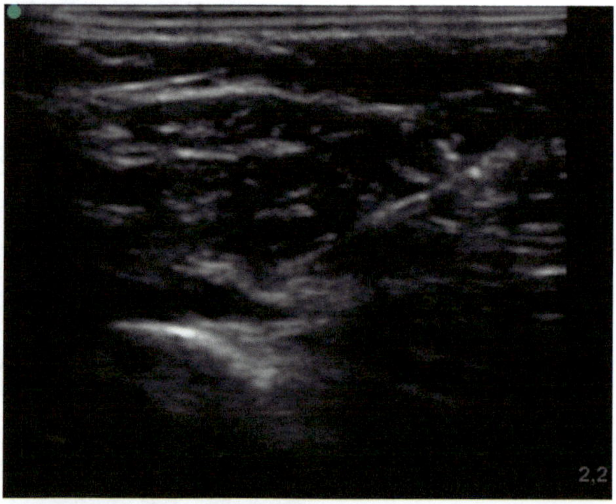

Fig. 10.25 LAX view of the progression of the puncture in the appropriate direction of the RSCV

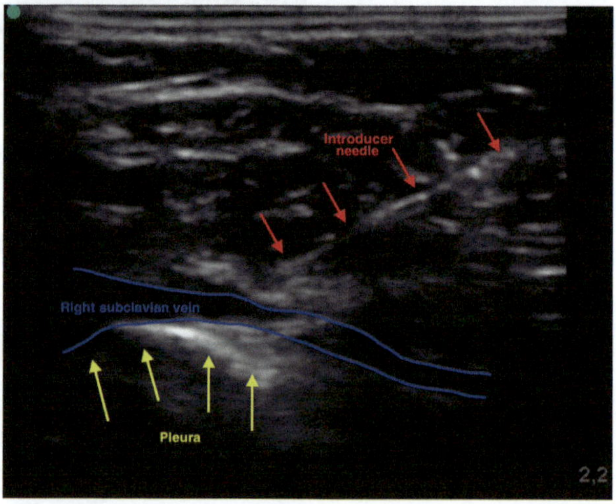

Fig. 10.26 Identifying structures
- The introducer needle is in the proper direction of the RSCV and is about to reach it
- To avoid incidents, it is important to always visualize the entire introducer needle at each moment of puncture progress

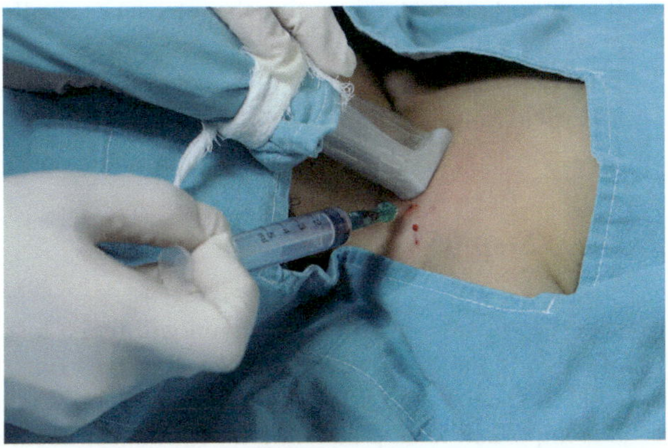

Fig. 10.27 Apply gentle negative pressure on the syringe plunger

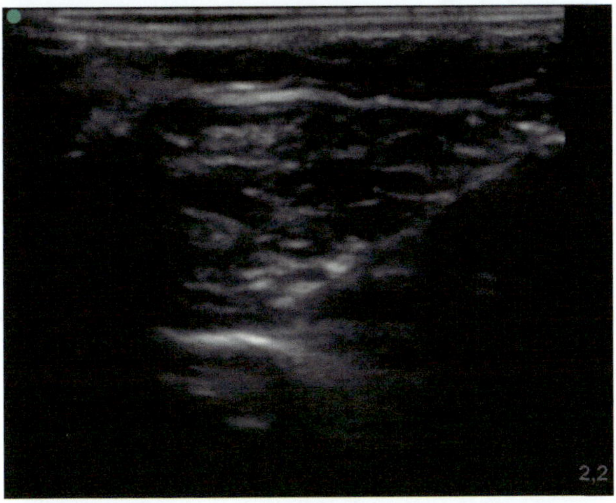

Fig. 10.28 LAX view of the cannulation of the RSCV

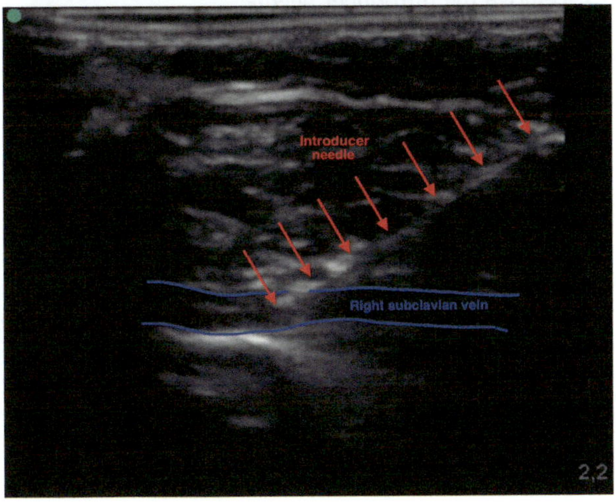

Fig. 10.29 Identifying structures

- The introducer needle is cannulating the RSCV

- It is important to stop inserting the introducer needle, so you do not penetrate the posterior wall.
- With experience, you will notice that resistance to the puncture is momentarily lost when you cannulate the vein.

10.4.5 Step 05

- When you cannulate the RSCV, you will feel a loss of resistance and the return of blood in the barrel of the syringe (Fig. 10.30).
- Hold the needle hub firmly with your left hand so the needle does not dislodge.
- It is important to stop inserting the introducer needle so you do not penetrate the posterior wall.

10.4.6 Step 06

- Hold the needle hub firmly and remove the syringe (Fig. 10.31).
- Insert the 0.18" guidewire, which should go through easily (Fig. 10.32).
- Verify the intravascular location of the guidewire by placing the transducer over the supraclavicular fossa (Fig. 10.33).
- LAX view of the intravascular guidewire within the RSCV (Figs. 10.34 and 10.35).

10.4.7 Step 07

- Remove the introducer needle.

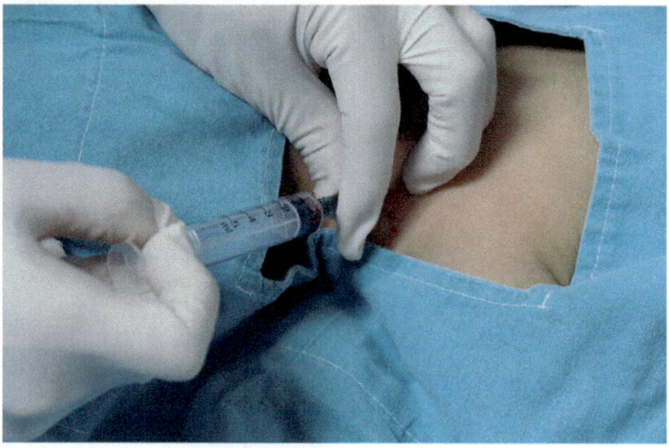

Fig. 10.30 Hold the needle hub and apply gentle negative pressure. Check for the return of blood in the barrel of the syringe

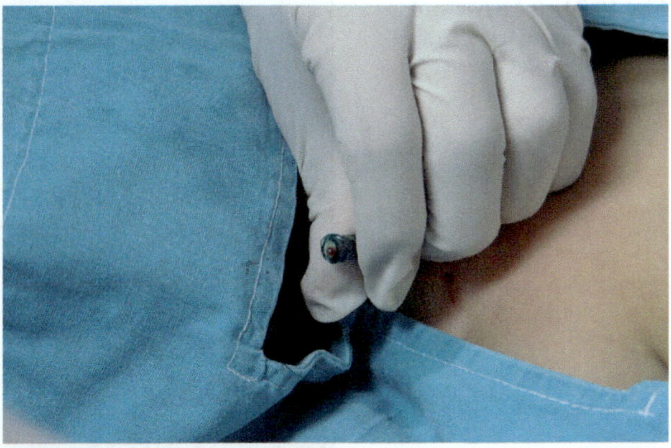

Fig. 10.31 Hold the needle hub firmly and remove the syringe

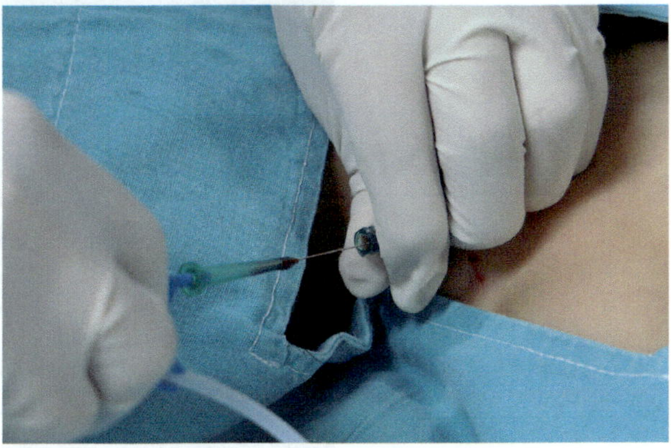

Fig. 10.32 Insert the guidewire

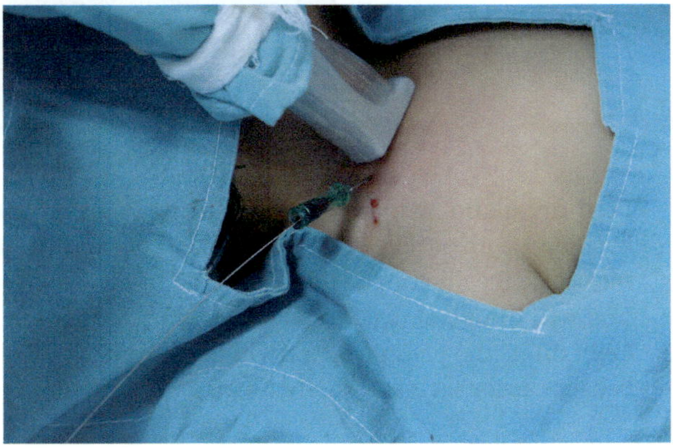

Fig. 10.33 Scan the supraclavicular fossa to verify the intravascular location of the guidewire

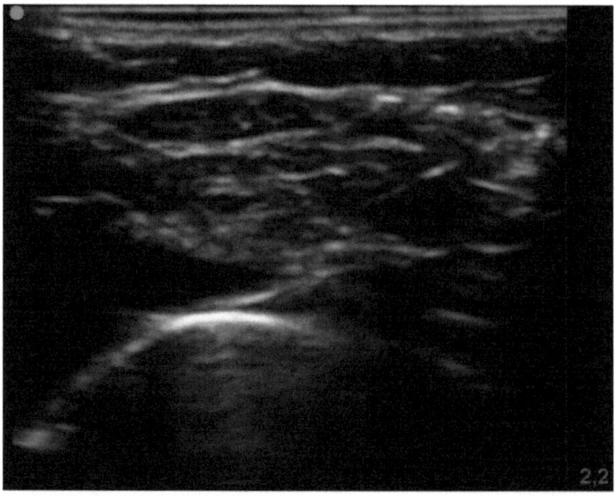

Fig. 10.34 LAX view of the intravascular guidewire within the RSCV

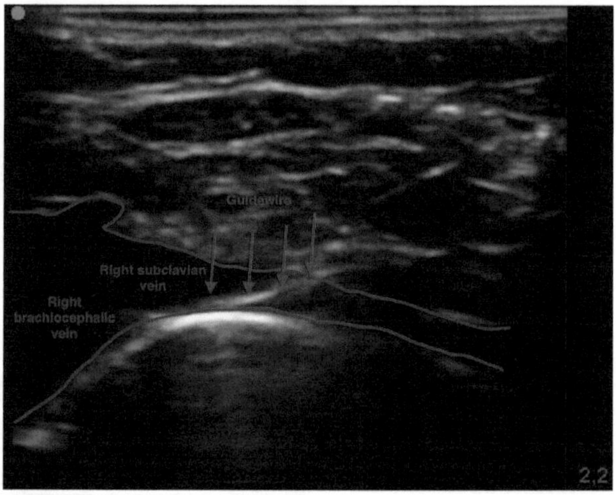

Fig. 10.35 Identifying structures
- The guidewire inside the RSCV

- Perform dilation with the right hand and countertraction of the skin with the left hand and with a "screw" maneuver. Try not to bend the guidewire.
- Introduce the dilator and dilate the path of the skin toward the RSCV (Fig. 10.36).
- You will often not need to make an incision to insert the dilator.
- Only dilate the path of the skin at the entrance of the RSCV. You will notice this because resistance is lost when you exert pressure with the dilator (Fig. 10.37).

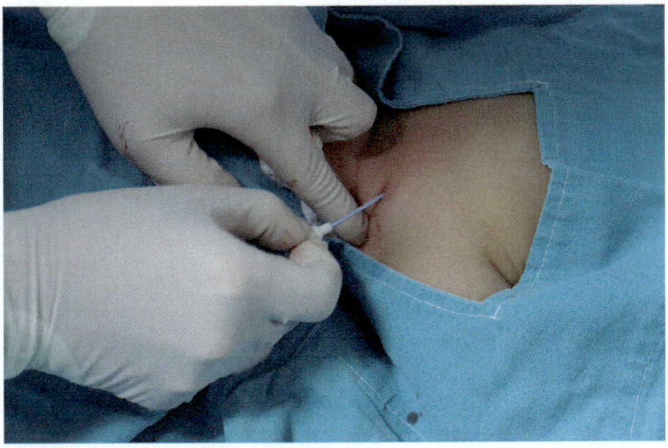

Fig. 10.36 Dilation of the skin

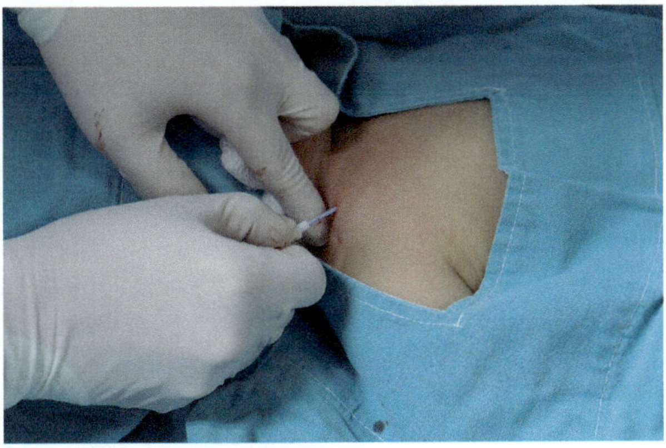

Fig. 10.37 Only dilate the path of the skin at the entrance of the RSCV

10.4.8 Step 08

- Introduce the central venous catheter using Seldinger's technique and remove the guidewire.
- The intravascular location of the catheter can also be checked (Fig. 10.38).
- LAX view of the catheter in the RSCV (Figs. 10.39 and 10.40).

10.4.9 Step 09

- Secure the catheter and place a sterile occlusive dressing according to the institutional protocol (Fig. 10.41).

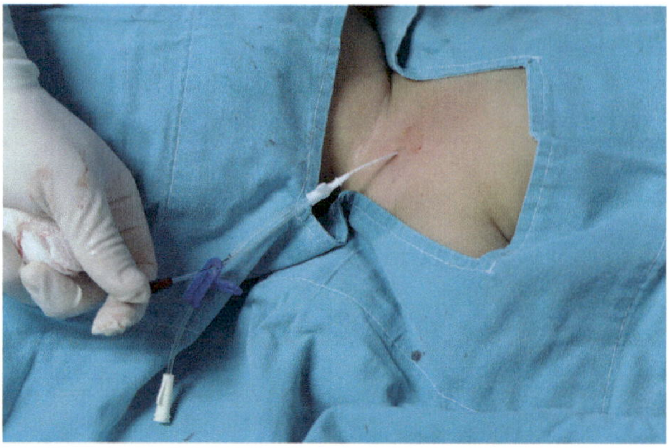

Fig. 10.38 Introduce the required intravascular catheter length

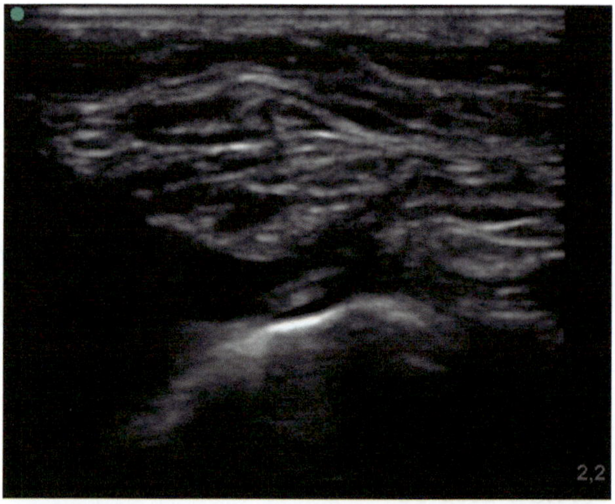

Fig. 10.39 LAX view of the intravascular catheter

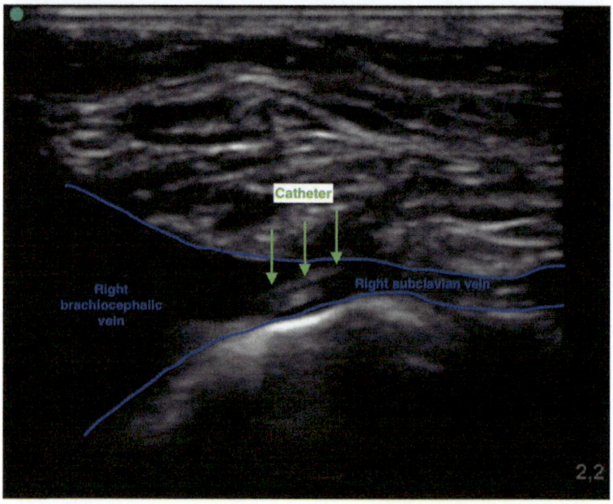

Fig. 10.40 Identifying structures

- The catheter enters the RSCV

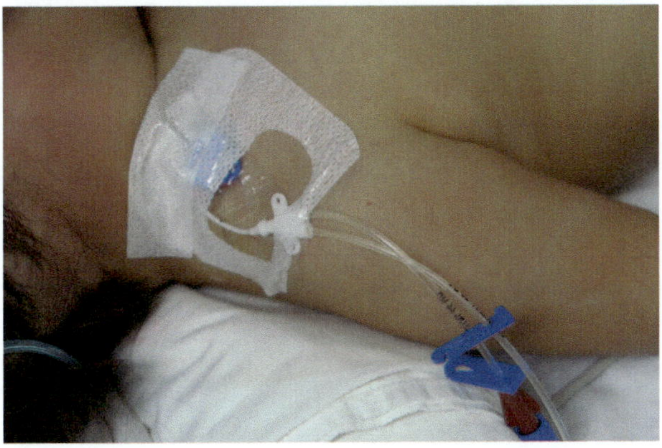

Fig. 10.41 Dressing according to the institutional protocol

Sources

1. Nardi N, Wodey E, Laviolle B, De La Brière F, Delahaye S, Engrand C, Gauvrit C, Dessard S, Defontaine A, Ecoffey C. Effectiveness and complications of ultrasound-guided subclavian vein cannulation in children and neonates. Anaesth Crit Care Pain Med. 2016;35(3):209–13. https://doi.org/10.1016/j.accpm.2015.09.007. Epub 2016 Feb 26. PMID: 26924612.
2. Guilbert AS, Xavier L, Ammouche C, Desprez P, Astruc D, Diemunsch P, Bientz J. Supraclavicular ultrasound-guided catheterization of the subclavian vein in pediatric and neonatal ICUs: a feasibility study. Pediatr Crit Care Med. 2013;14(4):351–5. https://doi.org/10.1097/PCC.0b013e3182745489. PMID: 23392376.
3. Byon HJ, Lee GW, Lee JH, Park YH, Kim HS, Kim CS, Kim JT. Comparison between ultrasound-guided supraclavicular and infraclavicular approaches for subclavian venous catheterization in children—a randomized trial. Br J Anaesth. 2013;111(5):788–92. https://doi.org/10.1093/bja/aet202. Epub 2013 Jun 10. PMID: 23756247.
4. Rhondali O, Attof R, Combet S, Chassard D, de Queiroz SM. Ultrasound-guided subclavian vein cannulation in infants: supraclavicular approach. Paediatr Anaesth. 2011;21(11):1136–41. https://doi.org/10.1111/j.1460-9592.2011.03614.x. Epub 2011 Jun 1. PMID: 21627714.
5. Attof R, Rhondali O, Combet S, Chassard D, De Queiroz M. Abord de la veine sous-clavière par voie sus-claviculaire sous échographie: une nouvelle approche en pédiatrie [Ultrasound-guided supraclavicular subclavian vein catheterization: a novel approach in children]. Ann Fr Anesth Reanim. 2010;29(9):651–4. https://doi.org/10.1016/j.annfar.2010.05.036. Epub 2010 Aug 14. PMID: 20709489.

Chapter 11
Supraclavicular Left Subclavian Vein in Pediatrics

11.1 Patient Positioning

- The patient is an 8-year-old weighing 24 kg.
- Position the patient on the left side of the bed.
- Place the patient's head to the right.
- Place a roll under the shoulders to extend the neck (Fig. 11.1).
- Gently hold the upper extremities with the arms caudal.
- The objective of positioning the patient is to increase the length of the cervical region and create a wider space between the clavicle and the jaw to access the supraclavicular fossae.

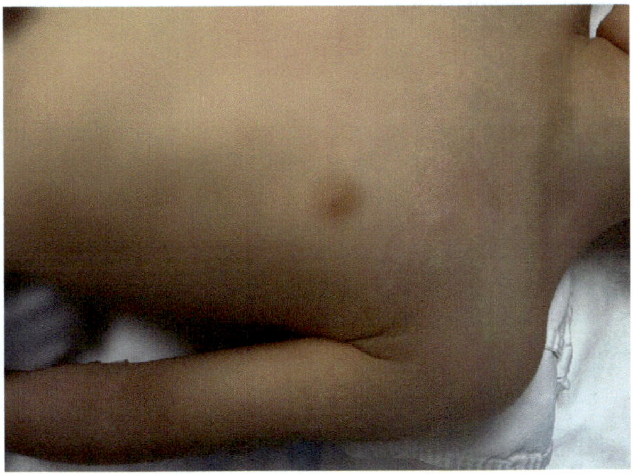

Fig. 11.1 Patient positioning

F. Montes-Tapia, *Atlas of Ultrasound-Guided Central Venous Catheter Placement*, https://doi.org/10.1007/978-3-031-61887-1_11

11.2 Scanning Technique

- Do a preliminary vascular assessment (non-sterile), known as rapid central vein assessment (RaCeVA).
- Stand on the left side of the bed or stretcher.
- Use a high-frequency linear transducer (13–6 MHz) with a hockey stick type or a larger probe.
- Place the ultrasound device in front of the operator at the right or left shoulder.
- Hold the transducer with your left hand and begin scanning with the transducer transverse to the neck and the tip of the hockey stick-type probe to the patient's right side.
- Start scanning in the middle of the neck and visualize the left internal jugular vein (LIJV) and the left carotid artery (LCA) in short-axis (SAX) view, and then sweep down to the supraclavicular fossae.
- When the lower edge of the transducer contacts the upper edge of the clavicle at the level of the middle third of the clavicle, begin to tilt posteriorly (Fig. 11.2).
- With this transducer position, the left subclavian artery (LSCA) will be visualized first.
- Perform a more posterior tilt and then the left subclavian vein (LSCV) will be visualized in long-axis (LAX) view (Figs. 11.3 and 11.4).
- Slide the transductor and scan from the middle to the inner third of the clavicle to see the LSCV and the left brachiocephalic vein (LBCV) (Figs. 11.5 and 11.6).
- Finally, slide the transductor to scan between the inner third of the clavicle and the sternal manubrium to visualize the LBCV (Figs. 11.7 and 11.8).

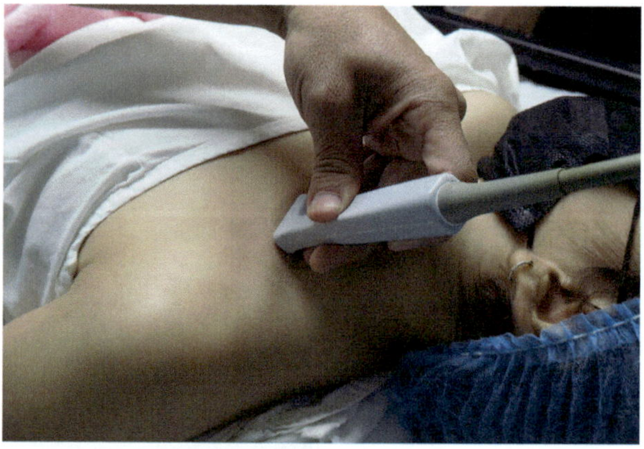

Fig. 11.2 Begin the scan at the level of the middle third of the clavicle

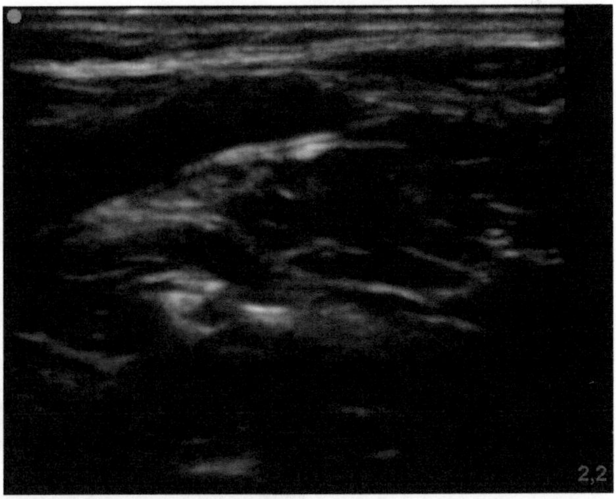

Fig. 11.3 Scan at the middle third of the clavicle. Supraclavicular LAX view of the left subclavian vein
- The scan depth is 2.2 cm

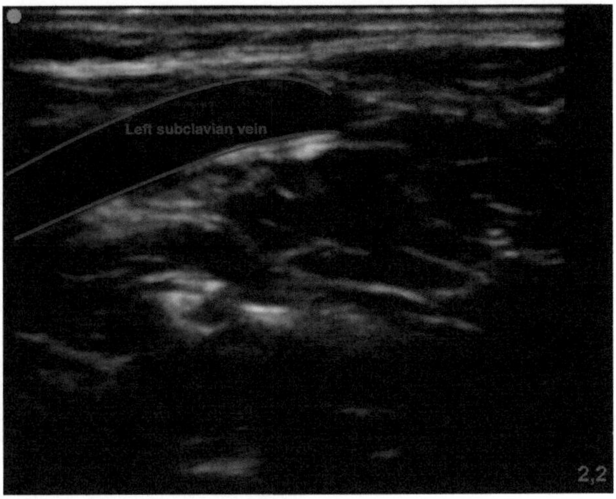

Fig. 11.4 Identifying structures
- The left subclavian vein has a diameter of 0.29 cm

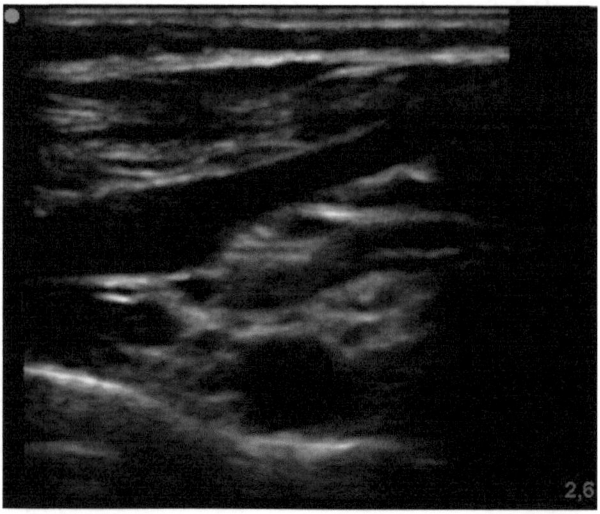

Fig. 11.5 Scan the inner third of the clavicle
- Supraclavicular vein view in LAX

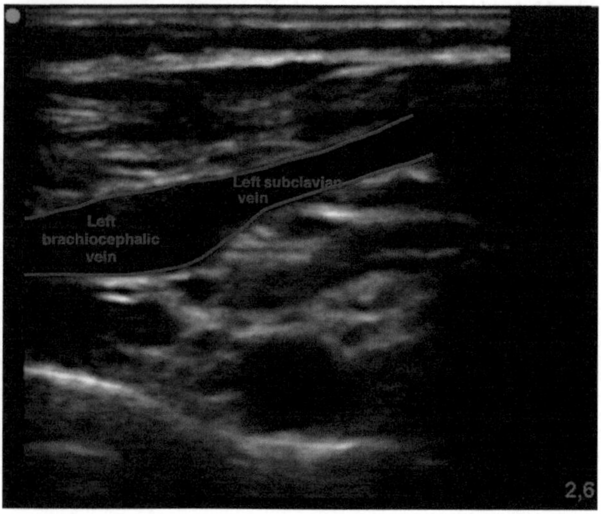

Fig. 11.6 Identifying structures
- The LSCV continues with the LBCV

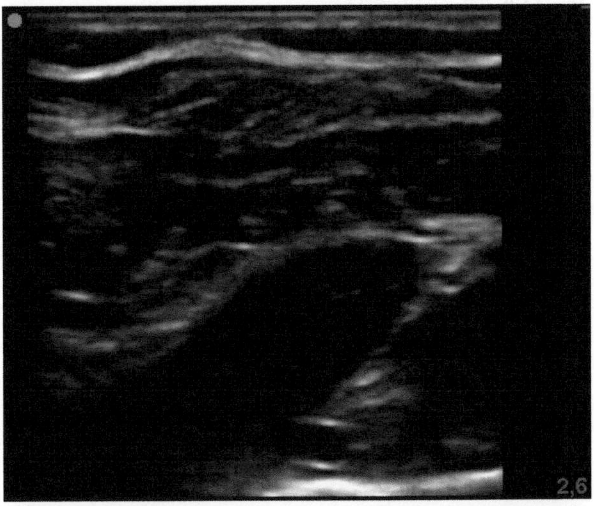

Fig. 11.7 Scan between the inner third of the clavicle and the sternal manubrium

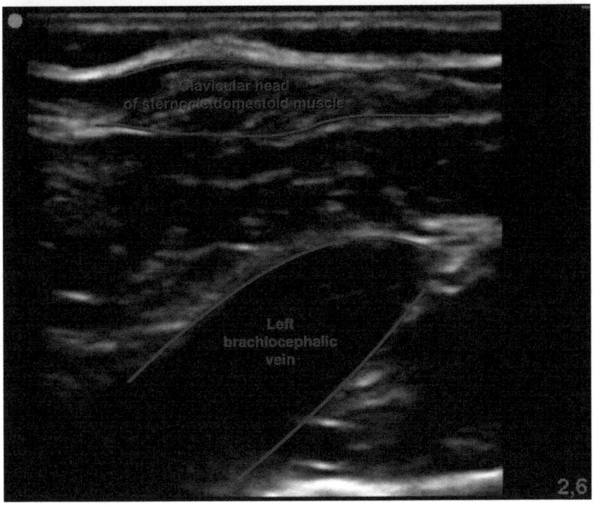

Fig. 11.8 Identifying structures
- The clavicular head of the sternocleidomastoid muscle is seen and, underneath, the LBCV as it courses obliquely downward to the superior vena cava (SVC)

11.3 Local Anesthesia Application

- The sterile field only leaves the cervical, upper pectoral, and left shoulder regions uncovered (Fig. 11.9).
- Real-time ultrasound-guided lidocaine infiltration.
- For infiltration, use a small needle 25–27 G.
- Use lidocaine 1%.
- Subcutaneous infiltration with lidocaine in the puncture tract 1.5–2 cm before the chosen venipuncture site to anesthetize the oblique puncture path as well as the fixation site of the catheter holder (Fig. 11.10).

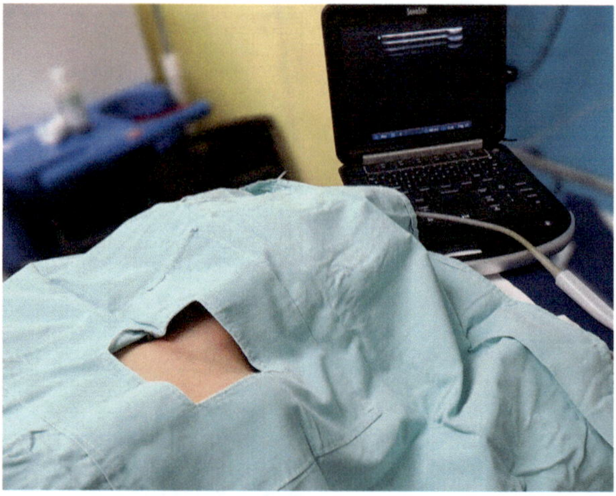

Fig. 11.9 The sterile field and the ultrasound device are in front of the operator

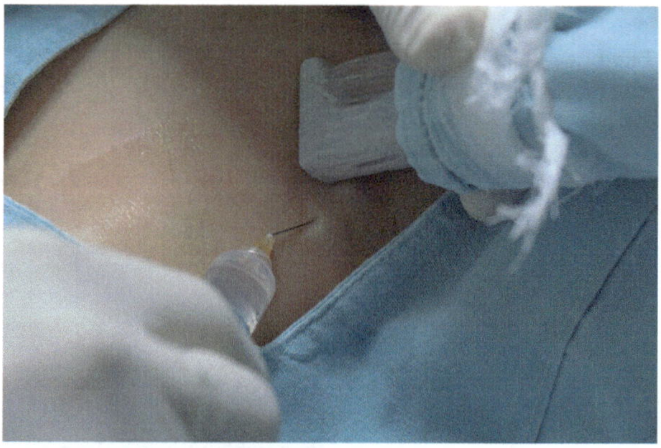

Fig. 11.10 Real-time ultrasound-guided lidocaine infiltration

11.4 Steps for Real-Time Ultrasound-Guided Access to Supraclavicular Left Subclavian Vein in Pediatrics

11.4.1 Step 01

- We will use an Arrow® 4 Fr, 13-cm, double-lumen catheter. This type of catheter has a 21-G introducer needle. You can also use a 22-G intravenous catheter for puncture.
- The operator stands on the left side of the bed (Fig. 11.11).
- Place the transducer at the level of the left supraclavicular fossae with the tip of the transducer to the right between the medial and the inner third of the clavicle (Fig. 11.12).
- Tilt the transducer posteriorly with the shaft almost in contact with the patient's mandible.

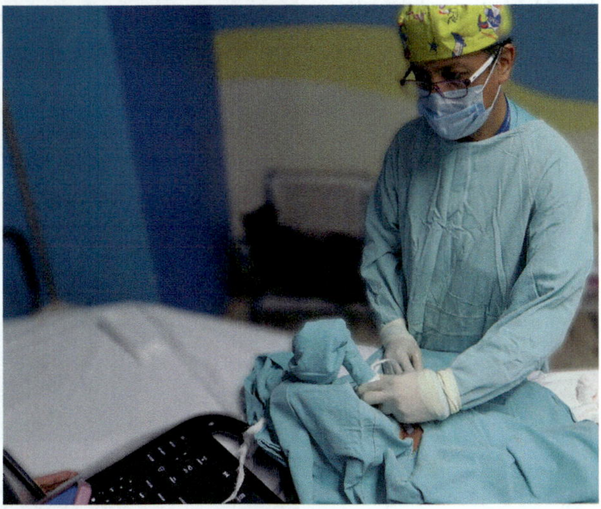

Fig. 11.11 The operator stands on the left side of the bed

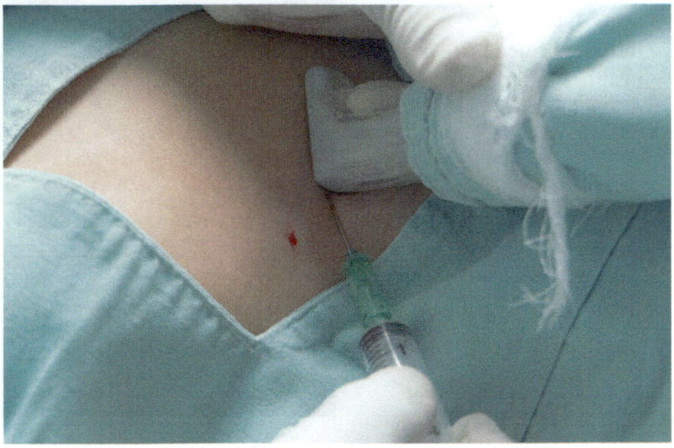

Fig. 11.12 The introducer needle is aligned to the central part of the thickness of the transducer following the direction of the tip of the hockey stick transducer at an angle of 10–20°

11.4.2 Step 02

- Once you identify the LSCV at LAX view on the screen, perform the puncture with a 21-G introducer needle, which comes with the central venous catheter kit.
- Start the puncture with a 10–20° angle to the skin from lateral to medial (Fig. 11.12).
- Place the introducer needle under the transducer following the path of the transducer and the central part of the thickness of the transducer.
- Begin with dynamic needle tracking (DNT), the basis of the ultrasound-guided puncture technique.

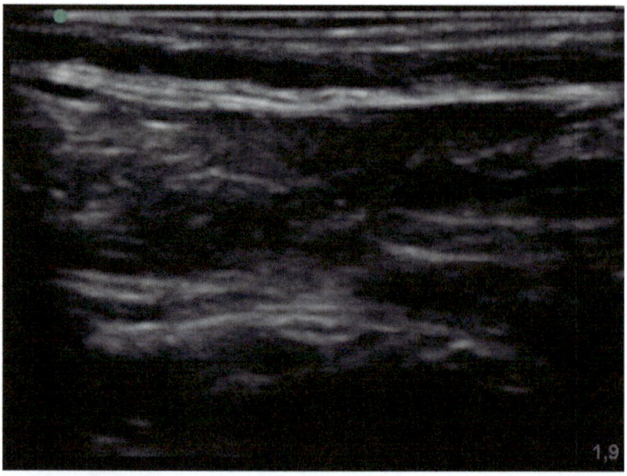

Fig. 11.13 Scan of the left supraclavicular fossae. LAX view at the start of the puncture

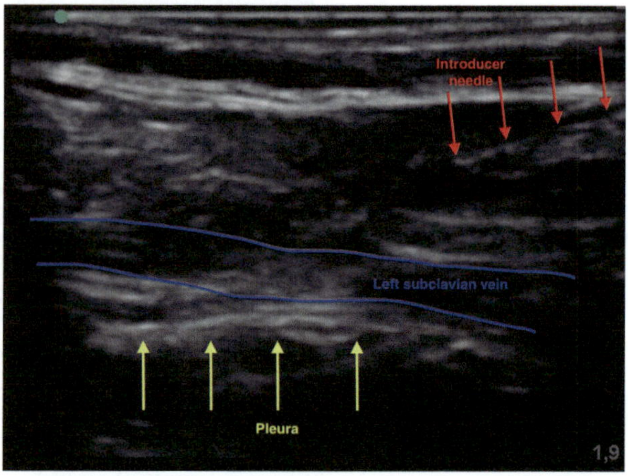

Fig. 11.14 Identifying structures

- The puncture has started, and the introducer needle is inserted in the direction of the LSCV

- It is important to visualize the entire introducer needle at each moment of puncture advancement to avoid incidents. The needle is visualized on the screen from the beginning of the puncture and is monitored throughout the procedure until venous cannulation.
- LAX view of the start of the puncture (Figs. 11.13 and 11.14).

11.4.3 Step 03

- Continue advancing the introducer needle under DNT (Fig. 11.15).
- LAX view of the introducer needle penetrating the anterior wall of the LSCV (Figs. 11.16 and 11.17).

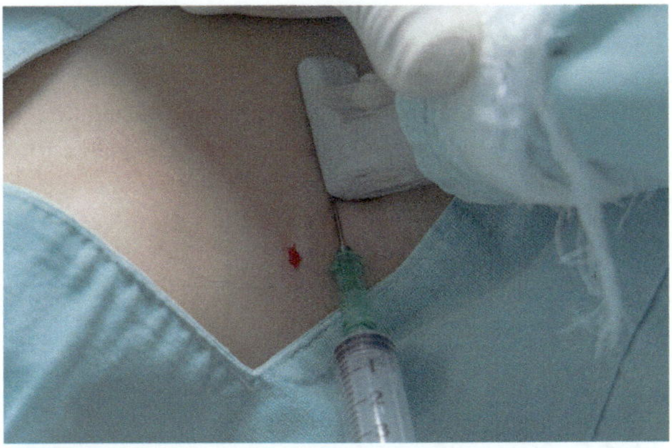

Fig. 11.15 Progression of the puncture following the path of the transducer and the central part of the thickness of the transducer

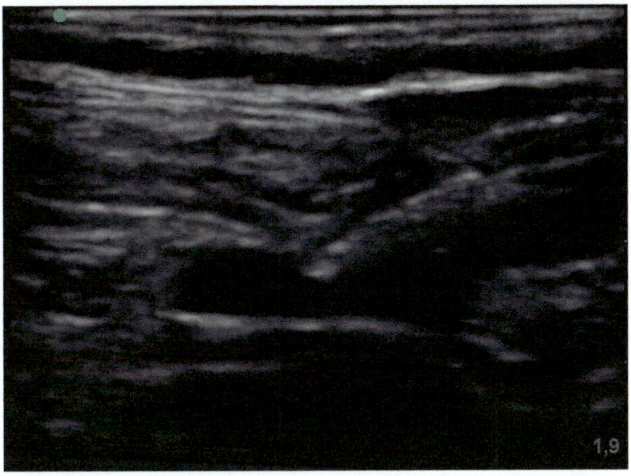

Fig. 11.16 LAX view of the introducer needle penetrating the anterior wall of the LSCV

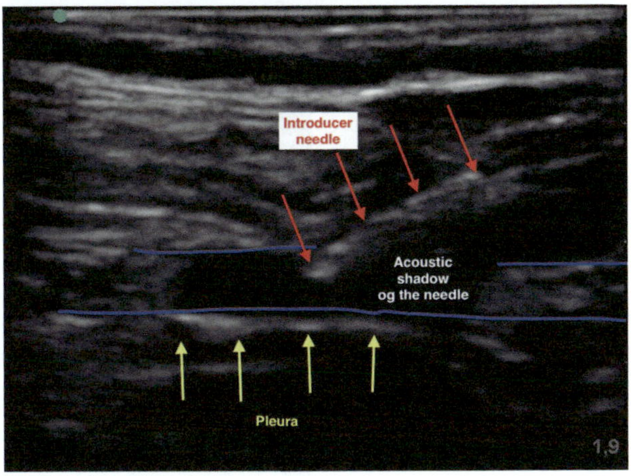

Fig. 11.17 Identifying structures
- The introducer needle penetrates the anterior wall of the LSCV
- The pleura lies inferior to the posterior wall of the LSCV

11.4.4 Step 04

- When you identify that you are penetrating the LSCV, apply gentle negative pressure on the syringe plunger as you advance the needle (Fig. 11.18).
- LAX view of the canalization of the LSCV (Figs. 11.19 and 11.20).
- It is important to stop inserting the introducer needle further so you do not penetrate the posterior wall.
- With experience, you will notice that resistance to the puncture is momentarily lost when you canalize a vein.

11.4.5 Step 05

- As soon as a flash of blood appears in the barrel of the syringe, stop advancing with the puncture and set the transducer aside.

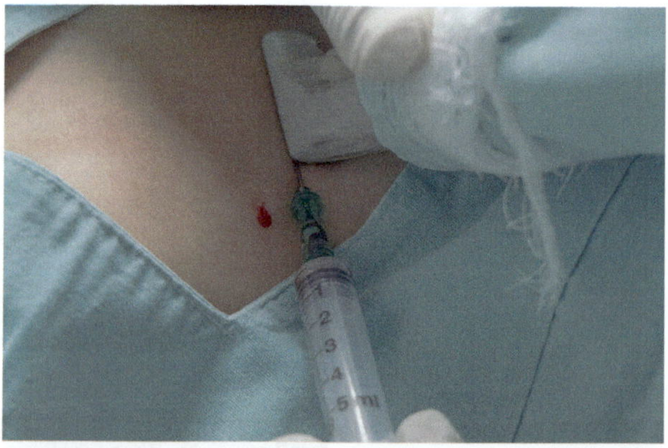

Fig. 11.18 Apply gentle negative pressure on the syringe plunger

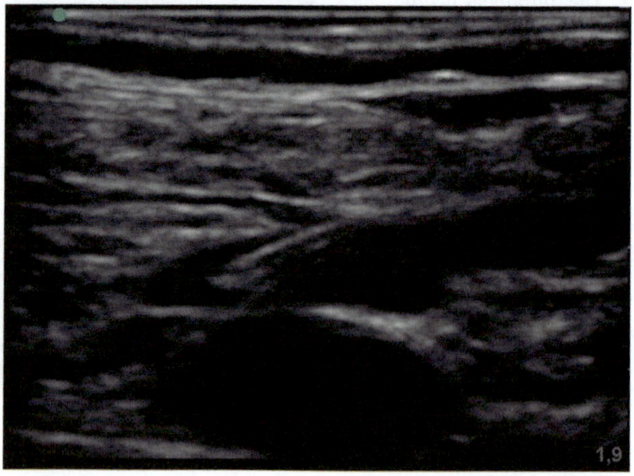

Fig. 11.19 LAX view of the canalization of the LSCV

- Remove the syringe (Fig. 11.21).
- Hold the needle hub firmly and insert the 0.18-inch guidewire, which should go through easily (Fig. 11.22).
- When you have inserted enough guidewire, withdraw the introducer needle.

11.4.6 Step 06

- Remove the introducer needle.
- Perform dilation with the right hand and countertract the skin with the left hand with a "screw" maneuver. Try not to bend the guidewire.
- Introduce the dilator and dilate the path of the skin toward the LSCV (Fig. 11.23).
- You will often not need to make an incision to insert the dilator.

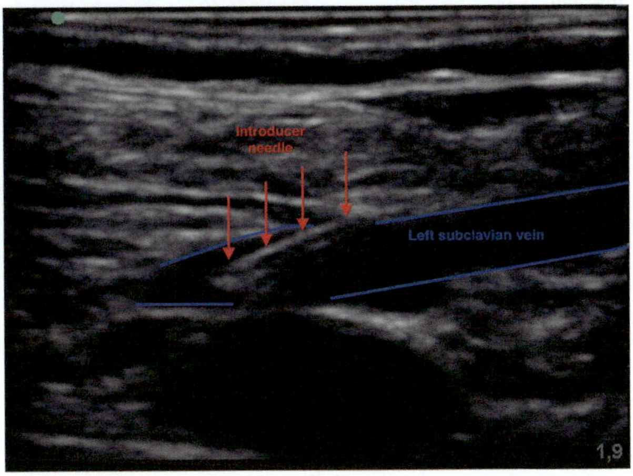

Fig. 11.20 Identifying structures
- The introducer needle has canalized the LSCV

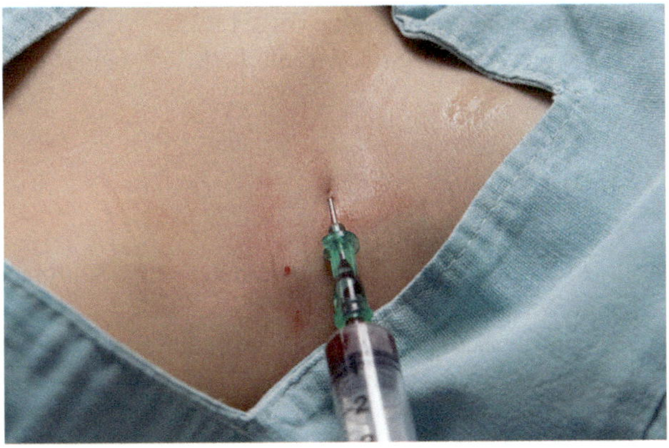

Fig. 11.21 Return of blood in the barrel of the syringe

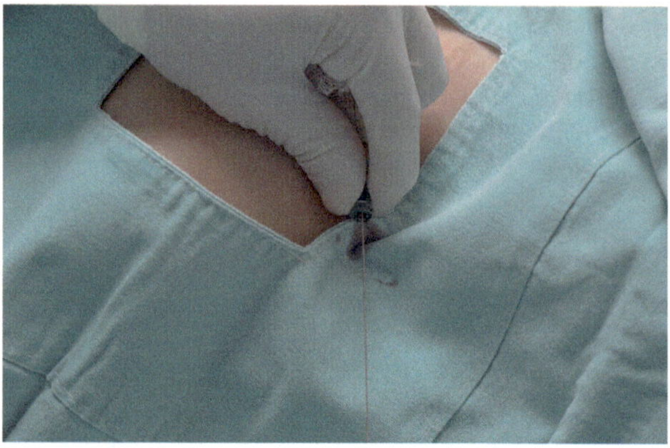

Fig. 11.22 Insert the guidewire

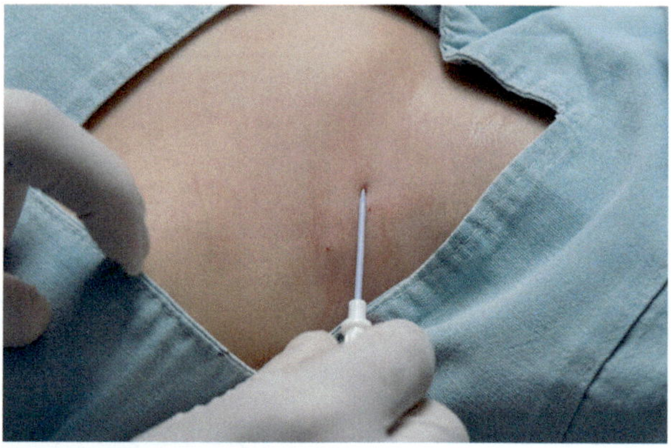

Fig. 11.23 Dilation of the skin

- Only dilate the path of the skin at the entrance of the RSCV. You will notice this because the resistance is lost when you exert pressure with the dilator (Fig. 11.24).
- Verify the intravascular location of the guidewire by placing the transducer over the supraclavicular fossae (Fig. 11.25).
- LAX view of the guidewire in the LSCV (Figs. 11.26 and 11.27).

11.4.7 Step 07

- Introduce the central venous catheter using Seldinger's technique and remove the guidewire (Fig. 11.28).
- The intravascular location of the catheter can also be checked.
- LAX view of the catheter in the LSCV (Figs. 11.29 and 11.30).

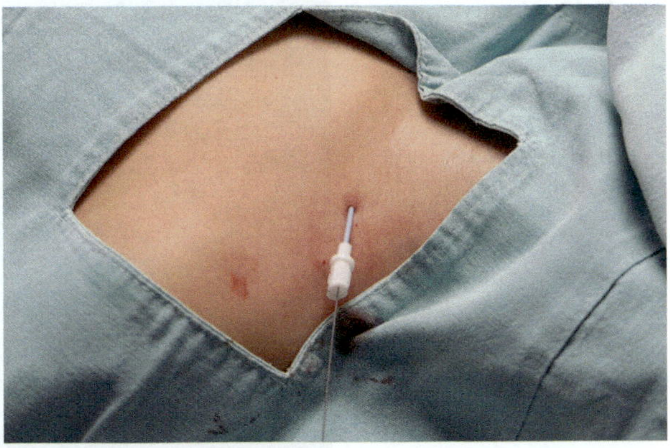

Fig. 11.24 Only dilate the path of the skin to the entrance of the LSCV

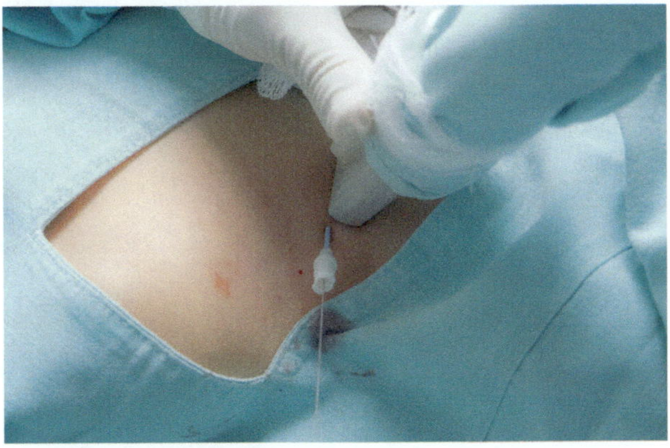

Fig. 11.25 Scan the supraclavicular fossa

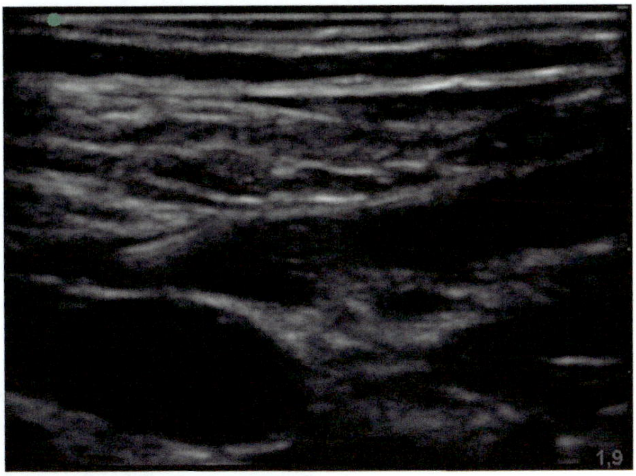

Fig. 11.26 LAX view of the guidewire in the LSCV

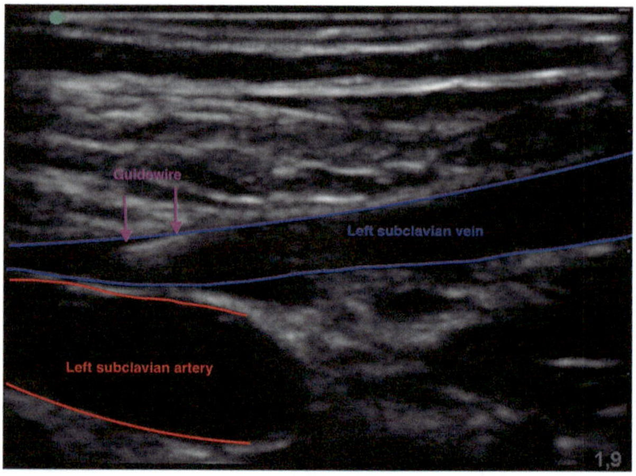

Fig. 11.27 Identifying structures

- The guidewire is located intravascularly in the LSCV
- In this view, you can see part of the LSCA

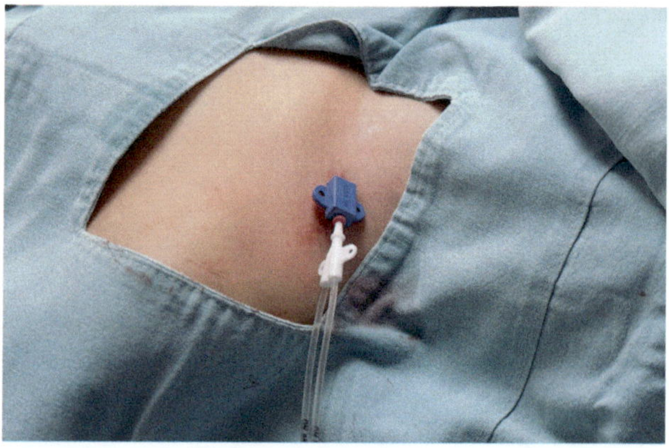

Fig. 11.28 Introduce the required intravascular catheter length

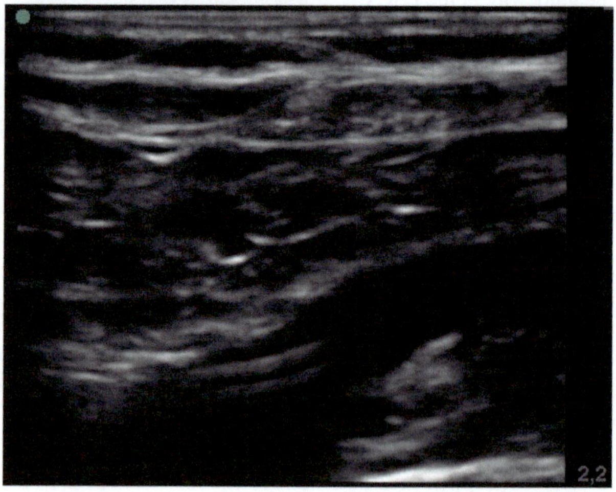

Fig. 11.29 LAX view of the intravascular catheter

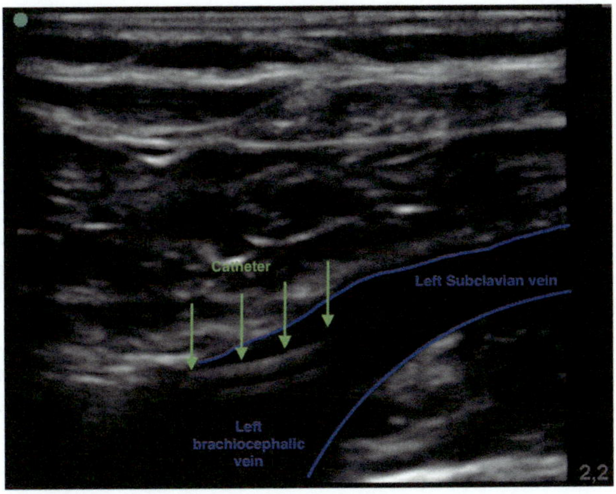

Fig. 11.30 Identifying structures
- The catheter enters the LBCV from the LSCV

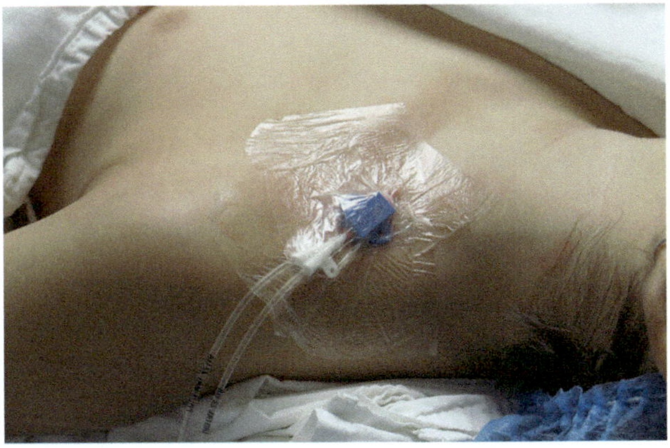

Fig. 11.31 Dressing according to the institutional protocol

11.4.8 Step 08

- Secure the catheter and place a sterile occlusive dressing according to the institutional protocol (Fig. 11.31).

Sources

1. Nardi N, Wodey E, Laviolle B, De La Brière F, Delahaye S, Engrand C, Gauvrit C, Dessard S, Defontaine A, Ecoffey C. Effectiveness and complications of ultrasound-guided subclavian vein cannulation in children and neonates. Anaesth Crit Care Pain Med. 2016;35(3):209–13. https://doi.org/10.1016/j.accpm.2015.09.007. Epub 2016 Feb 26. PMID: 26924612.

2. Guilbert AS, Xavier L, Ammouche C, Desprez P, Astruc D, Diemunsch P, Bientz J. Supraclavicular ultrasound-guided catheterization of the subclavian vein in pediatric and neonatal ICUs: a feasibility study. Pediatr Crit Care Med. 2013;14(4):351–5. https://doi.org/10.1097/PCC.0b013e3182745489. PMID: 23392376.
3. Byon HJ, Lee GW, Lee JH, Park YH, Kim HS, Kim CS, Kim JT. Comparison between ultrasound-guided supraclavicular and infraclavicular approaches for subclavian venous catheterization in children—a randomized trial. Br J Anaesth. 2013;111(5):788–92. https://doi.org/10.1093/bja/aet202. Epub 2013 Jun 10. PMID: 23756247.
4. Rhondali O, Attof R, Combet S, Chassard D, de Queiroz SM. Ultrasound-guided subclavian vein cannulation in infants: supraclavicular approach. Paediatr Anaesth. 2011;21(11):1136–41. https://doi.org/10.1111/j.1460-9592.2011.03614.x. Epub 2011 Jun 1. PMID: 21627714.
5. Attof R, Rhondali O, Combet S, Chassard D, De Queiroz M. Abord de la veine sous-clavière par voie sus-claviculaire sous échographie: une nouvelle approche en pédiatrie [Ultrasound-guided supraclavicular subclavian vein catheterization: a novel approach in children]. Ann Fr Anesth Reanim. 2010;29(9):651–4. https://doi.org/10.1016/j.annfar.2010.05.036. Epub 2010 Aug 14. PMID: 20709489.

Chapter 12
Extrathoracic Right Subclavian Vein in Pediatrics

12.1 Patient Positioning

- The patient is a 14-year-old weighing 81 kg.
- Position the patient supine close to the right side of the bed or stretcher.
- Position the patient's head to the left or center (Fig. 12.1).
- This procedure can be performed without a roll below the shoulders, as in this case.
- Gently hold the upper extremities, with the arms toward caudal.

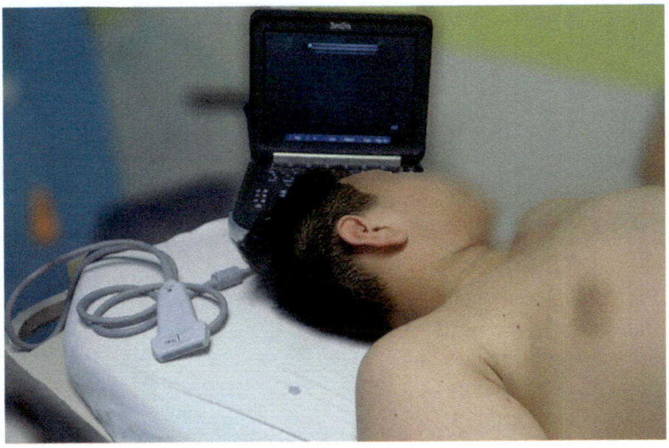

Fig. 12.1 Patient position

F. Montes-Tapia, *Atlas of Ultrasound-Guided Central Venous Catheter Placement*, https://doi.org/10.1007/978-3-031-61887-1_12

12.2 Scanning Technique

- Do a preliminary vascular assessment (non-sterile), known as rapid central vein assessment (RaCeVA).
- The operator stands on the right side of the patient (Fig. 12.2).
- Place the ultrasound in any of the following positions: on the side of the left shoulder, above the head, or at the right shoulder.
- We will use a high-frequency linear transducer (13–6 MHz) with a footprint of 5 cm.
- Scan the extrathoracic subclavian vessels in the short-axis (SAX) view, perpendicularly placing the transducer infraclavicular to the deltopectoral groove.
- Position the transducer position indicator toward the patient's left side (Fig. 12.3).
- The extrathoracic subclavian vessels run through the deltopectoral groove in an oblique course upward and from lateral to medial from the axillary fossa toward the middle third of the clavicle.

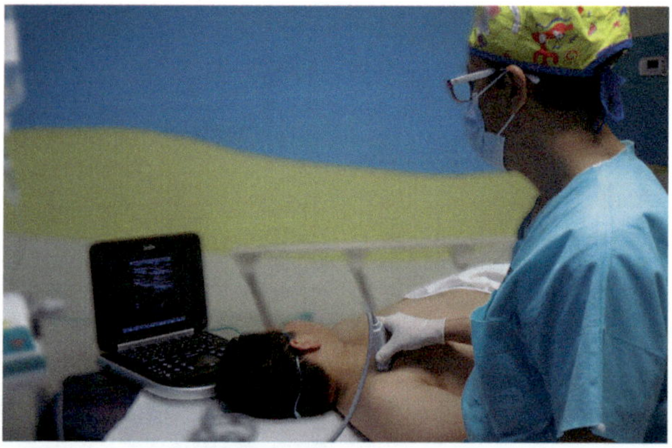

Fig. 12.2 The operator stands on the right side of the patient

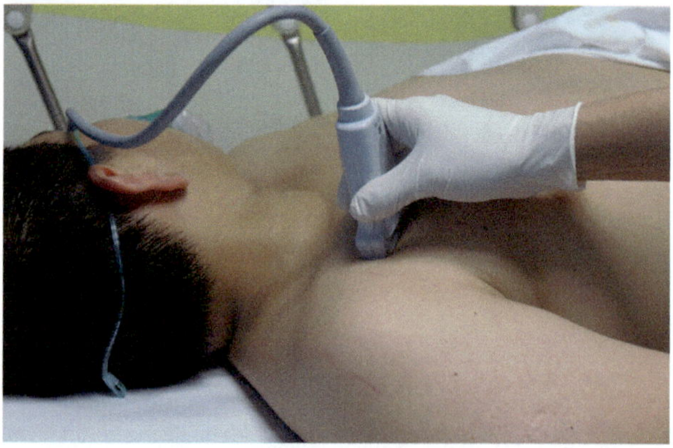

Fig. 12.3 Place the transducer in the right infraclavicular region and perpendicular to the deltopectoral groove

- Scan the groove from inferior to superior obliquely. The extrathoracic right subclavian vein (ETRSCV) begins after the junction of the axillary vein with the cephalic vein approximately midway through the deltopectoral groove.
- In the deltopectoral groove, the extrathoracic right subclavian artery (ETRSCA) is lateral, and the ETRSCV is medial. The vein varies in size with the respiratory cycle, while the artery maintains its constant beat. The vein can be compressed with the transducer to differentiate from the artery.
- SAX view of the extrathoracic subclavian vessels (Figs. 12.4, 12.5, 12.6 and 12.7).

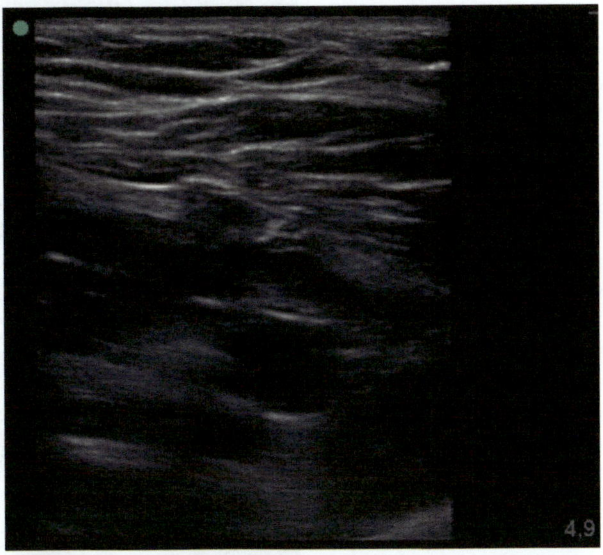

Fig. 12.4 Scan of the right infraclavicular region. SAX view of the extrathoracic subclavian vessels
- The transducer position indicator (aqua dot in the superior left corner of the image) points out the patient's left side
- Scan depth of 4,9 cm

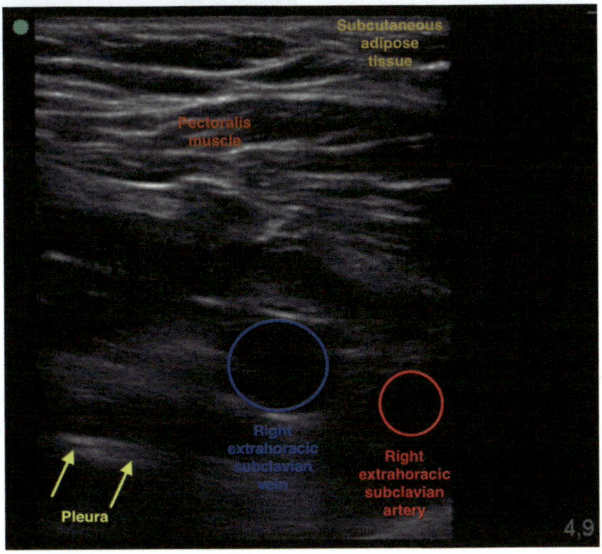

Fig. 12.5 Identifying structures
- Prominent subcutaneous adipose tissue
- The ETRSCA is lateral, and the ETRSCV is medial in the deltopectoral groove

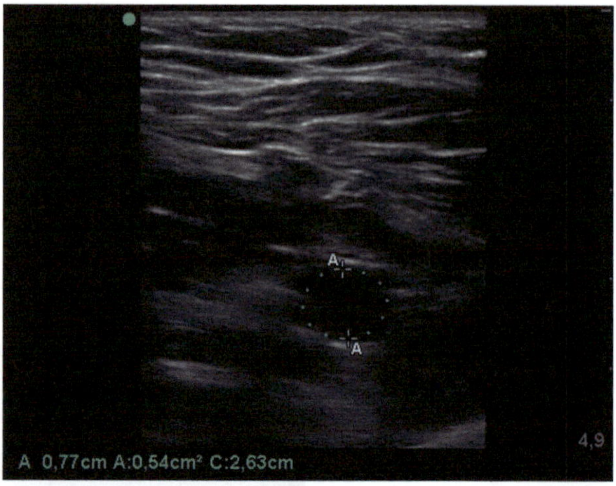

Fig. 12.6 SAX view of ETRSCV

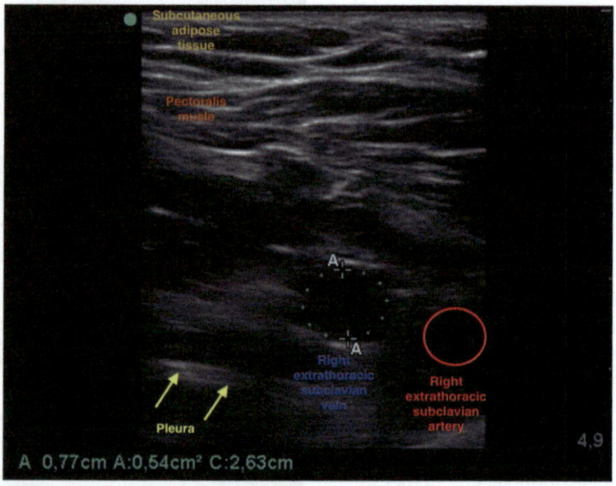

Fig. 12.7 Identifying structures

- The ETRSCV with an area of 0,54 cm^2 and a diameter of 0,77 cm

12.3 Local Anesthesia Application

- The sterile field only leaves the upper pectoral, right shoulder, and cervical regions uncovered.
- Real-time ultrasound-guided lidocaine infiltration.
- For infiltration, use a small needle 25–27 G.
- Use 1% lidocaine.
- Subcutaneous infiltration with lidocaine of the puncture tract 1,5–2 cm before the site chosen for ETRSCV puncture and the catheter fixation area (Fig. 12.8).

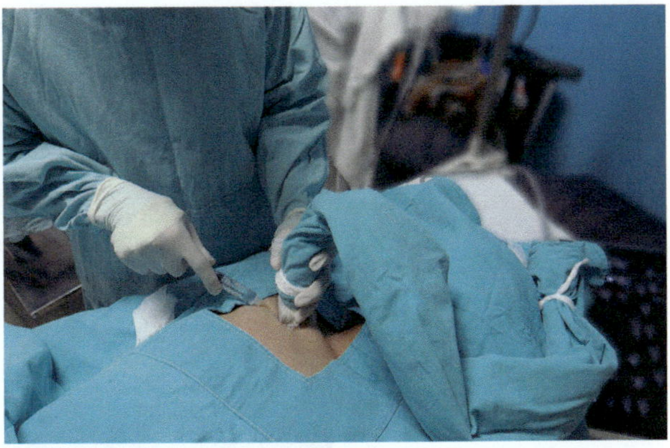

Fig. 12.8 Real-time ultrasound-guided lidocaine infiltration

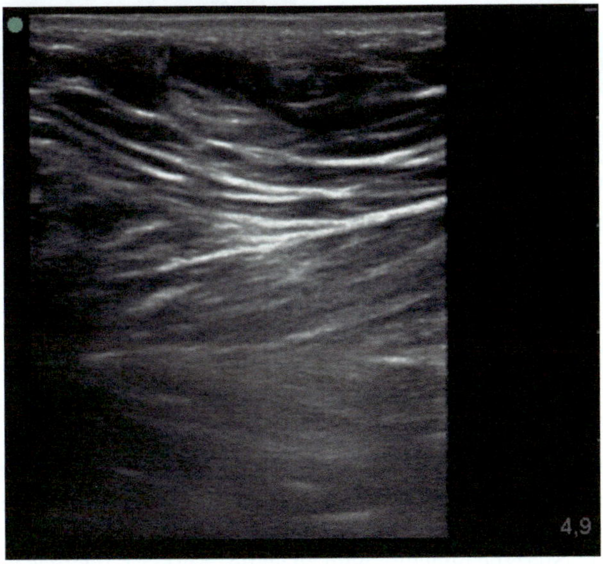

Fig. 12.9 Scan of the right infraclavicular region. SAX view of lidocaine infiltration

- The transducer position indicator (aqua dot in the superior left corner of the image) points out the patient's left side

- Scan of the right infraclavicular region. SAX view of lidocaine infiltration (Figs. 12.9 and 12.10).
- You can use the lidocaine infiltration puncture to guide where to perform the puncture with the introducer needle.

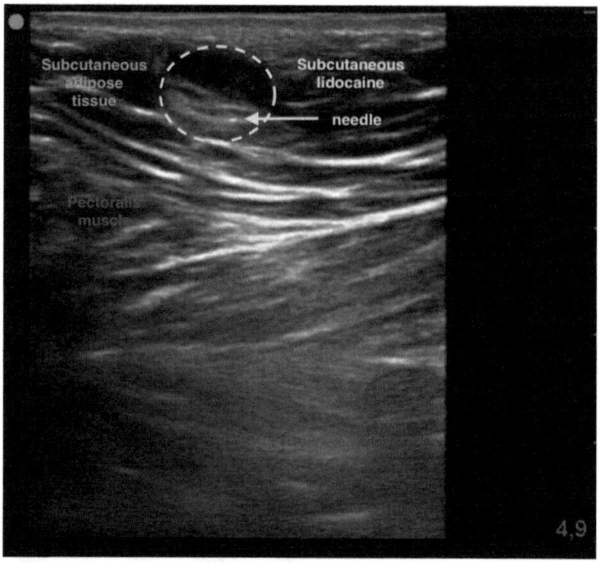

Fig. 12.10 Identifying structures
- The infiltration needle is identified as a hyperechogenic point
- Lidocaine infiltrates the subcutaneous adipose tissue
- The ETRSCV is compressed with the pressure applied to the needle

12.4 Steps for Real-Time Ultrasound-Guided Access to Extrathoracic Right Subclavian Vein in Pediatrics

12.4.1 Step 01

- We will use an Arrow® 7 Fr, 20-cm, double-lumen catheter.
- Place the transducer in the right infraclavicular region and perpendicular to the deltopectoral groove.
- Place the ETRSCV in the center of the transducer, and you will see the vein in the center of the screen on the ultrasound monitor. Therefore, the puncture directs the needle halfway down the length of the transducer.
- Start the puncture with an angle of 40–50° degrees in relation to the skin with the 18-G introducer needle on the Arrow® Raulerson Spring-Wire introductory syringe (Fig. 12.11).
- The puncture in SAX view requires beginning the ultrasound-guided dynamic needle tip positioning (DNTP) to guide the puncture in real time following the deltopectoral groove. So, you must sweep the transducer oblique upward and from lateral to medial from the axillary fossa toward the middle third of the clavicle, where the ETRSCV runs.
- SAX view of the start of the ETRSCV puncture (Figs. 12.12 and 12.13).

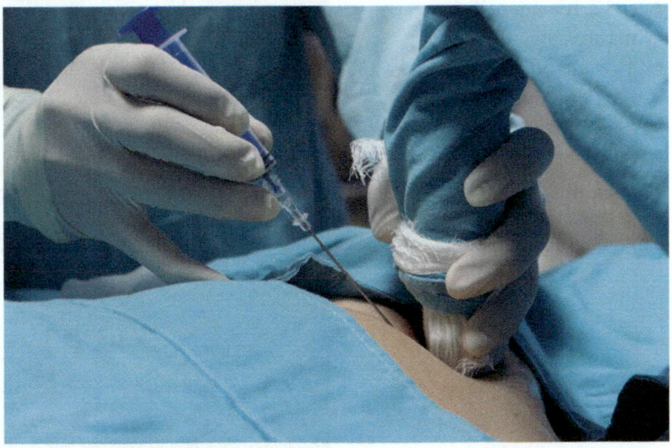

Fig. 12.11 The transducer in the right infraclavicular region and perpendicular to the deltopectoral groove. The puncture with an angle of 40–50°

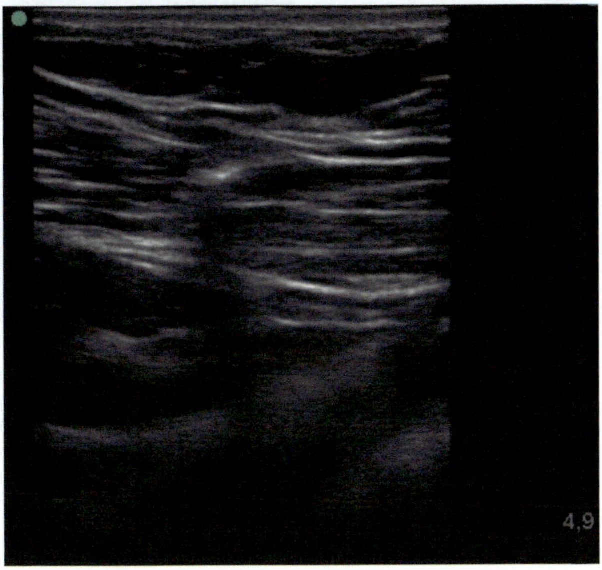

Fig. 12.12 Scan of the right infraclavicular region. SAX view of the start of the ETRSCV puncture

12.4.2 Step 02

- Perform DNTP; sweep the transducer toward the clavicle (Fig. 12.14).
- Keep the ETRSCV in the center of the screen.
- As the vein has an oblique trajectory, maintain the vein and the introducer needle in the center of the screen. The transducer will have to move perpendicular to the groove in an ascending manner.
- SAX view of the puncture progression. The introducer needle almost crosses all the muscles (Figs. 12.15 and 12.16).

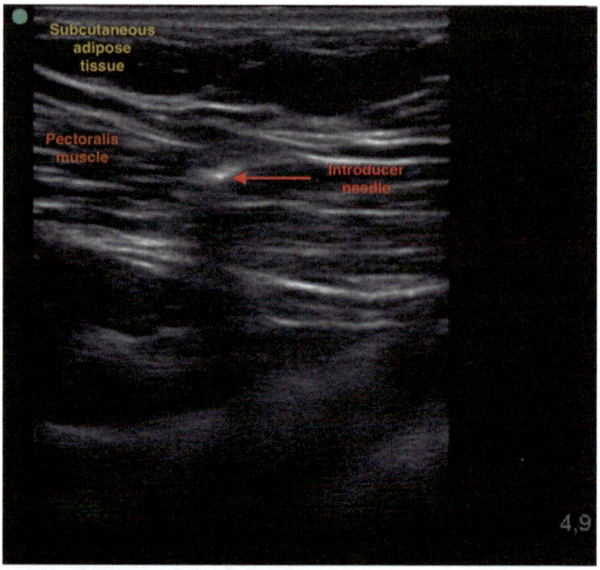

Fig. 12.13 Identifying structures
- The introducer needle is visualized as a bright hyperechoic (white) dot; it has passed through the subcutaneous tissue and penetrates the muscles

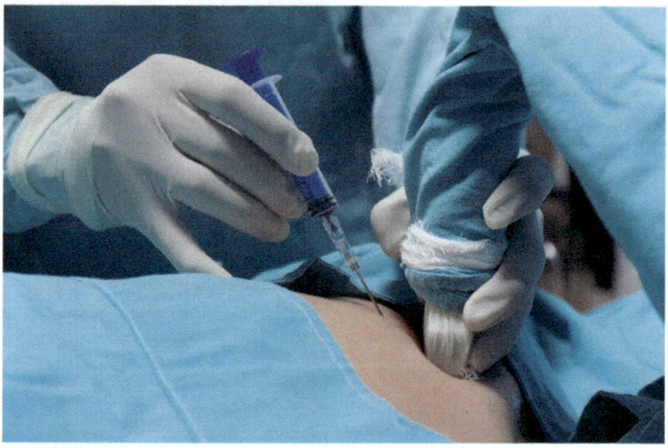

Fig. 12.14 Puncture progression: the transducer sweeps the deltopectoral groove from lateral to medial and inferior to superior

12.4.3 Step 03

- Modify the trajectory of the puncture slightly lateral, following the oblique course of the deltopectoral groove and with the transducer perpendicular to the groove (Fig. 12.17).
- View of the introducer needle close to the medial part of the ETRSCV (Figs. 12.18 and 12.19).
- Once you visualize the introducer needle inserted into the ETRSCV on the screen, stop the progression of the puncture so as not to penetrate the posterior wall (Figs. 12.20 and 12.21).
- Set the transducer aside.

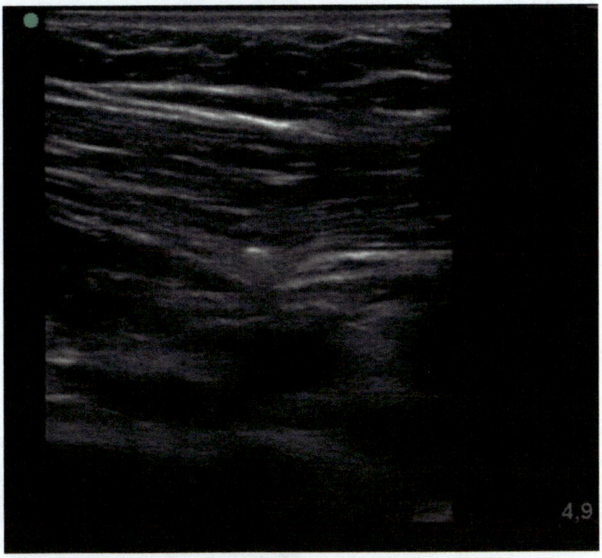

Fig. 12.15 SAX view of the DNTP as the puncture progresses toward the ETRSCV

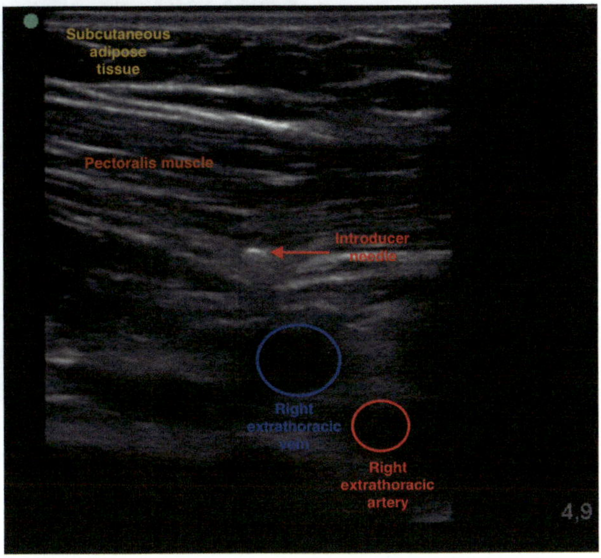

Fig. 12.16 Identifying structures

- The introducer needle follows a course medial to the direction of the ETRSCV, so the puncture is modified slightly lateral
- The introducer needle passes through almost all muscles

- Firmly fix the needle hub so the needle is not dislodged from its intravascular location.
- Maintain gentle negative pressure on the syringe plunger until a flash of blood appears in the barrel of the syringe, indicating the intravascular position of the introducer needle (Fig. 12.22).

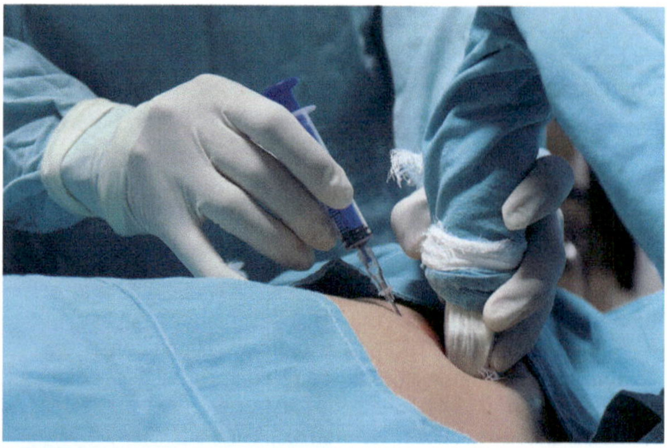

Fig. 12.17 Continue with the puncture in real-time DNTP toward the ETRSCV

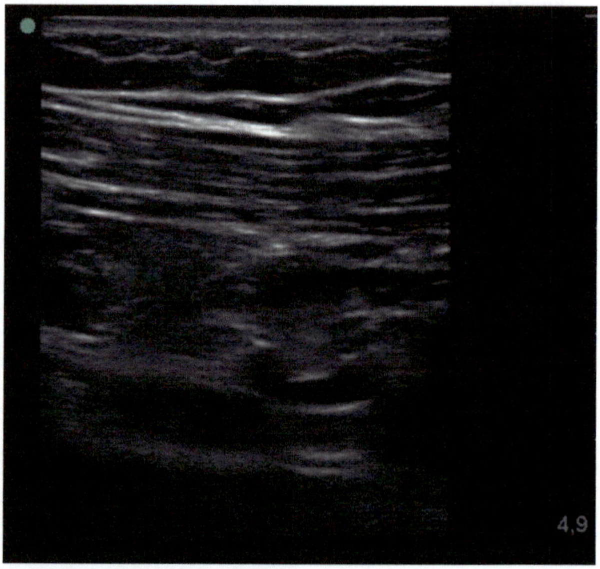

Fig. 12.18 SAX view of puncture advancement

12.4.4 Step 04

- Hold the hub of the introducer needle firmly so that the needle does not dislodge (Fig. 12.23).
- Introduce the guidewire through the Arrow® Raulerson Spring-Wire introductory syringe and 18-G introducer needle (Fig. 12.24).
- These two devices of this type of equipment will facilitate the maneuvers of canalization of the ETRSCV with the guidewire.
- Once you have introduced the appropriate length of guidewire to canalize the ETRSCV, remove the introducer needle and Raulerson syringe (Fig. 12.25).

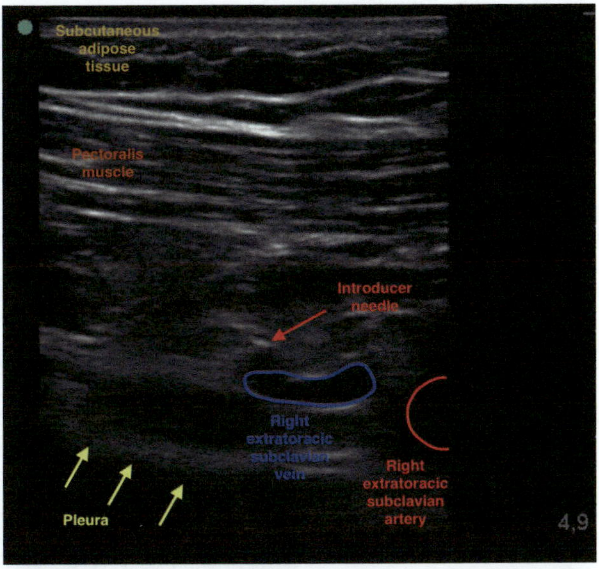

Fig. 12.19 Identifying structures
- The introducer needle is close to the medial part of the ETRSCV, which is beginning to deform due to direct compression by the needle

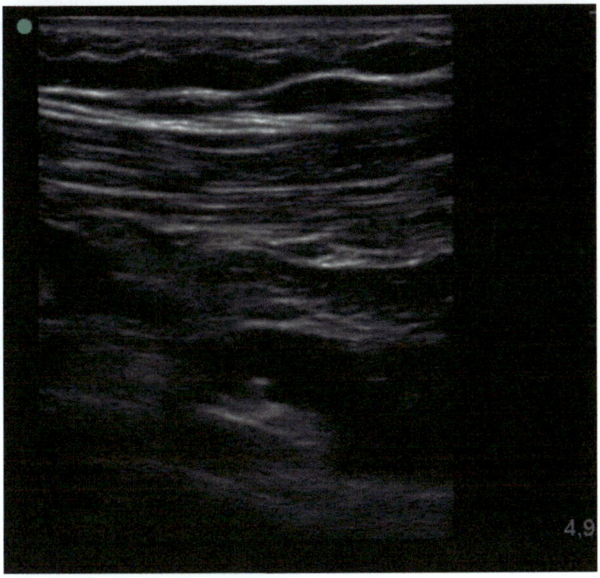

Fig. 12.20 LAX view of the ETRSCV cannulation

12.4.5 Step 05

- With your left hand, hold the entry of the guidewire firmly in the skin with gauze and fully withdraw the syringe and Raulerson syringe (Fig. 12.26).

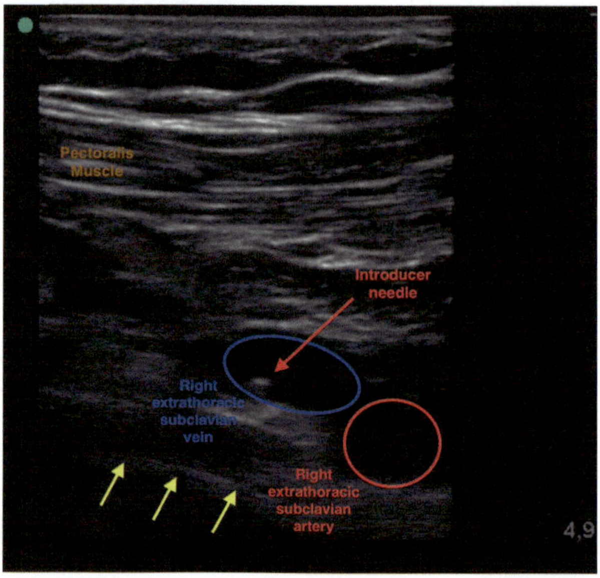

Fig. 12.21 Identifying structures
- The introducer needle is located inside the ETRSCV
- The vein recovers its diameter by stopping the progression of the puncture and, therefore, compression of the vein

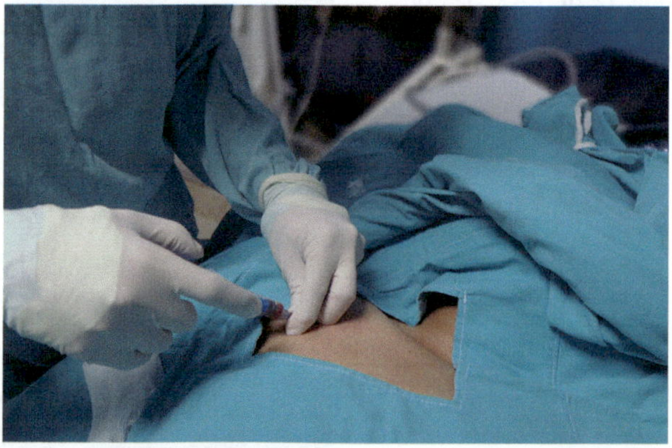

Fig. 12.22 Hold the needle hub, apply gentle negative pressure, and check for the return of blood in the barrel of the syringe

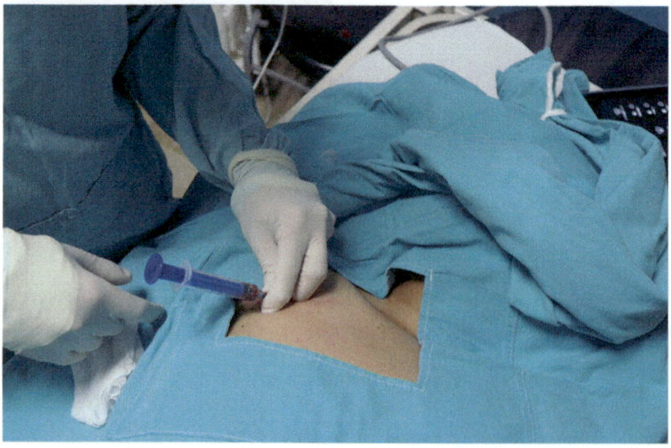

Fig. 12.23 Hold the hub of the introducer needle firmly with your left hand

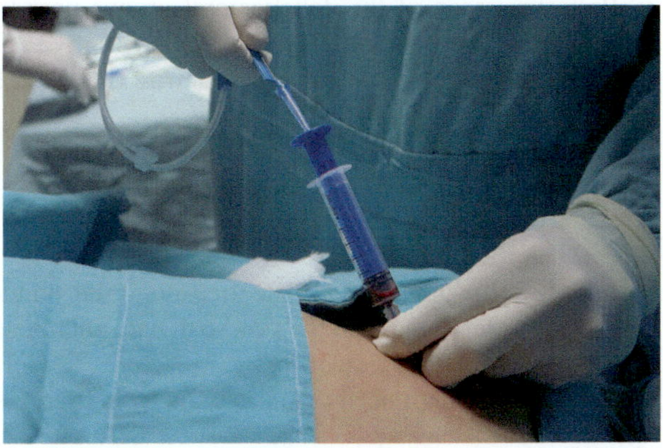

Fig. 12.24 Insert the guidewire

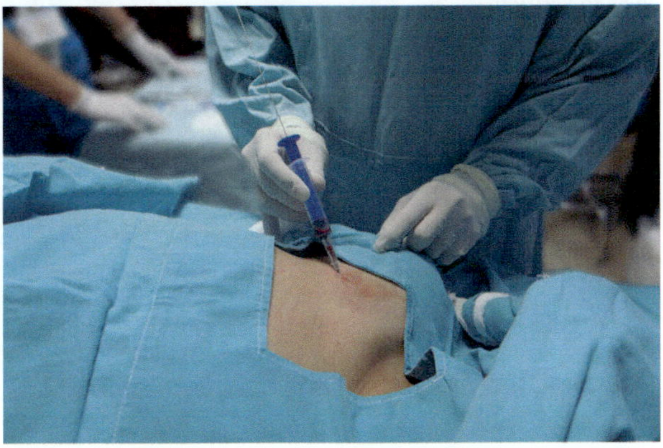

Fig. 12.25 Remove the introducer needle and the syringe

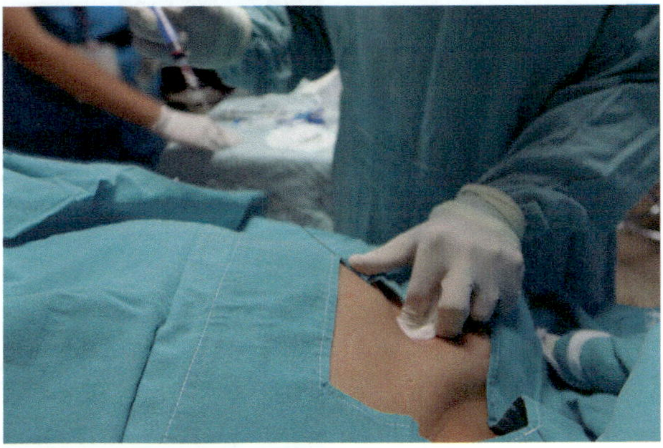

Fig. 12.26 Fully withdraw the syringe and Raulerson syringe

- Perform a scan of the deltopectoral groove near the clavicle in LAX view to verify that the guidewire is intravascular (Fig. 12.27).
- LAX view of the intravascular guidewire (Figs. 12.28 and 12.29).

12.4.6 Step 06

- Introduce the dilator and dilate the path of the skin toward the ETRSCV.
- With your left hand, pull the skin so that the dilator easily penetrates (Fig. 12.30).
- Try not to bend the guidewire.
- You will often not need to make an incision to insert the dilator.

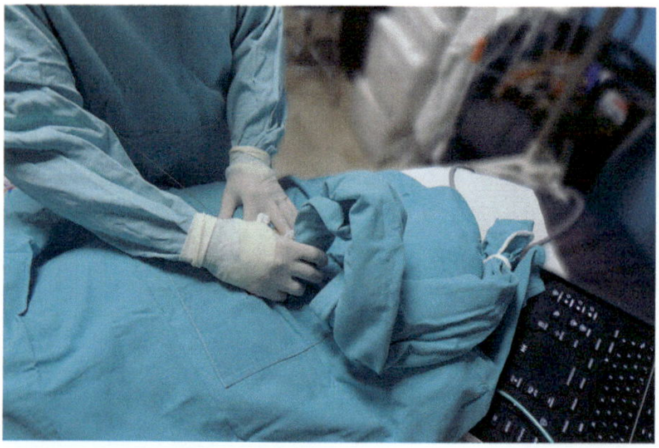

Fig. 12.27 Scan in LAX view to verify the intravascular location of the guidewire

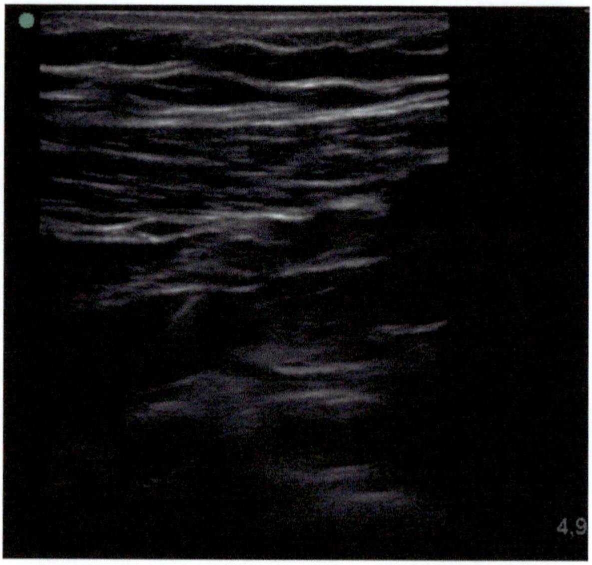

Fig. 12.28 Scan of the deltopectoral groove in LAX view

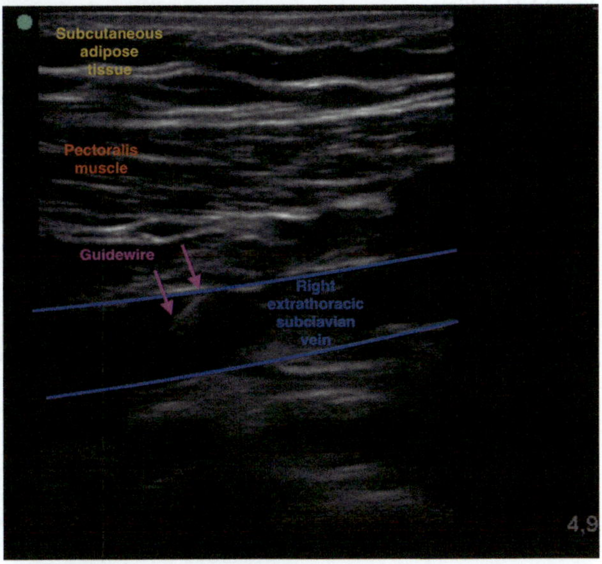

Fig. 12.29 Identifying structures
- The guidewire is inside the ETRSCV

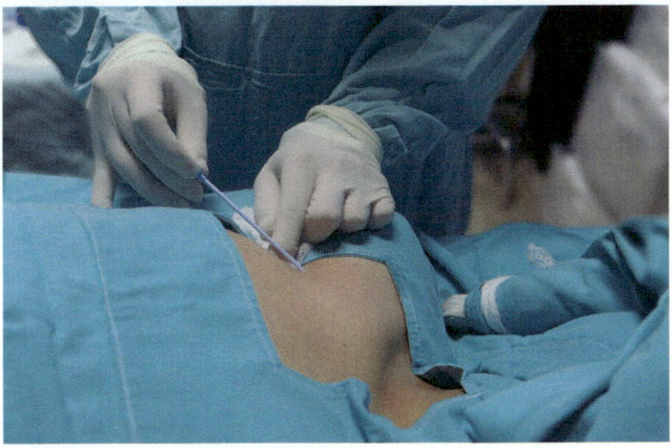

Fig. 12.30 Dilation of the skin

- The dilator insertion direction is also oblique toward the middle third of the clavicle. Only dilate the path of the skin at the entrance of the ETRSCV (Fig. 12.31).
- Remove the dilator, occlude the outlet with gauze, and apply gentle compression since a path is made with an 8,5 Fr dilator (Fig. 12.32).

12.4.7 Step 07

- With your left hand, block the outlet and hold the guidewire, as shown in the figure; with your right hand, insert the catheter over the guidewire (Fig. 12.33).

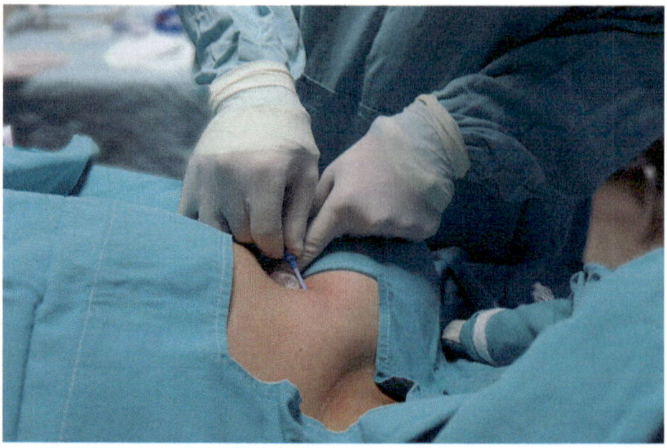

Fig. 12.31 Dilate following an oblique path toward the middle third of the clavicle

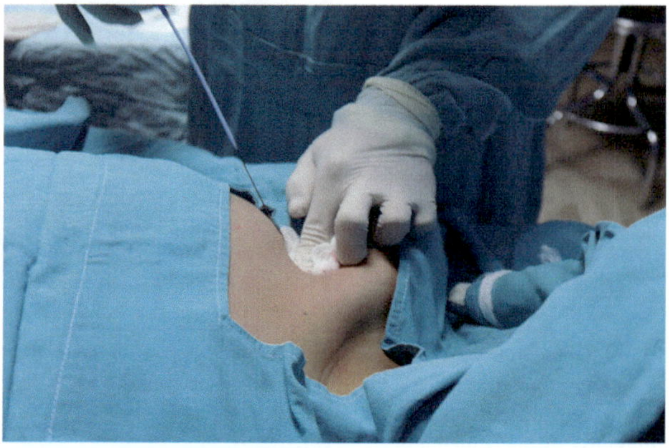

Fig. 12.32 Remove the dilator

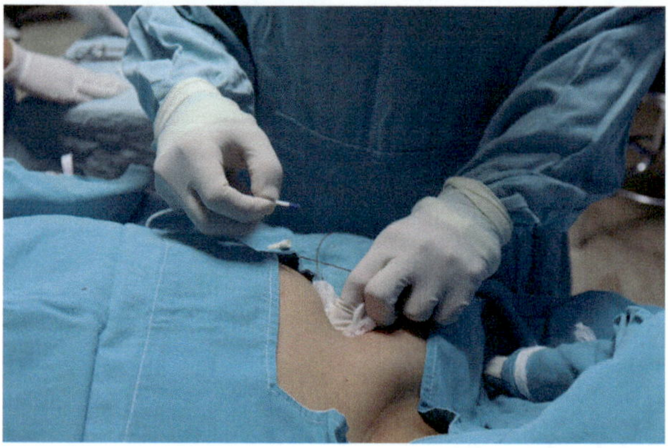

Fig. 12.33 Prepare to introduce the catheter over the guidewire

- Advance the catheter over the guidewire (Seldinger's technique), and then remove the guidewire (Fig. 12.34).
- Place the transducer longitudinally to the deltopectoral groove to perform the scan in LAX view and confirm the intravascular (ETSRCV) location of the catheter (Fig. 12.35).
- LAX view of the intravascular catheter in the ETRSCV (Figs. 12.36 and 12.37).
- In this subclavian extrathoracic access route, the guidewire or catheter sometimes tends to ascend to the ipsilateral jugular vein, so it is good to follow the path of the guidewire or catheter toward the ipsilateral brachiocephalic vein.
- Perform a scan of the region of the ipsilateral supraclavicular fossae or the cervical region to see that the guidewire or catheter is not in that vein (RIJV). If so, you must rearrange the guidewire or catheter in a central position (Fig. 12.38).
- LAX view of the catheter located within the right subclavian vein (Figs. 12.39 and 12.40).

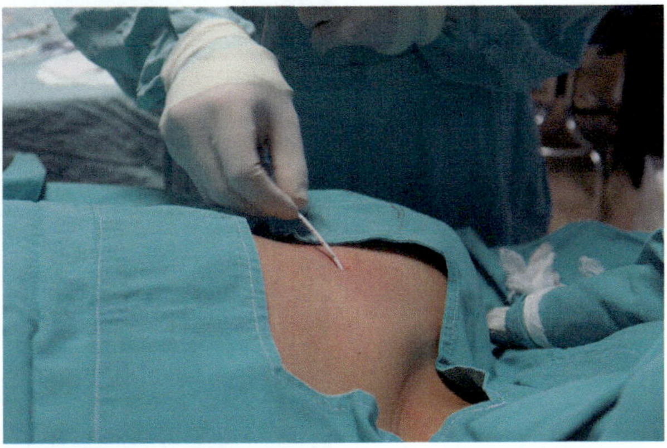

Fig. 12.34 Seldinger's technique: advance the catheter over the guidewire

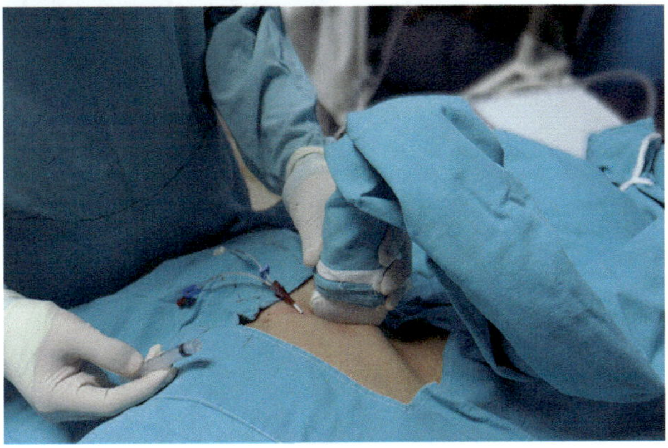

Fig. 12.35 Scan the intravascular location of the catheter in LAX view

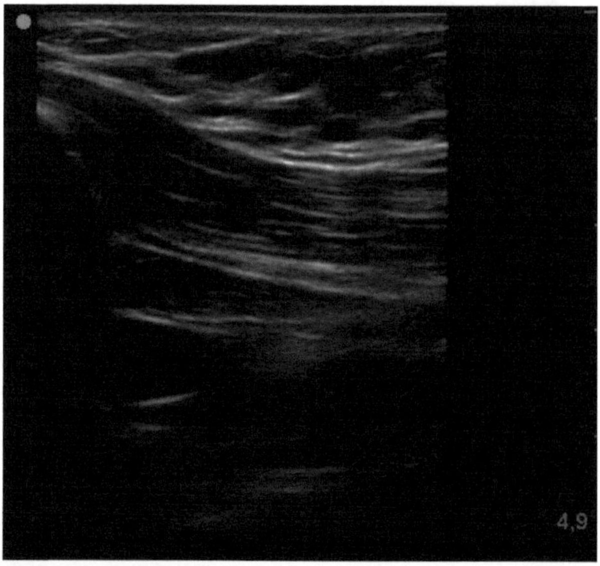

Fig. 12.36 LAX view of the intravascular catheter in the ETRSCV

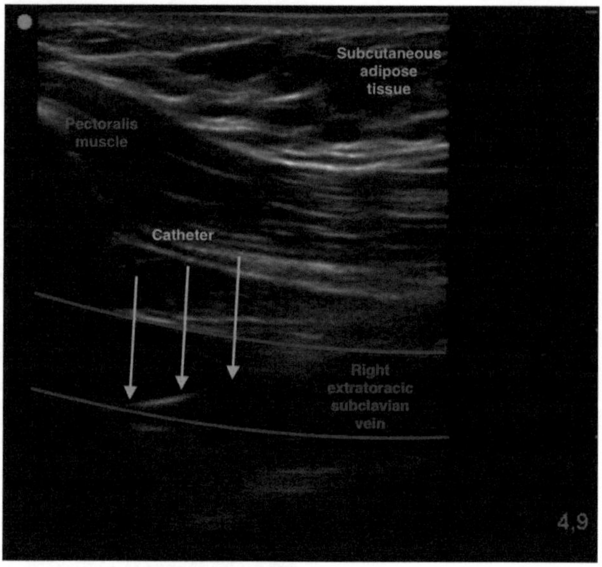

Fig. 12.37 Identifying structures

- The catheter is located within the ETRSCV

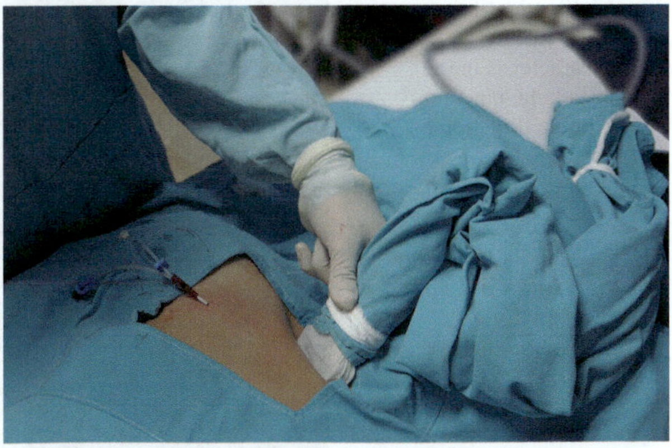

Fig. 12.38 Scan the right supraclavicular fossae

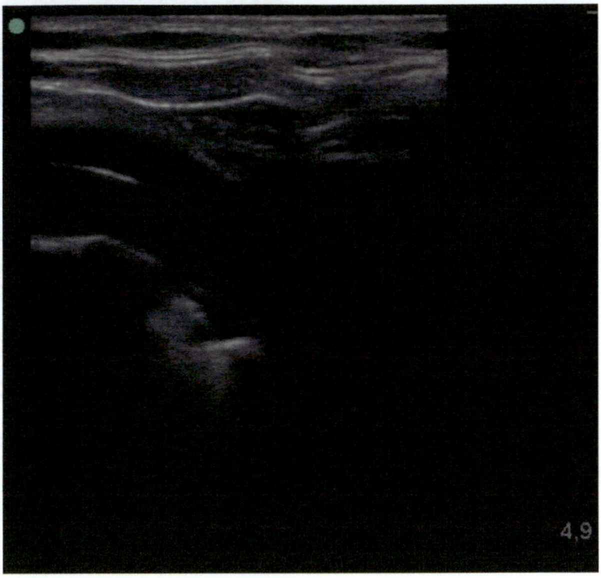

Fig. 12.39 Right supraclavicular scan. LAX view of the catheter path

12.4.8 Step 08

- Secure the catheter and place a sterile occlusive dressing according to the institutional protocol (Fig. 12.41).

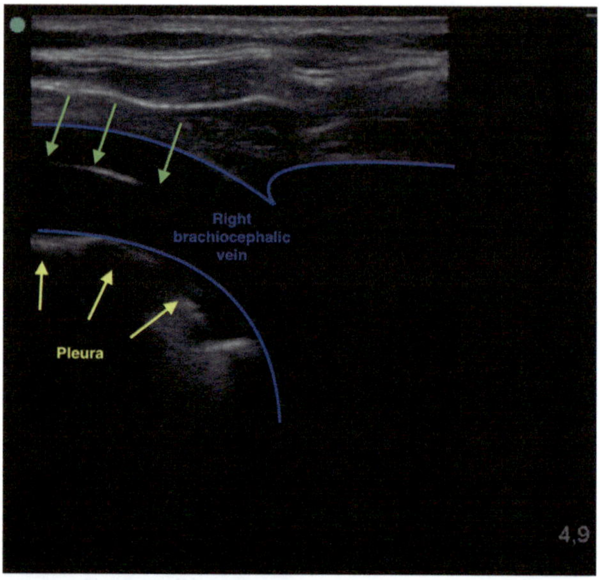

Fig. 12.40 Identifying structures

- The catheter is in the right subclavian vein and in the direction of the right brachiocephalic vein

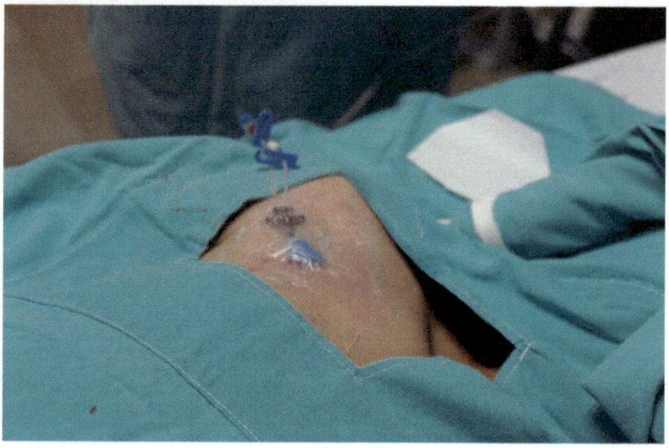

Fig. 12.41 Dressing according to the institutional protocol

Sources

1. Orihashi K, Sato K, Imai K, et al. Extrathoracic subclavian venipuncture under ultrasound guidance. Circ J. 2005;69(9):1111–5. https://doi.org/10.1253/circj.69.1111.
2. Sawasaki K, Sato T, Takayama Y, et al. Novel extrathoracic puncture techniques for pacemaker lead insertion: pitfalls of the conventional extrathoracic puncture method. J Arrhythmia. 2012;28(2):111–3. https://doi.org/10.1016/j.joa.2012.03.008.

3. Zei PC, Nasir J. Extrathoracic subclavian vein access. In: How-to manual for pacemaker and ICD devices; 2017. p. 9–16. https://doi.org/10.1002/9781118820674.ch2.
4. He Y, Yang W, Zhao Y, et al. Individualized blind techniques for puncture of intrathoracic and extrathoracic subclavian vein: three simple experience tips. Anatol J Cardiol. 2023;27(9):534–8. https://doi.org/10.14744/AnatolJCardiol.2023.2893. Publicado el 7 de junio de 2023
5. Brignole M, Deharo JC. Different techniques of venous access for CIEDs: advantages and disadvantages. Eur Heart J. 2023;44(46):4859–61. https://doi.org/10.1093/eurheartj/ehad749.

Chapter 13
Extrathoracic Left Subclavian Vein in Pediatrics

13.1 Patient Positioning

- The patient is 4 years old and weighs 17 kg.
- Position the patient in dorsal decubitus close to the left side of the bed or stretcher (Fig. 13.1).
- This procedure can be carried out without a roll under the shoulders, as in this case.
- Place the patient's head to the right or centered.
- Gently restrain the upper extremities with the arms caudal.
- Place the ultrasound device in any of these positions: next to the left shoulder, above the head, or the right shoulder.

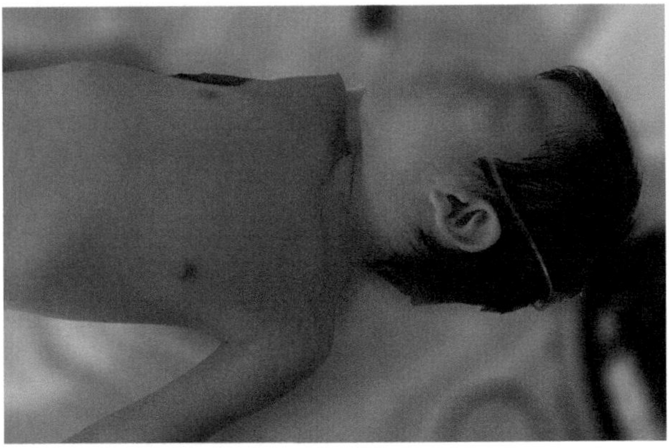

Fig. 13.1 Patient position

F. Montes-Tapia, *Atlas of Ultrasound-Guided Central Venous Catheter Placement*, https://doi.org/10.1007/978-3-031-61887-1_13

13.2 Scanning Technique

- Do a preliminary vascular assessment (non-sterile), known as rapid central vein assessment (RaCeVA).
- The operator stands on the left side of the patient.
- Place the ultrasound in any of the following positions: on the side of the left shoulder, above the head, or at the right shoulder (Fig. 13.2).
- We will use a high-frequency linear transducer (13–6 MHz) with a hockey stick-type probe.
- Scan the left extrathoracic subclavian vessels in the long-axis (LAX) view, and place the transducer longitudinally in the infraclavicular region (above the delto-pectoral groove), placing the tip of the transducer over the clavicle directed toward the ipsilateral neck (Fig. 13.3).
- The extrathoracic subclavian vessels run through the deltopectoral groove in an upward oblique direction from lateral to medial from the axillary fossa toward the middle third of the clavicle.

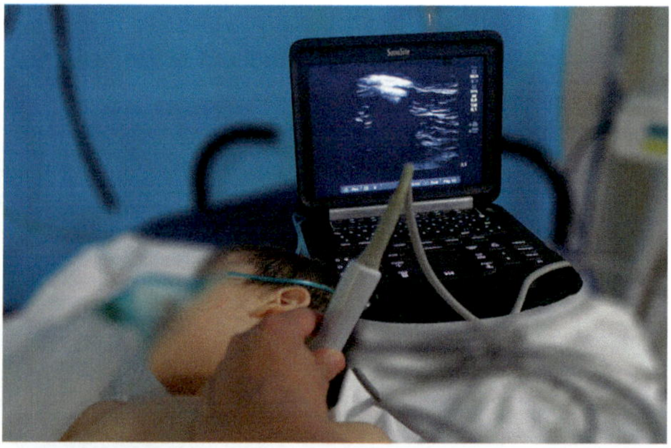

Fig. 13.2 Positioning of ultrasound equipment

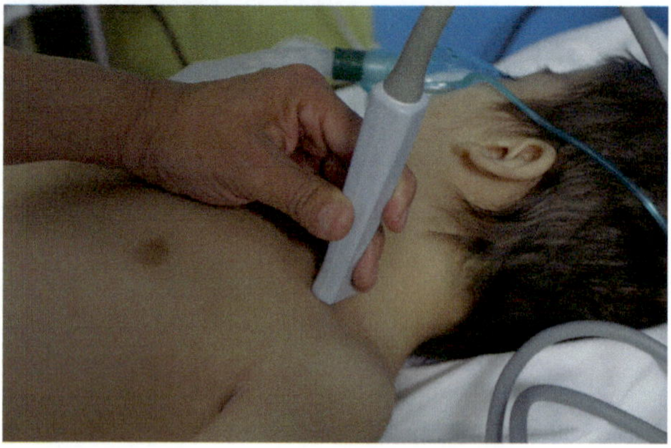

Fig. 13.3 Place the transducer in the left infraclavicular region and longitudinally to the deltopectoral groove (lateral scan)

- Scan the deltopectoral groove from lateral to medial in LAX view.
- In the deltopectoral groove, the extrathoracic left subclavian artery (ETLSCA) is lateral, and the extrathoracic left subclavian vein ETLSCV is medial. The vein varies in size with the respiratory cycle, while the artery maintains its constant beat. The vein can be compressed with the transducer to differentiate from the artery.
- Start by scanning the lateral edge of the deltopectoral groove (Fig. 13.3).
- LAX view of the left axillary and subclavian artery (Figs. 13.4 and 13.5).
- Slide the transducer medially (Fig. 13.6).
- LAX view of the ETLSCV begins after the confluence of the left axillary vein with the left cephalic vein (Figs. 13.7 and 13.8).
- LAX view of the ETLSCV diameter measurement (Figs. 13.9 and 13.10).

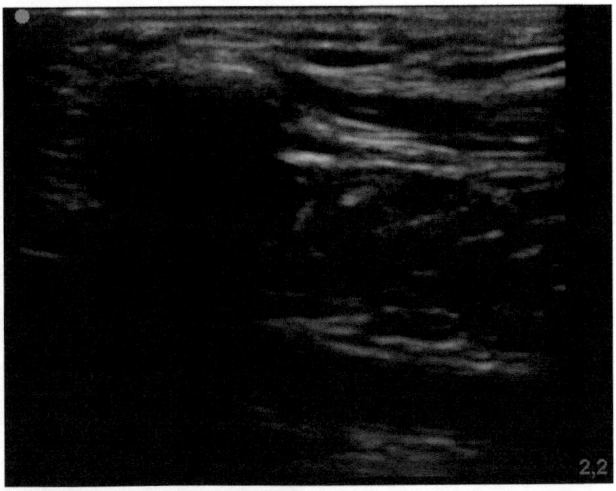

Fig. 13.4 Lateral scan of the deltopectoral groove
- The transducer position indicator (aqua dot in the superior left corner of the image) points out the patient's left neck (tip of the hockey stick transducer)
- Scan depth of 2,2 cm

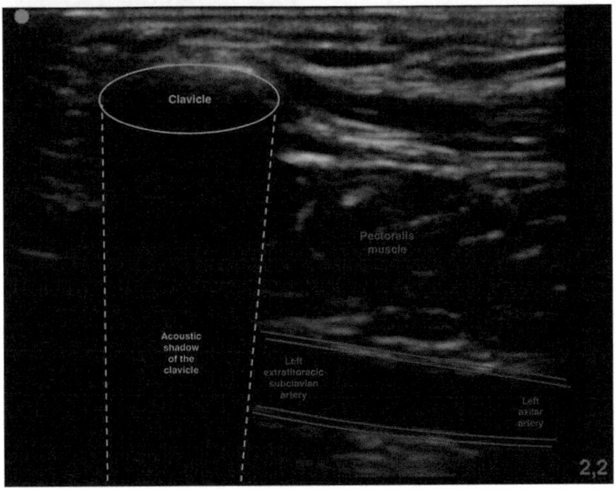

Fig. 13.5 Identifying structures
- The tip of the transducer is on the clavicle, and the rest of the transducer is on the infraclavicular region, which is why the clavicle and the pectoral region are visualized
- The pectoralis muscle over the left arterial vessels

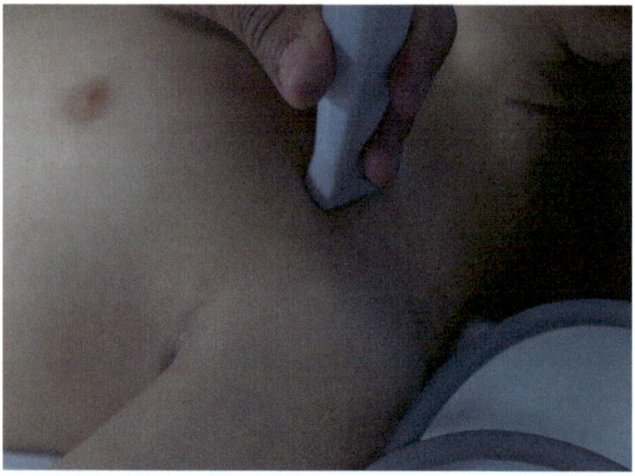

Fig. 13.6 Slide the transducer medially

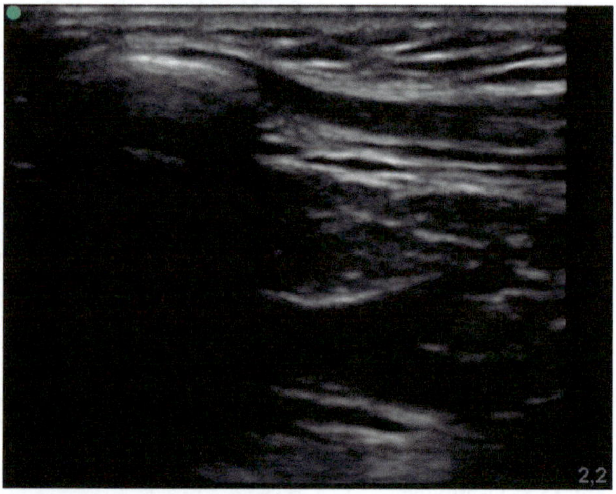

Fig. 13.7 Medial scan of the deltopectoral groove

- The transducer position indicator (aqua dot in the superior left corner of the image) points out the patient's left neck (tip of the hockey stick transducer)
- Scan depth of 2,2 cm

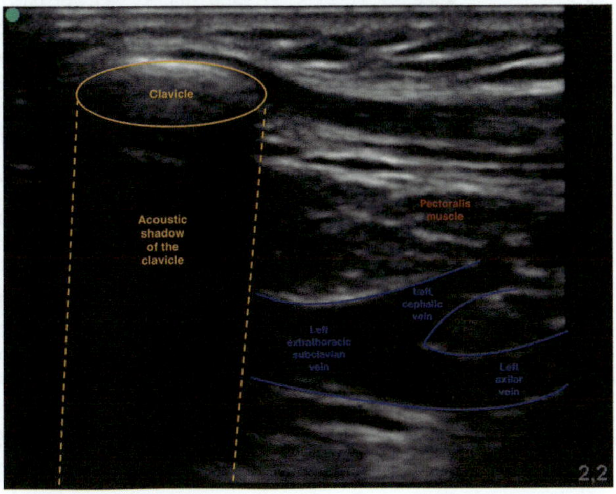

Fig. 13.8 Identifying structures

- The tip of the transducer is on the clavicle, and the rest of the transducer is on the infraclavicular region, which is why the clavicle and the pectoral region are visualized
- The pectoralis muscle over the left venous vessels
- The confluence of the left axillary and the left cephalic veins is visualized to form the subclavian vein. In this case, a small segment is called the left extrathoracic subclavian vein

Fig. 13.9 Medial scan of the deltopectoral groove

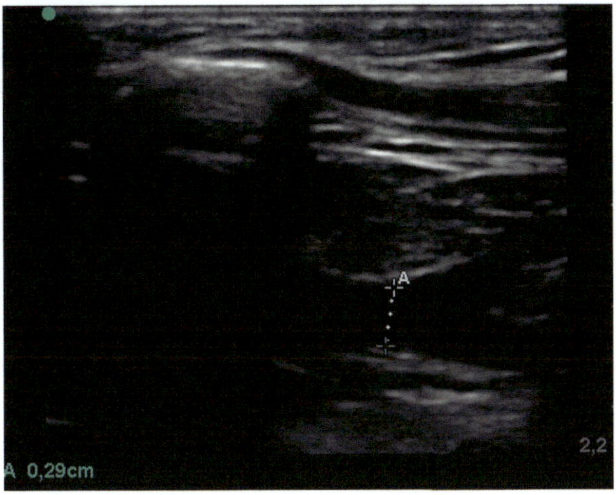

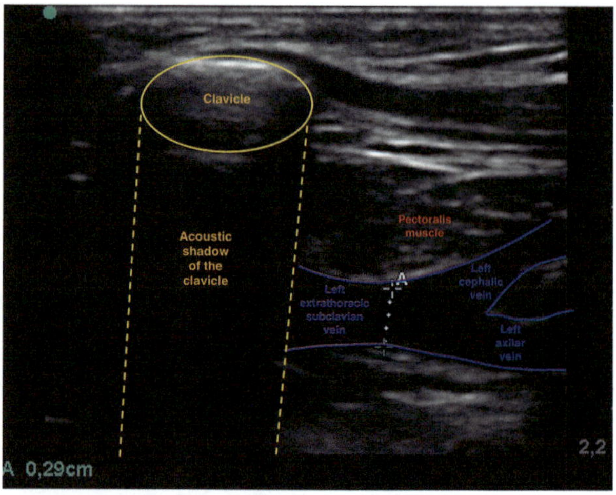

Fig. 13.10 Identifying structures
- The diameter of the ETLSCV is 0,29 cm

13.3 Local Anesthesia Application

- The sterile field only leaves the upper pectoral, right shoulder, and cervical regions uncovered (Fig. 13.11).
- Real-time ultrasound-guided lidocaine infiltration (Fig. 13.12).
- LAX view of the infiltration (Figs. 13.13 and 13.14).
- Subcutaneous infiltration with lidocaine in the puncture tract 1,5–2 cm before the site chosen for ETLSCV puncture and the catheter fixation area.
- You can use the lidocaine infiltration puncture to guide where to perform the puncture with the introducer needle.

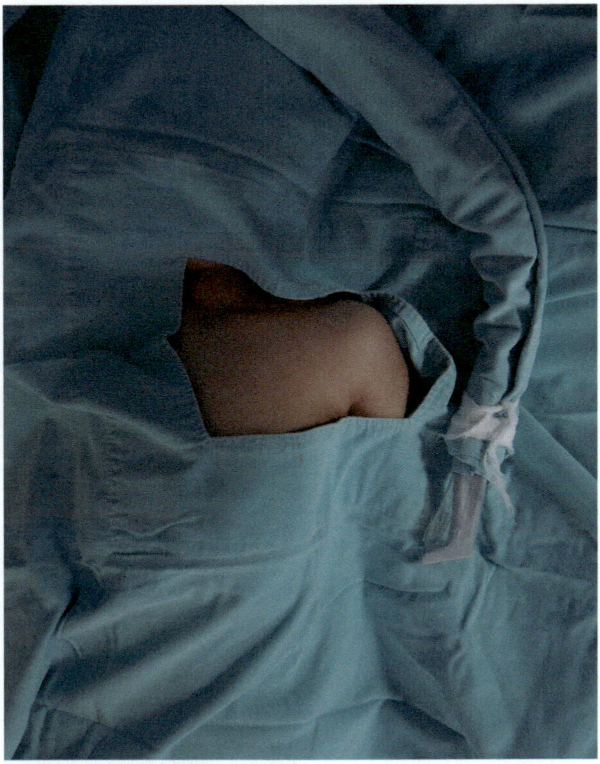

Fig. 13.11 Operator's view of the shoulder and the left infraclavicular region

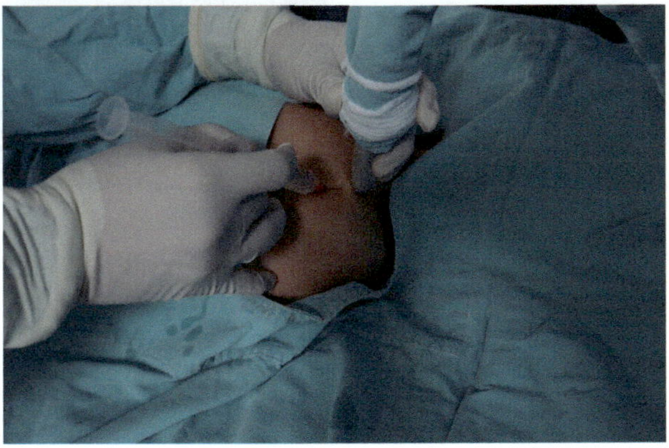

Fig. 13.12 Real-time ultrasound-guided lidocaine infiltration

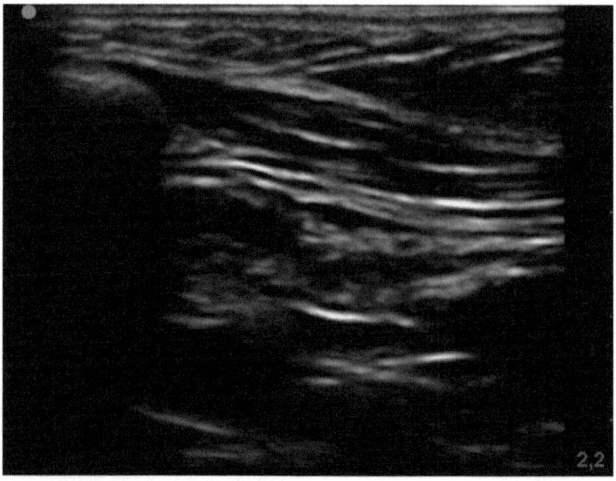

Fig. 13.13 LAX view of the infiltration

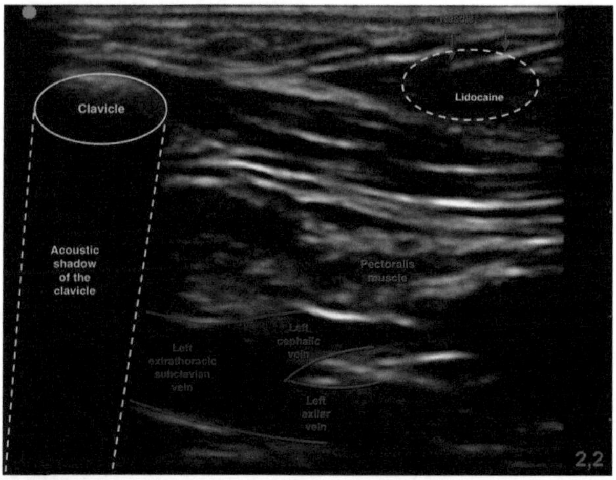

Fig. 13.14 Identifying structures
- The entry of the infiltration needle and the infiltration of lidocaine are visualized

13.4 Steps for Real-Time Ultrasound-Guided Access to Extrathoracic Left Subclavian Vein in Pediatrics

13.4.1 Step 01

- We will use a Medadv® 4 Fr, 13-cm, double-lumen catheter.
- The operator stands on the left side of the patient.
- Place the transducer longitudinally in the infraclavicular region (above the delto-pectoral groove), placing the tip of the transducer over the clavicle directed toward the ipsilateral neck.
- Once you identify the ETLSCV at the LAX view on the screen, start the puncture with an angle of 50–60° in relation to the skin, with a 21-G introducer needle.

The puncture is performed following the central part of the thickness of the hockey stick-type probe (Fig. 13.15).

- The puncture in LAX view requires beginning the ultrasound-guided dynamic needle tracking (DNT) to guide the puncture in real time. As it is a very short segment of the vein, to track the needle, the transducer movement will be carried out with lateral or medial displacements to keep the needle below the insonation area.
- LAX view of the start of the ETLSCV puncture (Figs. 13.16 and 13.17).

13.4.2 Step 02

- Continue with the puncture at the same angle of inclination (Fig. 13.18).
- Maintain visualization of the introducer needle and the ETLSCV and continue with the puncture.

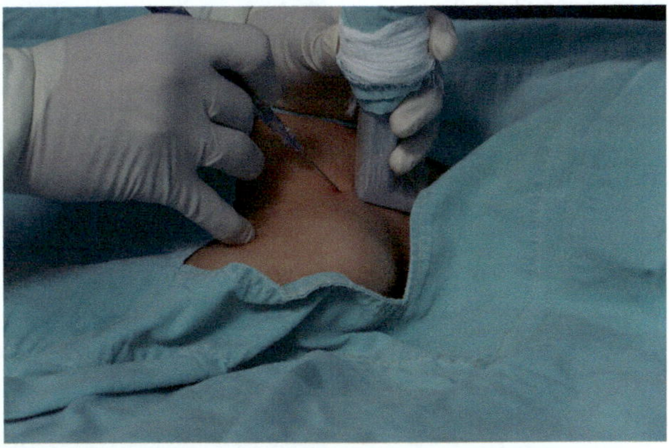

Fig. 13.15 The introducer needle is aligned to the central part of the thickness of the transducer and follows the direction of the tip of the hockey stick transducer at an angle of 50°–60°

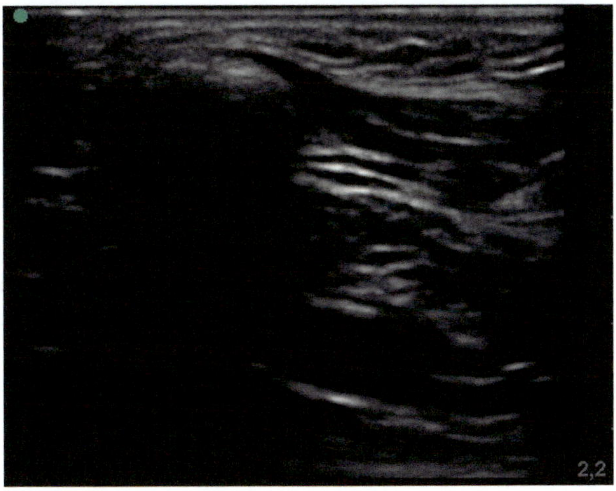

Fig. 13.16 Scan of the left infraclavicular region. LAX view of introducer needle entry into the subcutaneous tissue

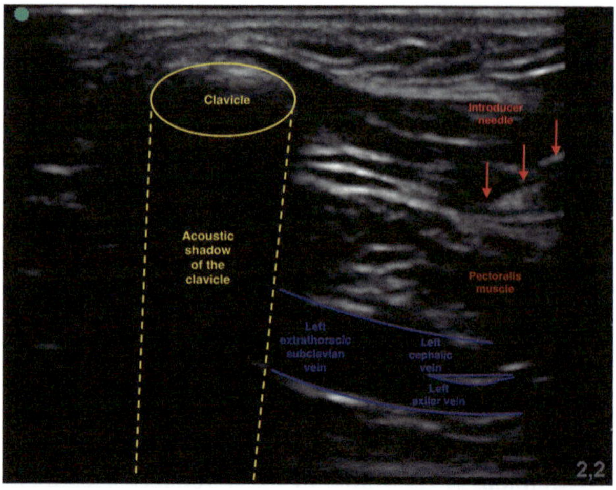

Fig. 13.17 Identifying structures
- The acoustic shadow of the clavicle hides the course at this level of the ETLSCV
- The introducer needle is aligned with the disposition of the ETLSCV
- ETLSCV changes with respiration

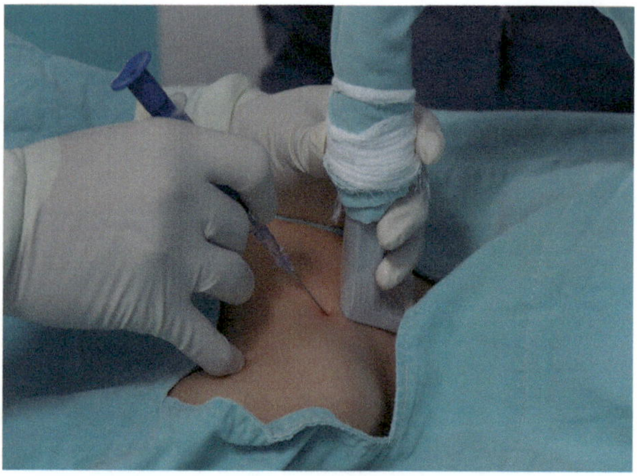

Fig. 13.18 Progression of the puncture: keep the puncture in the middle part of the thickness of the transducer following the direction of the tip of the hockey stick probe

- LAX view of the progression of the puncture; the introducer needle almost crosses through all the muscles (Figs. 13.19 and 13.20).

13.4.3 Step 03

- Modify the puncture angle to 40–50° and continue with the trajectory of the puncture in the direction of the ETLSCV. Once it is identified that it is approaching the anterior wall of the vein, suction will be applied to the syringe (Fig. 13.21).
- Keep the introducer needle and the ETLSCV in the center of the screen.
- LAX view of the introducer needle crossing the pectoral muscles (Figs. 13.22 and 13.23).

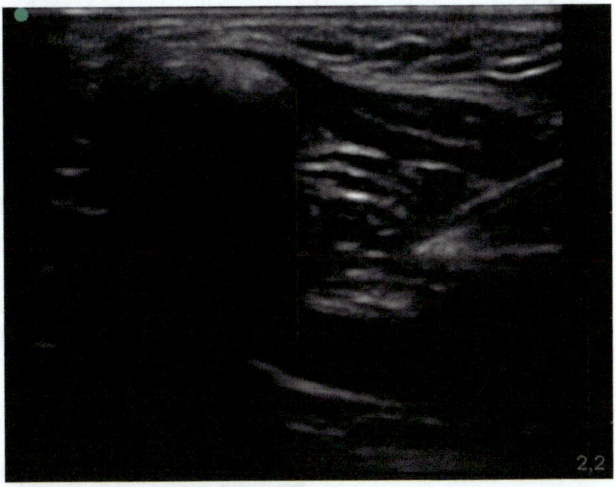

Fig. 13.19 LAX view of the puncture progresses toward the ETLSCV

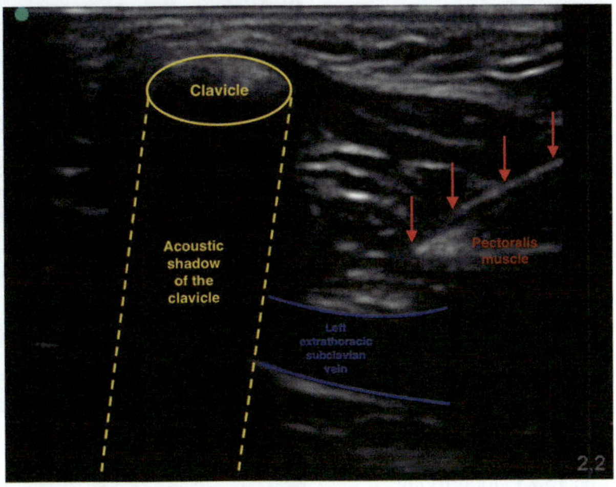

Fig. 13.20 Identifying structures

- The introducer needle follows a suitable course in the direction of the ETLSCV, lying just above the vein
- The introducer needle almost crossed through all the muscles

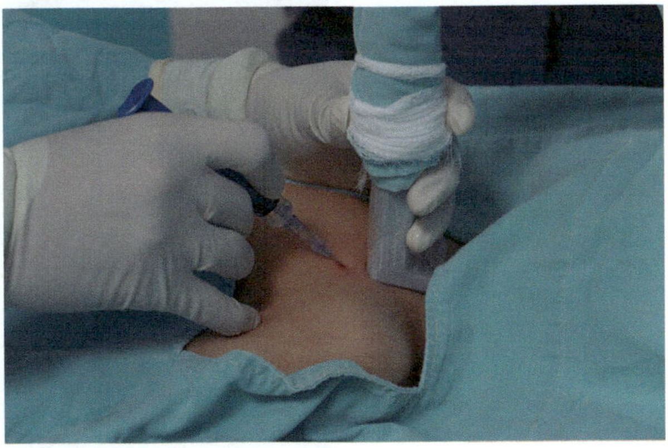

Fig. 13.21 Continue with the puncture in real-time DNTP toward the ETLSCV

- LAX view of the introducer needle almost completely passing through the pectoral muscles (Figs. 13.24 and 13.25).
- Once you visualize the introducer needle inserted into the ETLSCV on the screen, apply gentle negative pressure on the syringe plunger (Fig. 13.26).
- Always perform this step under DNTP so as not to cross the posterior wall of the vein.
- LAX view of ETLSCV cannulation (Figs. 13.27 and 13.28).
- Once you visualize the intravascular needle inserted into the ETLSCV on the screen, set the transducer aside.
- Hold the hub of the introducer needle firmly and maintain gentle negative pressure on the syringe plunger until blood appears in the barrel of the syringe (Fig. 13.29).

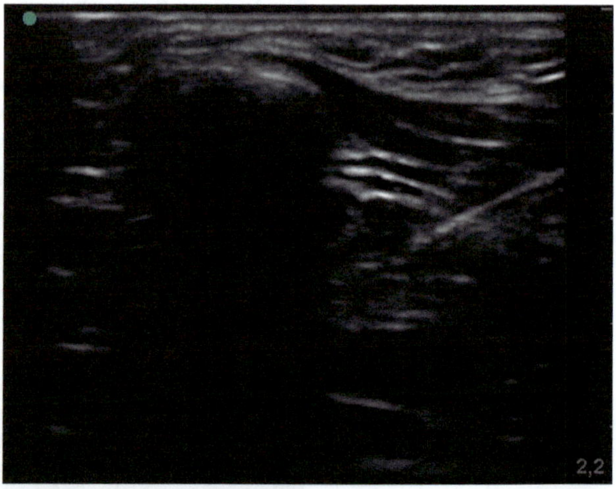

Fig. 13.22 LAX view of the puncture progression

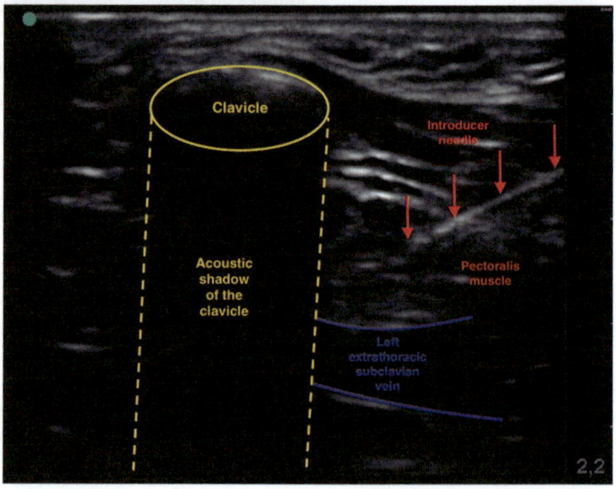

Fig. 13.23 Identifying structures
- The introducer needle crossing the pectoral muscles

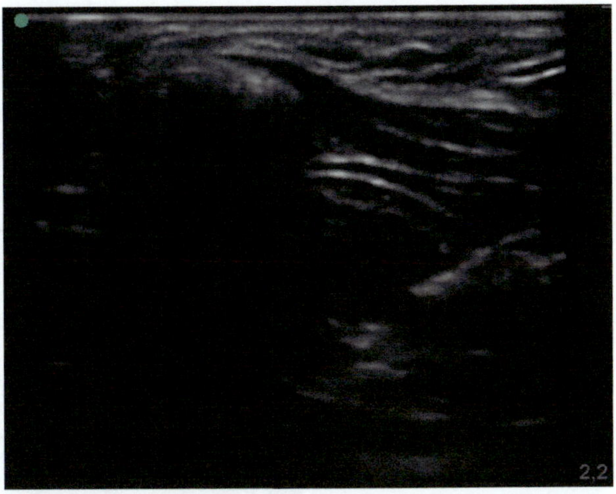

Fig. 13.24 LAX view of the introducer needle

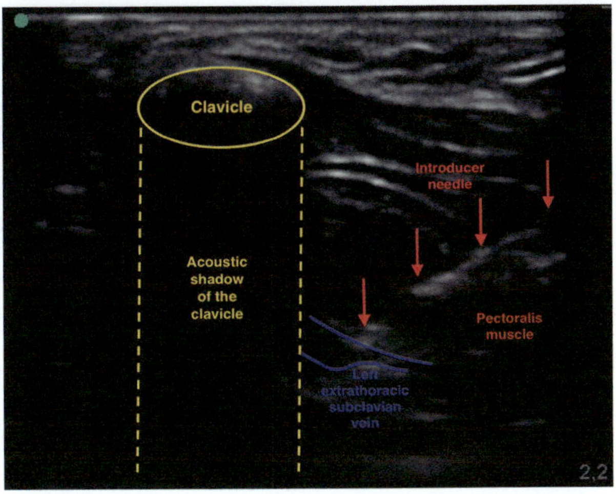

Fig. 13.25 Identifying structures

- Decrease in caliber and deformation of the ETLSCV
  - The increase in compression produces these changes in the vein as the puncture advances in the correct direction of the vein

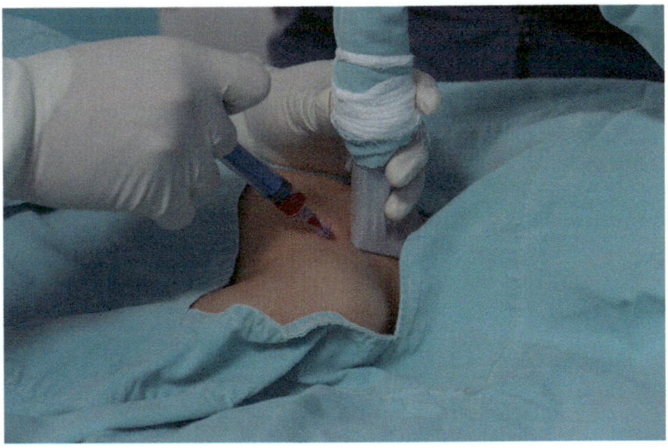

Fig. 13.26 Apply gentle negative pressure on the syringe plunger

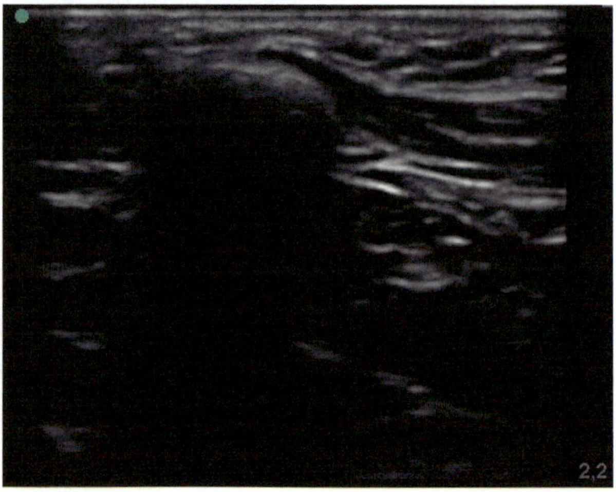

Fig. 13.27 LAX view of the ETLSCV cannulation

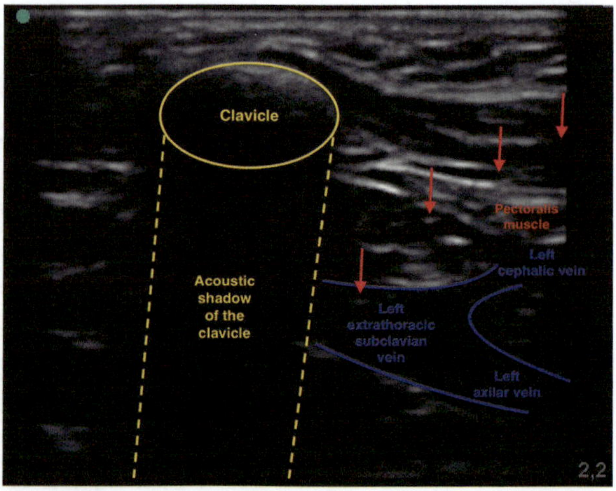

Fig. 13.28 The tip of the introducer needle is penetrating the lumen of the ETLSCV; while puncture is being performed, it is aspirated. Blood will immediately enter the syringe

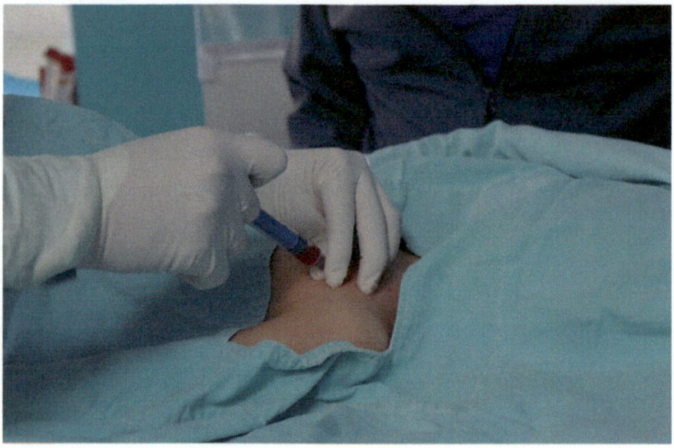

Fig. 13.29 Hold the needle hub, apply gentle negative pressure, and check for the return of blood in the barrel of the syringe

13.4.4 Step 04

- Hold the hub of the introducer needle firmly so that the needle does not dislodge (Fig. 13.30).
- Introduce the 0.018" guidewire through the introducer needle (Fig. 13.31).
- Withdraw the introducer needle once the proper length of the guidewire has been inserted (Fig. 13.32).
- Perform a scan of the deltopectoral groove near the clavicle in LAX view to verify that the guidewire is intravascular (Fig. 13.33).
- SAX view of the guidewire in the ETLSCV (Figs. 13.34 and 13.35).
- The cannulation of the left and right extrathoracic veins tends to go to the ipsilateral internal jugular vein; therefore, the location of the guidewire should always be scanned in SAX view of the cervical vessels (Figs. 13.36, 13.37 and 13.38) and LAX view of the left brachiocephalic vein (LBCV) in the left supraclavicular fossae (Figs. 13.39, 13.40 and 13.41).
  - If the guidewire is in the LIJV, you must rearrange the guidewire to the LBCV. This procedure can also be done under ultrasound guidance without fluoroscopy.

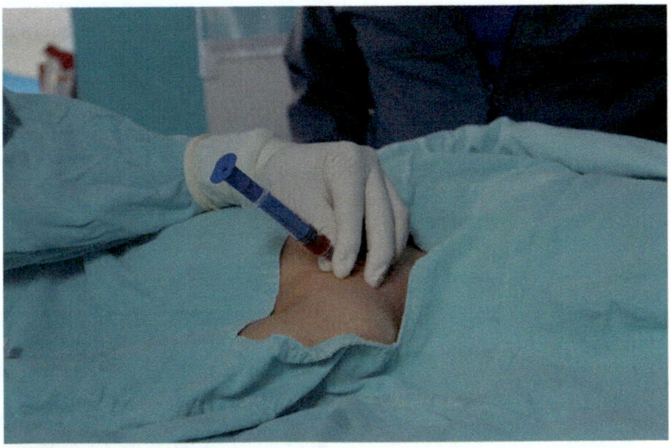

Fig. 13.30 Remove the syringe

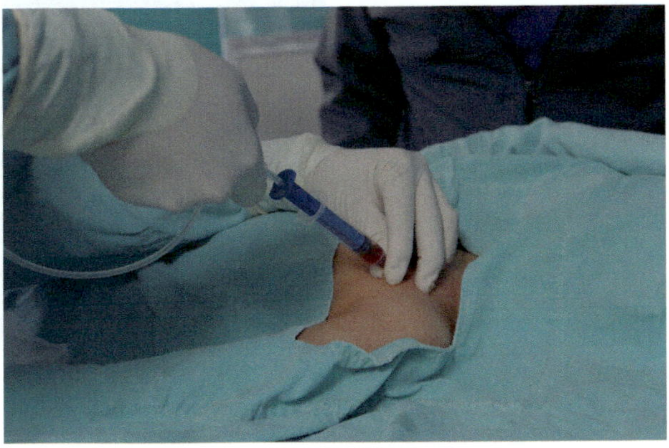

Fig. 13.31 Insert the guidewire

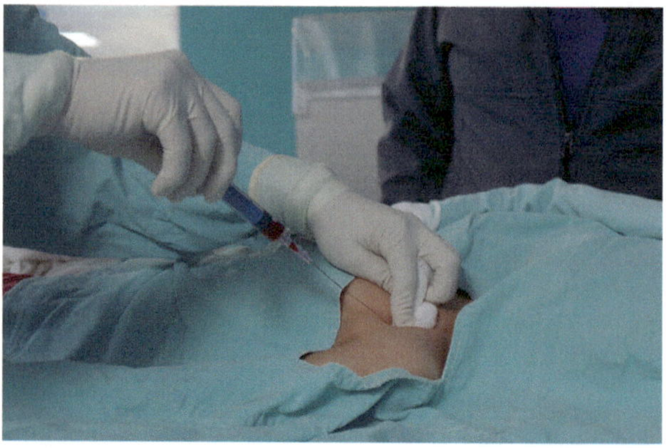

Fig. 13.32 Remove the introducer needle

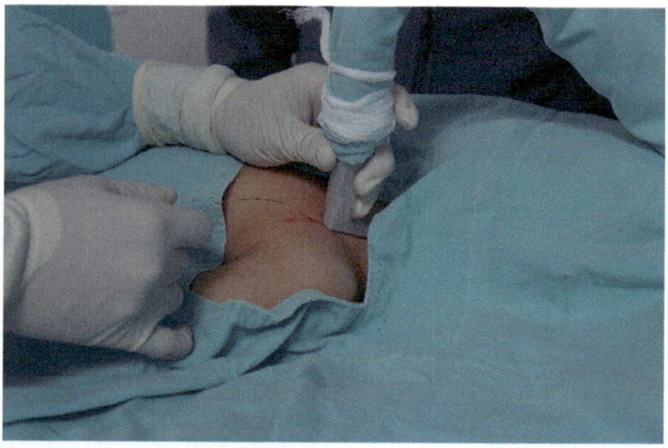

Fig. 13.33 Scan of the deltopectoral groove

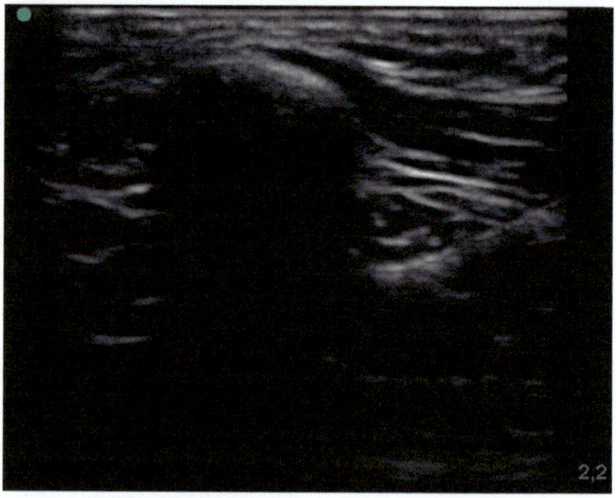

Fig. 13.34 Scan of the deltopectoral groove

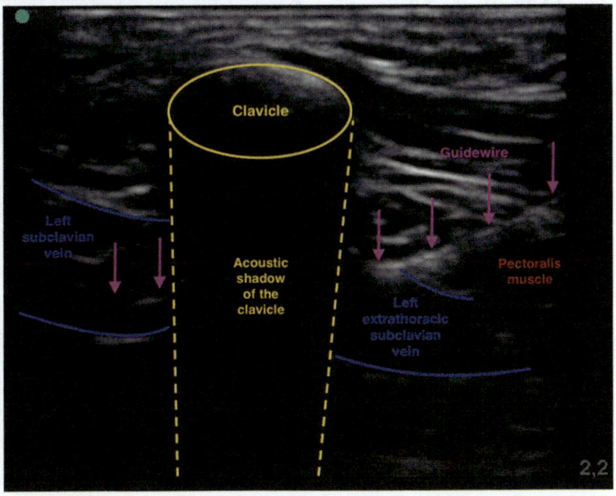

Fig. 13.35 Identifying structures
- LAX view of the guidewire in the ETLSCV

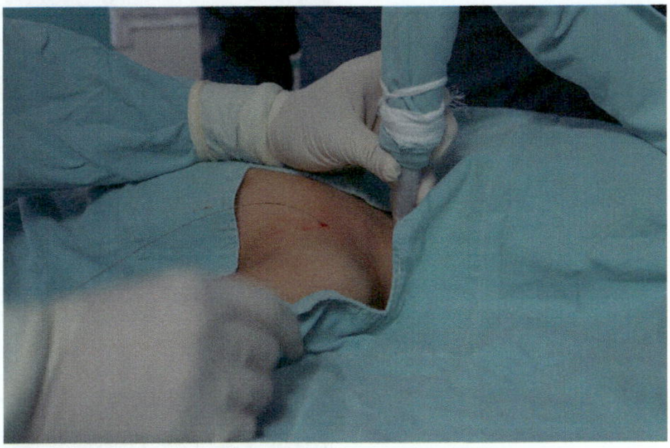

Fig. 13.36 Scan of the cervical vessels

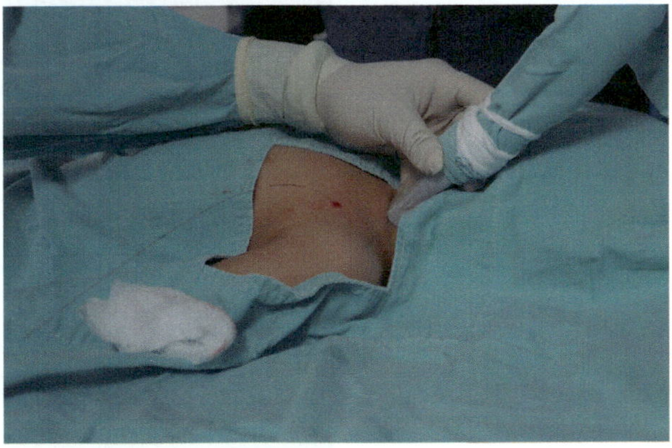

Fig. 13.37 Scan of the supraclavicular fossae

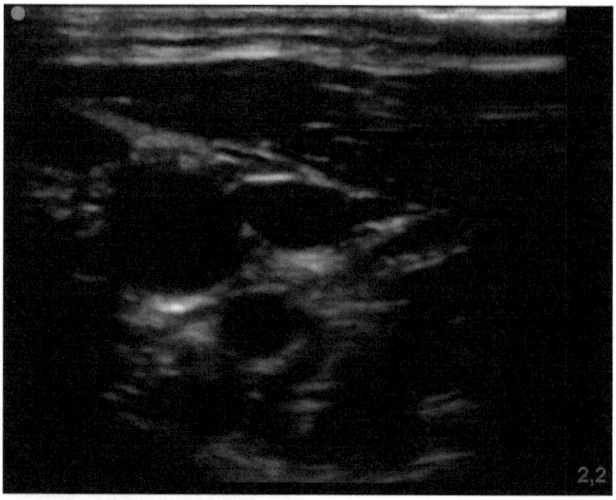

Fig. 13.38 Scan of the cervical region. SAX view

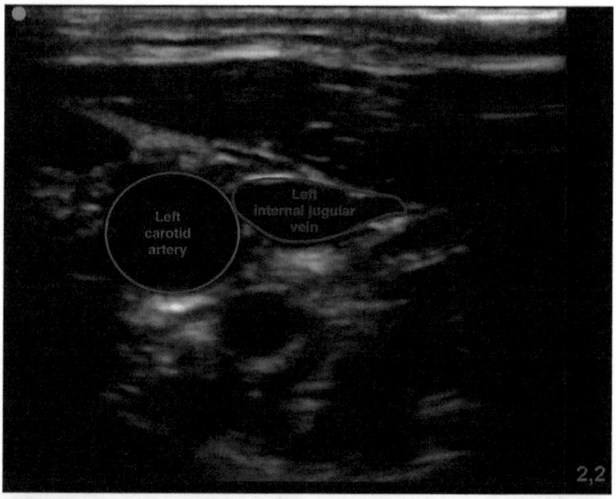

Fig. 13.39 Identifying structures
- LIJV and LCA without guidewire inside

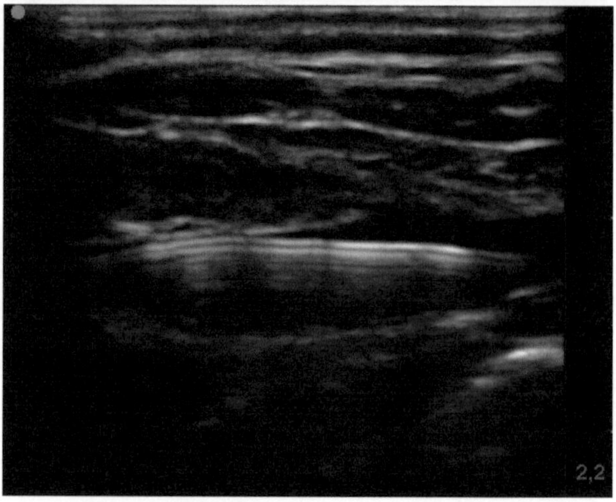

Fig. 13.40 Scan of the supraclavicular fossae

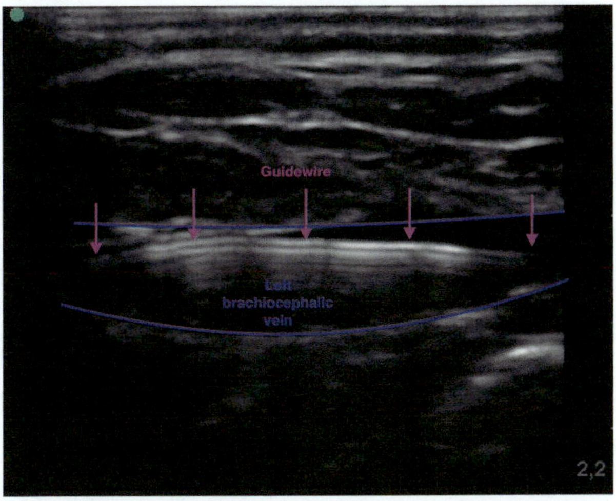

Fig. 13.41 The guidewire is inside the left brachiocephalic vein

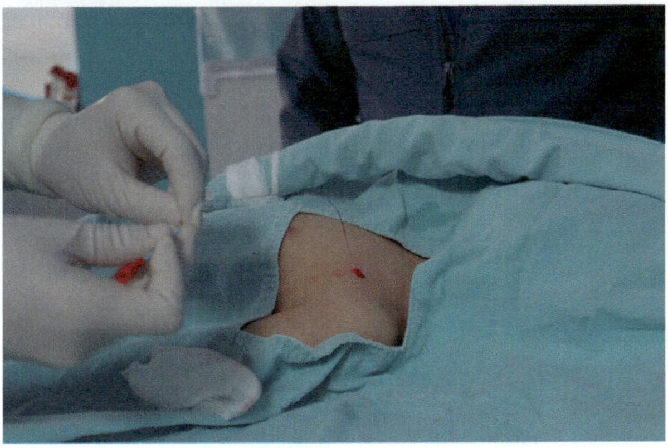

Fig. 13.42 Introduce the dilator over the guidewire

13.4.5 Step 05

- Introduce the dilator over the guidewire (Fig. 13.42).
- Dilate the path of the skin toward the ETLSCV (Fig. 13.43).
- With your left hand, pull the skin so that the dilator can easily penetrate the skin (Fig. 13.44).
- Try not to bend the guidewire.
- You will often not need to make an incision to insert the dilator.
- Remove the dilator, and with your left hand and a piece of gauze, occlude the exit of the skin so that the dilated hole does not bleed (Fig. 13.45).

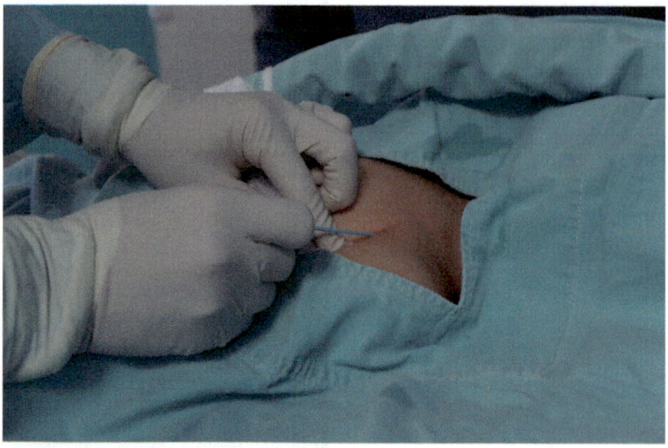

Fig. 13.43 Dilation of the skin

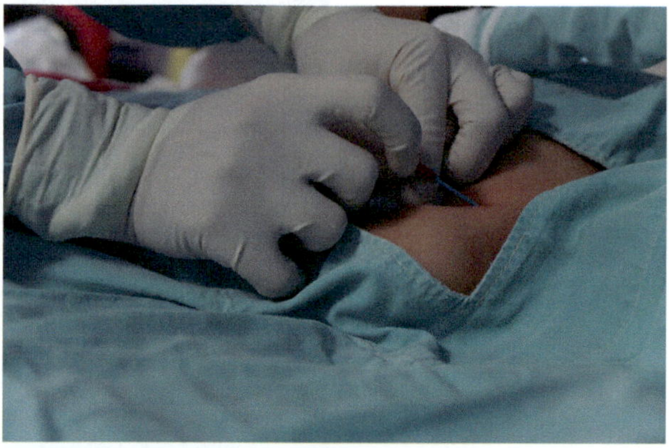

Fig. 13.44 With your left hand, contract the skin

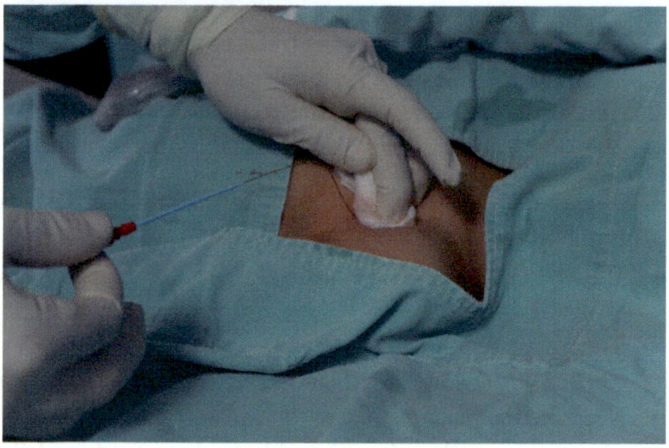

Fig. 13.45 Occlude the exit of the skin

13.4.6 Step 06

- Introduce the catheter over the guidewire (Fig. 13.46).
- Advance the catheter over the guidewire (Seldinger's technique) (Fig. 13.47).
- Insert the appropriate length of the catheter (Fig. 13.48).
- Confirms the patency of the catheter (Fig. 13.49).
- Place the transducer longitudinally in the deltopectoral groove (Fig. 13.50) to perform the scan in LAX view and confirm the intravascular (ETLSCV) location of the catheter (Figs. 13.51 and 13.52).
- In this subclavian extrathoracic access route, the guidewire or catheter sometimes tends to ascend to the ipsilateral jugular vein, so it is good to follow the path of the guidewire or catheter toward the ipsilateral LBCV.
- You can also scan the ipsilateral supraclavicular fossae to see the catheter in the LBCV toward the vena cava (Fig. 13.53).
- LAX view of the catheter within the LBCV (Figs. 13.54 and 13.55).

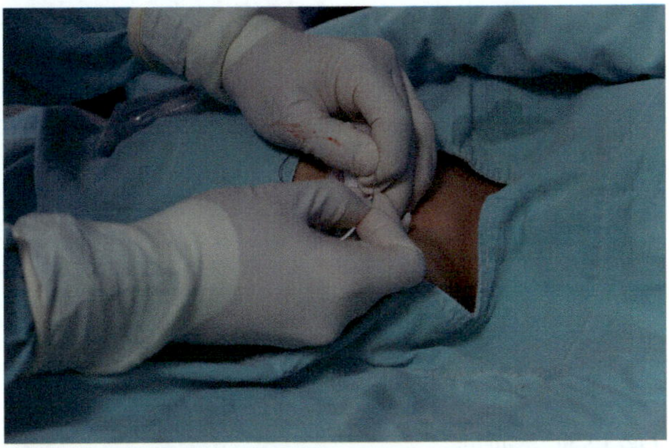

Fig. 13.46 Insert the catheter over the guidewire

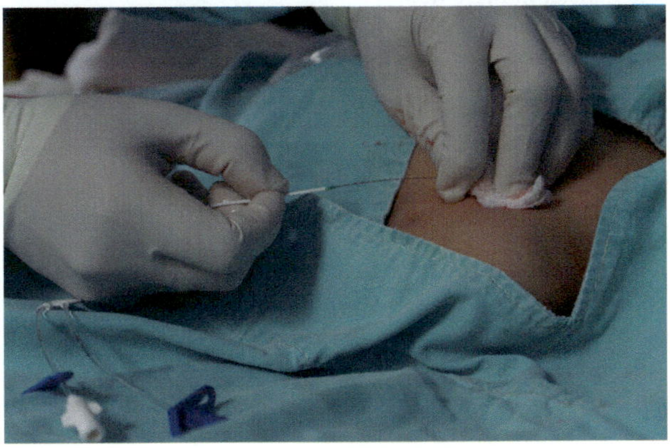

Fig. 13.47 Seldinger's technique: advance the catheter over the guidewire

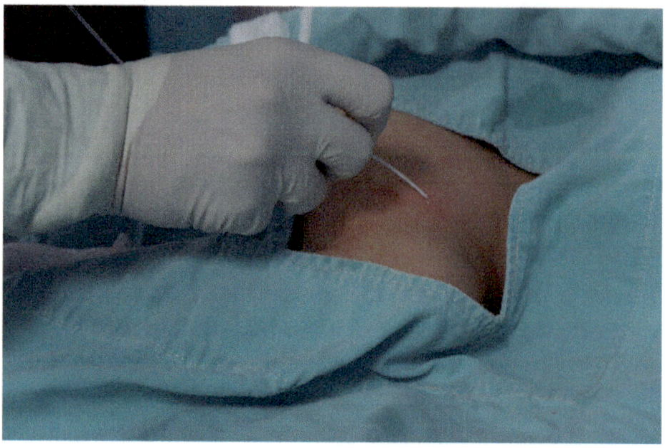

Fig. 13.48 Insert the appropriate length of catheter

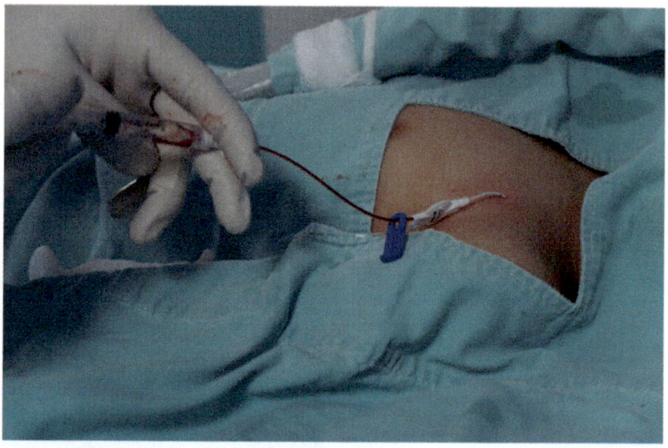

Fig. 13.49 Confirms the patency of the catheter

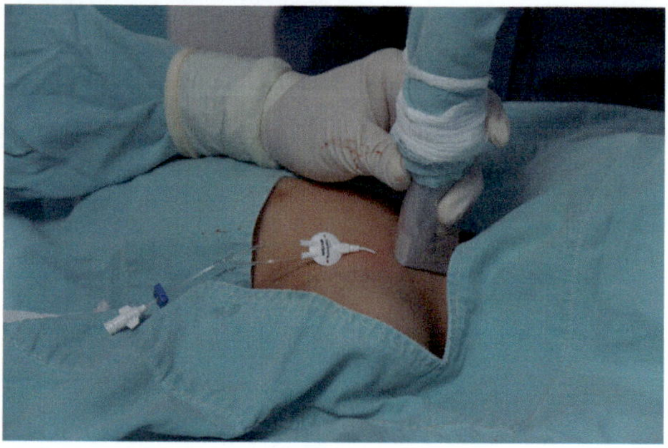

Fig. 13.50 Scan the intravascular location of the catheter in LAX view

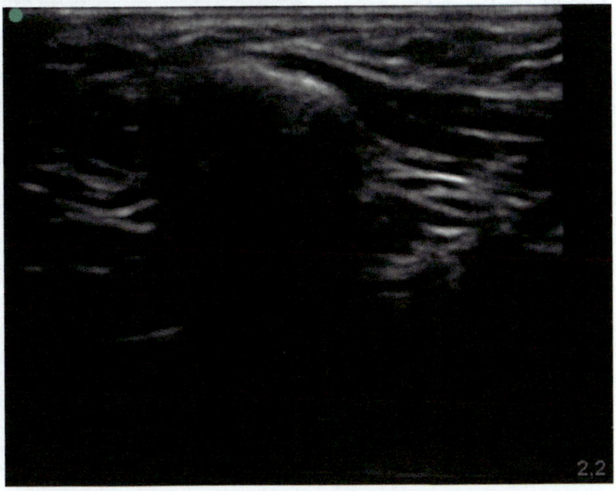

Fig. 13.51 LAX view of ETLSCV

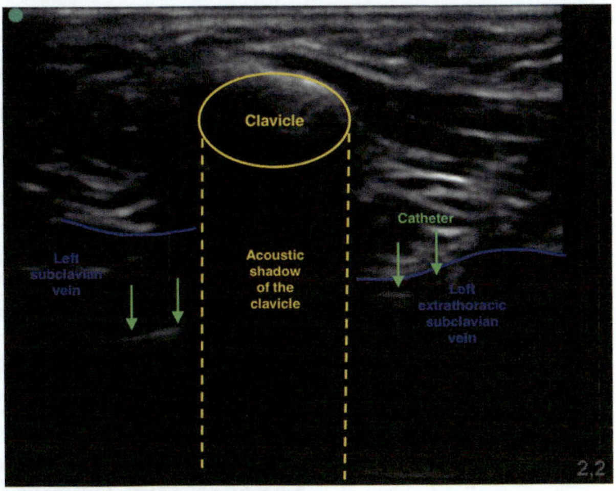

Fig. 13.52 Identifying structures

- Catheter inside ETLSCV following the course toward the left subclavian vein

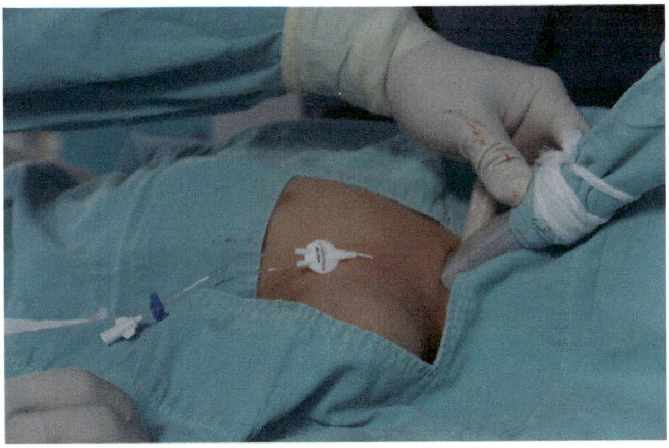

Fig. 13.53 Scan of the left supraclavicular fossae

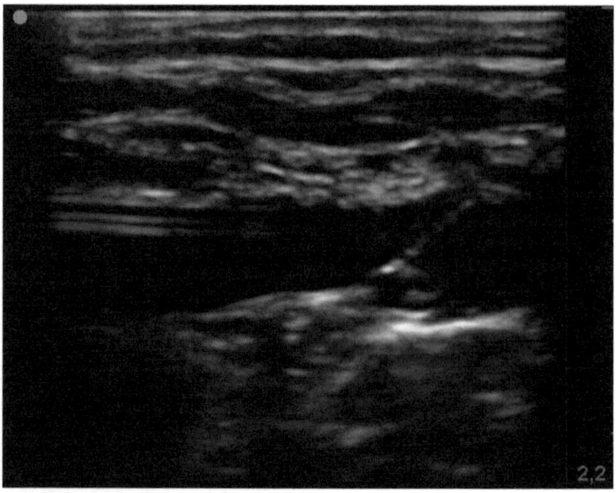

Fig. 13.54 Scan of the left supraclavicular fossae. LAX view of the LBCV

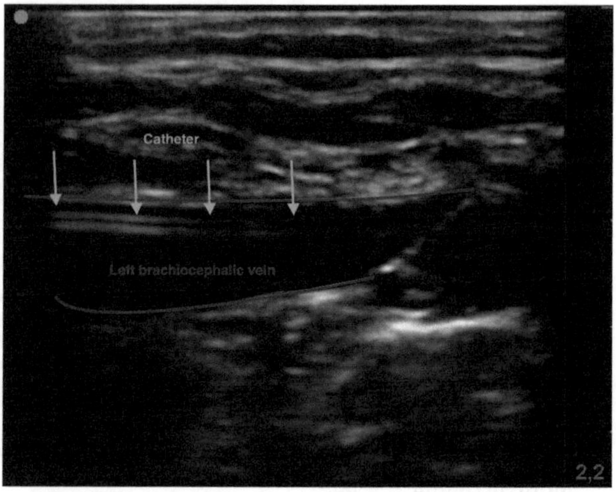

Fig. 13.55 Identifying structures

- The catheter is in the LBCV toward the vena cava

13.4.7 Step 07

- Secure the catheter and place a sterile occlusive dressing according to the institutional protocol (Fig. 13.56).

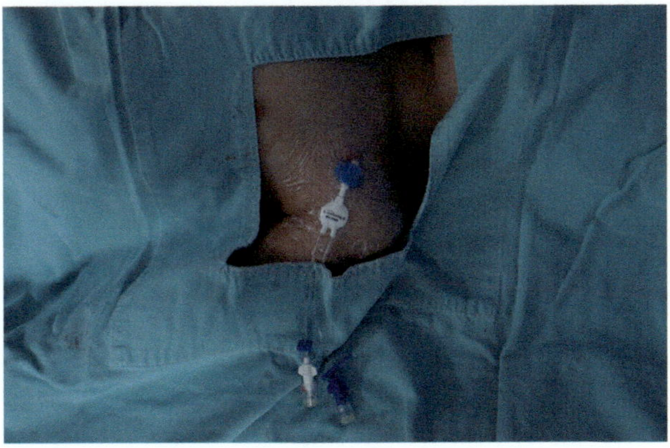

Fig. 13.56 Dressing according to the institutional protocol

Sources

1. Orihashi K, Sato K, Imai K, et al. Extrathoracic subclavian venipuncture under ultrasound guidance. Circ J. 2005;69(9):1111–5. https://doi.org/10.1253/circj.69.1111.
2. Sawasaki K, Sato T, Takayama Y, et al. Novel extrathoracic puncture techniques for pacemaker lead insertion: pitfalls of the conventional extrathoracic puncture method. J Arrhythmia. 2012;28(2):111–3. https://doi.org/10.1016/j.joa.2012.03.008.
3. Zei PC, Nasir J. Extrathoracic subclavian vein access. In: How-to manual for pacemaker and ICD devices; 2017. p. 9–16. https://doi.org/10.1002/9781118820674.ch2.
4. He Y, Yang W, Zhao Y, et al. Individualized blind techniques for puncture of intrathoracic and Extrathoracic subclavian vein: three simple experience tips. Anatol J Cardiol. 2023;27(9):534–8. https://doi.org/10.14744/AnatolJCardiol.2023.2893. Publicado el 7 de junio de 2023
5. Brignole M, Deharo JC. Different techniques of venous access for CIEDs: advantages and disadvantages. Eur Heart J. 2023;44(46):4859–61. https://doi.org/10.1093/eurheartj/ehad749.

Chapter 14
Right Brachiocephalic Vein in Pediatrics

14.1 Patient Positioning

- The patient is a 3-year-old weighing 9 kg.
- Position the patient supine close to the head of the bed.
- Position the patient's head to the left.
- Place a roll under the shoulders to extend the neck, placing the head lower than the left shoulder (Fig. 14.1).
- The goal of patient positioning for this procedure is to increase the cervical area between the mandible and clavicle to gain access to the supraclavicular fossae.
- Gently hold the upper extremities with the arms toward caudal.

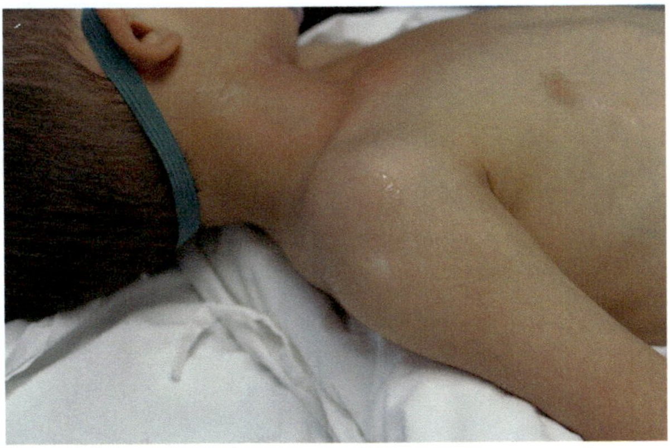

Fig. 14.1 Patient position

F. Montes-Tapia, *Atlas of Ultrasound-Guided Central Venous Catheter Placement*, https://doi.org/10.1007/978-3-031-61887-1_14

14.2 Scanning Technique

- Do a preliminary vascular assessment (non-sterile), known as rapid central vein assessment (RaCeVA).
- The operator stands at the head of the patient, on the right side.
- A high-frequency linear transducer (13–6 MHz), with a hockey stick-type or 5-cm footprint probe, can be used.
- The ultrasound is placed at the patient's feet in front of the operator or to the side of the right shoulder (Fig. 14.2).
- Start the scan in the middle of the right neck with the transducer transverse and the tip of the hockey stick transducer to the patient's left side (Fig. 14.3).
- Begin the scan of the vessels in short-axis (SAX) view and sweep down to the clavicle.
- SAX view of the cervical vessels (Figs. 14.4 and 14.5).
- Continue sweeping downward, and before entering in contact with the clavicle, scan the cervical vessels again (Fig. 14.6).

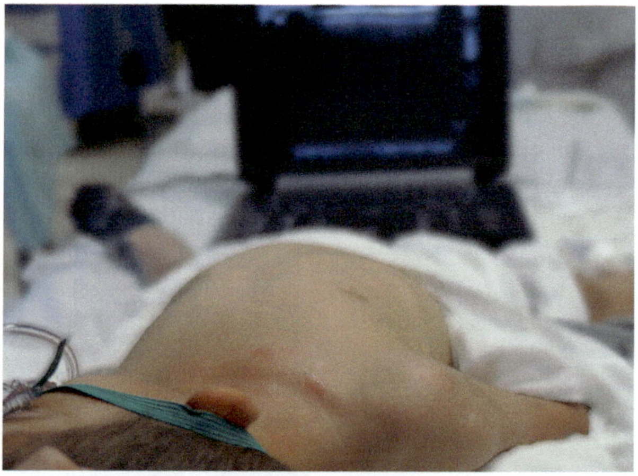

Fig. 14.2 The ultrasound is placed at the patient's feet in front of the operator

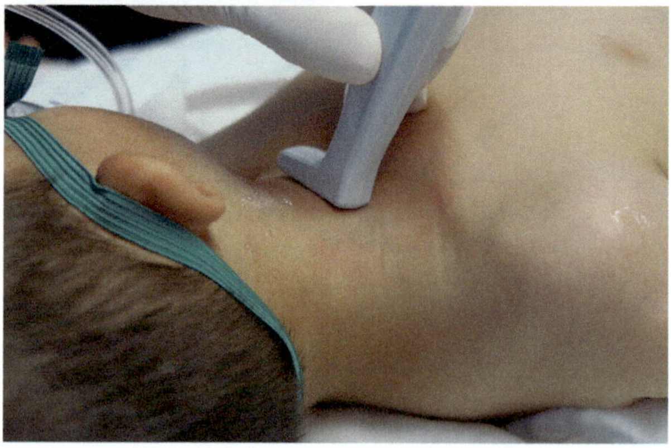

Fig. 14.3 Start the scan in the middle of the right neck

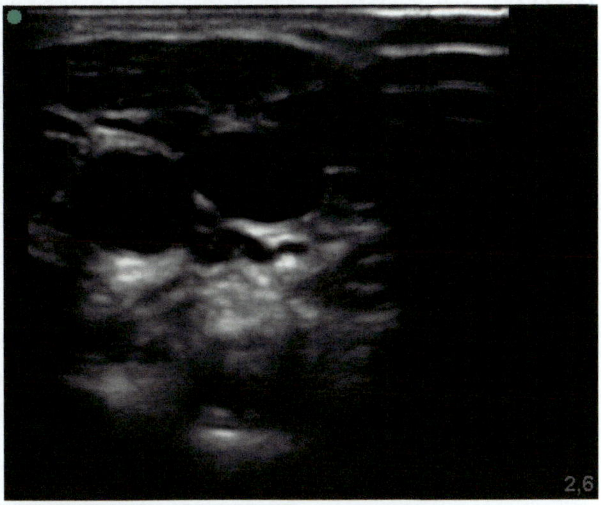

Fig. 14.4 Scan of the right cervical region. SAX view of cervical vessels
- The probe indicator is on the patient's left side, identified on the screen as the aqua dot at the top left of the image
- The scan depth is 2,6 cm

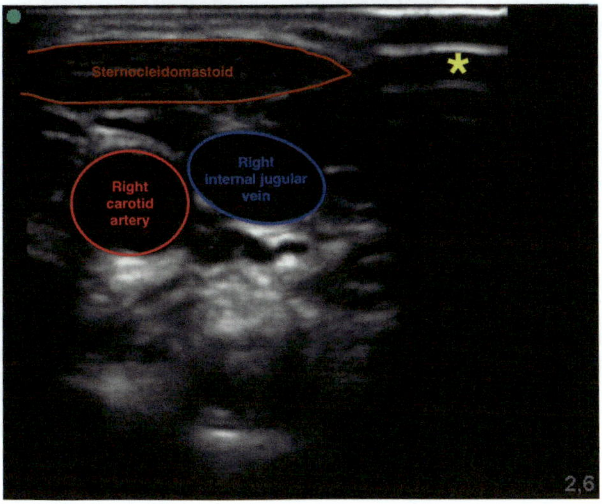

Fig. 14.5 Identifying structures
- The right internal jugular vein (RIJV) and right carotid artery (RCA) under the sternocleidomastoid muscle
- The RIJV is lateral to the RCA
- * Indicates the lack of contact of the transducer on the patient's skin
  - See in Fig. 14.3 that the transducer's lateral part (right of the patient) is not in contact with the patient. This view is translated in this ultrasonographic image by transverse lines as barcodes that indicate this lack of contact of the transducer

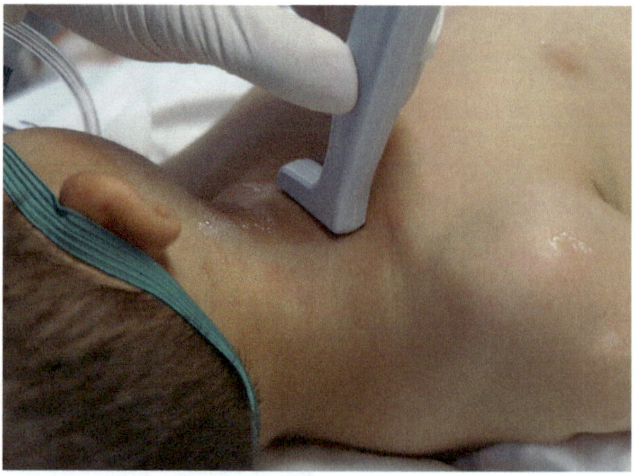

Fig. 14.6 Lower cervical scan, transducer almost in contact with the clavicle

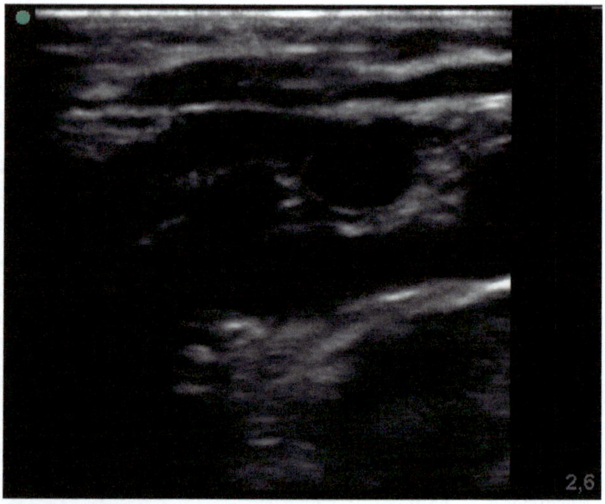

Fig. 14.7 Visualization of vessels at the base of the neck

- Visualization of the cervical vessels in SAX view (Figs. 14.7 and 14.8).
- Place the transducer in contact with the clavicle in the right supraclavicular fossae between the inner third of the clavicle and the sternal notch. Maintain the tip of the hockey stick transducer to the left (Fig. 14.9).
- Then, tilt the transducer to posterior:
  - The aim of tilting the transducer is to visualize the retroclavicular and thoracic inlet area to identify the right brachiocephalic vein (RBCV) in LAX view and perform the puncture in this view.
  - LAX view of the RBCV, left brachiocephalic vein (LBCV), and the superior vena cava (SVC) (Figs. 14.10 and 14.11).

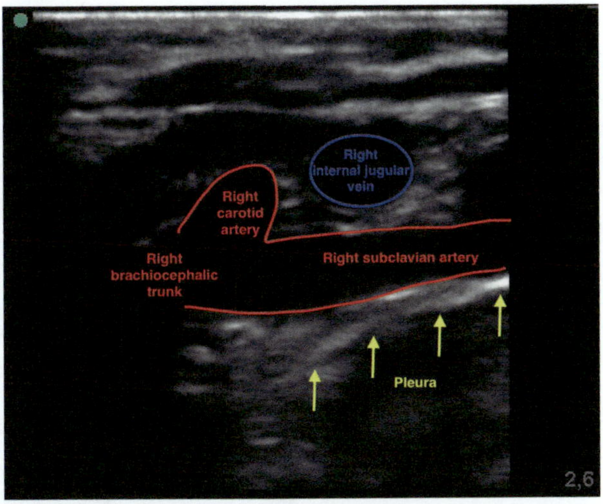

Fig. 14.8 Identifying structures

- The right brachiocephalic trunk originates the right carotid artery (RCA) and the right subclavian artery (RSCA), which is displayed longitudinally (LAX view)
- At this level of scanning, the RIJV is still visualized in a cross section (SAX view)
- The pleura is in contact with the inferior wall of the RSCA

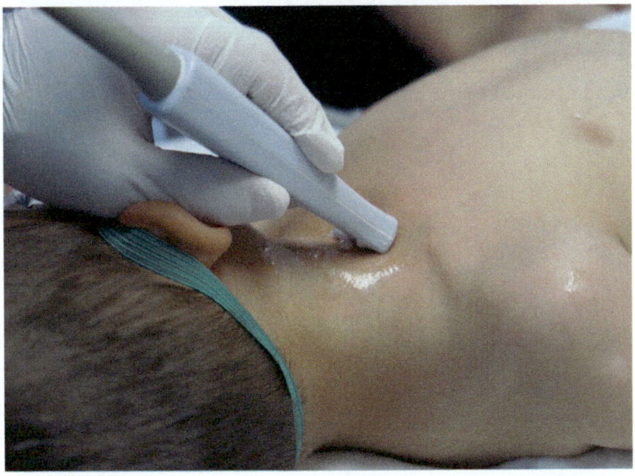

Fig. 14.9 Transducer in the right supraclavicular fossae with the tip to the left, between the inner third of the clavicle and the sternal notch, tilting to posterior

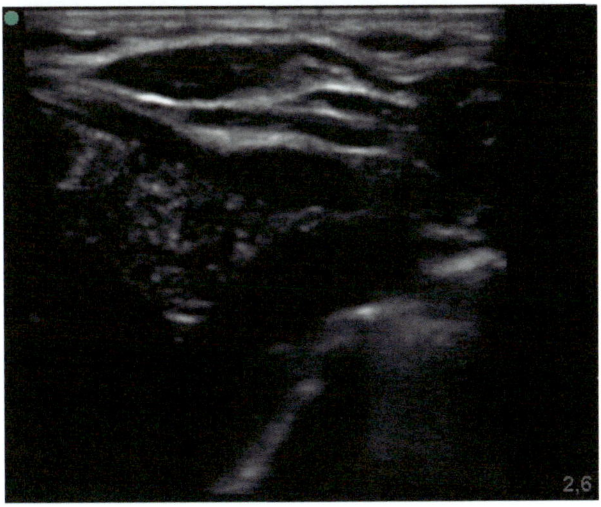

Fig. 14.10 LAX view of the thoracic vessels

- The diameter of the RBCV is 5,2 cm
- Scan depth is 2,6 cm

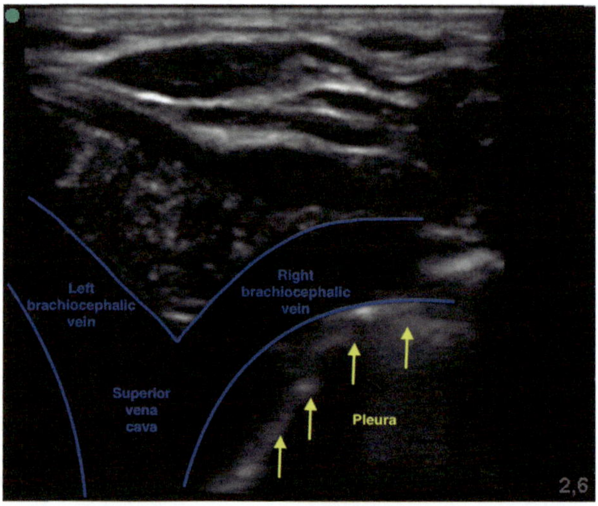

Fig. 14.11 Identifying structures

- The formation of the superior vena cava from the inflow of the RBCV and LBCV

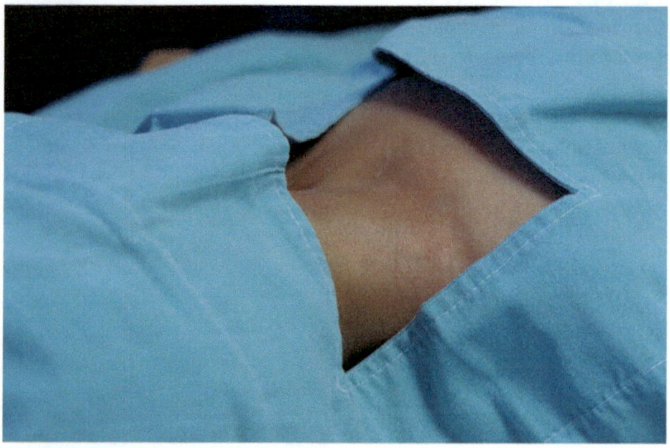

Fig. 14.12 Right cervicothoracic area. The head is turned to the left

14.3 Local Anesthesia Application

- The sterile field only leaves the right cervical and upper pectoral regions uncovered.
- Operator's view of the right cervicothoracic area. The head is turned to the left (Fig. 14.12).
- Real-time ultrasound-guided lidocaine infiltration.
- For infiltration, use a small needle 25 to 27 G.
- Use lidocaine 1%.

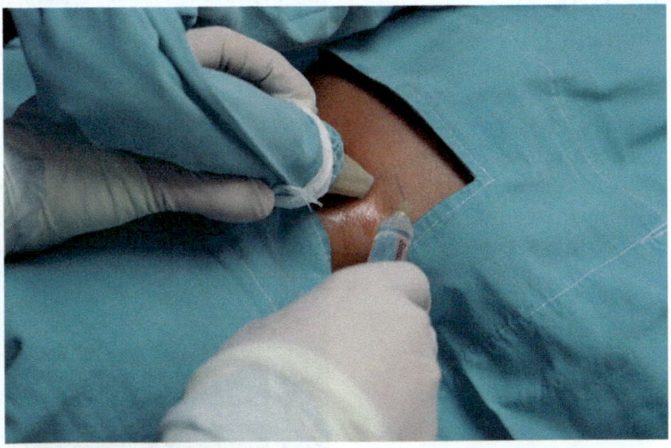

Fig. 14.13 Real-time ultrasound-guided lidocaine infiltration

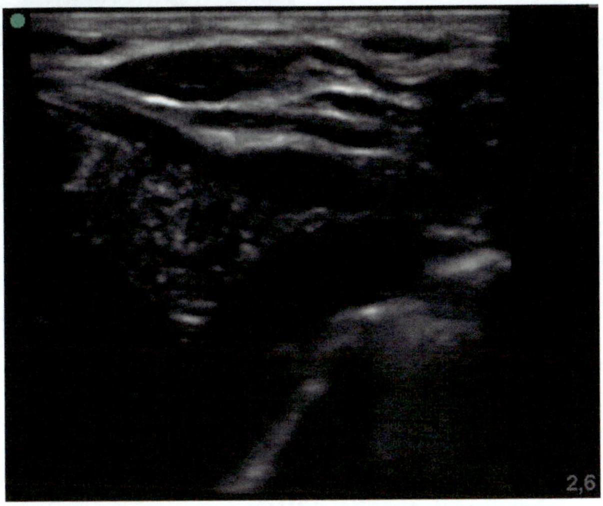

Fig. 14.14 Scan of the retroclavicular and thoracic inlet veins. LAX view of subcutaneous infiltration of lidocaine

- Subcutaneous infiltration with lidocaine in the puncture tract 1,5 to 2 cm before the site chosen for RBCV puncture and the catheter fixation area (Fig. 14.13).
- Scan of the retroclavicular and thoracic inlet veins. SAX view of lidocaine infiltration (Figs. 14.14 and 14.15).
- You can use the lidocaine infiltration puncture to guide where to perform the puncture with the introducer needle.

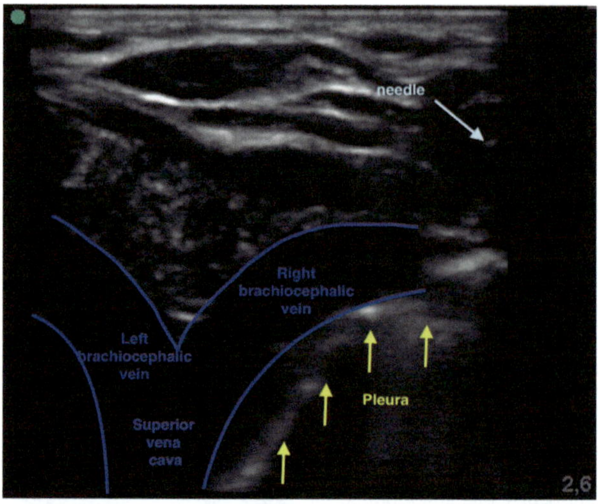

Fig. 14.15 Identifying structures
- The tip of the infiltration needle is seen as a bright hyperechoic (white) dot on the subcutaneous tissue; the movement of this hyperechoic point is seen in real time

14.4 Steps for Real-Time Ultrasound-Guided Access to Right Brachiocephalic Vein in Pediatrics

14.4.1 Step 01

- We will use a Medadv® 7 Fr, 20-cm, double-lumen catheter.
- This type of catheter has an 18-G introducer needle on the Raulerson Spring-Wire introductory syringe. You can also use a 18-G intravenous catheter for the puncture.
- Place the transducer in the right supraclavicular fossae.
- Perform the puncture in LAX.
- Start the puncture at an angle of 60°–70° to penetrate the skin and enter the subcutaneous tissue (Fig. 14.16).
- Puncture from lateral to medial and posterior to anterior to visualize the introducer needle.
- Introduce the needle slowly, as it is a short distance from the skin to the vein.
- Because the RBCV has a more vertical trajectory, the introducer needle will not be displayed transversely on the screen but rather obliquely.
- LAX view of the start of the puncture (Figs. 14.17 and 14.18).

14.4.2 Step 02

- Modify the puncture angle to 50–60° to visualize the introducer needle so the needle will be below the insonation area of the transducer (Fig. 14.19).
- Always perform the puncture with dynamic needle tracking (DNT).

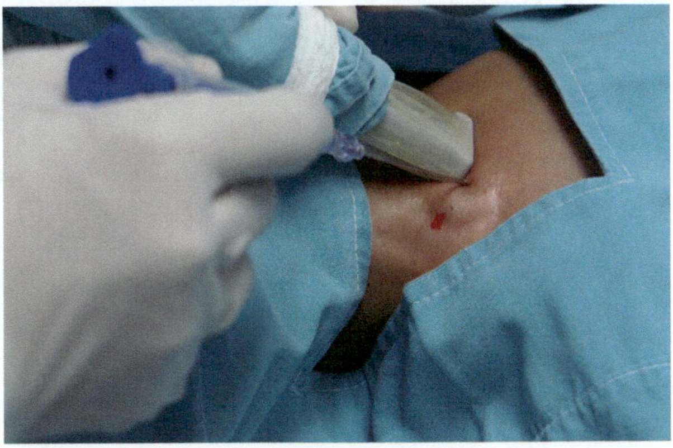

Fig. 14.16 Start the puncture at an angle of 60°–70°

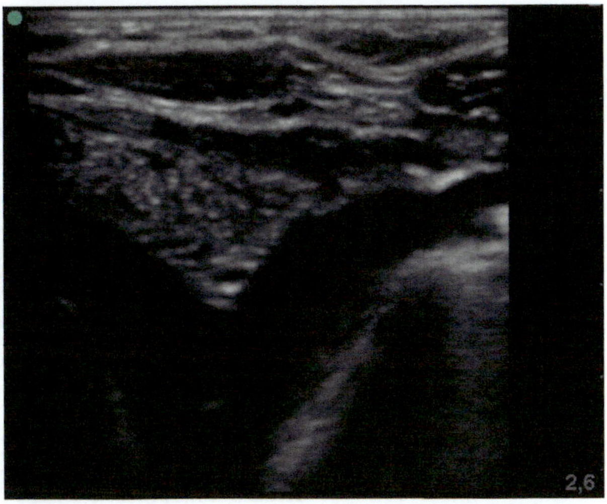

Fig. 14.17 LAX view of the start of the RBCV puncture

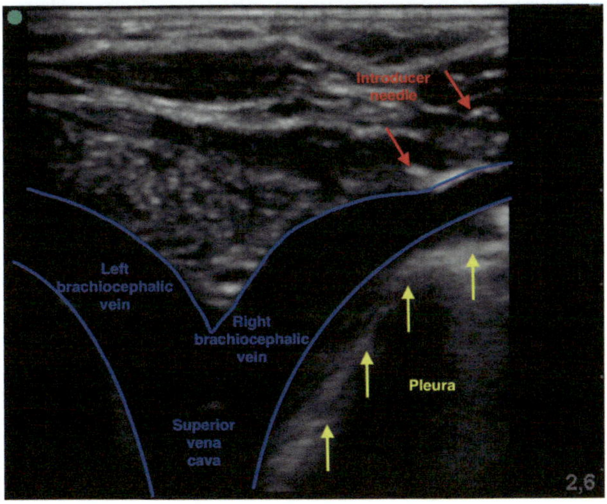

Fig. 14.18 Identifying structures

- The introducer needle has an oblique direction located on the anterior wall of the RBCV
- Compression of the anterior wall of the RBCV is visualized due to the pressure exerted by the puncture

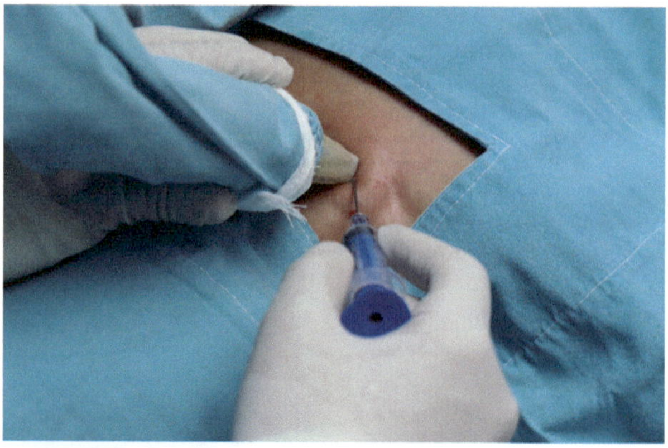

Fig. 14.19 Modify the puncture angle to 50–60°

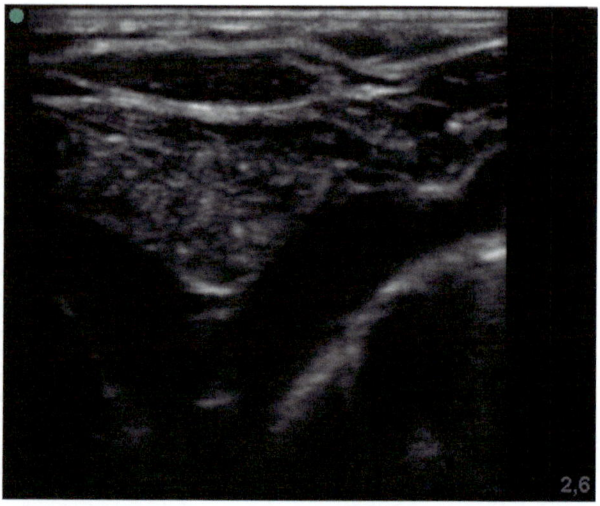

Fig. 14.20 LAX view of the compression of the anterior wall of the RBCV

- LAX view of the arrival of the needle to the anterior wall of the RBCV (Figs. 14.20 and 14.21).
- Follow the puncture path to cannulate the vein (Fig. 14.22).
- Visualization of the deformation of the anterior wall of the RBCV caused by the compression of the introducer needle demonstrating the correct path of the puncture toward the vein (Figs. 14.23 and 14.24).

14.4.3 Step 03

- RBCV cannulation. When you feel the loss of puncture resistance (indicating vein cannulation), you will also show the intravascular location of the needle on the monitor in real time (Fig. 14.25).

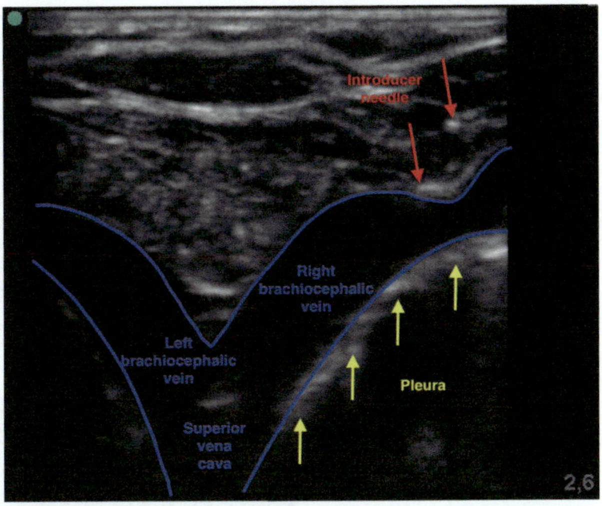

Fig. 14.21 Identifying structures
- The deformation of the anterior wall of the RBCV caused by compression of the puncture caused by the introducer needle indicates that we are on the right track
- Continue the path of the puncture

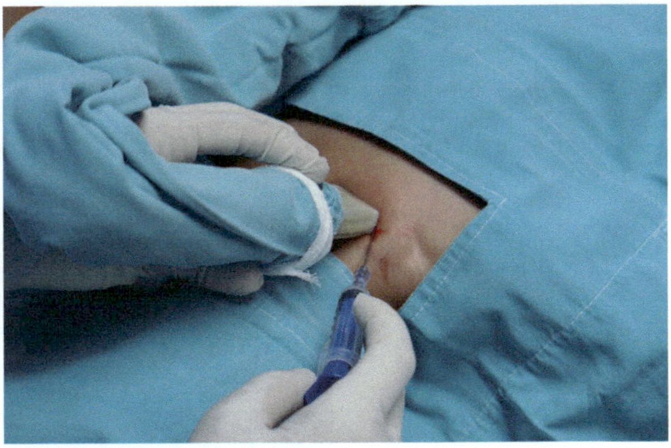

Fig. 14.22 Continue with the puncture in DNT toward the RBCV

- LAX view of the RBCV cannulation (Figs. 14.26 and 14.27).
- Set the transducer aside.
- Firmly fix the needle hub with your left hand so the needle is not dislodged from its intravascular location.
- Make a gentle negative pressure on the syringe plunger until a flash of blood appears in the barrel of the syringe, indicating the intravascular position of the introducer needle (Fig. 14.28).

14.4.4 Step 04

- Hold the needle hub firmly and insert the 0.032" guidewire through the Raulerson syringe and the introducer needle (Fig. 14.29).

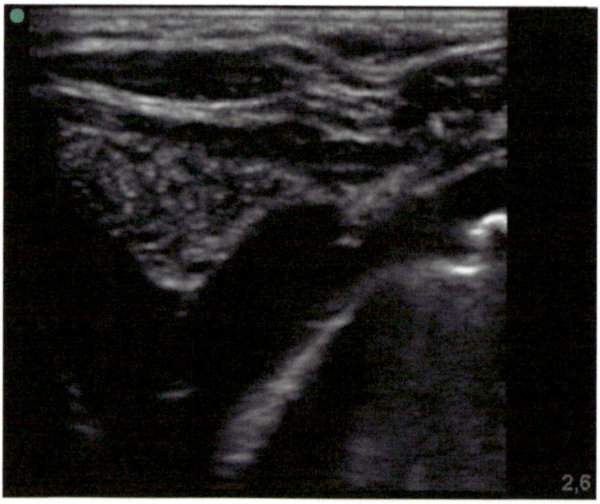

Fig. 14.23 LAX view of the start of the RBCV cannulation

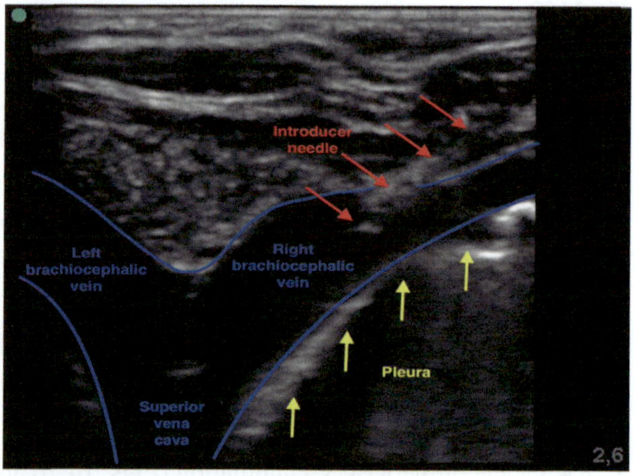

Fig. 14.24 Identifying structures

- The introducer needle initiates the penetration of the anterior wall of the RBCV

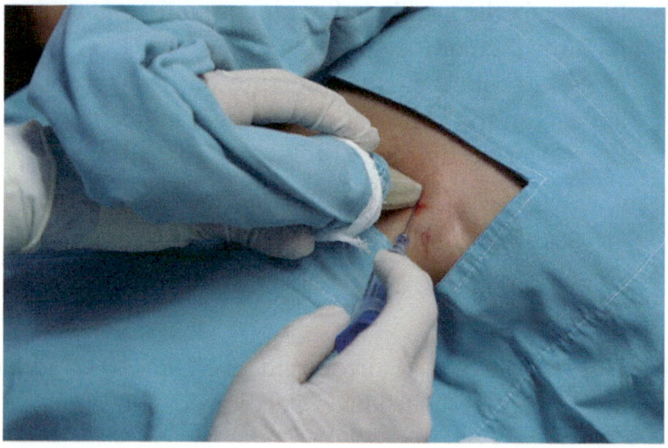

Fig. 14.25 Continue the puncture trajectory and cannulate the RBCV

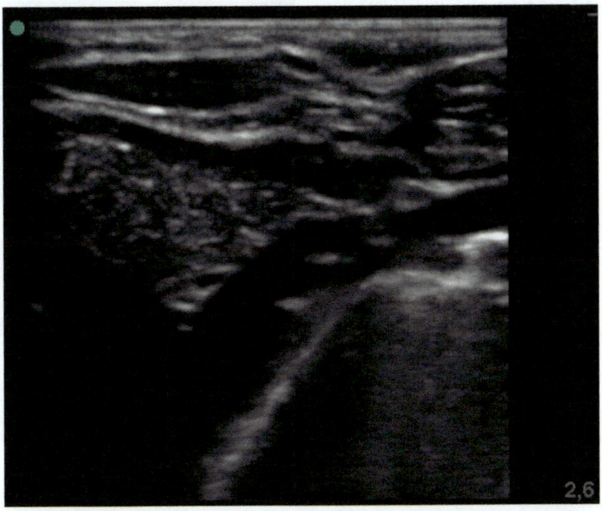

Fig. 14.26 LAX view of the RBCV cannulation

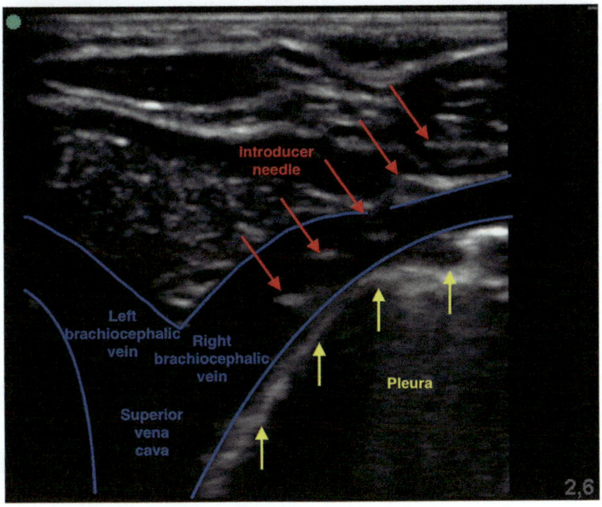

Fig. 14.27 Identifying structures
- The oblique trajectory of the introducer needle and not being echogenic cannot be easily identified
- The pleura in the inferior and lateral wall of the vein

- Remove the introducer needle and the Raulerson syringe.
- Place the transducer in the supraclavicular fossae to identify the intravascular guidewire (Fig. 14.30).
- LAX view of the intravascular guidewire (Figs. 14.31 and 14.32).

14.4.5 Step 05

- Introduce the dilator and dilate the path of the skin toward the RBCV.

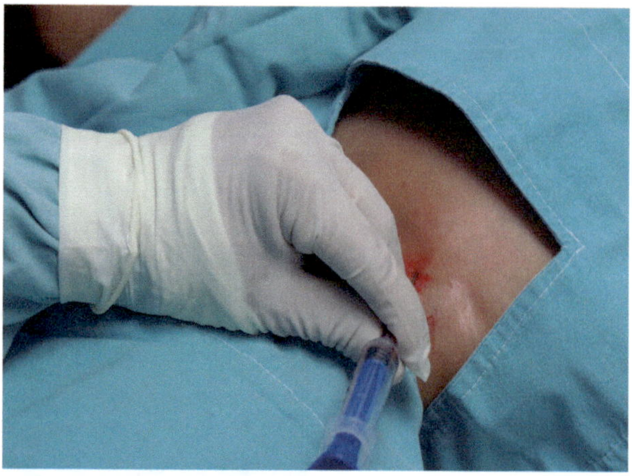

Fig. 14.28 Apply gentle negative pressure and check for the return of blood in the barrel of the syringe

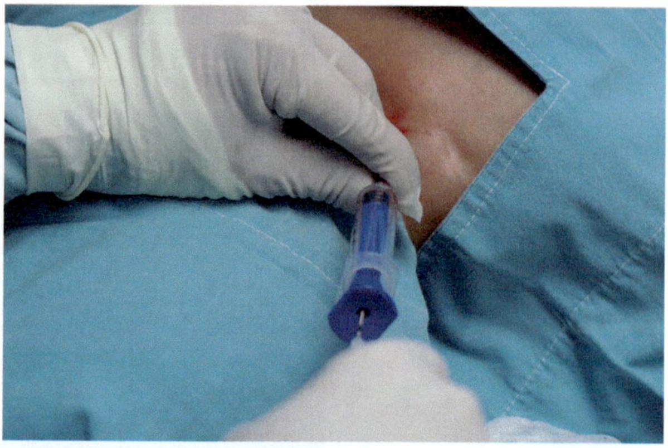

Fig. 14.29 Insert the guidewire

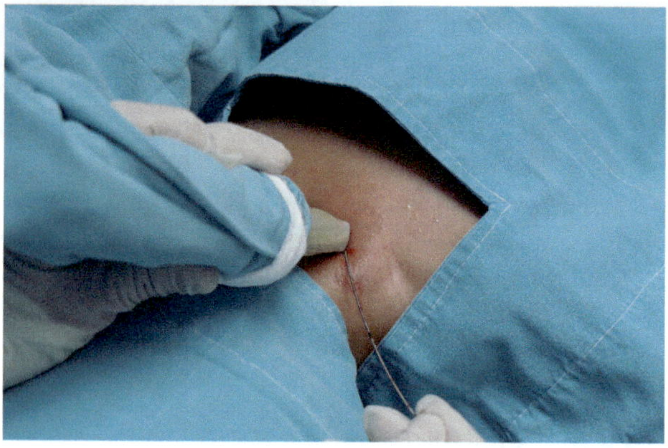

Fig. 14.30 Scan the supraclavicular fossae to verify the intravascular location of the guidewire

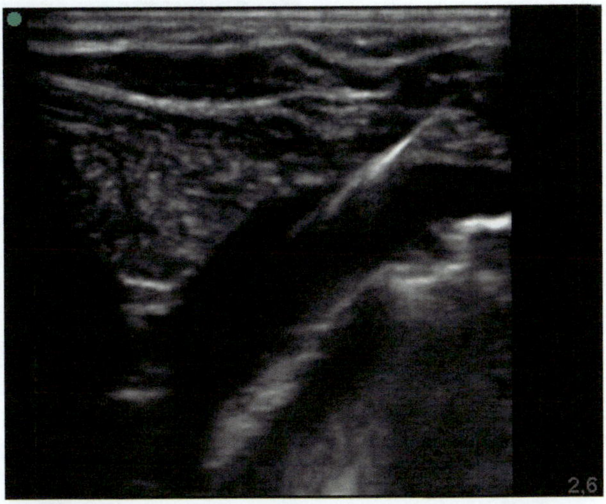

Fig. 14.31 LAX view of the intravascular guidewire

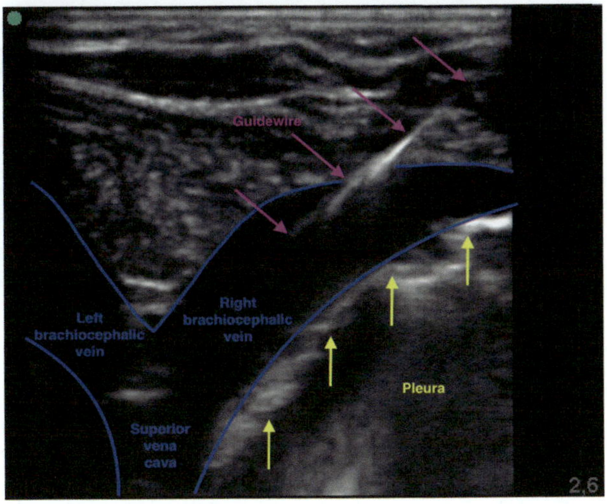

Fig. 14.32 Identifying structures
- Guidewire in the RBCV descending toward the SVC

- With your left hand, pull the skin so that the dilator can easily penetrate the skin (Fig. 14.33).
- Try not to bend the guidewire.
- You will often not need to make an incision to insert the dilator.
- When you finish dilating, occlude the already dilated puncture entry site with gauze and your left hand so it does not bleed (Fig. 14.34).

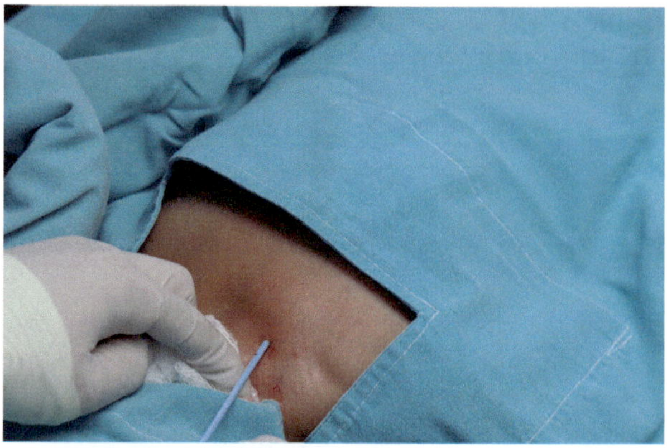

Fig. 14.33 Dilation of the skin

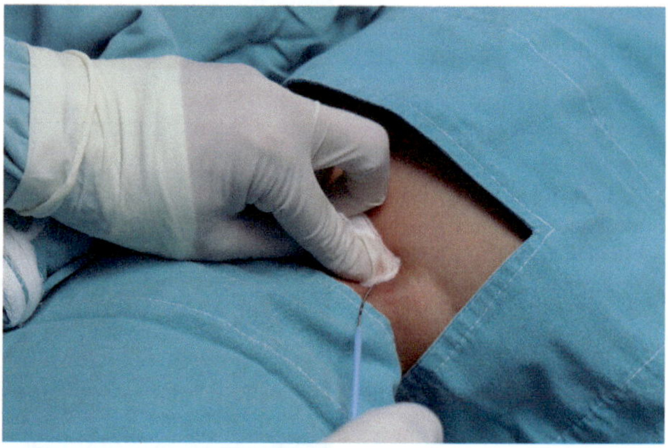

Fig. 14.34 Remove the dilator

14.4.6 Step 06

- Advance the catheter over the guidewire (Seldinger's technique) and remove the guidewire (Fig. 14.35).
- Scan the intravascular location of the catheter by placing the transducer over the supraclavicular fossae (Fig. 14.36).
- LAX view of the intravascular catheter (Figs. 14.37 and 14.38).

14.4.7 Step 07

- Secure the catheter and place a sterile occlusive dressing according to the institutional protocol (Fig. 14.39).

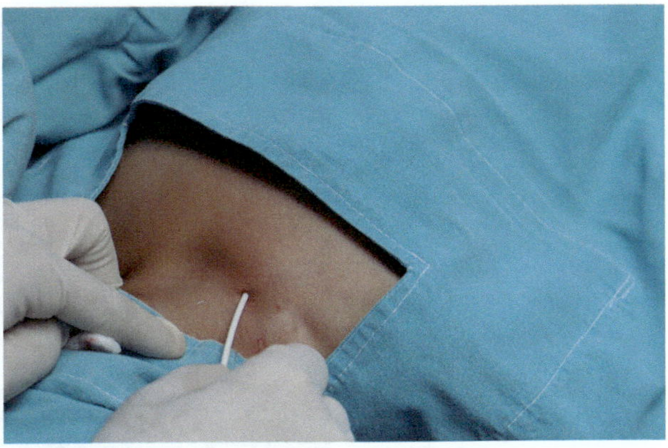

Fig. 14.35 Seldinger's technique: advance the catheter over the guidewire

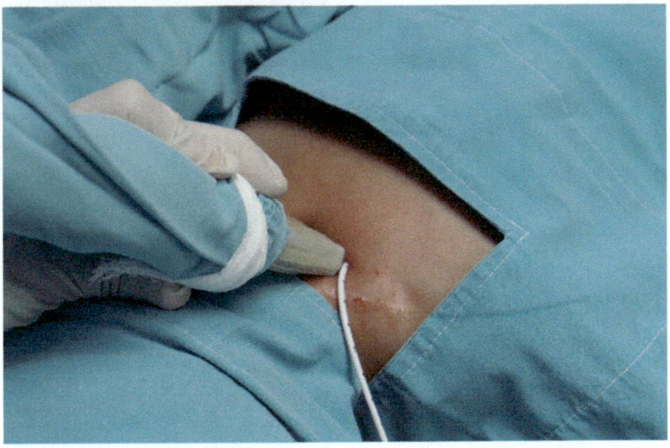

Fig. 14.36 Scan the intravascular location of the catheter

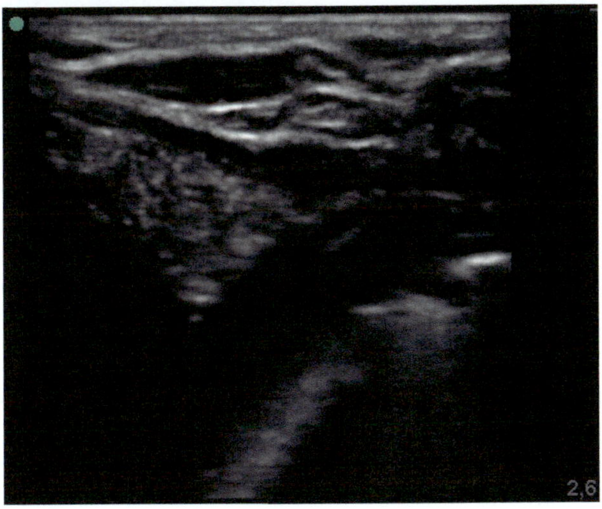

Fig. 14.37 LAX view of the intravascular catheter

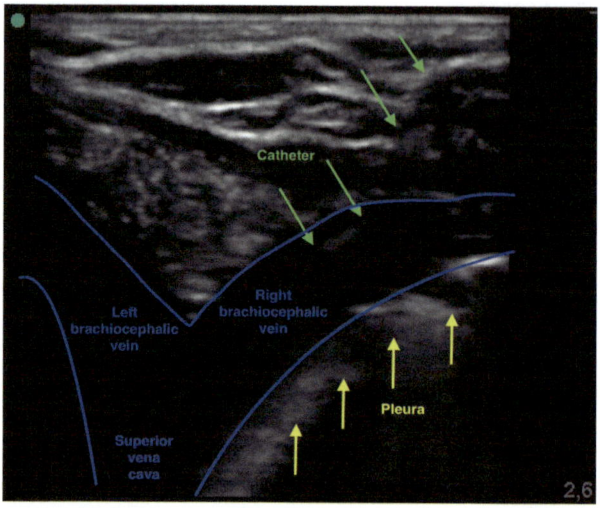

Fig. 14.38 Identifying structures

- The catheter with a descending path toward the SVC is identified

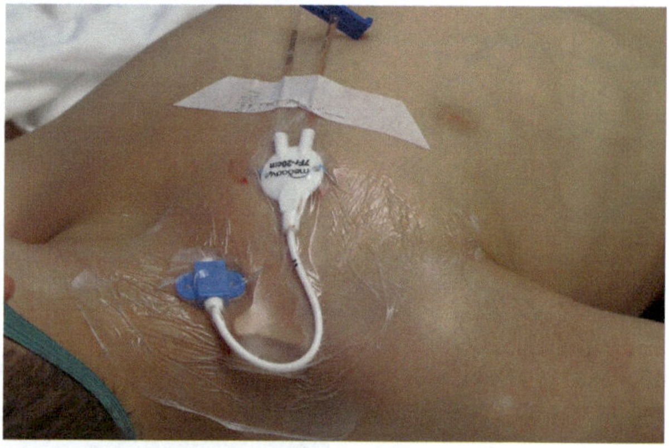

Fig. 14.39 Dressing according to the institutional protocol

Sources

1. Breschan C, Platzer M, Jost R, Stettner H, Beyer AS, Feigl G, Likar R. Consecutive, prospective case series of a new method for ultrasound-guided supraclavicular approach to the brachiocephalic vein in children. Br J Anaesth. 2011;106(5):732–7. https://doi.org/10.1093/bja/aer031. Epub 2011 Mar 17
2. Aytekin C, Özyer U, Harman A, Boyvat F. Ultrasound-guided brachiocephalic vein catheterization in infants weighing less than five kilograms. J Vasc Access. 2015;16(6):512–4. https://doi.org/10.5301/jva.5000385. Epub 2015 May 30
3. Breschan C, Graf G, Jost R, Stettner H, Feigl G, Goessler A, Neuwersch S, Koestenberger M, Likar R. Ultrasound-guided supraclavicular cannulation of the right brachiocephalic vein in small infants: a consecutive, prospective case series. Paediatr Anaesth. 2015;25(9):943–9. https://doi.org/10.1111/pan.12700. Epub 2015 Jun 17

4. Oulego-Erroz I, Alonso-Quintela P, Terroba-Seara S, Jiménez-González A, Rodríguez-Blanco S, Vázquez-Martínez JL. Ultrasound-guided cannulation of the brachiocephalic vein in neonates and preterm infants: a prospective observational study. Am J Perinatol. 2018;35(5):503–8. https://doi.org/10.1055/s-0037-1608803. Epub 2017 Nov 28
5. Spagnuolo F, Vacchiano T. Ultrasound-guided cannulation of the brachiocephalic vein in newborns: a novel approach with a supraclavicular view for tip navigation and tip location. J Vasc Access. 2022;23(4):515–23. https://doi.org/10.1177/11297298211001159. Epub 2021 Mar 16
6. Breschan C, Graf G, Arneitz C, Stettner H, Neuwersch S, Stadik C, Koestenberger M, Holasek S, Likar R. Retrospective evaluation of 599 brachiocephalic vein cannulations in neonates and preterm infants. Br J Anaesth. 2022;129(5):e138–40. https://doi.org/10.1016/j.bja.2022.08.006. Epub 2022 Sep 13

Chapter 15
Right Brachiocephalic Vein in Neonates

15.1 Patient Positioning

- The patient is a newborn weighing 2480 g.
- Position the patient supine near the head of the thermic crib.
- Position the patient's head to the left.
- Place a roll under the shoulders to extend the neck, placing the head lower than the left shoulder (Fig. 15.1).
- The goal of patient positioning for this procedure is to increase the cervical area between the jaw and clavicle to gain access to the supraclavicular fossae.
- Gently hold the upper extremities with the arm caudal.

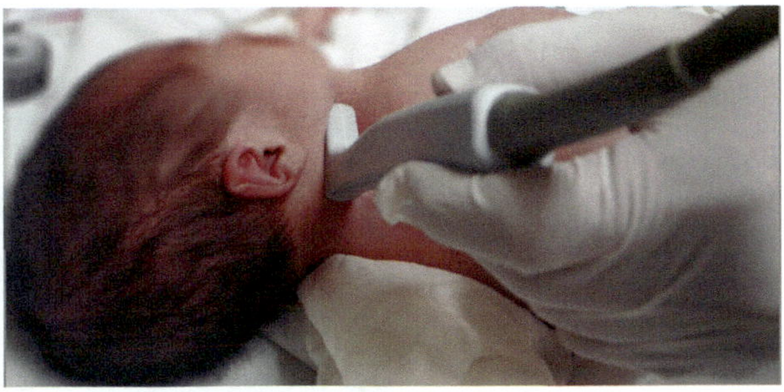

Fig. 15.1 Patient position. Start the scan in the middle of the right neck

F. Montes-Tapia, *Atlas of Ultrasound-Guided Central Venous Catheter Placement*, https://doi.org/10.1007/978-3-031-61887-1_15

15.2 Scanning Technique

- Do a preliminary vascular assessment (non-sterile), known as rapid central vein assessment (RaCeVA).
- The operator stands at the patient's head on the right side.
- Since the supraclavicular fossa at this age is very small, it is recommended to use a high-frequency linear transducer (13–6 MHz) with a hockey stick type.
- The ultrasound is placed at the patient's feet in front of the operator or to the side of the right shoulder.
- Scan the middle of the right neck with the transducer transverse and the tip of the hockey stick to the patient's left side (Fig. 15.1).
- View of cervical vessels in short-axis (SAX) view (Figs. 15.2 and 15.3).
- Sweep down to the clavicle.
- Place the transducer in contact with the clavicle in the right supraclavicular fossae between the inner third of the clavicle and the sternal notch. Maintain the tip of the hockey stick transducer to the left (Fig. 15.4).
- Tilt posteriorly, and with the shaft of the transducer almost in contact with the patient's mandible, the right brachiocephalic vein (RBCV) will be visible following the right subclavian vein (RSCV) (Fig. 15.5).
  - The aim of tilting the transducer is to visualize the retroclavicular and thoracic inlet area to identify the RBCV in the long-axis (LAX) view and perform the puncture in this view.
  - LAX view of the right internal jugular vein (RIJV), right subclavian vein (RSCV), RBCV, left brachiocephalic vein (LBCV), and superior vena cava (SVC) (Figs. 15.6 and 15.7).

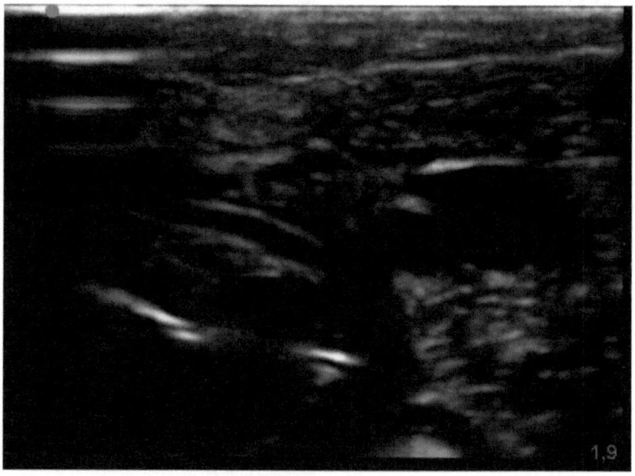

Fig. 15.2 Scan in the middle of the right neck. SAX view of cervical vessels
- The probe indicator is on the patient's left side, identified on the screen as the aqua dot at the top left of the image
- The scan depth is 1,9 cm

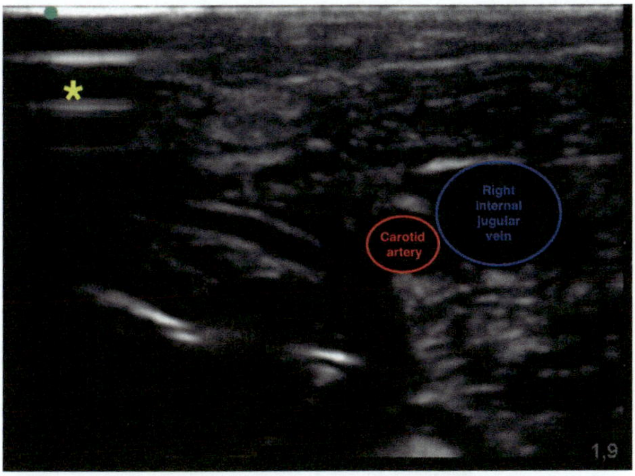

Fig. 15.3 Identifying structures

- The right internal jugular vein (RIJV) is lateral to the right carotid artery (RCA)
- *Indicates the lack of contact of the transducer on the patient's skin. The medial part of the transducer (left of the patient) is not in contact with the patient. This view is translated in this ultrasonographic image by transverse lines as barcodes that indicate this lack of contact of the transducer

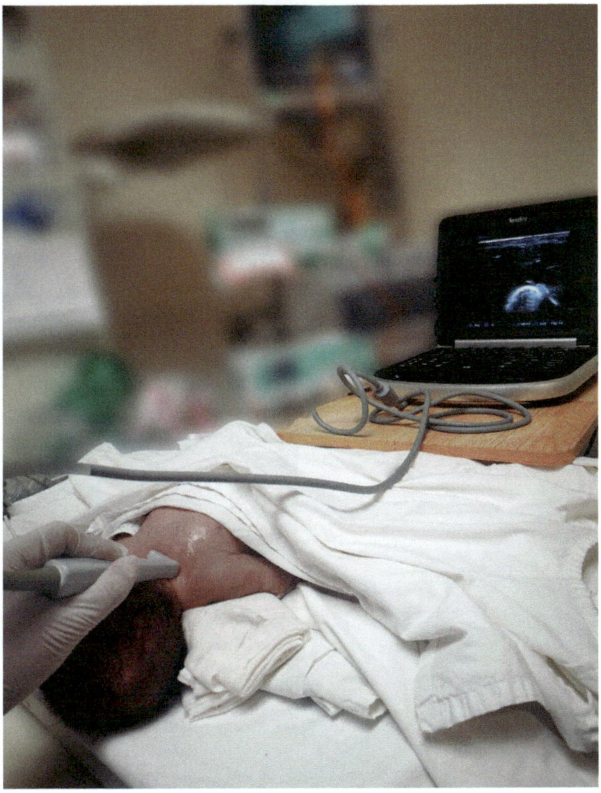

Fig. 15.4 Transducer in the right supraclavicular fossae with the tip to the left

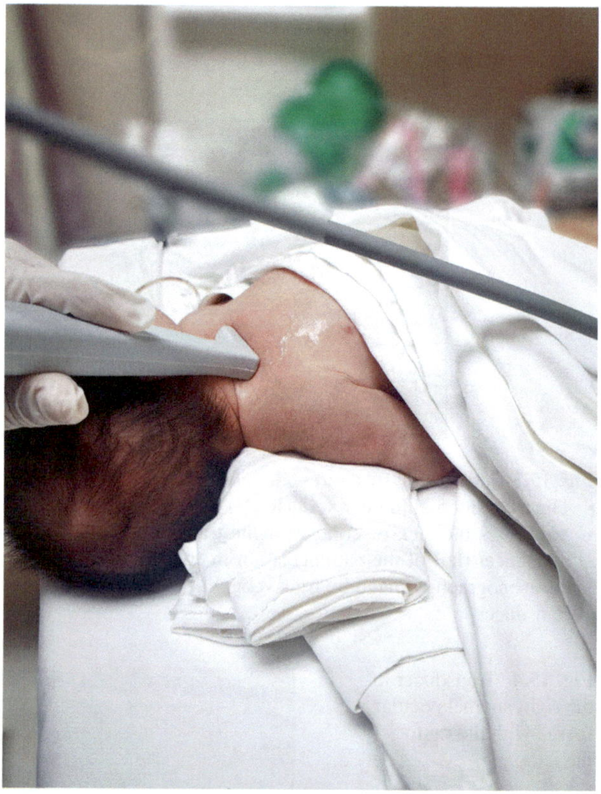

Fig. 15.5 Place the transducer between the inner third of the clavicle and the sternal notch and tilt to posterior

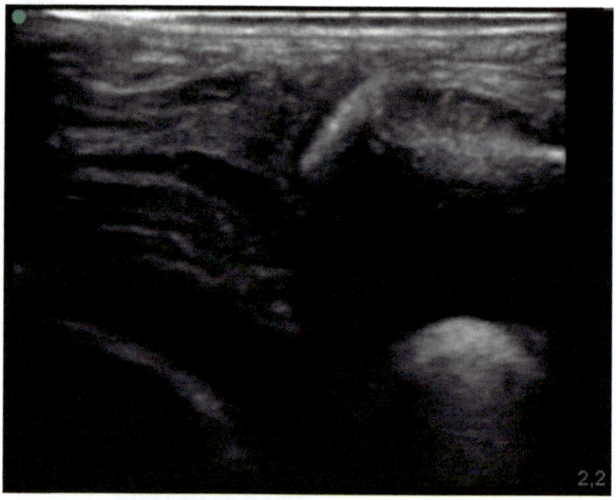

Fig. 15.6 Scan of the retroclavicular and thoracic inlet veins. LAX view

- The diameter of the RBCV is 4,0 cm
- Scan depth is 2,2 cm

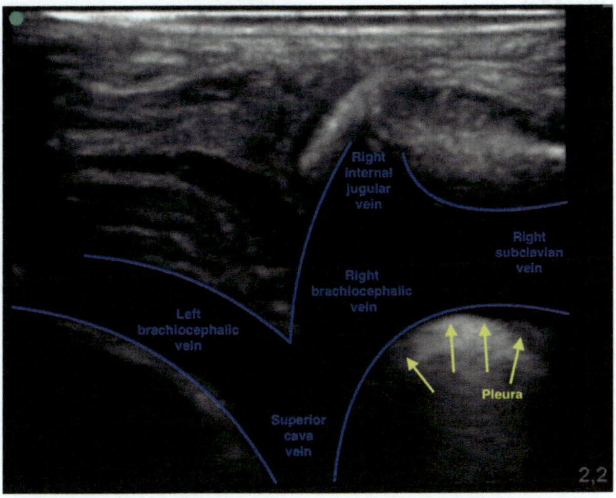

Fig. 15.7 Identifying structures—two confluences are identified
- The formation of the RBCV from the influx of the RIJV and the RSCV
- The formation of the SVC from the inflow of the RBCV and LBCV

15.3 Local Anesthesia Application

- The sterile field only leaves the cervical and upper pectoral regions uncovered.
- Operator's view of the right cervicothoracic area. The head is turned to the left (Fig. 15.8).
- Real-time ultrasound-guided lidocaine infiltration.
- For infiltration, use a small needle 25- 27-G.
- Use 1% lidocaine.
- Subcutaneous infiltration with lidocaine in the puncture tract 1,5–2 cm before the site chosen for RBCV puncture and the catheter fixation area.

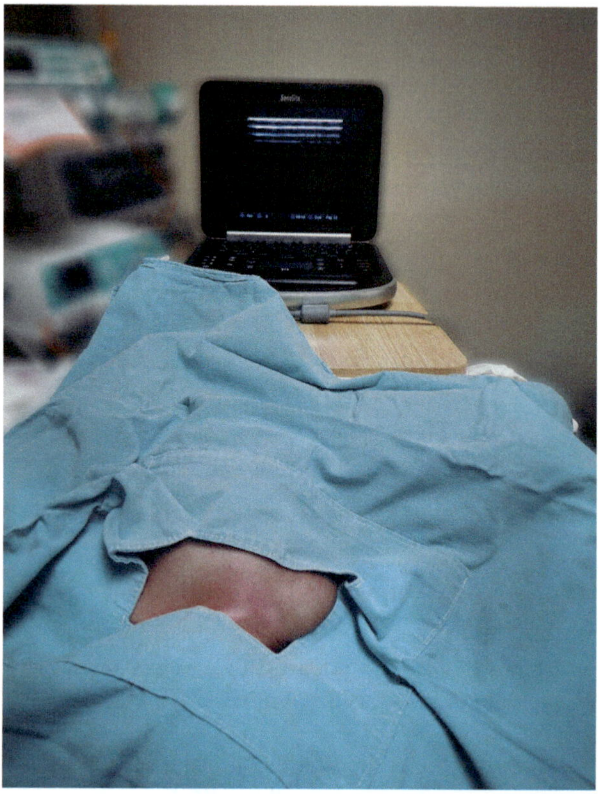

Fig. 15.8 Operator's view with the ultrasound at the feet of the patient

15.4 Steps for Real-Time Ultrasound-Guided Access to Right Brachiocephalic Vein in Neonates

15.4.1 Step 01

- We will use a Vygon® 3 Fr, 6-cm, double-lumen catheter. This type of catheter has a 21-G echogenic introducer needle, which helps better visualize, although you can also use a 24-G intravenous catheter.
- Place the transducer at the level of the right supraclavicular fossae with the tip of the transducer to the left between the inner third of the clavicle and the sternal notch.
- Tilt posteriorly and with the transducer shaft almost in contact with the patient's mandible to visualize the RBCV (Fig. 15.9).
- LAX view of retroclavicular and thoracic inlet veins (Figs. 15.10 and 15.11).
- Perform the puncture at an angle of 60°–70° to penetrate the skin and enter the subcutaneous tissue (Fig. 15.12).

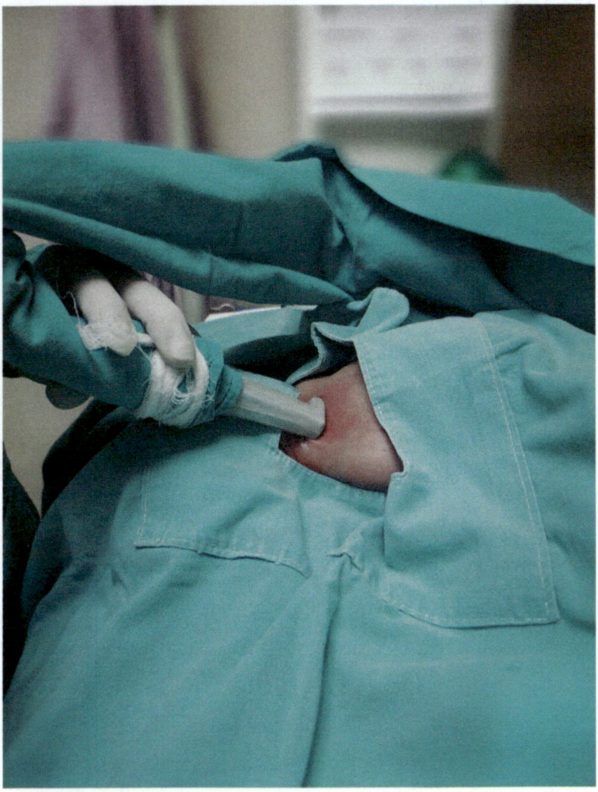

Fig. 15.9 Place the transducer at the level of the right supraclavicular fossae and tilt posteriorly, with the shaft of the transducer almost in contact with the patient's mandible

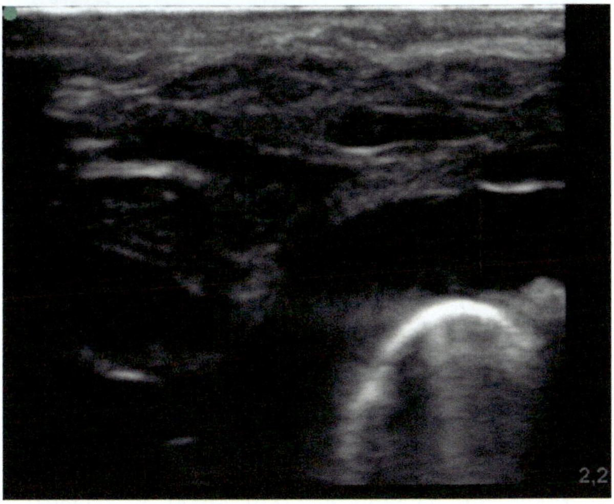

Fig. 15.10 Scan of the retroclavicular and thoracic inlet area. LAX view from the right supraclavicular fossae

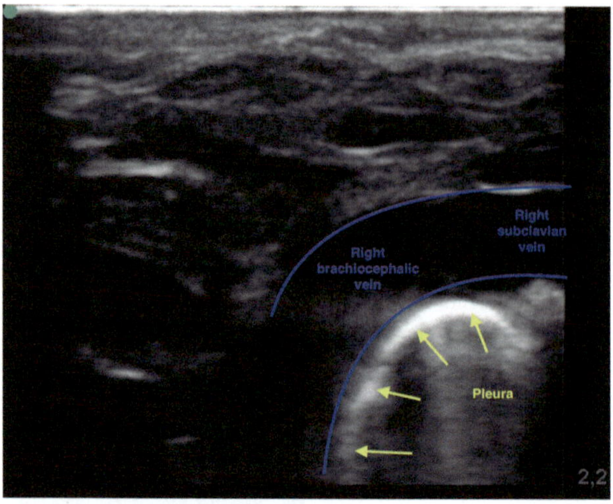

Fig. 15.11 Identifying structures
- The RSCV and its continuation with the RBCV
- The pleura in the inferior wall of the RSCV and the lateral wall of the RBCV

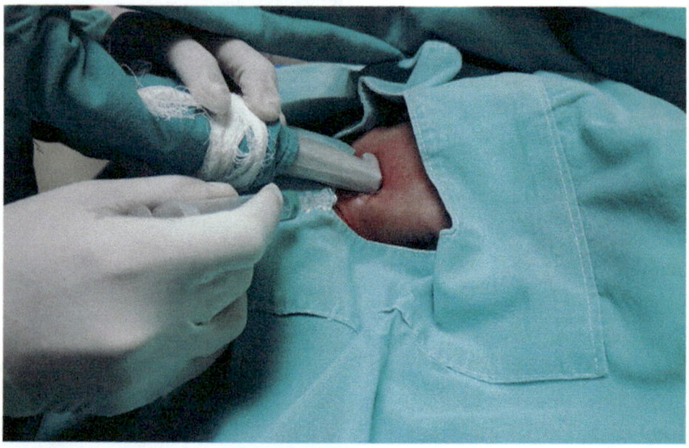

Fig. 15.12 Start the puncture at an angle of 60° to 70°

- Start the puncture of the posterior angle of the transducer, from lateral to medial and from posterior to anterior, to visualize the introducer needle in LAX.
- Since it is a short distance from the skin to the vein, introduce the needle slowly.
- Because the RBCV has a more vertical trajectory, the LAX introducer needle will not be displayed transversely on the screen but rather obliquely (Figs. 15.13 and 15.14).

15.4.2 Step 02

- Modify the puncture angle to 50–60° to visualize the introducer needle so the needle will be below the insonation area of the transducer (Fig. 15.15).
- Always perform the puncture with dynamic needle tracking (DNT).
- Follow the path of the oblique puncture toward the RBCV.

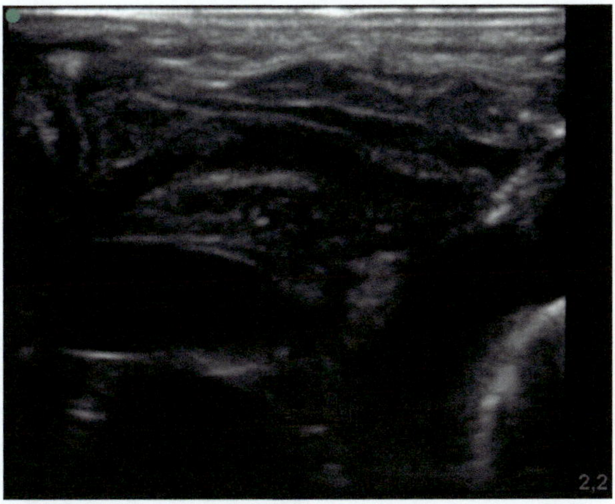

Fig. 15.13 LAX view of the start of the RBCV puncture

- The echogenic introducer needle helps better visualize it

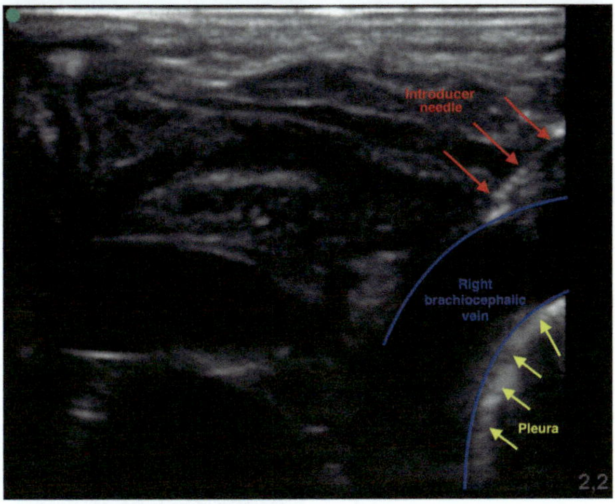

Fig. 15.14 Identifying structures

- The introducer needle has an oblique direction located on the anterior wall of the RBCV

- Visualization of the deformation of the anterior wall of the RBCV caused by compression of the introducer needle demonstrates the correct path of the puncture toward the vein (Figs. 15.16 and 15.17).

15.4.3 Step 03

- Follow the puncture path to penetrate the vein. When you feel a loss of resistance (indicating vein cannulation), you will also see the intravascular location of the introducer needle on the screen in real time (Fig. 15.18).
- LAX view of the cannulation of the RBCV (Figs. 15.19 and 15.20).

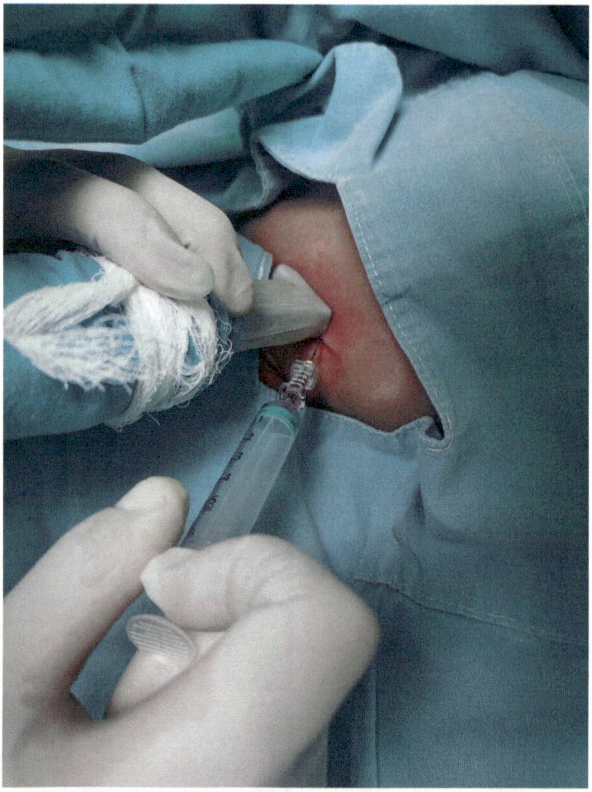

Fig. 15.15 Follow the path of the oblique puncture with DNT

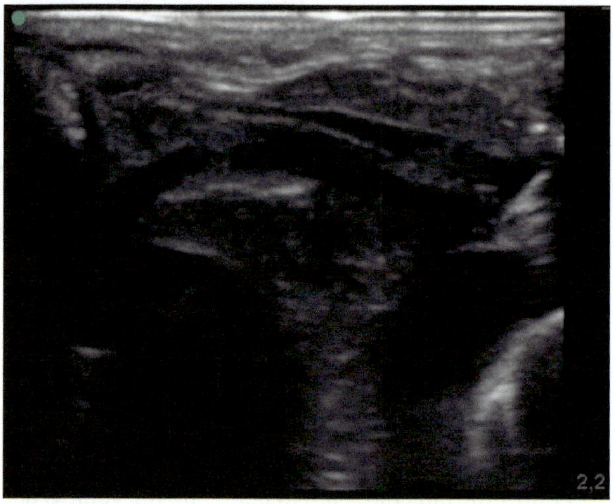

Fig. 15.16 LAX view of the compression of the anterior wall of the RBCV

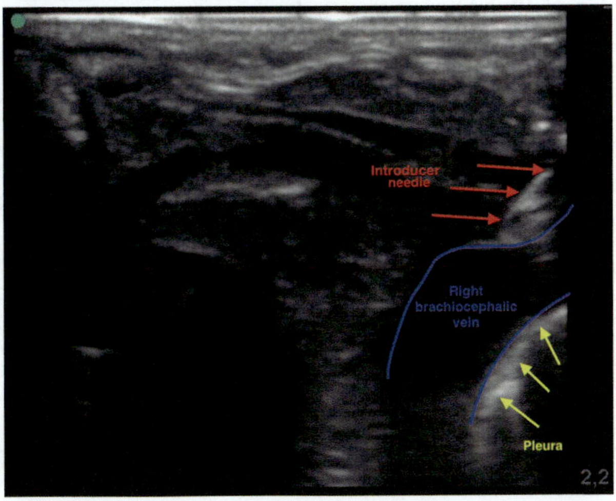

Fig. 15.17 Identifying structures

- The deformation of the anterior wall of the RBCV caused by compression of the puncture caused by the introducer needle indicates that we are on the right track
- Continue the path of the puncture

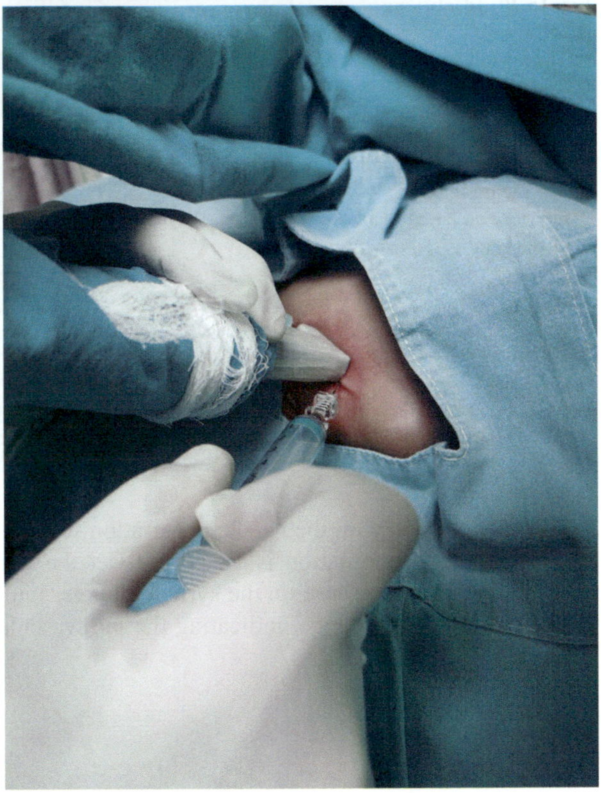

Fig. 15.18 Continue the puncture trajectory and cannulate the RBCV

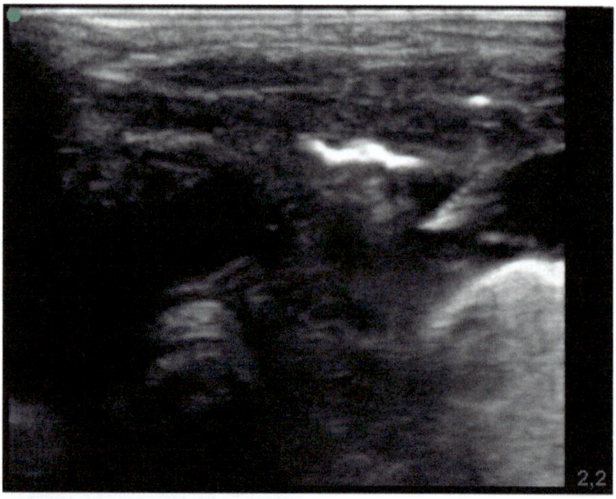

Fig. 15.19 LAX view of the cannulation of the RBCV

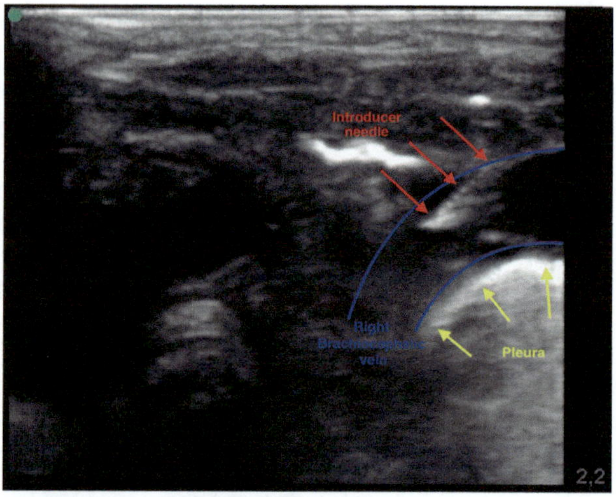

Fig. 15.20 Identifying structures
- The introducer needle, in its oblique course, is intravascular. Since it is an echogenic needle, it can be easily identified
- The pleura in the inferior and lateral wall of the vein

- Do not continue with the needle penetration so as not to cross the vein.
- Once RBCV cannulation is visualized, set the transducer aside and maintain gentle negative pressure on the syringe plunger until a flash of blood appears in the barrel of the syringe, indicating the intravascular location of the introducer needle (Fig. 15.21).

15.4.4 Step 04

- Insert the 0,3-mm nitinol guidewire, which should pass easily (Fig. 15.22).

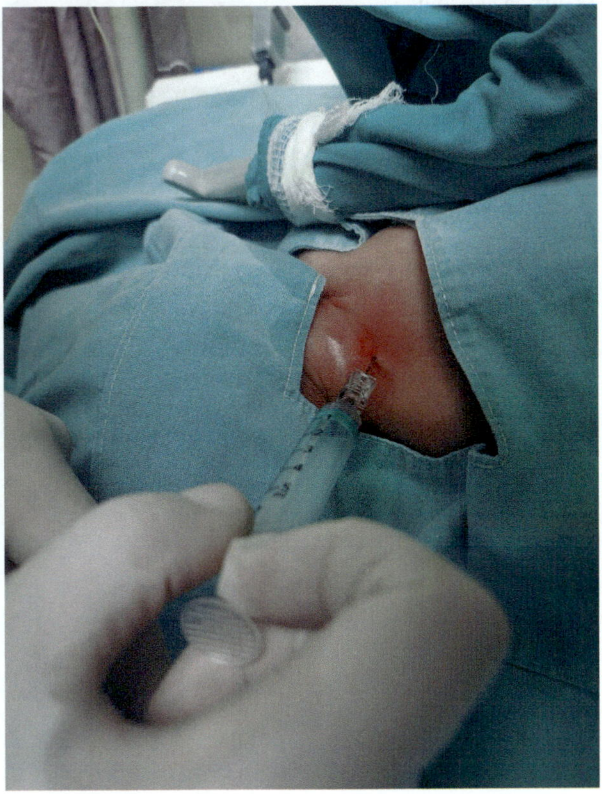

Fig. 15.21 Set the transducer aside, apply gentle negative pressure, and check for the return of blood in the barrel of the syringe

- This type of guidewire is marked every 10 cm, so the guidewire should not go beyond the first 5 cm.
- Place the transducer in the supraclavicular fossae to identify the intravascular guidewire (Fig. 15.23).
- LAX view of the intravascular guidewire (Figs. 15.24 and 15.25).

15.4.5 Step 05

- Once you corroborate the guidewire canalizing the RBCV, dilation of the skin toward the RBCV is performed.
- With your left hand, pull the skin so that the dilator can easily penetrate the skin (Fig. 15.26).

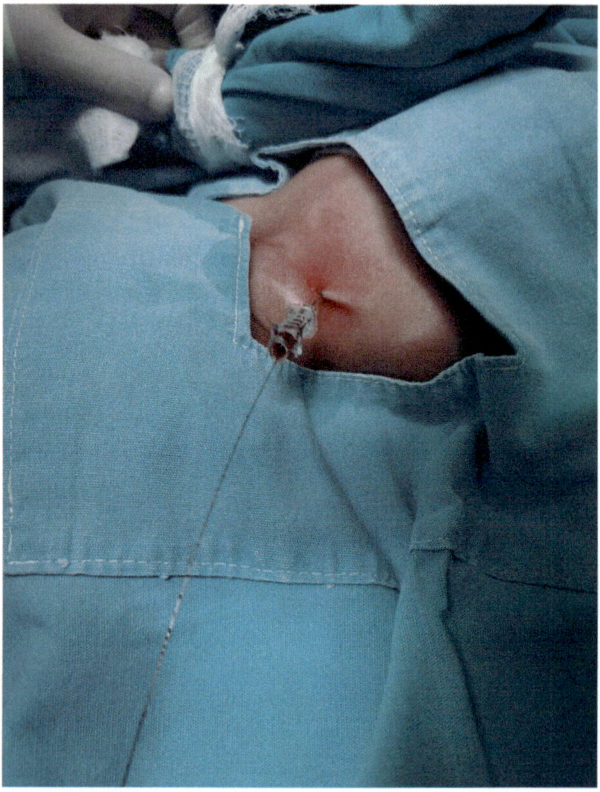

Fig. 15.22 Insert the guidewire

15.4.6 Step 06

- Introduce the 3 Fr, 6-cm, double-lumen catheter with Seldinger's technique and remove the guidewire (Fig. 15.27).
- Verify the intravascular location of the catheter by placing the transducer over the supraclavicular fossae (Fig. 15.28).
- LAX view of the intravascular catheter (Figs. 15.29 and 15.30).

15.4.7 Step 07

- Secure the catheter and place a sterile occlusive dressing according to the institutional protocol (Fig. 15.31).

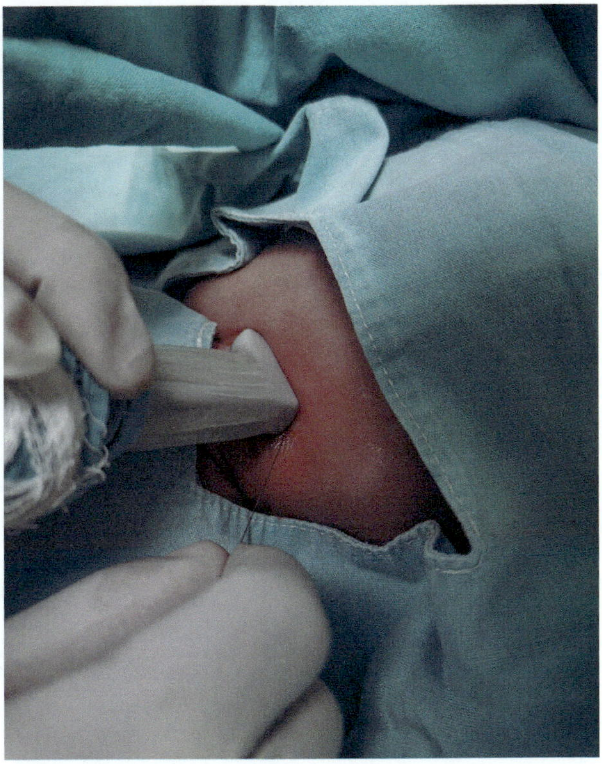

Fig. 15.23 Scan the supraclavicular fossae to verify the intravascular location of the guidewire

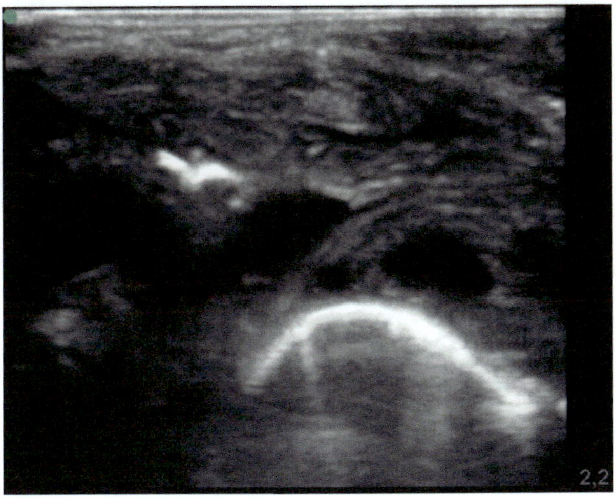

Fig. 15.24 LAX view of the intravascular guidewire

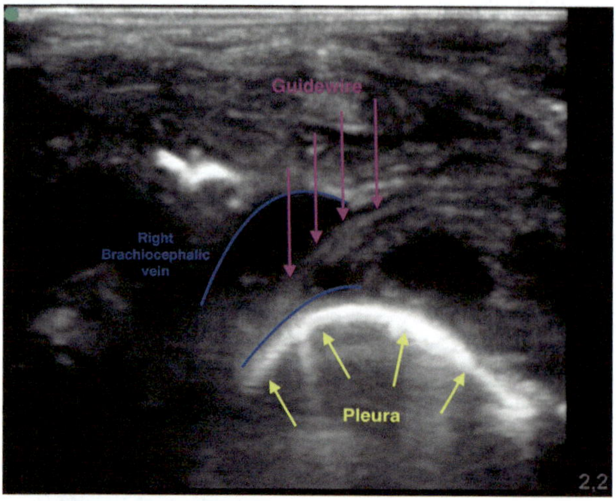

Fig. 15.25 Identifying structures

- The guidewire presents a downward path in the direction of the SVC

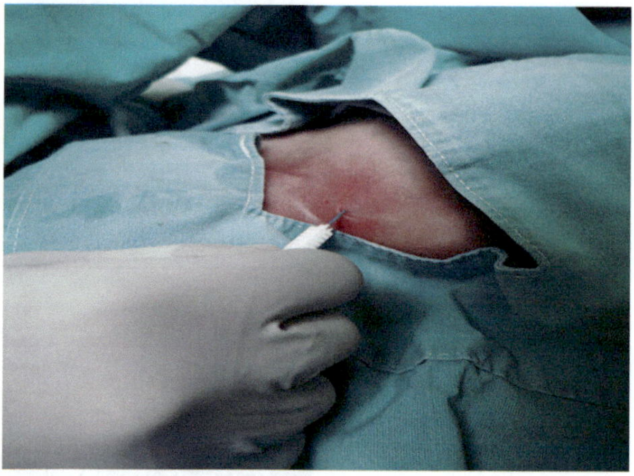

Fig. 15.26 Dilation of the skin

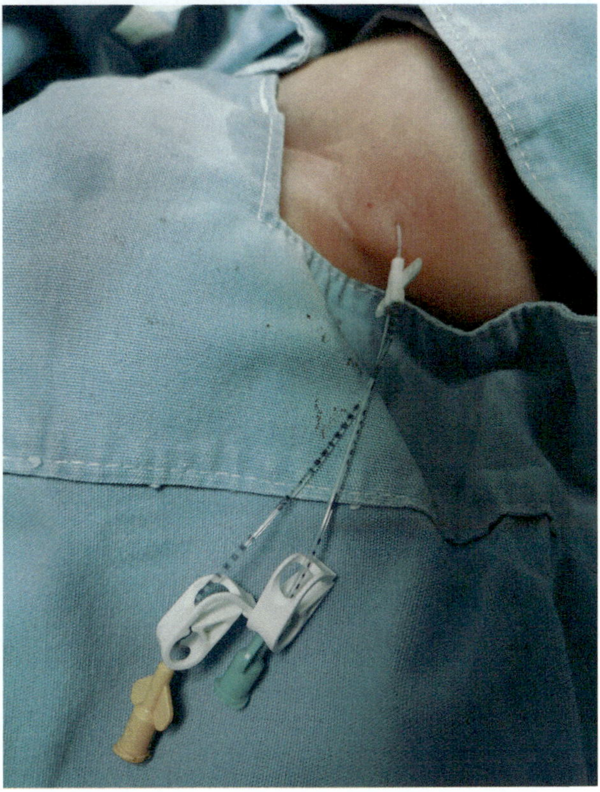

Fig. 15.27 Seldinger's technique: advance the catheter over the guidewire

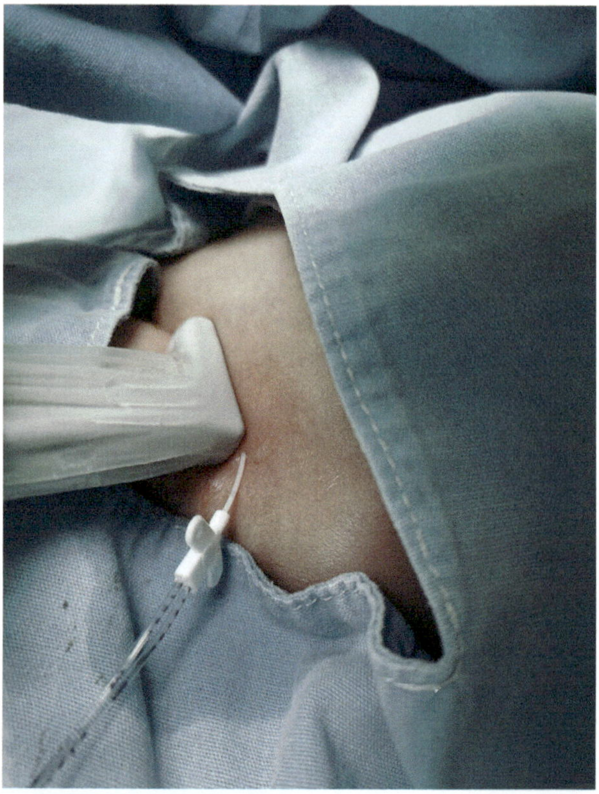

Fig. 15.28 Scan the intravascular location of the catheter

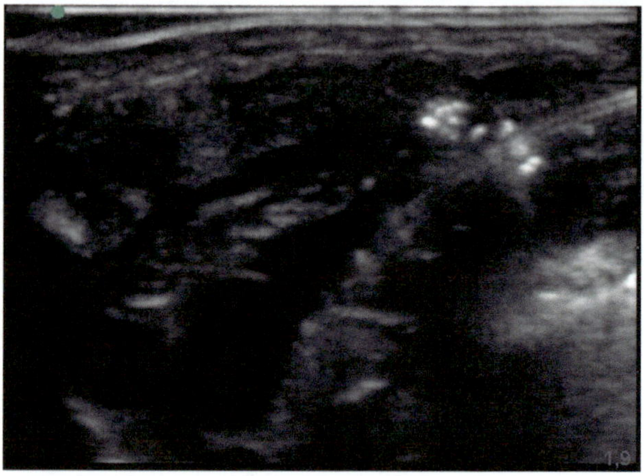

Fig. 15.29 LAX view of the intravascular catheter

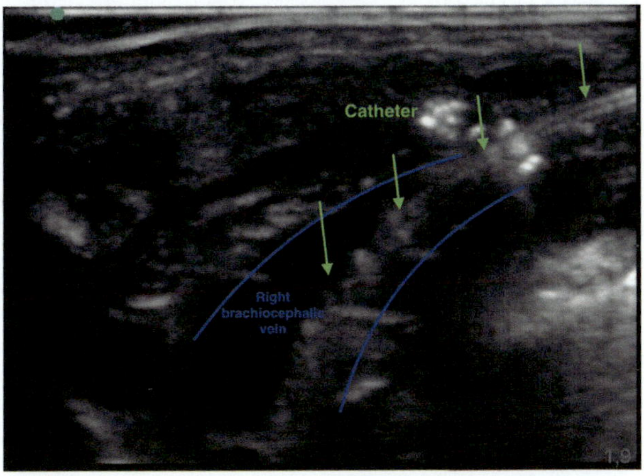

Fig. 15.30 Identifying structures

- We have decreased the scan depth to 1,9 cm, and the descending path of the catheter toward the SVC is identified

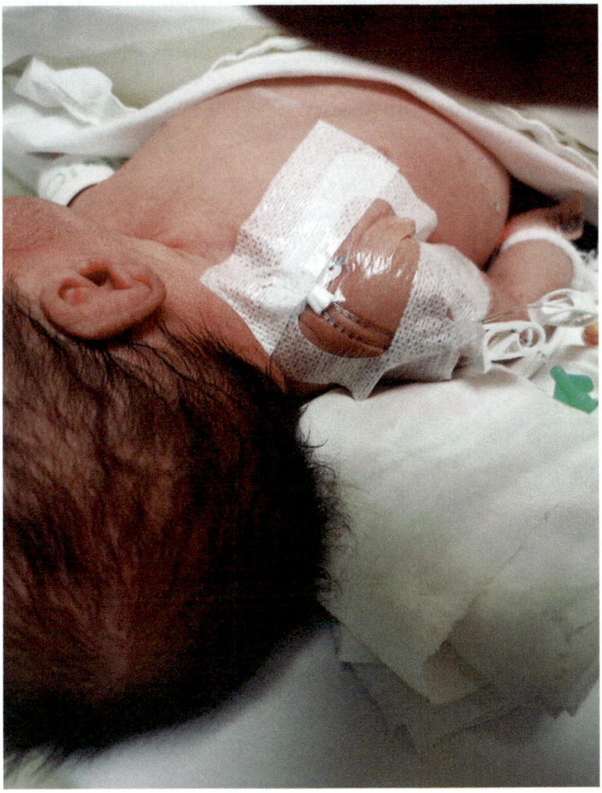

Fig. 15.31 Dressing according to the institutional protocol

Sources

1. Breschan C, Platzer M, Jost R, Stettner H, Beyer AS, Feigl G, Likar R. Consecutive, prospective case series of a new method for ultrasound-guided supraclavicular approach to the brachiocephalic vein in children. Br J Anaesth. 2011;106(5):732–7. https://doi.org/10.1093/bja/aer031. Epub 2011 Mar 17
2. Aytekin C, Özyer U, Harman A, Boyvat F. Ultrasound-guided brachiocephalic vein catheterization in infants weighing less than five kilograms. J Vasc Access. 2015;16(6):512–4. https://doi.org/10.5301/jva.5000385. Epub 2015 May 30
3. Breschan C, Graf G, Jost R, Stettner H, Feigl G, Goessler A, Neuwersch S, Koestenberger M, Likar R. Ultrasound-guided supraclavicular cannulation of the right brachiocephalic vein in small infants: a consecutive, prospective case series. Paediatr Anaesth. 2015;25(9):943–9. https://doi.org/10.1111/pan.12700. Epub 2015 Jun 17
4. Oulego-Erroz I, Alonso-Quintela P, Terroba-Seara S, Jiménez-González A, Rodríguez-Blanco S, Vázquez-Martínez JL. Ultrasound-guided cannulation of the brachiocephalic vein in neonates and preterm infants: a prospective observational study. Am J Perinatol. 2018;35(5):503–8. https://doi.org/10.1055/s-0037-1608803. Epub 2017 Nov 28
5. Spagnuolo F, Vacchiano T. Ultrasound-guided cannulation of the brachiocephalic vein in newborns: a novel approach with a supraclavicular view for tip navigation and tip location. J Vasc Access. 2022;23(4):515–23. https://doi.org/10.1177/11297298211001159. Epub 2021 Mar 16
6. Breschan C, Graf G, Arneitz C, Stettner H, Neuwersch S, Stadik C, Koestenberger M, Holasek S, Likar R. Retrospective evaluation of 599 brachiocephalic vein cannulations in neonates and preterm infants. Br J Anaesth. 2022;129(5):e138–40. https://doi.org/10.1016/j.bja.2022.08.006. Epub 2022 Sep 13

Chapter 16
Left Brachiocephalic Vein in Pediatrics

16.1 Patient Positioning

- The patient is a 10-year-old weighing 52 kg.
- Position the patient supine, close to the left side of the bed or stretcher.
- Position the patient's head to the right.
- Place a roll under the shoulders to extend the neck, placing the head lower than the left shoulder (Fig. 16.1).
- The goal of patient positioning for this procedure is to increase the cervical area between the mandible and clavicle to gain access to the supraclavicular fossae.
- Gentle support of the upper extremities is performed with the arm caudal.

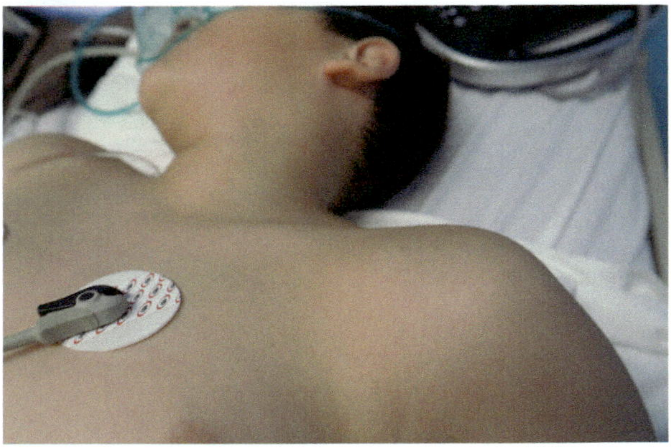

Fig. 16.1 Patient position

F. Montes-Tapia, *Atlas of Ultrasound-Guided Central Venous Catheter Placement*, https://doi.org/10.1007/978-3-031-61887-1_16

16.2 Scanning Technique

- Do a preliminary vascular assessment (non-sterile), known as rapid central vein assessment (RaCeVA).
- The operator stands on the left side of the patient at shoulder level.
- Place the ultrasound device above the patient's head or in front of the operator (Fig. 16.2).
- A high-frequency linear transducer (13–6 MHz) with a 5-cm footprint probe can be used.
- Star the scan in the middle of the left neck with the transducer transverse and the probe indicator to the patient's right side (Fig. 16.3).
- Begin the scan of the vessels in short-axis (SAX) view and sweep down to the clavicle.
- Scan view of cervical vessels in the middle of the neck (Figs. 16.4 and 16.5).
- Continue sweeping downward, and before entering in contact with the clavicle, scan the cervical vessels again (Fig. 16.6).

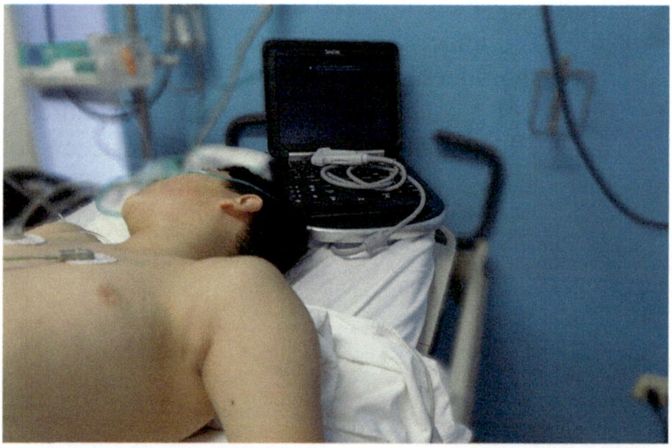

Fig. 16.2 Place the ultrasound device above the patient's head

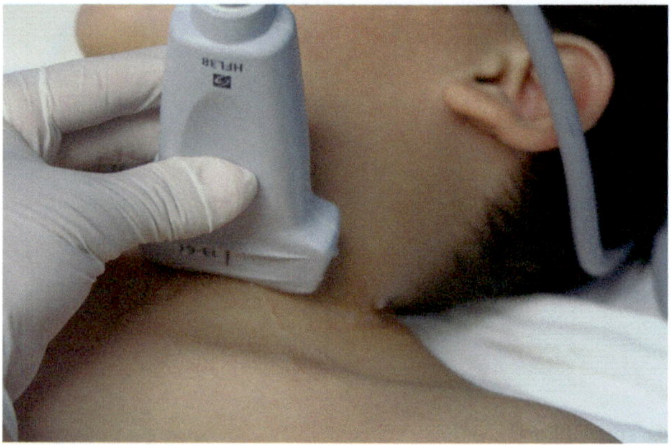

Fig. 16.3 Star the scan in the middle of the left neck

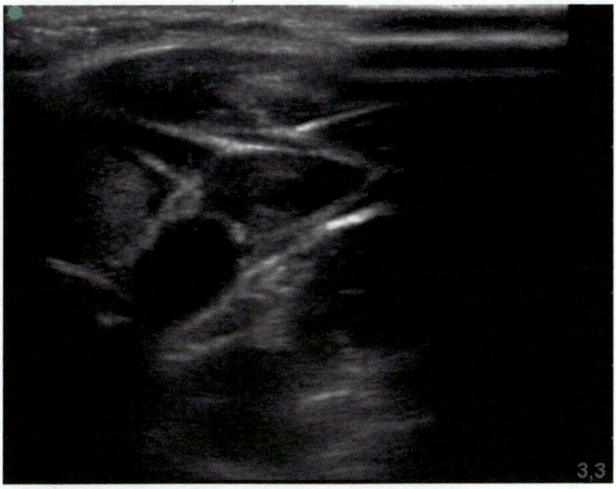

Fig. 16.4 Scan of the middle of the neck. SAX view of cervical vessels

- The probe indicator is on the patient's right side, identified on the screen as the aqua dot at the top left of the image
- The scan depth is 3,3 cm

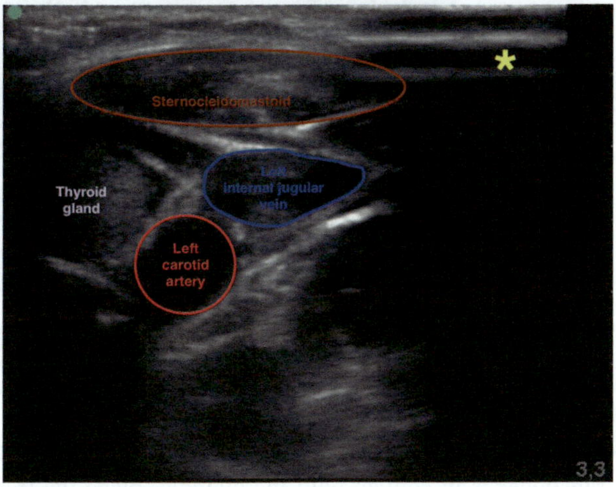

Fig. 16.5 Identifying structures

- The left internal jugular vein (LIJV) and left carotid artery (LCA) are under the sternocleidomastoid muscle
- The LIJV is lateral and anterior to the LCA
- The LIJV differs from the artery on compression since the vein will change to oval but not the artery
- *Indicates the lack of contact of the transducer on the patient's skin – See in Fig. 16.3 that the transducer's lateral part (left of the patient) is not in contact with the patient. This view is translated in this ultrasonographic image by transverse lines as barcodes that indicate this lack of contact of the transducer
- The thyroid gland is medial to the cervical vessels

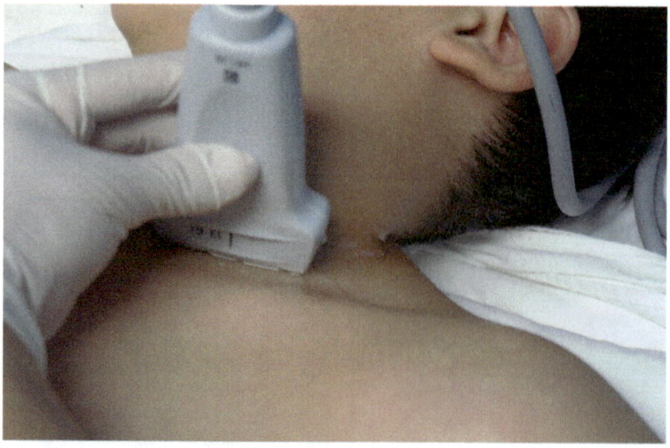

Fig. 16.6 Lower cervical scan before entering in contact with the clavicle

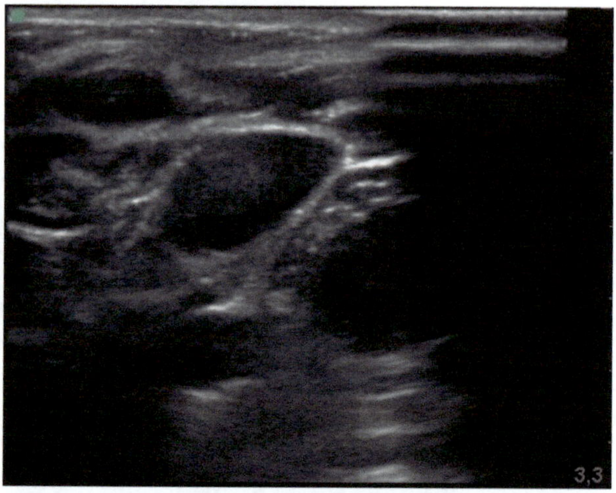

Fig. 16.7 Lower cervical scan. SAX view of cervical vessels

- Lower cervical scan. SAX view of cervical vessels (Figs. 16.7 and 16.8).
- When the transducer is in contact with the clavicle, place the transducer in the left supraclavicular fossae between the inner third of the clavicle and the sternal notch.
- Tilt the transducer back slightly (Fig. 16.9).
  - The aim of tilting the transducer is to visualize the retroclavicular area to identify the left brachiocephalic vein (LBCV) in LAX view and perform the puncture in this view (Figs. 16.10 and 16.11).
- From school age, the LBCV is more superficial behind the clavicle, so it does not require a lot of backward tilt to locate it. On the contrary, at lower ages, more tilt is required to access the LBCV.

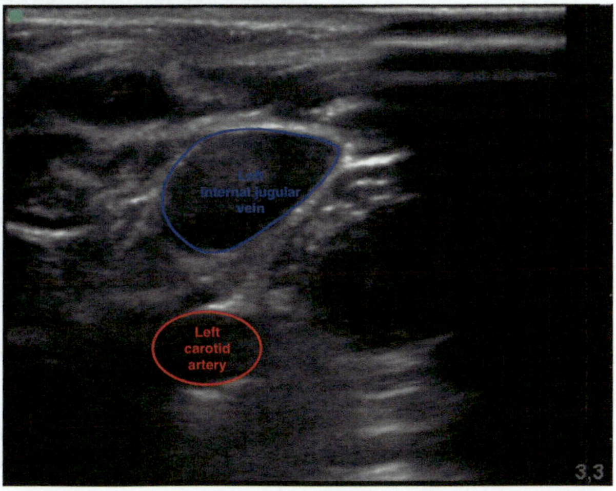

Fig. 16.8 Identifying structures
- The LCA becomes deep relative to the LIJV

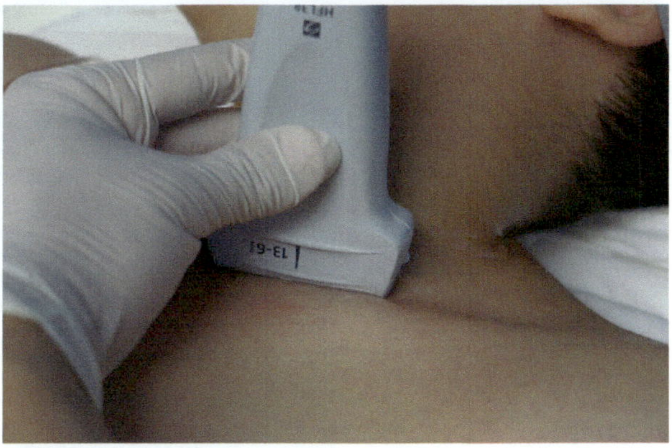

Fig. 16.9 Scan in the left supraclavicular fossae. Tilt the transducer back slightly

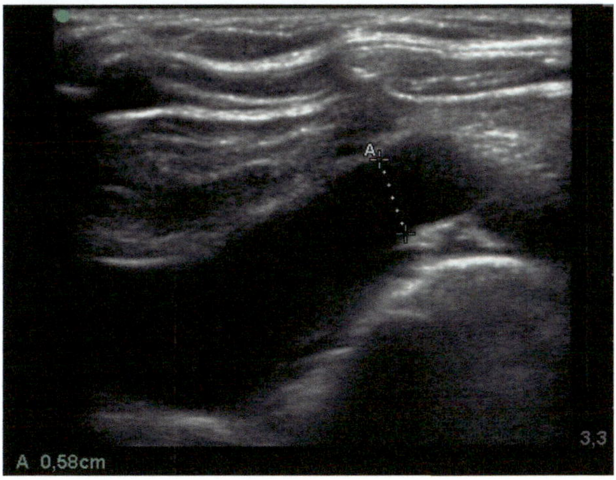

Fig. 16.10 Left supraclavicular fossae scan. LAX view of the left brachiocephalic vein
- The diameter of the LBCV is 0,58 cm

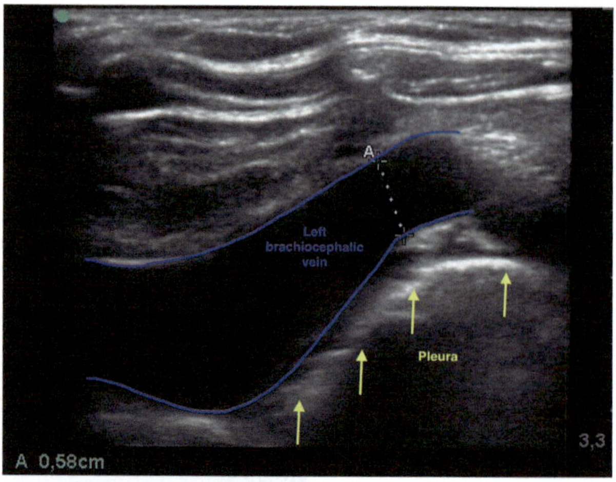

Fig. 16.11 Identifying structures
- The LBCV and its transverse trajectory toward the patient's right in the superior mediastinum
- The pleura is in contact with the posterior wall of the LBCV

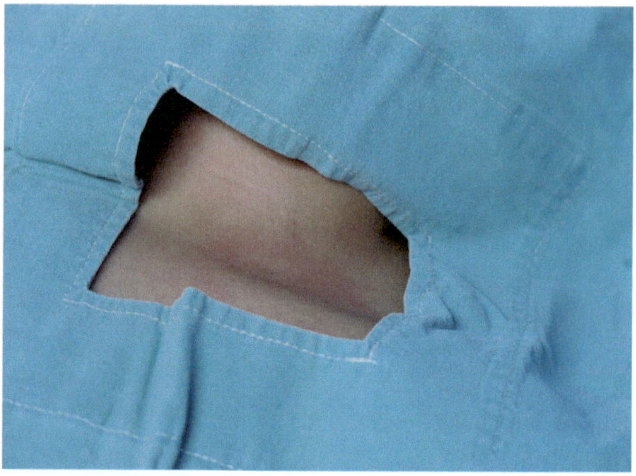

Fig. 16.12 Left supraclavicular region uncovered. The head is turned to the right

16.3 Local Anesthesia Application

- Real-time ultrasound-guided lidocaine infiltration.
- The sterile field only leaves the left supraclavicular region uncovered. The head is turned to the right (Fig. 16.12).
- The operator stands on the left side of the patient at shoulder level (Fig. 16.13).
- Align the transducer in the left supraclavicular fossae between the inner third of the clavicle and the sternal notch (Fig. 16.14).
- For infiltration, use a small needle 25 to 27 G.
- Use lidocaine 1%.
- Subcutaneous infiltration with lidocaine in the puncture tract 1,5–2 cm before the site chosen for LBCV puncture and the catheter fixation area (Fig. 16.15).

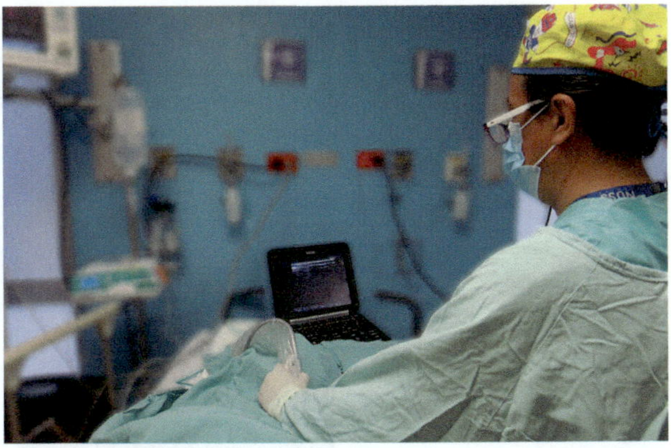

Fig. 16.13 Operator position

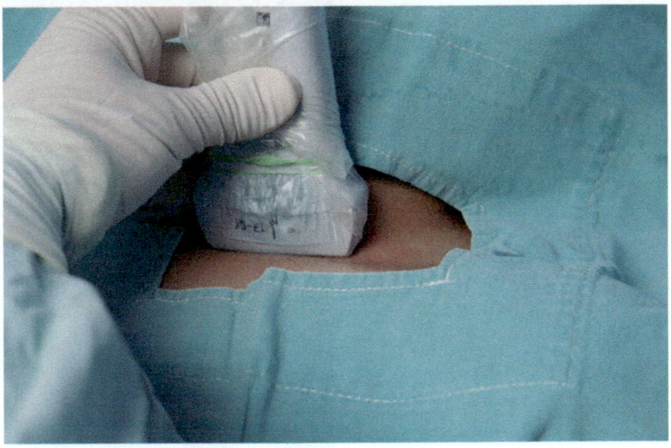

Fig. 16.14 Scan the left supraclavicular fossae. The head is turned to the right. Tilt the transducer back slightly

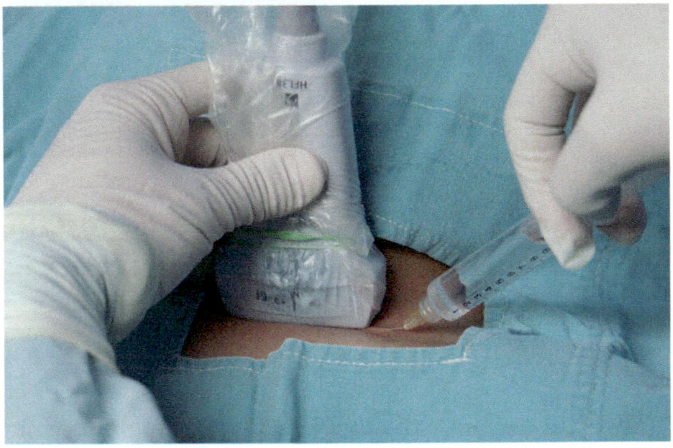

Fig. 16.15 Real-time ultrasound-guided lidocaine infiltration

- Scan of the retroclavicular and thoracic inlet veins. LAX view of lidocaine infiltration (Figs. 16.16 and 16.17).
- You can use the lidocaine infiltration puncture to guide where to perform the puncture with the introducer needle.

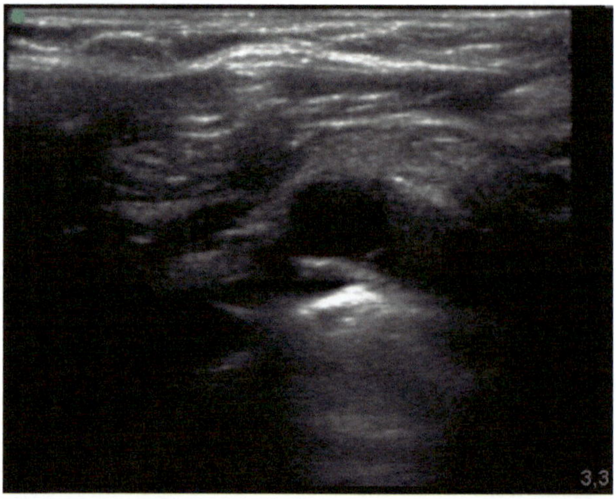

Fig. 16.16 Scan of the retroclavicular and thoracic inlet veins. LAX view of subcutaneous infiltration of lidocaine

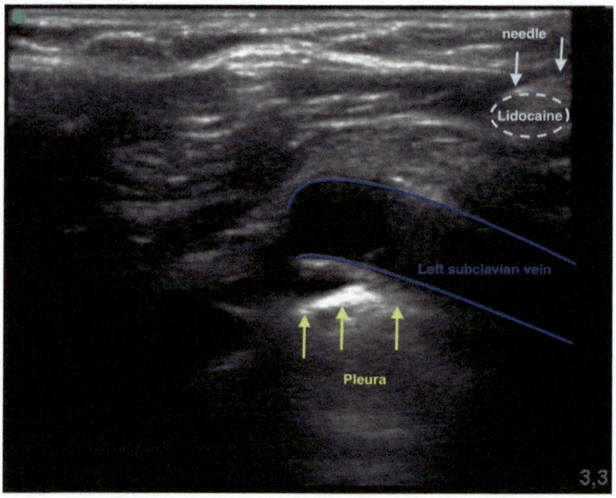

Fig. 16.17 Identifying structures
- LAX view of the infiltration in the subcutaneous tissue
- However, there is still no good alignment of the infiltration needle with the LBCV. Only the LSCV can be seen

16.4 Steps for Real-Time Ultrasound-Guided Access to Left Brachiocephalic Vein in Pediatrics

16.4.1 Step 01

- We will use an Arrow® 7 Fr, 20-cm, double-lumen catheter.
- Perform the puncture in LAX view in the left supraclavicular fossae (Fig. 16.18).
- Use an 18-G introducer needle with an Arrow® Raulerson spring-wire introduction syringe.
- Place the transducer in the left supraclavicular fossae.
- Perform the puncture in LAX.

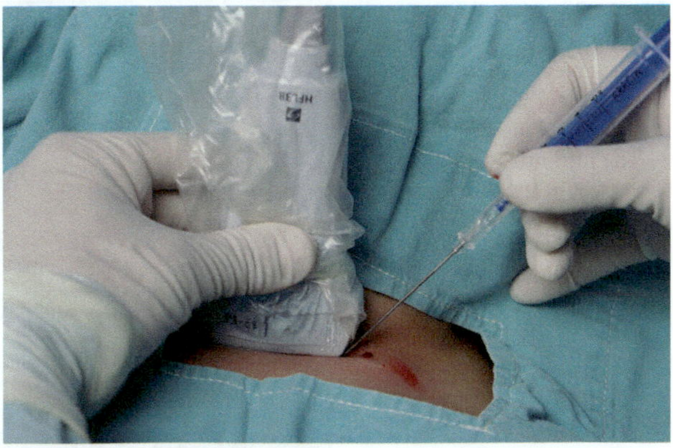

Fig. 16.18 Start the puncture at an angle of 60°–70°

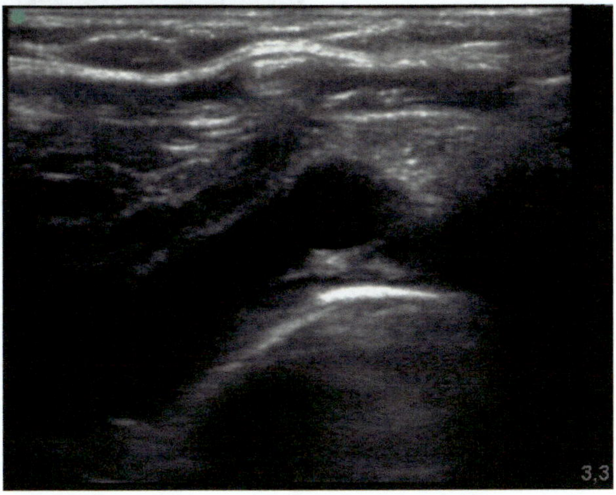

Fig. 16.19 LAX view of the start of the LBCV puncture

- Start the puncture at an angle of 50°–60° to penetrate below the footprint.
- Puncture from lateral to medial and posterior to anterior to visualize the introducer needle.
- Since it is a short distance from the skin to the vein, introduce the needle slowly.
- LAX view of the start of the puncture (Figs. 16.19 and 16.20).

16.4.2 Step 02

- The key point when puncturing any structure in LAX is to align the needle with the direction of the transducer; to achieve this, you need to puncture in the middle of the width of the transducer following the trajectory of the footprint (Fig. 16.21).

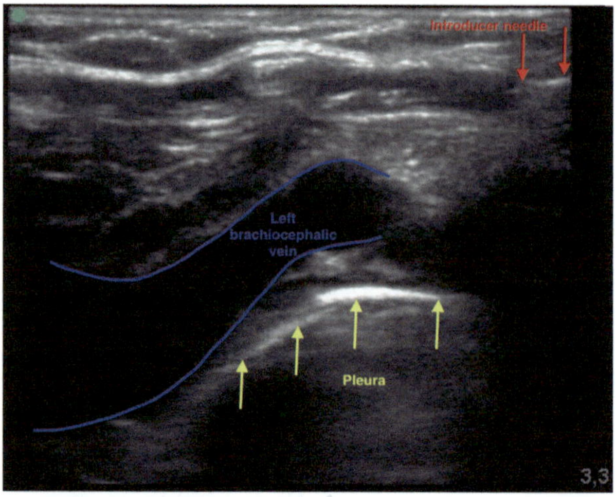

Fig. 16.20 Identifying structures

- The entry of the introducer needle into the subcutaneous tissue
- The introducer needle is not yet in the direction of the LBCV
- The pleura is in contact with the posterior wall of the LBCV

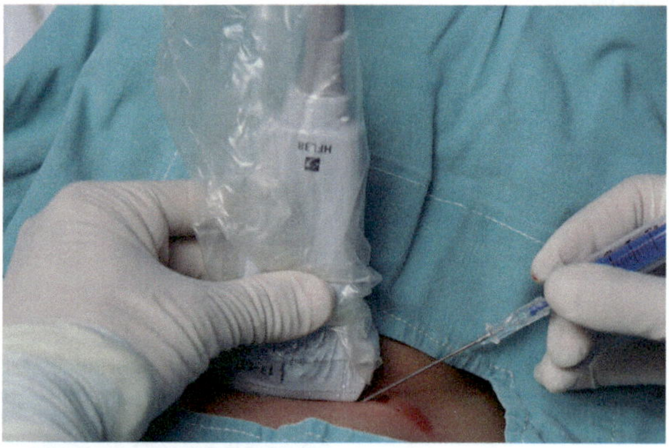

Fig. 16.21 Modify the puncture angle to 40–50°

- Always perform the puncture with dynamic needle tracking (DNT).
- Modify the puncture angle to 40°–50° in the direction of the LBCV.
- LAX view of puncture progression with modification of the puncture angle (Figs. 16.22 and 16.23).
- Advance the puncture, always in DNT (Fig. 16.24).
- LAX view of the puncture progression (Figs. 16.25 and 16.26).

16.4.3 Step 03

- Continue puncture in the same direction to cannulate the LBCV (Fig. 16.27).
- LAX view of the start of the anterior wall puncture of the LBCV (Figs. 16.28 and 16.29).

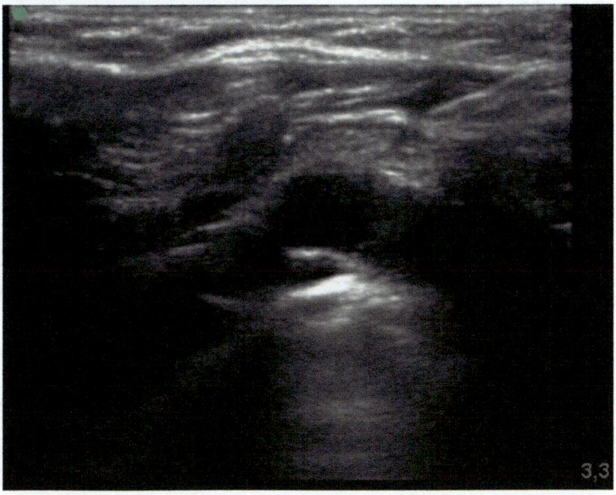

Fig. 16.22 LAX view of puncture progression with modification of the puncture angle

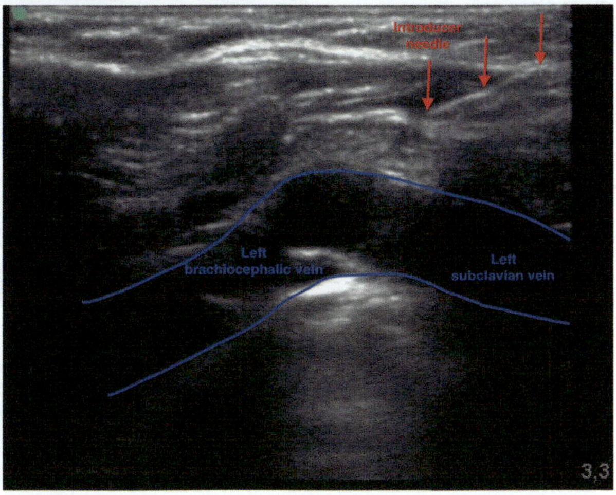

Fig. 16.23 Identifying structures

- Now, the introducer needle is in the direction of the LBCV

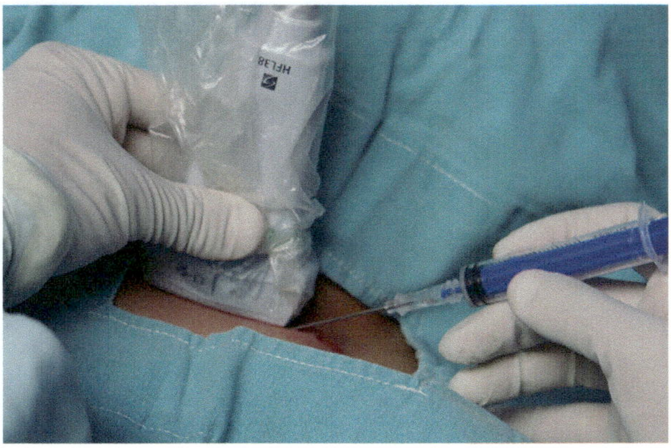

Fig. 16.24 Continue with the puncture in DNT

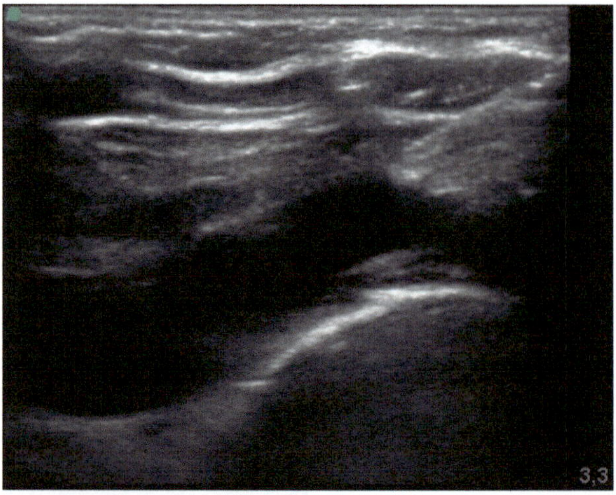

Fig. 16.25 LAX view of the puncture progression

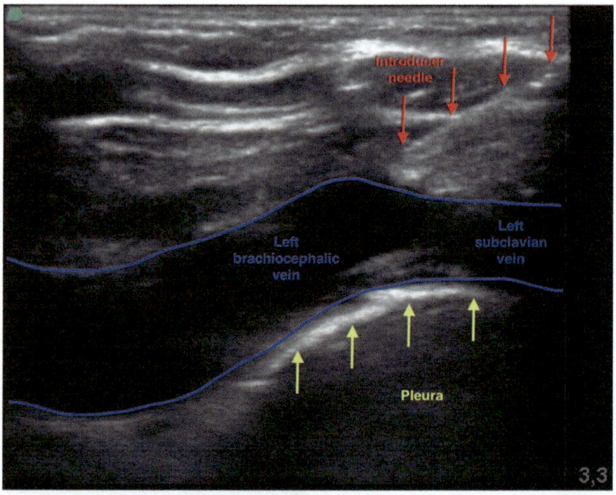

Fig. 16.26 Identifying structures
- LAX view of the introducer needle near the anterior wall of the LBCV

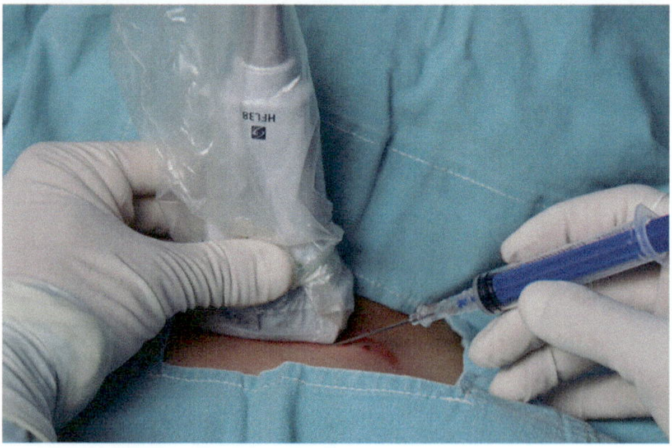

Fig. 16.27 Follow the puncture path to cannulate the vein

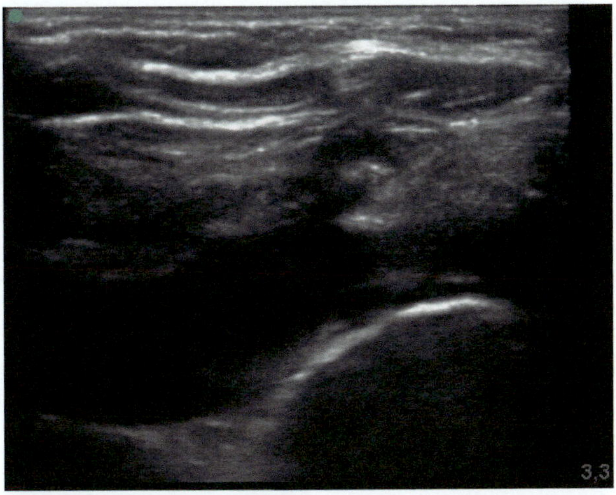

Fig. 16.28 LAX view of the start of the anterior wall puncture of the LBCV

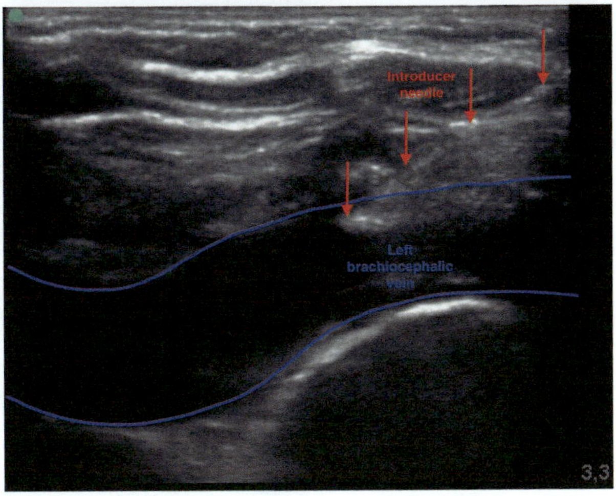

Fig. 16.29 Identifying structures
- The introducer needle initiates the penetration of the anterior wall of the LBCV

- Insert the introducer needle more deeply to adequately cannulate the LBCV (Fig. 16.30).
- Cannulation of the LBCV (Figs. 16.31 and 16.32).
- As soon as cannulation of the LBCV is visualized, aspirate the syringe, and when it returns blood, stop advancing the puncture (Fig. 16.33).
- LAX view of the LBCV cannulation (Figs. 16.34 and 16.35).
- Set the transducer aside.
- Apply gentle negative pressure on the syringe plunger until a flash of blood appears in the barrel of the syringe, indicating the intravascular position of the introducer needle (Fig. 16.36).

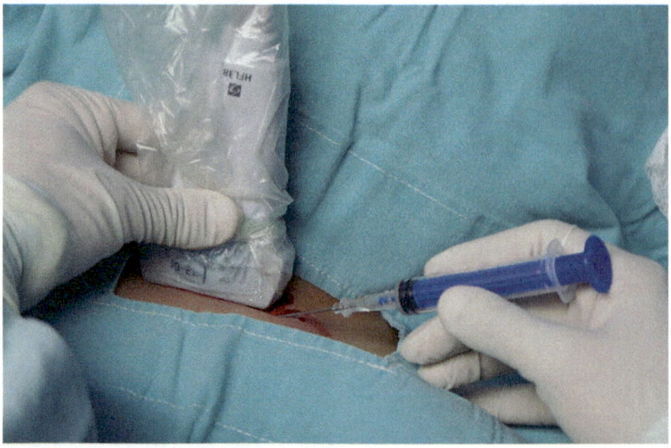

Fig. 16.30 Insert the introducer needle deeply to adequately cannulate the LBCV

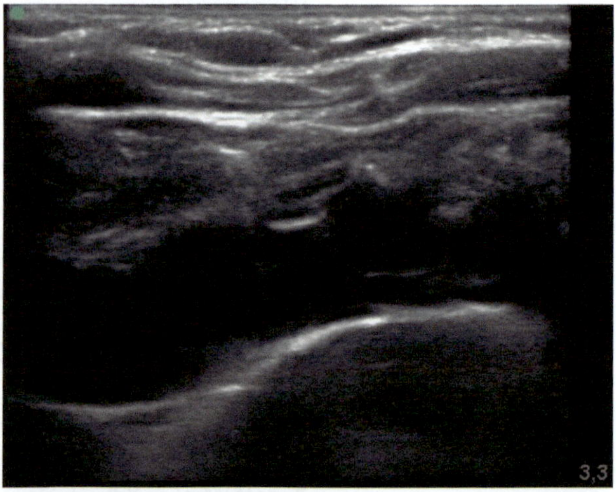

Fig. 16.31 LAX view of the cannulation of the LBCV

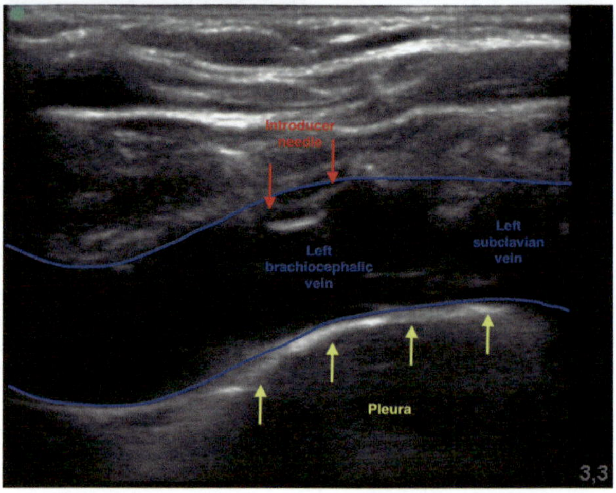

Fig. 16.32 Identifying structures

- The tip of the introducer needle penetrates the LBCV intravascularly

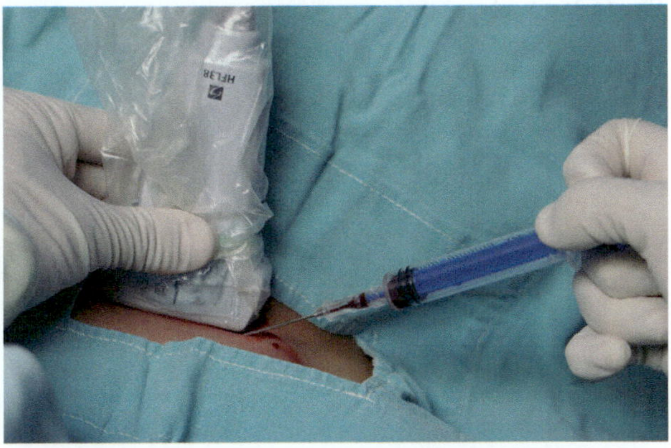

Fig. 16.33 Aspirate the syringe as soon the cannulation of the LBCV is visualized and stop advancing the puncture

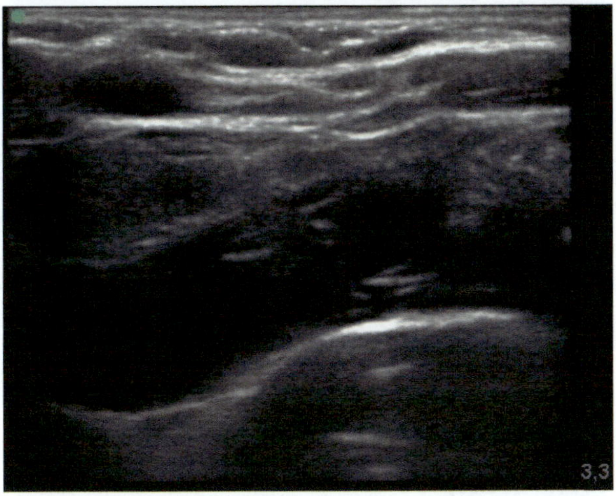

Fig. 16.34 LAX view of the LBCV cannulation

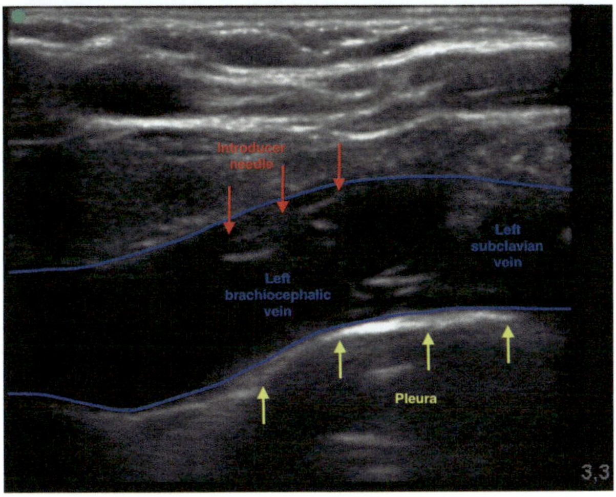

Fig. 16.35 Identifying structures

- The introducer needle is cannulating the LBCV, so the introduction of the needle is stopped
- The pleura is identified in the posterior wall of the LBCV and is parallel to the trajectory of the needle puncture

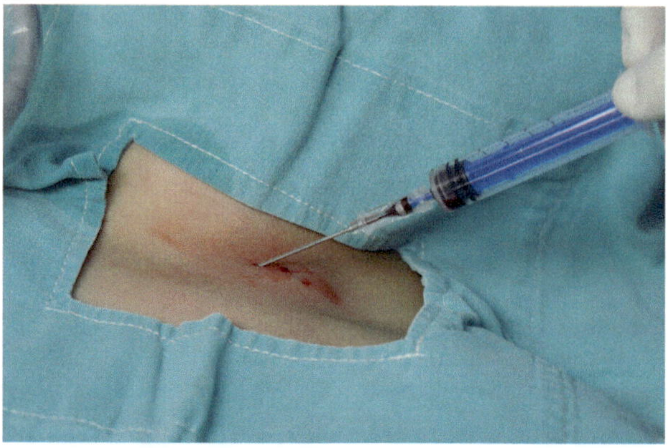

Fig. 16.36 Apply gentle negative pressure and check for the return of blood in the barrel of the syringe

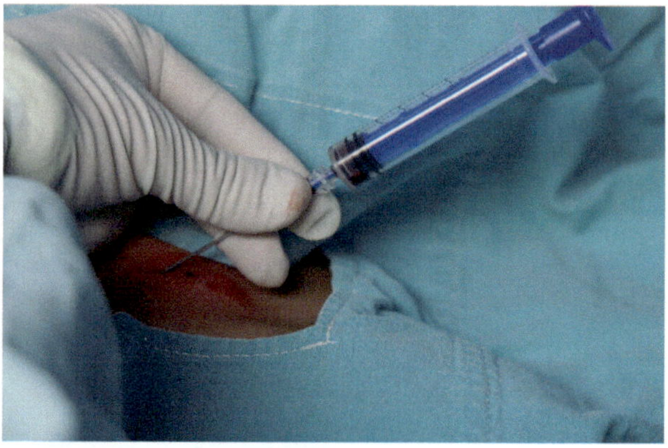

Fig. 16.37 Hold the needle hub firmly with your left hand

16.4.4 Step 04

- Hold the needle hub firmly with your left hand so the needle is not dislodged from its intravascular location (Fig. 16.37).
- Insert the 0.032" guidewire through the Arrow® Raulerson syringe and the introducer needle (Fig. 16.38).
- Once you have passed enough guidewire, remove the introducer needle and the ARROW® Raulerson syringe.
- With the left hand, a gauze covers the entry in the skin of the guidewire (Fig. 16.39).
- Place the transducer in the supraclavicular fossae to identify the intravascular guidewire (Fig. 16.40).
- LAX view of the intravascular guidewire (Figs. 16.41 and 16.42).

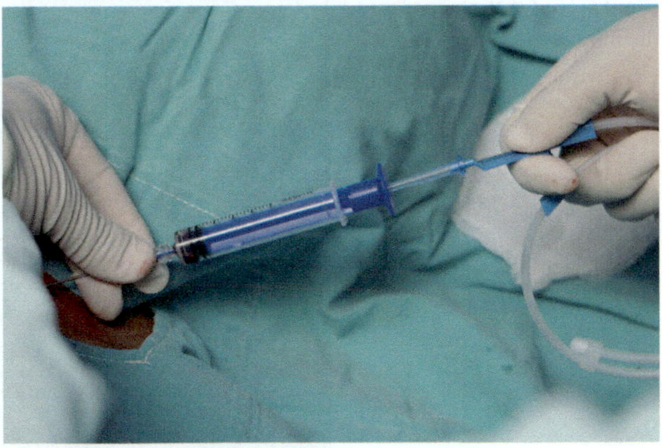

Fig. 16.38 Insert the guidewire

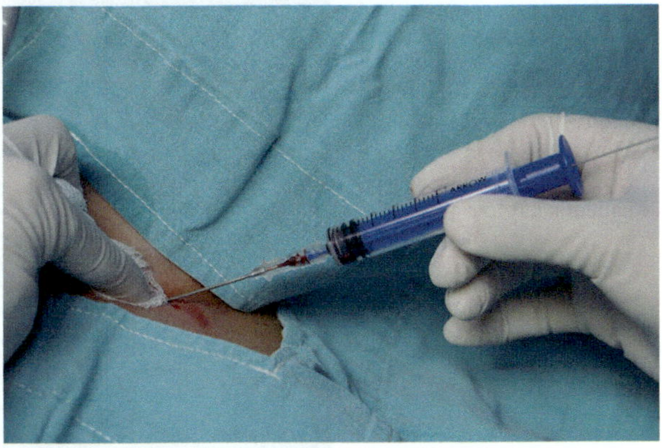

Fig. 16.39 Remove the introducer needle and the ARROW® Raulerson syringe

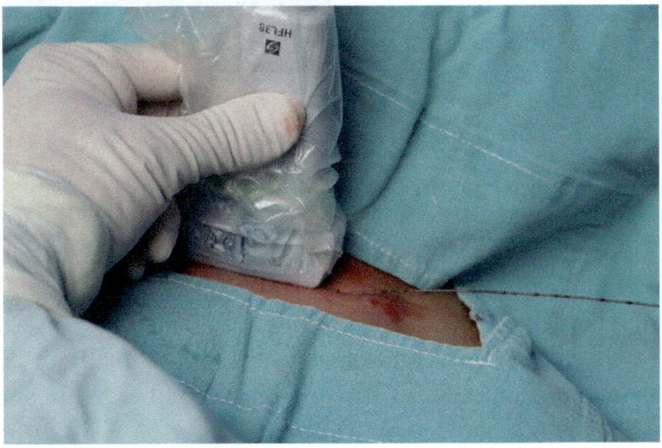

Fig. 16.40 Scan the supraclavicular fossae to verify the intravascular location of the guidewire

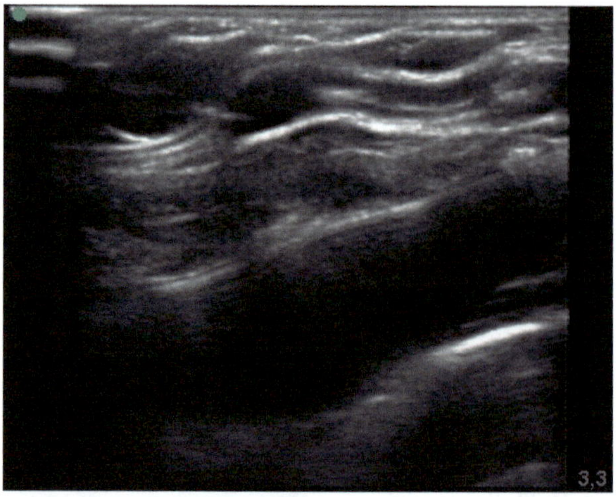

Fig. 16.41 LAX view of the intravascular guidewire

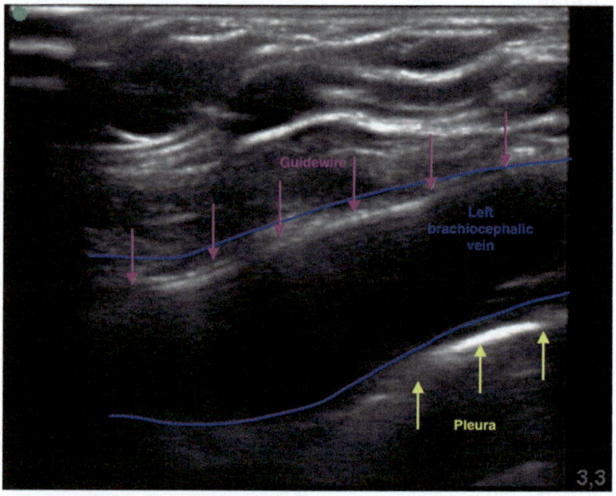

Fig. 16.42 Identifying structures
- The guidewire in the LBCV runs from the patient's left to right

16.4.5 Step 05

- It begins with the dilatation of the path of the skin toward the LBCV, contracting the skin with the index finger of the left hand so that the dilator can easily penetrate (Fig. 16.43).
- You will often not need to make an incision to insert the dilator.
- Use a corkscrew motion as needed to gradually insert the dilator (Fig. 16.44).
- The introduction of the dilator should be gentle so that the guidewire will not be bent.
- When you finish dilating, occlude the already dilated puncture entry site with gauze and your left hand so it does not bleed (Fig. 16.45).

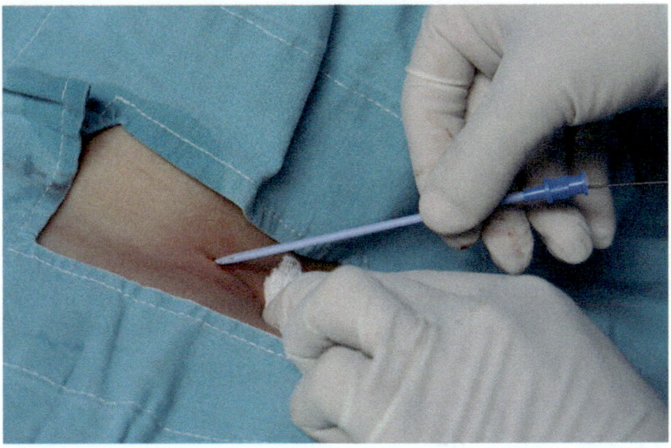

Fig. 16.43 Dilation of the skin

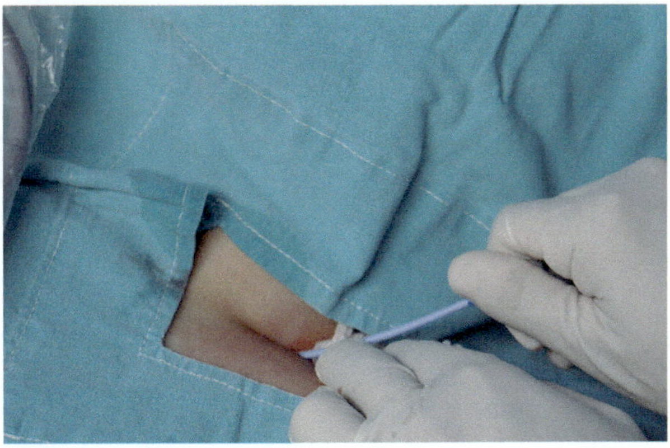

Fig. 16.44 Gentle introduction of the dilator

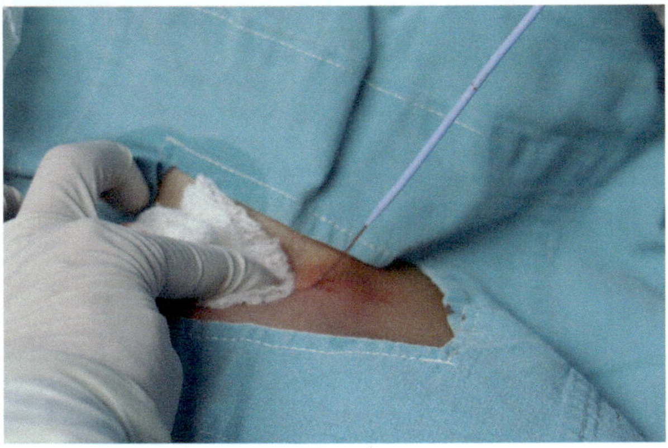

Fig. 16.45 Remove the dilator

16.4.6 Step 06

- With the left hand, hold the guidewire and insert the catheter over it (Fig. 16.46).
- Advance the catheter over the guidewire (Seldinger's technique) (Fig. 16.47).
- Remove the guidewire, check the venous return of the lines, and clean them with saline (Fig. 16.48).
- Verify the intravascular location of the catheter by placing the transducer over the supraclavicular fossae.
- LAX view of the central venous catheter inside the LBCV (Figs. 16.49 and 16.50).

16.4.7 Step 07

- Secure the catheter and place a sterile occlusive dressing according to the institutional protocol (Fig. 16.51).

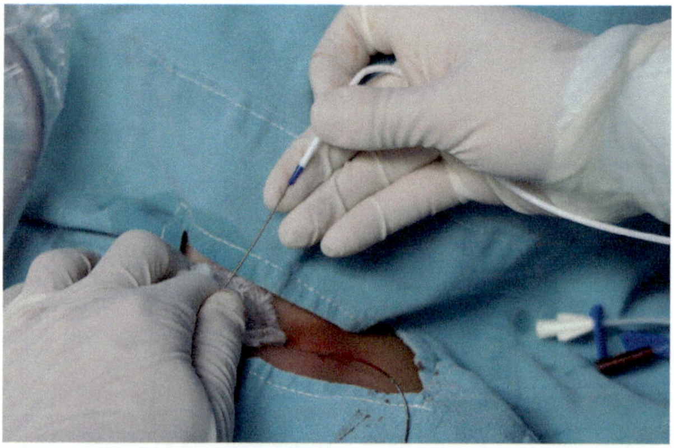

Fig. 16.46 Hold the guidewire and insert the catheter over this

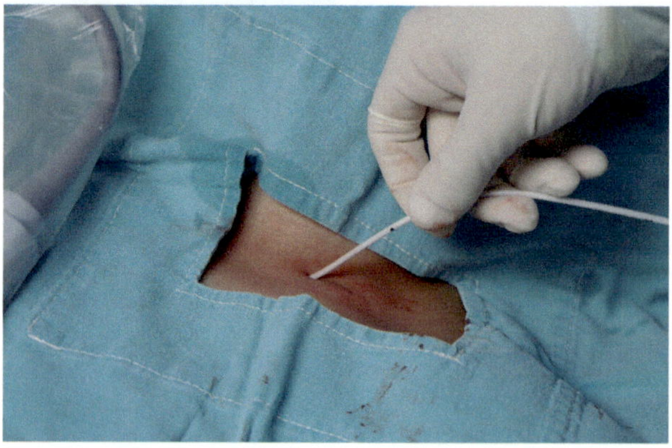

Fig. 16.47 Seldinger's technique: advance the catheter over the guidewire

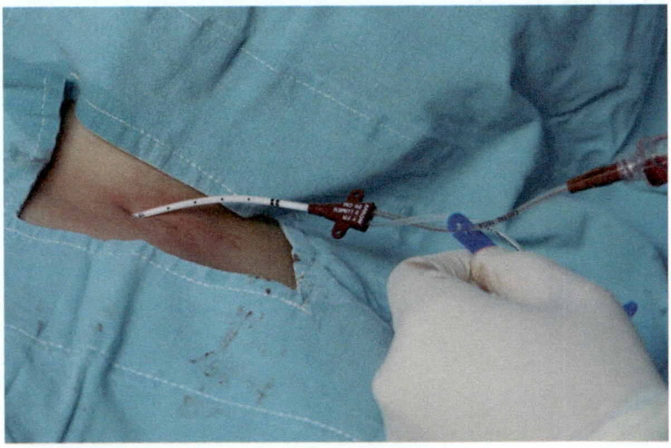

Fig. 16.48 Check the venous return of the lines and clean them with saline

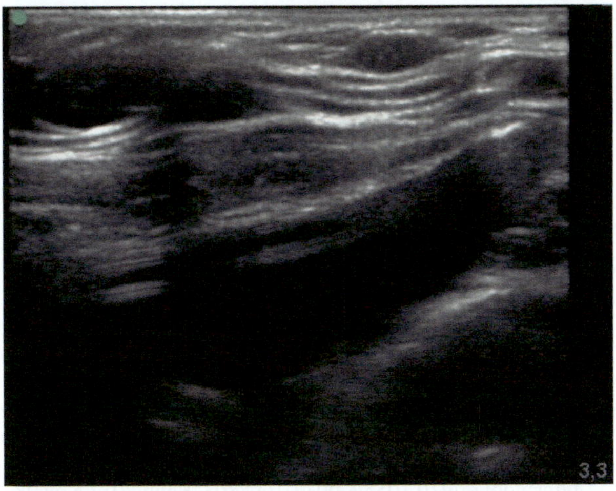

Fig. 16.49 Scan of supraclavicular fossae. LAX view of the central venous catheter inside the LBCV

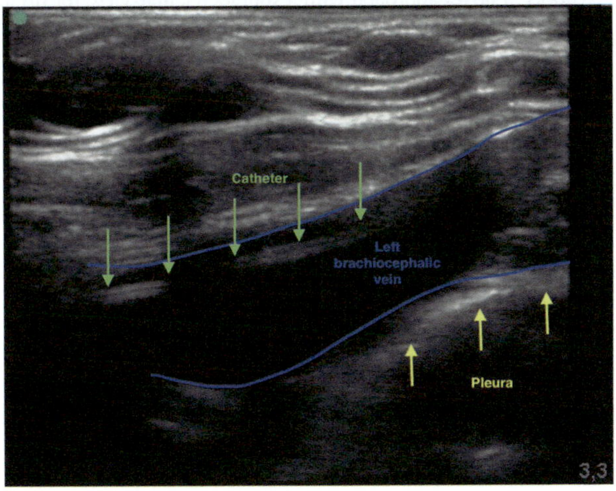

Fig. 16.50 Identifying structures

- Catheter inside the LBCV
- The catheter runs from the patient's left to right

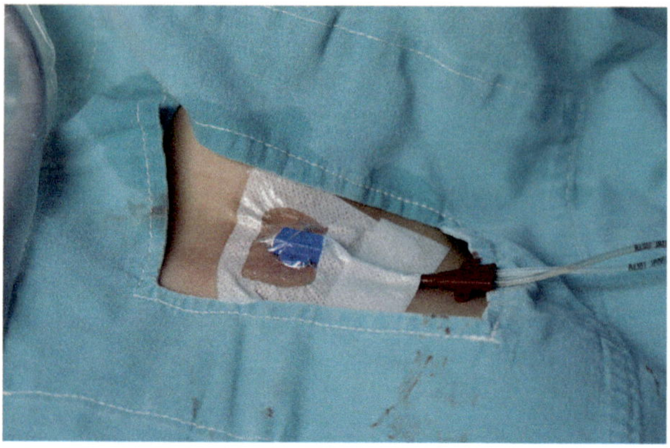

Fig. 16.51 Dressing according to the institutional protocol

Sources

1. Breschan C, Platzer M, Jost R, Stettner H, Beyer AS, Feigl G, Likar R. Consecutive, prospective case series of a new method for ultrasound-guided supraclavicular approach to the brachiocephalic vein in children. Br J Anaesth. 2011;106(5):732–7. https://doi.org/10.1093/bja/aer031. Epub 2011 Mar 17
2. Aytekin C, Özyer U, Harman A, Boyvat F. Ultrasound-guided brachiocephalic vein catheterization in infants weighing less than five kilograms. J Vasc Access. 2015;16(6):512–4. https://doi.org/10.5301/jva.5000385. Epub 2015 May 30
3. Breschan C, Graf G, Jost R, Stettner H, Feigl G, Goessler A, Neuwersch S, Koestenberger M, Likar R. Ultrasound-guided supraclavicular cannulation of the right brachiocephalic vein in small infants: a consecutive, prospective case series. Paediatr Anaesth. 2015;25(9):943–9. https://doi.org/10.1111/pan.12700. Epub 2015 Jun 17
4. Oulego-Erroz I, Alonso-Quintela P, Terroba-Seara S, Jiménez-González A, Rodríguez-Blanco S, Vázquez-Martínez JL. Ultrasound-guided cannulation of the brachiocephalic vein in neonates and preterm infants: a prospective observational study. Am J Perinatol. 2018;35(5):503–8. https://doi.org/10.1055/s-0037-1608803. Epub 2017 Nov 28
5. Spagnuolo F, Vacchiano T. Ultrasound-guided cannulation of the brachiocephalic vein in newborns: a novel approach with a supraclavicular view for tip navigation and tip location. J Vasc Access. 2022;23(4):515–23. https://doi.org/10.1177/11297298211001159. Epub 2021 Mar 16
6. Breschan C, Graf G, Arneitz C, Stettner H, Neuwersch S, Stadik C, Koestenberger M, Holasek S, Likar R. Retrospective evaluation of 599 brachiocephalic vein cannulations in neonates and preterm infants. Br J Anaesth. 2022;129(5):e138–40. https://doi.org/10.1016/j.bja.2022.08.006. Epub 2022 Sep 13

Chapter 17
Left Brachiocephalic Vein in Neonates

17.1 Patient Positioning

- The patient is a newborn weighing 3200 g.
- Position the patient supine, close to the left side of the crib.
- Position the patient's head to the right.
- Place a roll under the shoulders to extend the neck, placing the head lower than the left shoulder (Fig. 17.1).
- The goal of patient positioning for this procedure is to increase the cervical area between the mandible and clavicle to gain access to the supraclavicular fossae.
- Gentle support of the upper extremities is performed with the arm caudal.

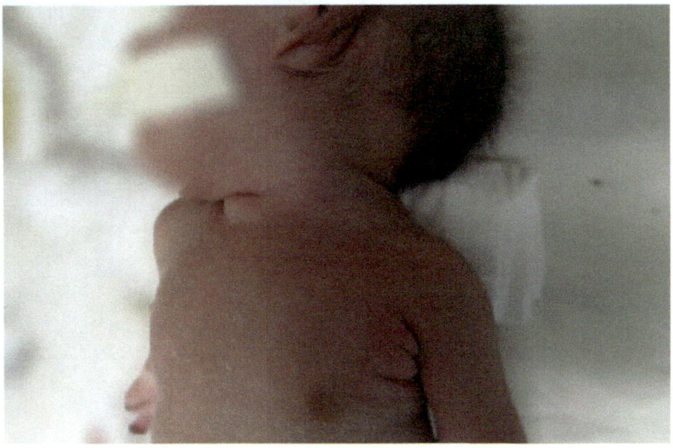

Fig. 17.1 Patient position

F. Montes-Tapia, *Atlas of Ultrasound-Guided Central Venous Catheter Placement*, https://doi.org/10.1007/978-3-031-61887-1_17

17.2 Scanning Technique

- Do a preliminary vascular assessment (non-sterile), known as rapid central vein assessment (RaCeVA).
- The operator stands on the left side of the patient at shoulder level.
- Place the ultrasound device in any of these positions: in front of the operator or above the patient's head (Fig. 17.2).
- Because the supraclavicular fossae at this age is very small, a high-frequency linear (13–6 Mhz) hockey stick transducer will be used.
- Scan in the middle of the left neck with the transducer transverse and the tip of the hockey stick transducer to the patient's right side (Fig. 17.3).
- Begin the scan of the vessels in SAX view of the right carotid artery (LCA) and the left internal jugular vein (LIJV) and sweep down to the clavicle.
- When the transducer is in contact with the clavicle, align the transducer in the left supraclavicular fossae between the inner third of the clavicle and the sternal notch. Maintain the tip of the transducer to the right.
- Tilt the transducer back (Fig. 17.4).
  - The aim of tilting the transducer is to visualize the retroclavicular area to identify the left brachiocephalic vein (LBCV) in the long-axis (LAX) view and perform the puncture in this view (Figs. 17.5 and 17.6).

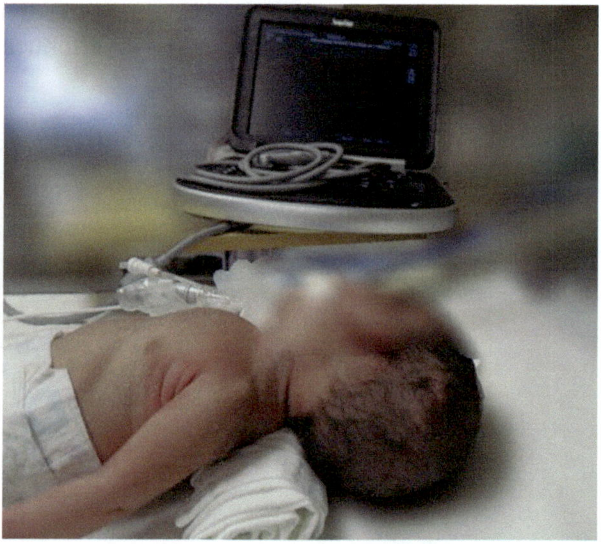

Fig. 17.2 Place the ultrasound device on the patient's right side

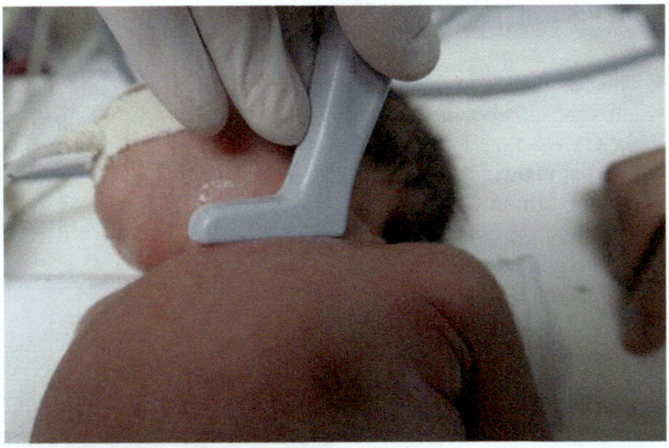

Fig. 17.3 Star the scan in the middle of the left neck

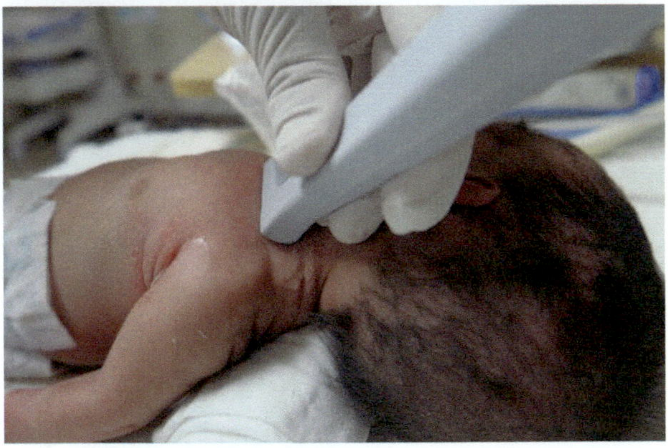

Fig. 17.4 Scan in the left supraclavicular fossae. Tilt the transducer back

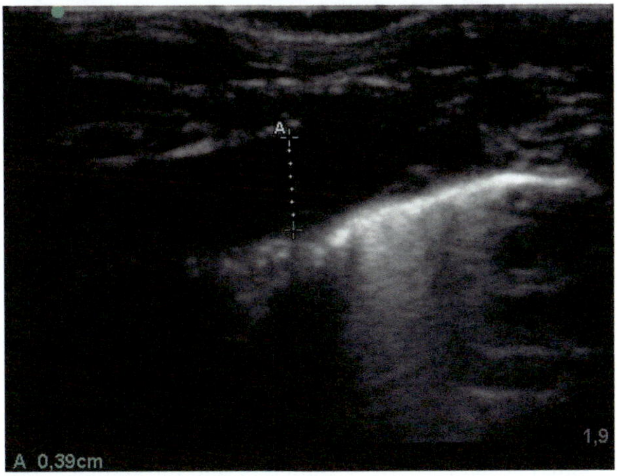

Fig. 17.5 Left supraclavicular fossae scan. LAX view of the LBCV

- The diameter of the LBCV is 0,39 cm
- Scan depth is 1,9 cm

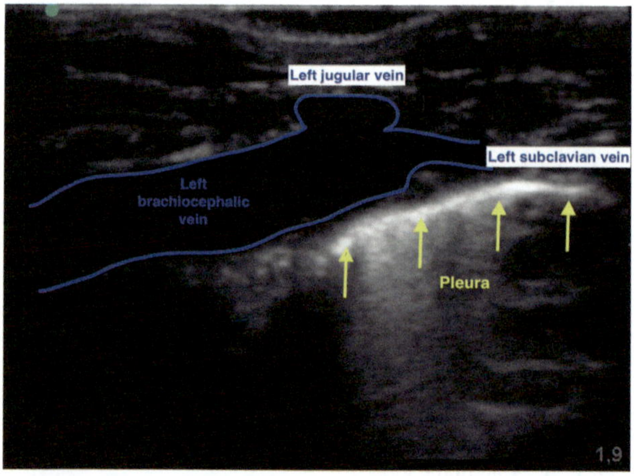

Fig. 17.6 Identifying structures
- The confluence of the left subclavian vein (LSCV) and the left internal jugular vein (LIJV) form the LBCV
- The pleura is in close contact with the inferior wall of the LSCV and the LBCV

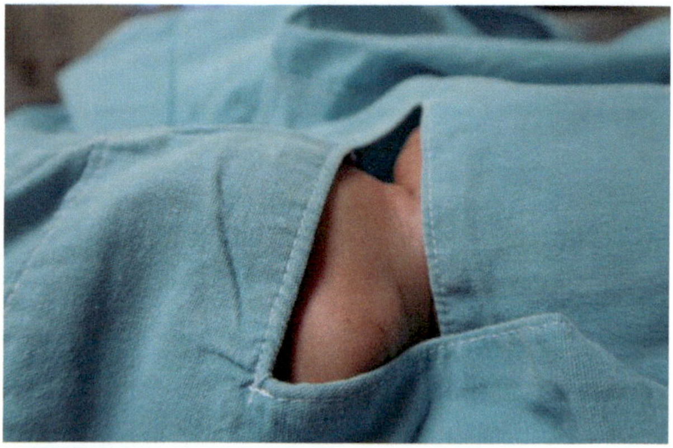

Fig. 17.7 Operator view from the patient's left side at left shoulder level

17.3 Local Anesthesia Application

- Real-time ultrasound-guided lidocaine infiltration.
- The sterile field only leaves the left cervical and upper pectoral regions uncovered. The head is turned to the right (Fig. 17.7).
- The operator stands on the left side of the patient at shoulder level (Fig. 17.8).
- Hold the transducer with your left hand and begin scanning the left supraclavicular fossae between the inner third of the clavicle and the sternal notch and the tip of the hockey stick transducer to the patient's right side.
- For infiltration, use a small needle 25–27 G.
- Use lidocaine 1%.
- Subcutaneous infiltration with lidocaine in the puncture tract 1,5–2 cm before the site chosen for LBCV puncture and the catheter fixation area (Fig. 17.9).
- LAX view of the infiltration (Figs. 17.10 and 17.11).

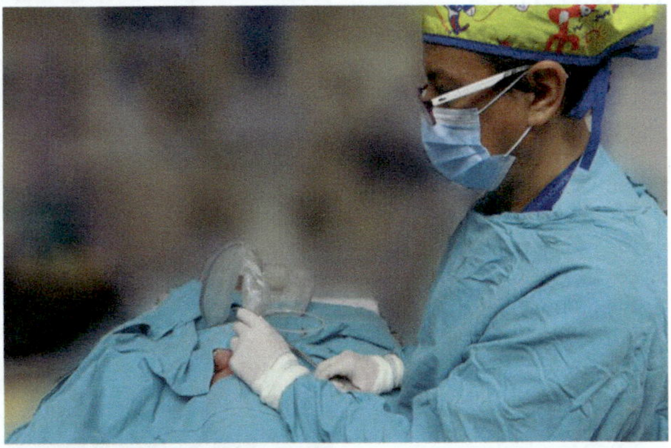

Fig. 17.8 The operator stands on the left side of the patient at shoulder level

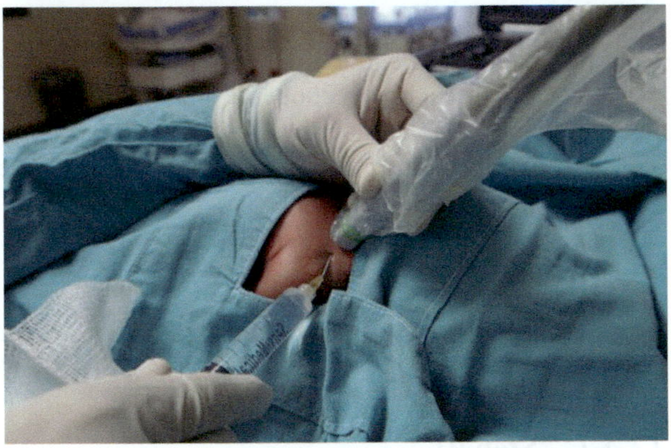

Fig. 17.9 Real-time ultrasound-guided lidocaine infiltration

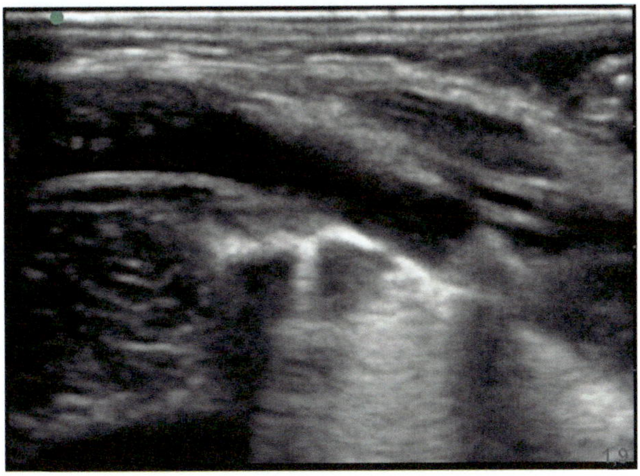

Fig. 17.10 Scan of the left supraclavicular fosse. LAX view of lidocaine infiltration

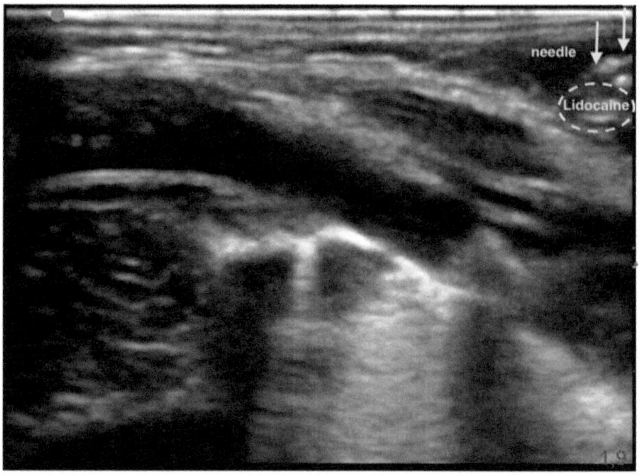

Fig. 17.11 Identifying structures
- The infiltration needle (25 G) is identified between the subcutaneous tissue for infiltration of the skin and the path that will follow the puncture of the LBCV
- This moment of the procedure can be used to determine if the site of choice for the puncture is in the plane of the LBCV, as in this case

- In premature babies, due to the scant subcutaneous tissue, infiltration with lidocaine can cause a hyperechogenic area that will hide the structures below it, so it would be advisable to perform puncture only with good sedation and analgesia. Then, before dilating the skin and the path to the vein, it is infiltrated with lidocaine.

17.4 Steps for Real-Time Ultrasound-Guided Access to the Left Brachiocephalic Vein in Neonates

17.4.1 Step 01

- We will use a Vygon® 3 Fr, 10-cm (or 6-cm), double-lumen catheter.
- Perform the puncture in LAX view of the left supraclavicular fossa (Fig. 17.12).
- Use a 24-G intravenous catheter.
- The key point when puncturing any structure in LAX view is to align the needle with the direction of the transducer; to achieve this, you need to puncture in the middle of the width of the hockey stick transducer and follow its trajectory.
- Start the puncture at an angle of 40°–50° to penetrate the skin and enter the subcutaneous tissue.
- LAX view of the start of the LBCV puncture (Figs. 17.13 and 17.14).
- Due to the superficiality of the vessels in the neonatal stage:
  - The puncture movements must always be guided by ultrasound in real time.
  - The puncture movements must be short so as not to cross the vessels or puncture surrounding structures.

Fig. 17.12 LAX view of the start of the LBCV puncture

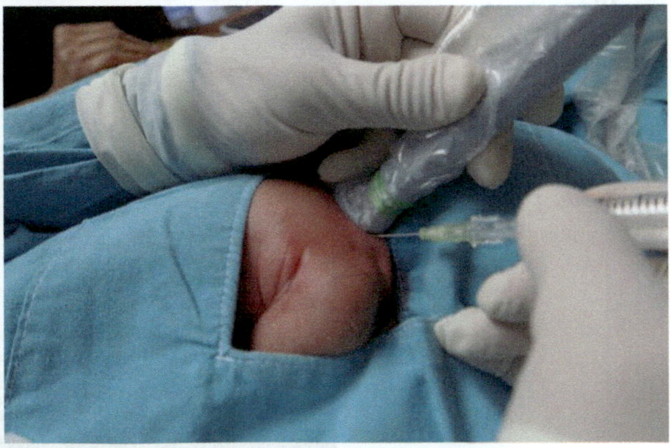

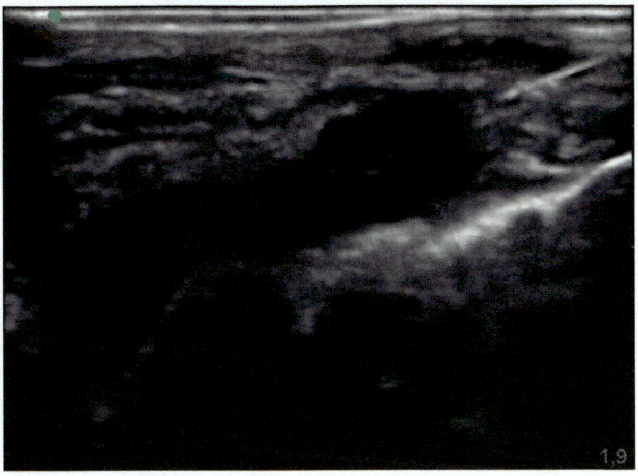

Fig. 17.13 Identifying structures

- The entry of the intravenous catheter in the subcutaneous tissue view in LAX
- A good trajectory of the intravenous catheter is visualized in relation to the LBCV
- The LBCV and right brachiocephalic vein (RBCV) are visualized as forming the superior vena cava (SVC)
- The pleura, which is in contact with the posterior wall of the LBCV, is identified
- The relationship between the intravenous catheter and the pleura will be kept in a parallel plane. This relationship is a safety measure to avoid injuring the pleura and forming a pneumothorax

  – You should always visualize the tip of the puncture needle.
  – If you cannot see the tip, do not proceed with the puncture; first, find it or remove the needle and restart the puncture.

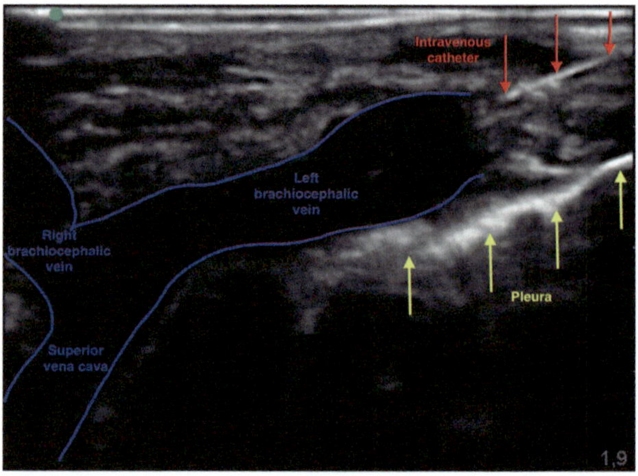

Fig. 17.14 Start the puncture at an angle of 40°–50°

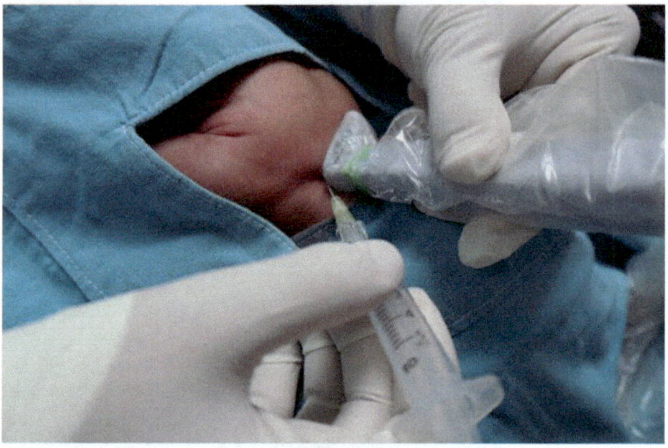

Fig. 17.15 Continue with the puncture in DNT

17.4.2 Step 02

- Continue the puncture by dynamic needle tracking (DNT) in the same direction (Fig. 17.15).
- LAX view of the start of the LBCV cannulation (Figs. 17.16 and 17.17).

17.4.3 Step 03

- Carry out the cannulation of the LBCV since you identified the entrance of the intravenous catheter in the vein (Fig. 17.18).
- LAX view of the LBCV cannulation (Figs. 17.19 and 17.20)
- Always check the trajectory of the puncture on the ultrasound screen, viewing the entire length of the intravenous catheter from the tip and body. If you cannot

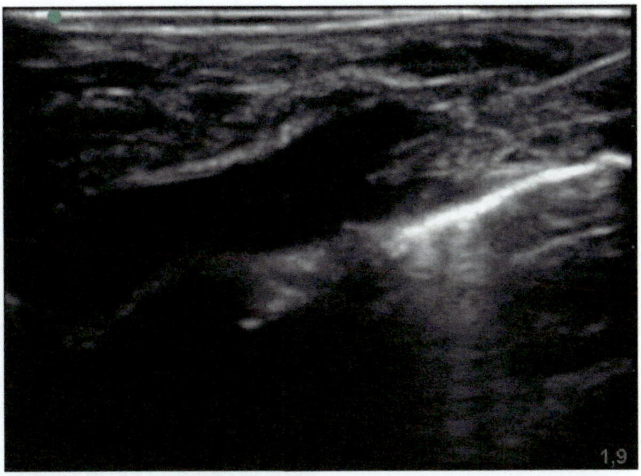

Fig. 17.16 LAX view of the LBCV puncture

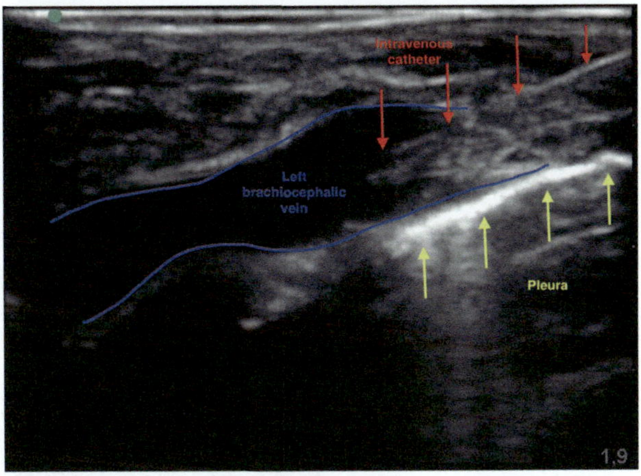

Fig. 17.17 Identifying structures

- The intravenous catheter initiates the cannulation of the LBCV

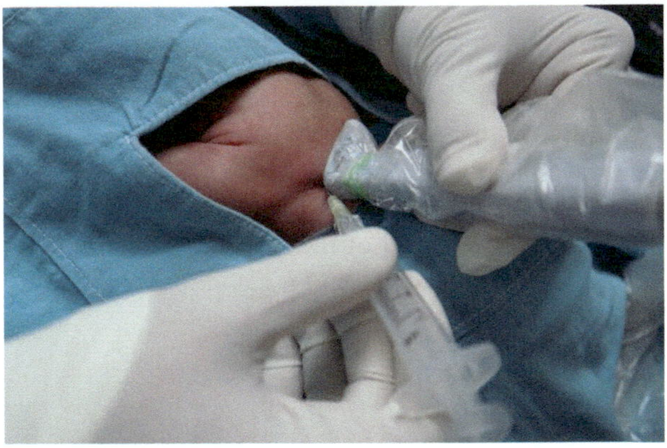

Fig. 17.18 Cannulation of the LBCV

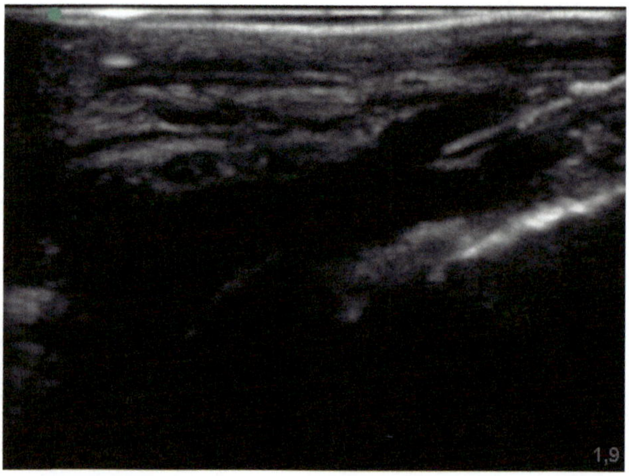

Fig. 17.19 LAX view of the LBCV cannulation

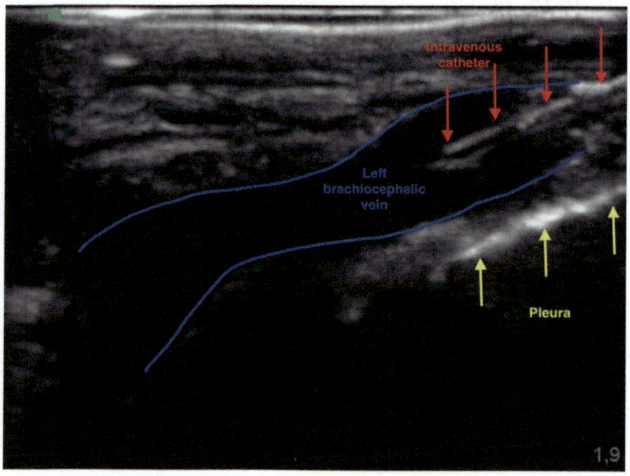

Fig. 17.20 Identifying structures
- The intravenous catheter is reliably intravascular

visualize it completely, search for the intravenous catheter with the transducer, scanning medial or lateral to locate it.

- Once the LBCV cannulation is visualized, set the transducer aside (Fig. 17.21).
- Firmly fix the intravenous catheter hub so the needle is not dislodged from its intravascular location.
- Maintain gentle negative pressure on the syringe plunger until a flash of blood appears in the barrel of the syringe, indicating the intravascular location of the intravenous catheter (Fig. 17.22).

17.4.4 Step 04

- Remove the puncture needle and move the catheter tube inside the LBCV to cannulate the vein with the catheter tube.

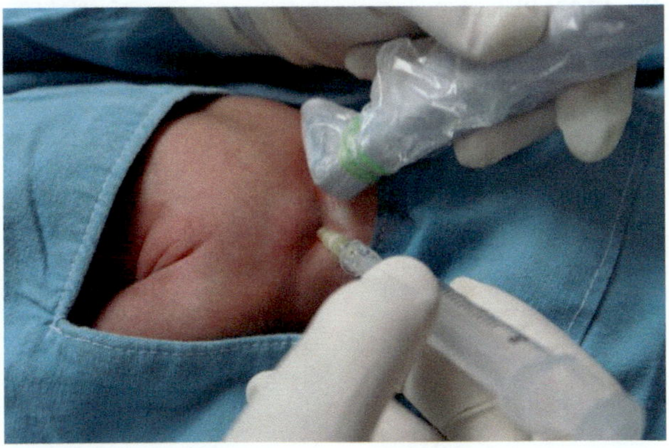

Fig. 17.21 Leave the transducer when the LBCV cannulation is visualized

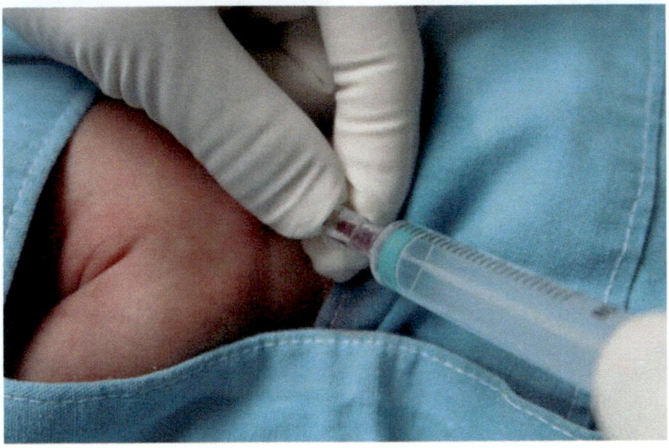

Fig. 17.22 Maintain gentle negative pressure on the syringe plunger

- Once the catheter tube is inserted, the needle is removed. This skill must be practiced to not accidentally remove the catheter (Fig. 17.23).
- Hold the catheter hub firmly with your left hand.
- Insert the 0,3-mm nitinol guidewire, which should pass easily (Fig. 17.24).
- This type of guidewire is marked every 10 cm, so the guidewire should not go beyond the first 5 cm.
- Place the transducer in the supraclavicular fossae to identify the intravascular guidewire (Fig. 17.25).
- LAX view of the intravascular guidewire (Figs. 17.26, 17.27, 17.28 and 17.29).
- Another method to identify the guidewire (or catheter) within the LBCV is to scan the suprasternal notch. Place the transducer vertically over the sternal notch with half of it over the suprasternal notch and half over the sternum (Fig. 17.30). The LBCV will be identified in SAX view. This scan provides a better view of LBCV when the thymus is prominent.
- SAX view of LBCV at the suprasternal notch (Figs. 17.31 and 17.32).

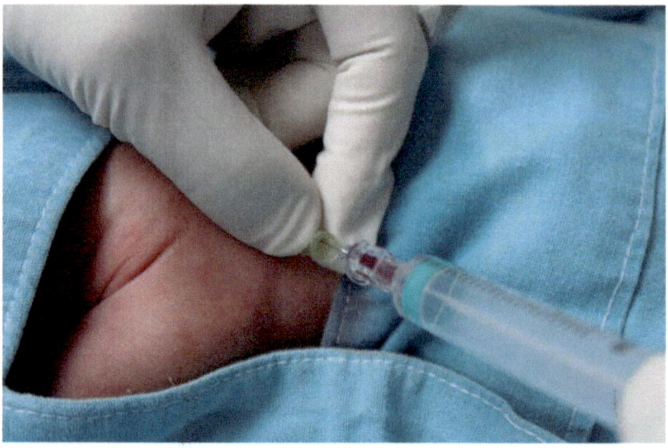

Fig. 17.23 Remove the puncture needle and leave the catheter tube inside the LBCV

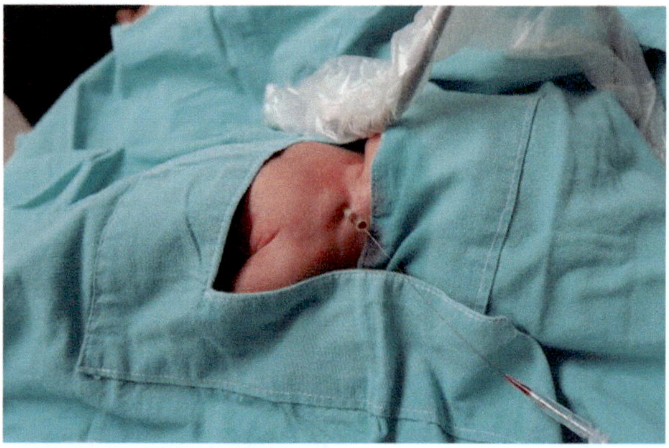

Fig. 17.24 Insert the guidewire

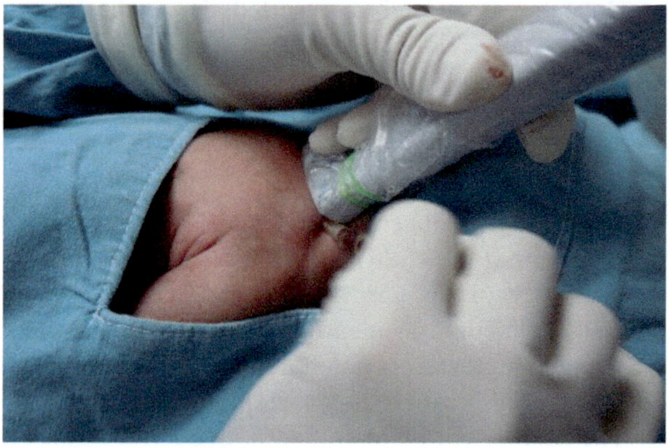

Fig. 17.25 Scan the supraclavicular fossae to verify the intravascular location of the guidewire

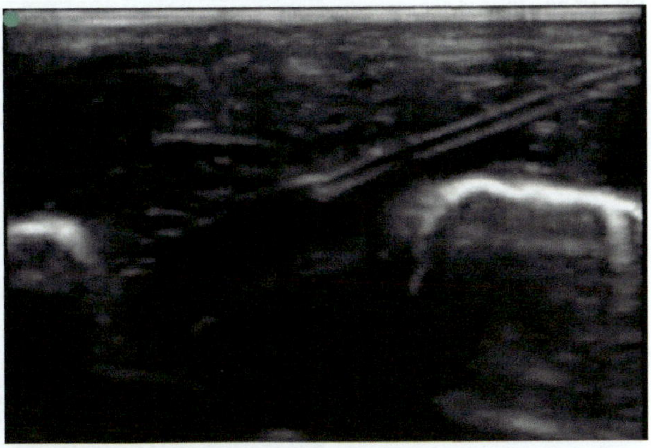

Fig. 17.26 LAX view of the catheter tube in the LBCV

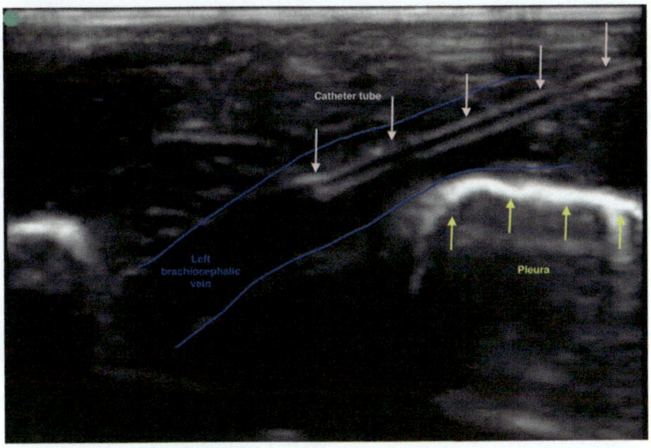

Fig. 17.27 Identifying structures

- The intravenous catheter tube remains cannulating the LBCV without the needle

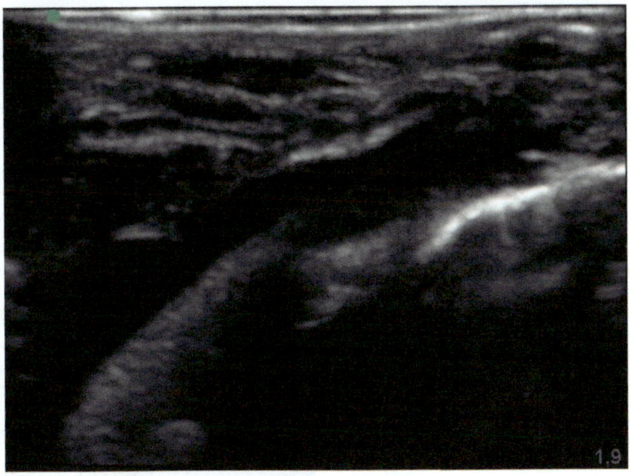

Fig. 17.28 LAX view of the intravascular guidewire

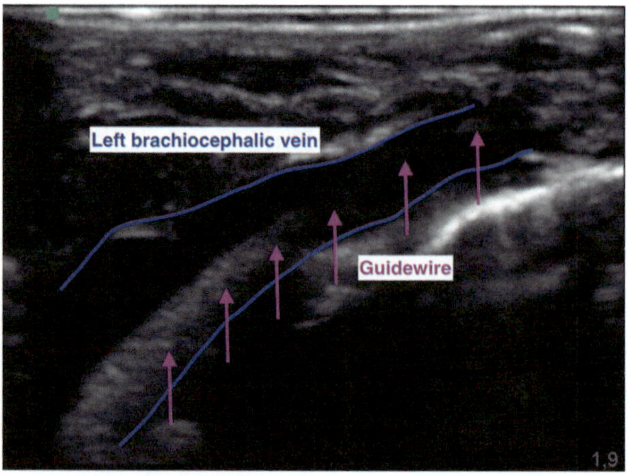

Fig. 17.29 Identifying structures

- Guidewire in the LBCV, which descends toward the SVC

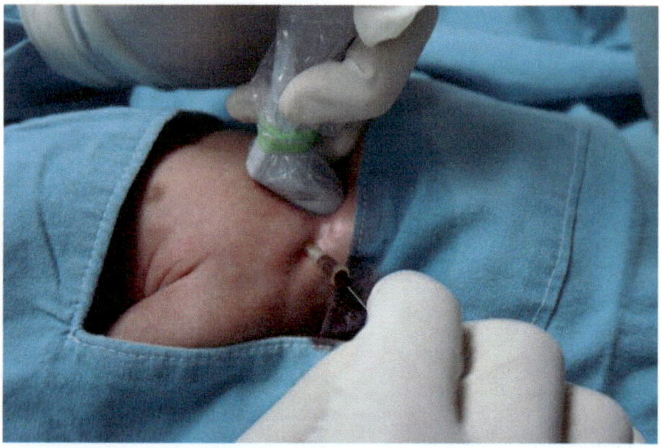

Fig. 17.30 Scan of the suprasternal notch

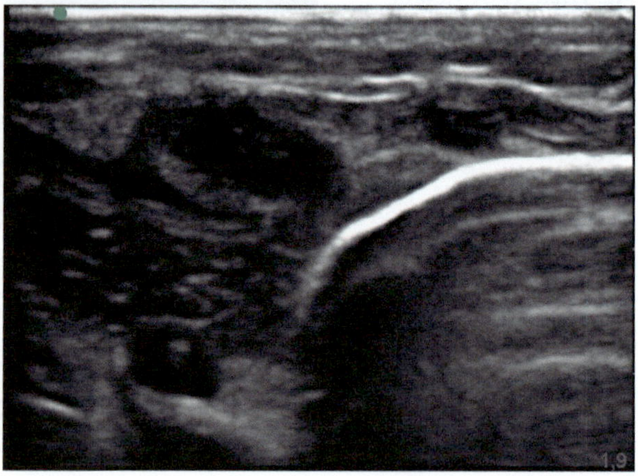

Fig. 17.31 SAX view of LBCV at the suprasternal notch

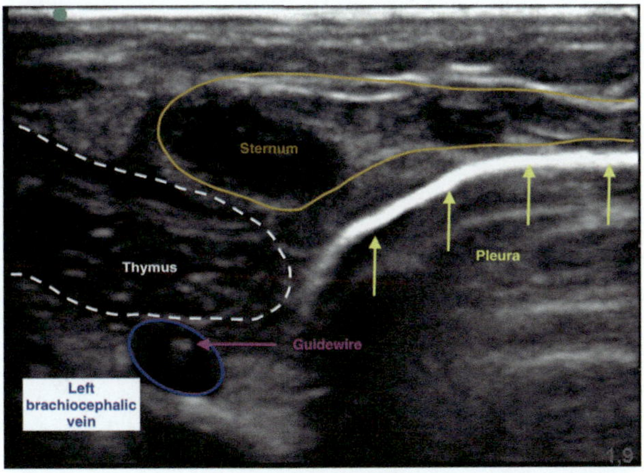

Fig. 17.32 Identifying structures
- The LBCV is located below the thymus
- The guidewire is identified as a hyperechogenic dot within the LBCV

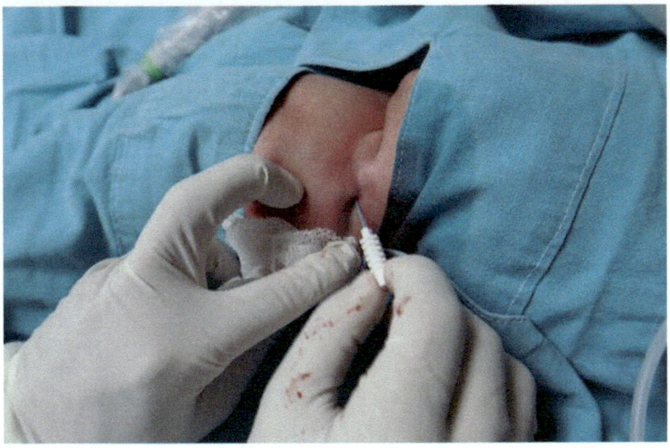

Fig. 17.33 Dilation of the skin

17.4.5 Step 05

- Once you corroborate the guidewire cannulating the LBCV, dilation of the skin toward the LBCV is performed (Fig. 17.33).
- Pull the skin with the index finger of the left hand so that the dilator can easily penetrate.

17.4.6 Step 06

- Introduce the 3 Fr, 10-cm, double-lumen catheter with Seldinger's technique and remove the guidewire.
- Remove the guidewire, check the venous return of the lines, and clean them with saline (Fig. 17.34).

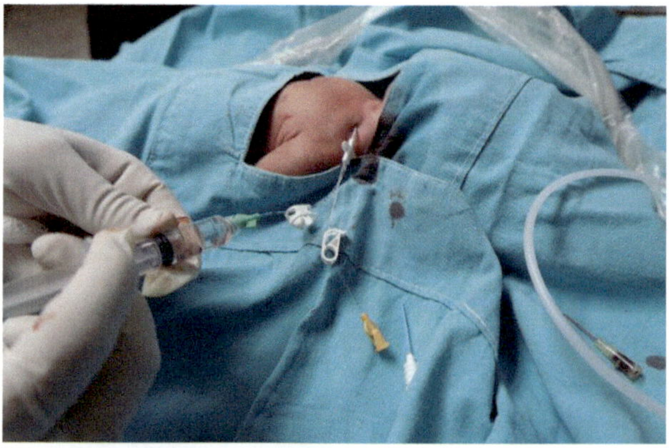

Fig. 17.34 Check the venous return of the lines and clean them with saline

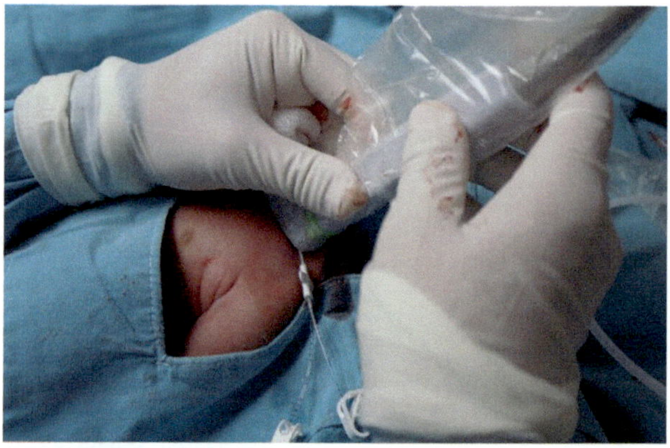

Fig. 17.35 Scan of the supraclavicular fossae

- Verify the intravascular location of the catheter by placing the transducer over the supraclavicular fossae (Fig. 17.35).
- LAX view of the central venous catheter inside the LBCV (Figs. 17.36 and 17.37).

17.4.7 Step 07

- Secure the catheter and place a sterile occlusive dressing according to the institutional protocol (Fig. 17.38).

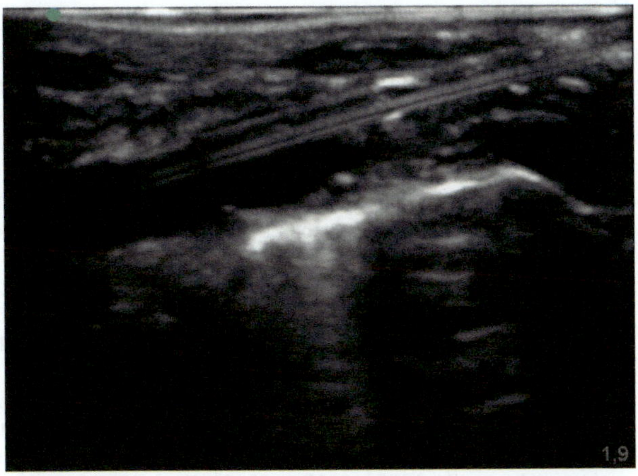

Fig. 17.36 LAX view of the intravascular catheter

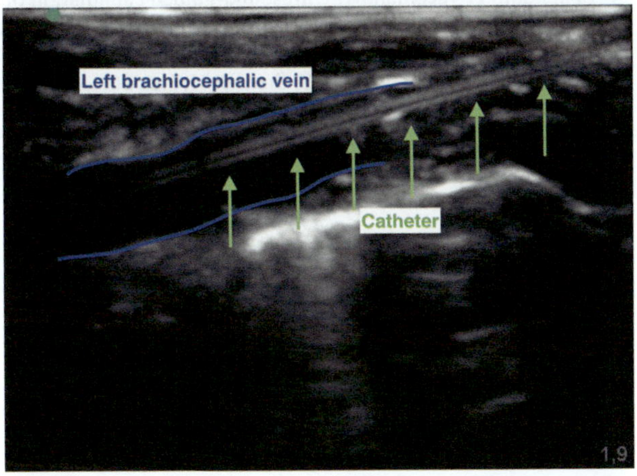

Fig. 17.37 Identifying structures

- Catheter inside the LBCV

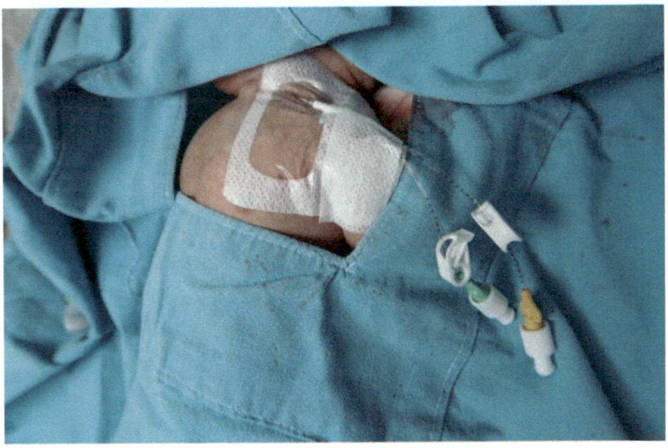

Fig. 17.38 Dressing according to the institutional protocol

Sources

1. Breschan C, Platzer M, Jost R, Stettner H, Beyer AS, Feigl G, Likar R. Consecutive, prospective case series of a new method for ultrasound-guided supraclavicular approach to the brachiocephalic vein in children. Br J Anaesth. 2011;106(5):732–7. https://doi.org/10.1093/bja/aer031. Epub 2011 Mar 17
2. Aytekin C, Özyer U, Harman A, Boyvat F. Ultrasound-guided brachiocephalic vein catheterization in infants weighing less than five kilograms. J Vasc Access. 2015;16(6):512–4. https://doi.org/10.5301/jva.5000385. Epub 2015 May 30
3. Breschan C, Graf G, Jost R, Stettner H, Feigl G, Goessler A, Neuwersch S, Koestenberger M, Likar R. Ultrasound-guided supraclavicular cannulation of the right brachiocephalic vein in small infants: a consecutive, prospective case series. Paediatr Anaesth. 2015;25(9):943–9. https://doi.org/10.1111/pan.12700. Epub 2015 Jun 17
4. Oulego-Erroz I, Alonso-Quintela P, Terroba-Seara S, Jiménez-González A, Rodríguez-Blanco S, Vázquez-Martínez JL. Ultrasound-guided cannulation of the brachiocephalic vein in neonates and preterm infants: a prospective observational study. Am J Perinatol. 2018;35(5):503–8. https://doi.org/10.1055/s-0037-1608803. Epub 2017 Nov 28
5. Spagnuolo F, Vacchiano T. Ultrasound-guided cannulation of the brachiocephalic vein in newborns: a novel approach with a supraclavicular view for tip navigation and tip location. J Vasc Access. 2022;23(4):515–23. https://doi.org/10.1177/11297298211001159. Epub 2021 Mar 16
6. Breschan C, Graf G, Arneitz C, Stettner H, Neuwersch S, Stadik C, Koestenberger M, Holasek S, Likar R. Retrospective evaluation of 599 brachiocephalic vein cannulations in neonates and preterm infants. Br J Anaesth. 2022;129(5):e138–40. https://doi.org/10.1016/j.bja.2022.08.006. Epub 2022 Sep 13

Chapter 18
Right Femoral Vein in Pediatrics

18.1 Patient Positioning

- The patient is a 2-year-old weighing 13 kg.
- Position the patient on the right side with their leg near the border of the bed.
- Position the patient supine with the legs extended, separated from the midline, and with gentle restraint at the ankles.
- Place a roll under the hip (Fig. 18.1).

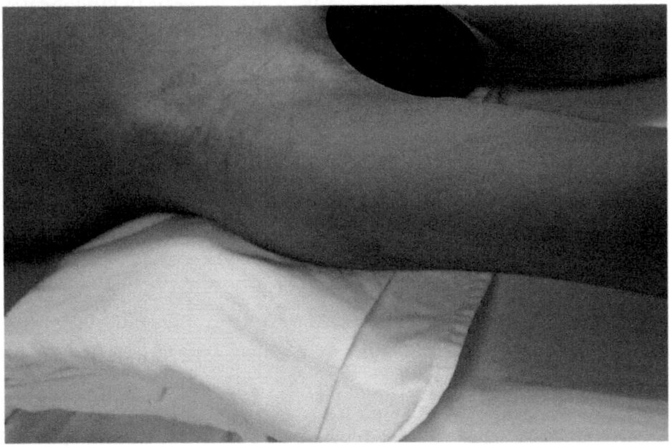

Fig. 18.1 Place a roll under the hip

F. Montes-Tapia, *Atlas of Ultrasound-Guided Central Venous Catheter Placement*, https://doi.org/10.1007/978-3-031-61887-1_18

18.2 Scanning Technique

- Do a preliminary vascular assessment (non-sterile), known as rapid femoral vein assessment (RaFeVA).
- The operator stands on the right side of the bed (Fig. 18.2).
- The ultrasound is placed at the level of the left or right shoulder or above the patient's head.
- A high-frequency linear transducer (13–6 MHz) with a hockey stick transducer can be used.
- The transducer is placed at the level of the inguinal ligament with the tip toward the patient's right side, which will be marked on the screen as the left side, corresponding to the operator's left. This is done to correlate the operator's movements with those of the screen (Fig. 18.3).
- Scan in short-axis (SAX) view to identify the arteriovenous bundle (Figs. 18.4 and 18.5).
- Elevate the hip with a roll to keep the transducer in contact with the lower abdominal wall and inguinal region. If the hip is not elevated, the inguinal region would be in a depression, and contact of the transducer with this region could not occur.

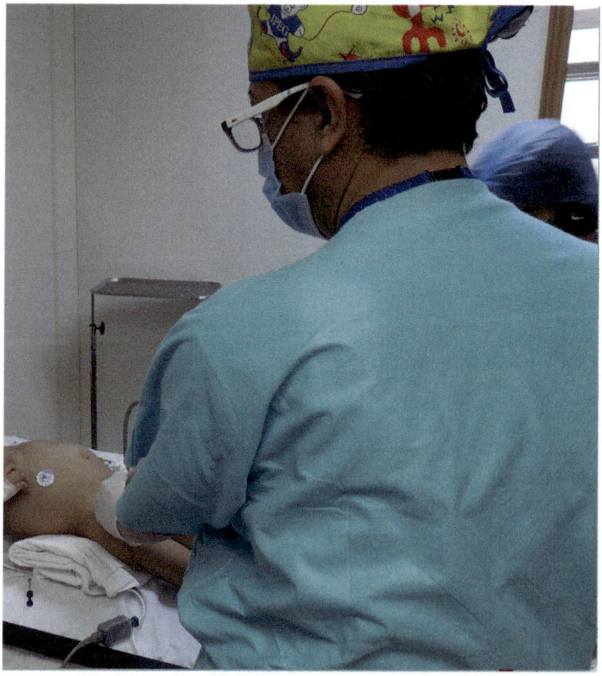

Fig. 18.2 Operator position

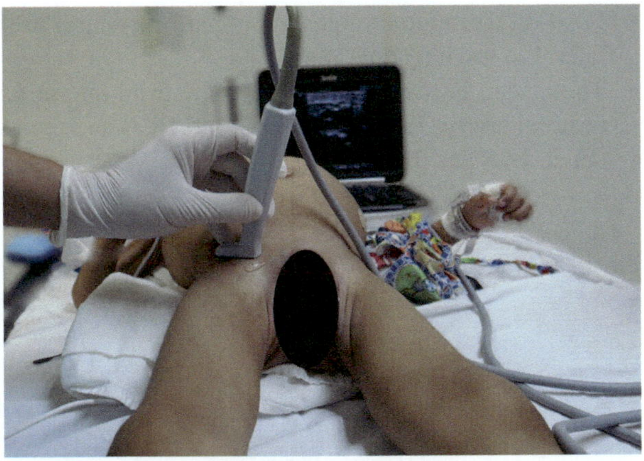

Fig. 18.3 Scan in SAX view

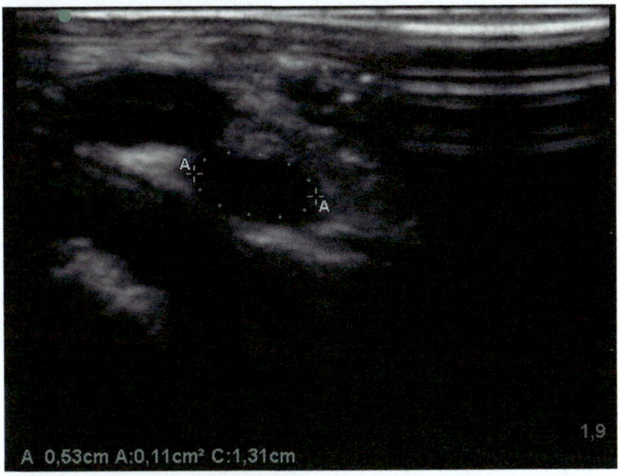

Fig. 18.4 Inguinal scan. SAX view of the right femoral bundle

- Scan depth is 1,9 cm

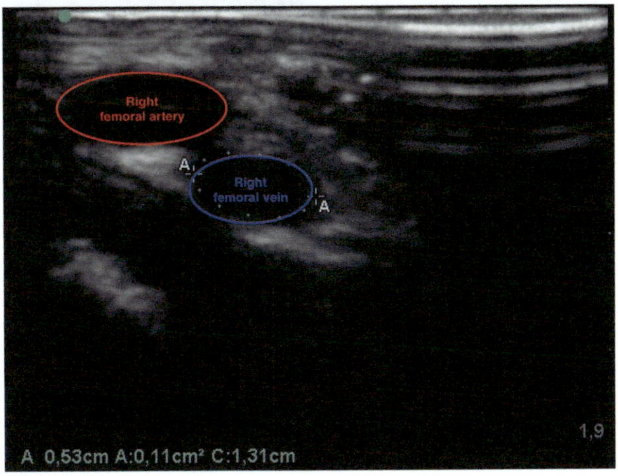

Fig. 18.5 Identifying structures

- The right femoral vein (RFV) diameter is 0,53 cm, with an area of 0,11 cm^2

- Position the inguinal ligament at half the length of the transducer and scan from lateral to medial (Fig. 18.6).
- Then, scan in long-axis (LAX) view from lateral to medial to identify the right femoral artery (RFA) (Figs. 18.7 and 18.8) and then the right femoral vein (RFV) (Figs. 18.9 and 18.10).

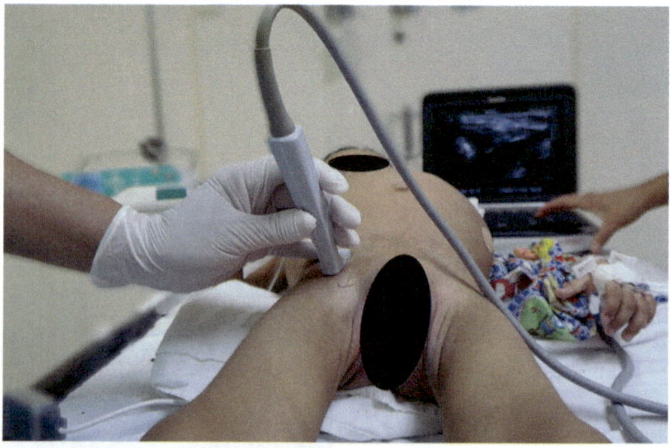

Fig. 18.6 Scan in LAX view

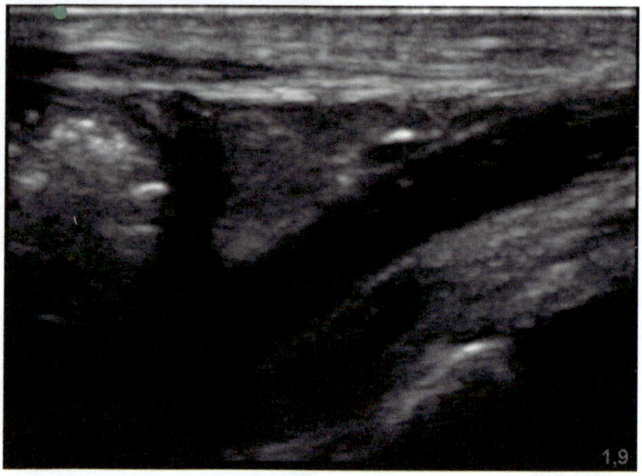

Fig. 18.7 Lateral scan of the right leg. LAX view of the RFA

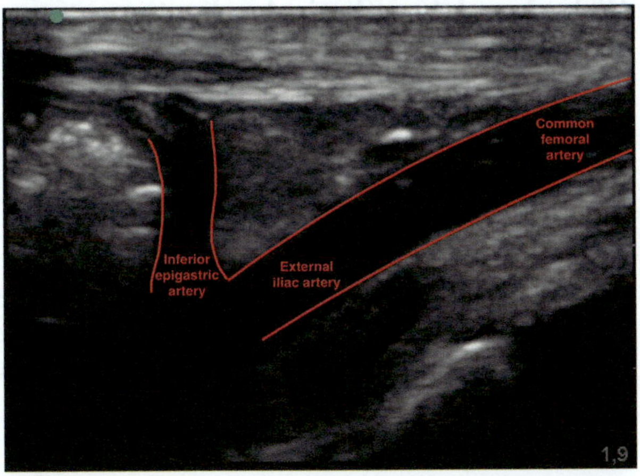

Fig. 18.8 Identifying structures
- The common RFA is seen in LAX view
- The external iliac artery and the emergence of the inferior epigastric artery are also visualized

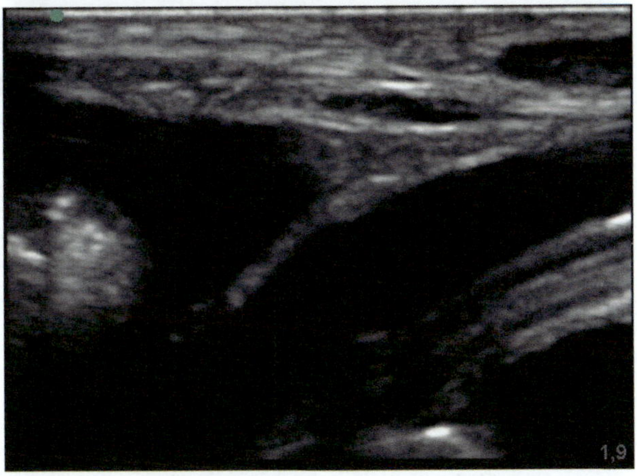

Fig. 18.9 Medial scan of the leg. LAX view of the common LFV

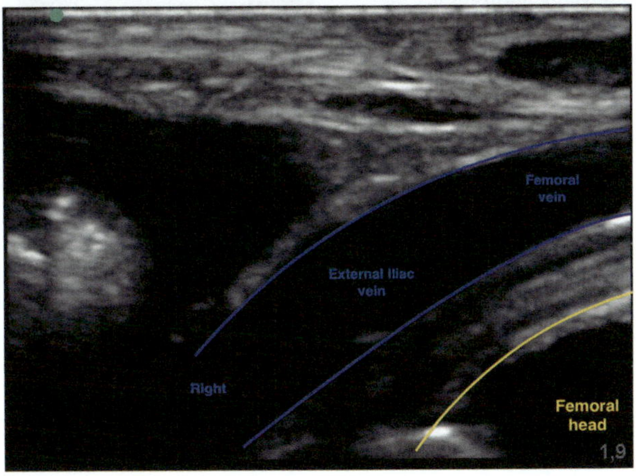

Fig. 18.10 Identifying structures
- The common RFV and the external iliac vein are also visualized

18.3 Local Anesthesia Application

- The sterile field leaves the lower right abdomen, inguinal, and anterior thigh regions uncovered (Fig. 18.11).
- Position the patient with leg extension.
- Real-time ultrasound-guided lidocaine infiltration.
- For infiltration, use a small needle 25- 27-G.
- Use 1% lidocaine.
- Subcutaneous infiltration with lidocaine in the puncture tract 1,5–2 cm before the site chosen for RFV puncture and the catheter fixation area (Fig. 18.12).
- LAX view of lidocaine infiltration in the subcutaneous tissue (Figs. 18.13, 18.14, 18.15 and 18.16).

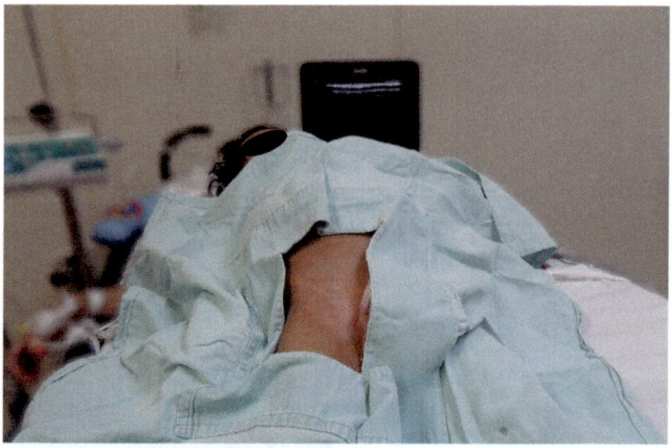

Fig. 18.11 Operator view

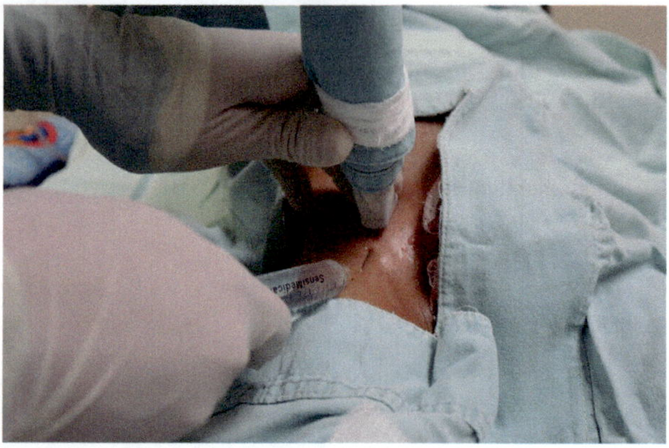

Fig. 18.12 Real-time ultrasound-guided lidocaine infiltration

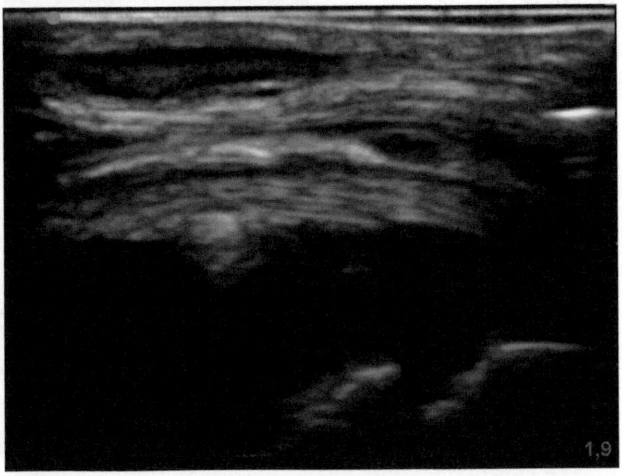

Fig. 18.13 Scan of the inguinal area. LAX view of infiltration of lidocaine

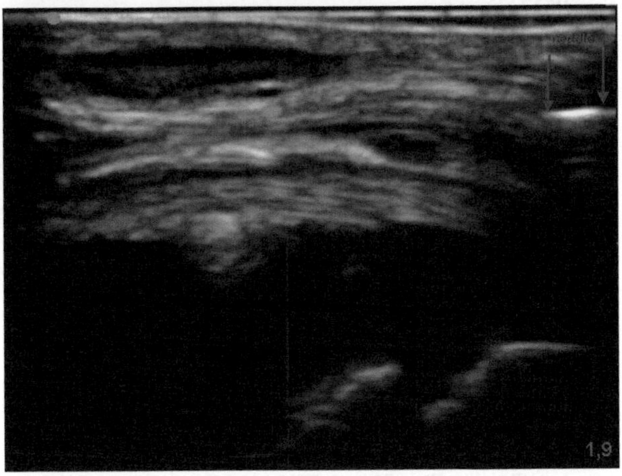

Fig. 18.14 Identifying structures

- The infiltration needle (25 G) is identified in the subcutaneous tissue
- This procedure moment can be used to determine if the site of choice for the puncture is in the plane of the RFV

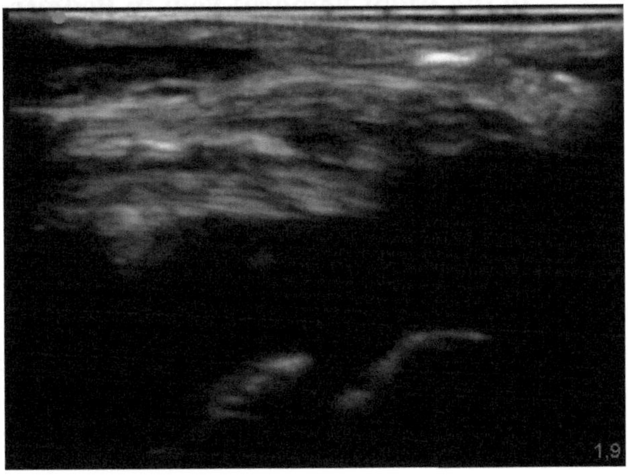

Fig. 18.15 LAX view of lidocaine in the subcutaneous tissue

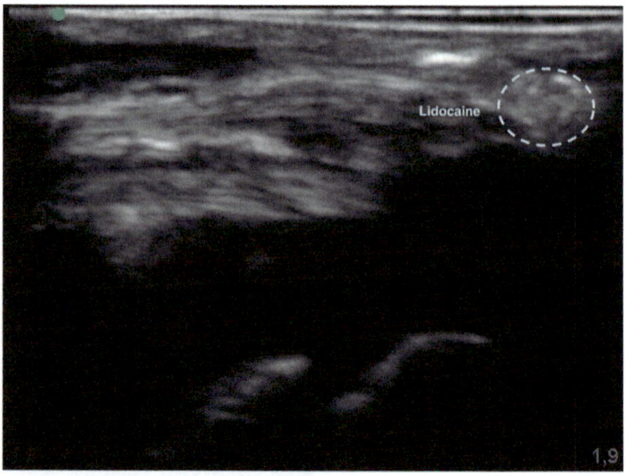

Fig. 18.16 Identifying structures
- Lidocaine will form a hyperechoic area

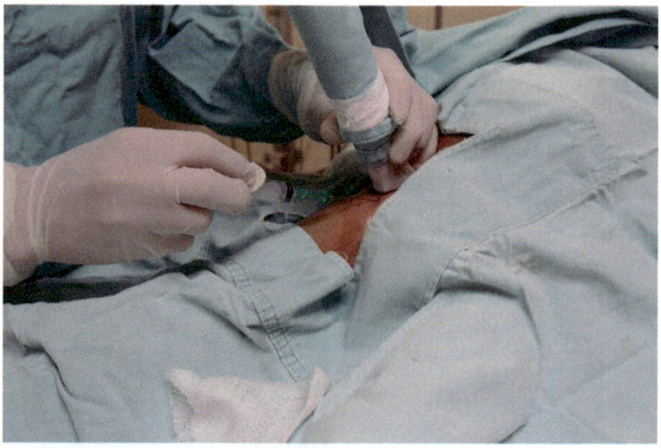

Fig. 18.17 Start the puncture at an angle of 10°–20°

18.4 Steps for Real-Time Ultrasound-Guided Access to the Right Femoral Vein in Pediatrics

18.4.1 Step 01

- We will use a 30-cm, double-lumen Arrow® 4 Fr catheter.
- Perform the puncture in LAX view, below the inguinal ligament, using a 21-G introducer needle.
- Begin the ultrasound-guided dynamic needle tracking (DNT) to guide the puncture in real time.
- Start the puncture with an angle between 10° and 20°. The objective is to penetrate under the skin and first identify the location of the introducer needle and then over the vein (Fig. 18.17).

  - Puncture in the middle of the thickness of the transducer so that the introducer needle can be visualized along the path aligned with the vein (Figs. 18.18 and 18.19).

- This patient has little subcutaneous tissue. A higher angle of puncture can cause you to penetrate more deeply or incidentally traverse the vein or artery.

18.4.2 Step 02

- In DNT, slightly increase the puncture angle to less than 30° to cannulate the RFV (Fig. 18.20).
- LAX view of modification of the angle of puncture (Figs. 18.21 and 18.22).
- Continue with the puncture since the puncture angle and the RFV are aligned (Fig. 18.23).

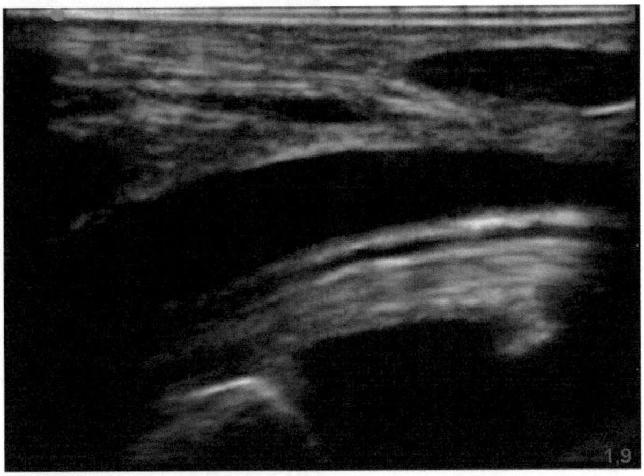

Fig. 18.18 LAX view of the entry of the introducer needle into the subcutaneous tissue

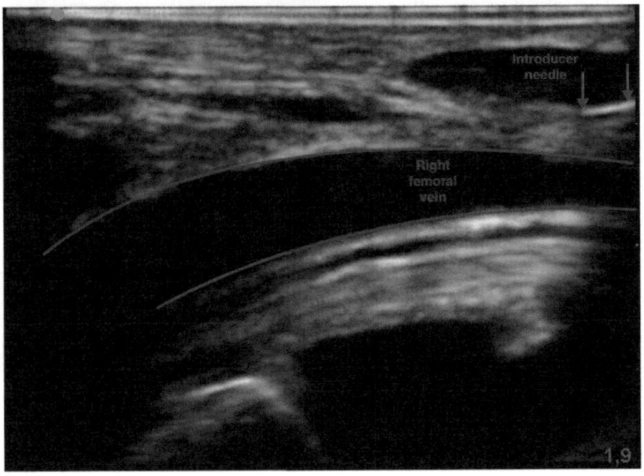

Fig. 18.19 Identifying structures
- The introducer needle with a puncture angle between 10° and 20° and good alignment with the RFV

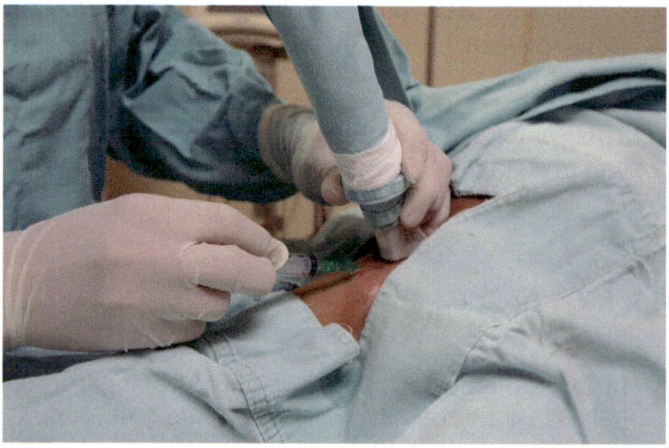

Fig. 18.20 Modify the puncture to 30°

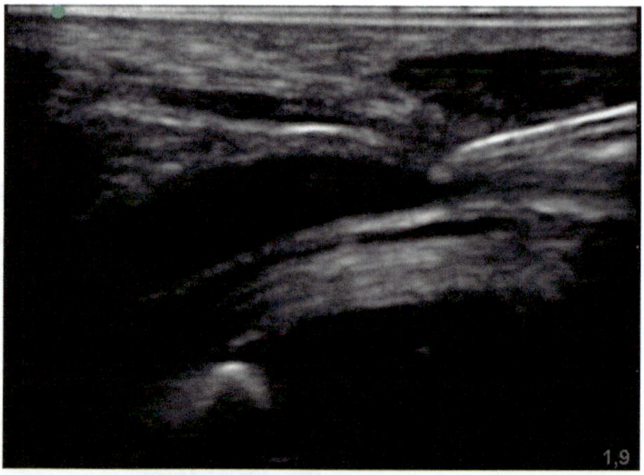

Fig. 18.21 LAX view of the correct direction of the puncture to 30°

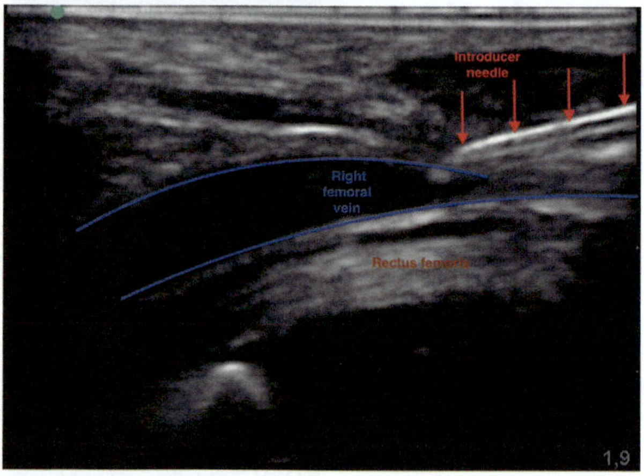

Fig. 18.22 Identifying structures

- The introducer needle reaches the anterior wall of the RFV

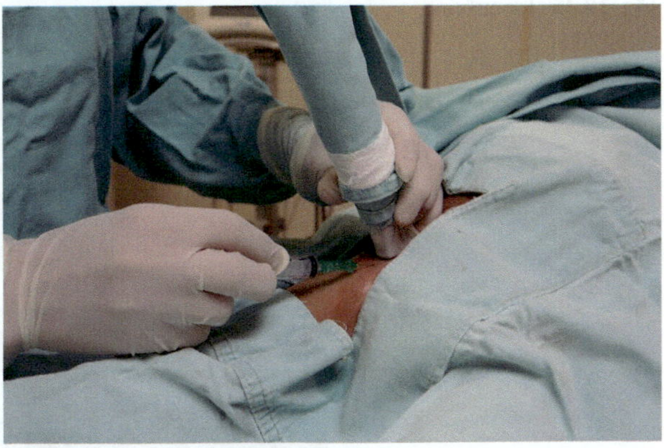

Fig. 18.23 Continue the puncture trajectory

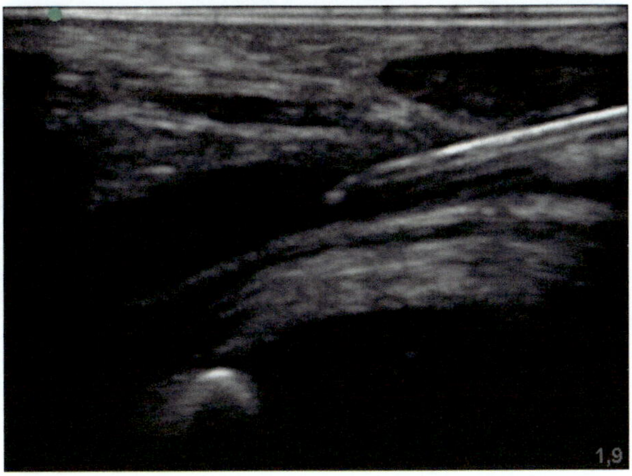

Fig. 18.24 LAX view of the cannulation of the RFV

- LAX view of the arrival of the introducer needle to the anterior wall of the RFV (Figs. 18.24 and 18.25).

18.4.3 Step 03

- Advance the introducer needle further while maintaining gentle negative pressure on the syringe plunger as you advance the needle (Fig. 18.26).
- LAX view of the beginning of the entry of the introducer needle into the RFV (Figs. 18.27 and 18.28).
- Identify the complete cannulation of the vein on the ultrasound screen.
- Maintain gentle negative pressure on the syringe plunger until a flash of blood appears in the barrel of the syringe (Fig. 18.29).
- Set the transducer aside.
- Check for free blood flow through the introducer needle cannulating the RFV (Fig. 18.30).

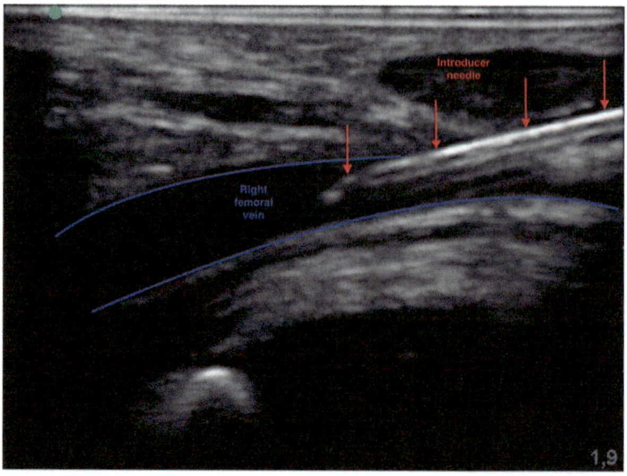

Fig. 18.25 Identifying structures

- The introducer needle has entered the RFV

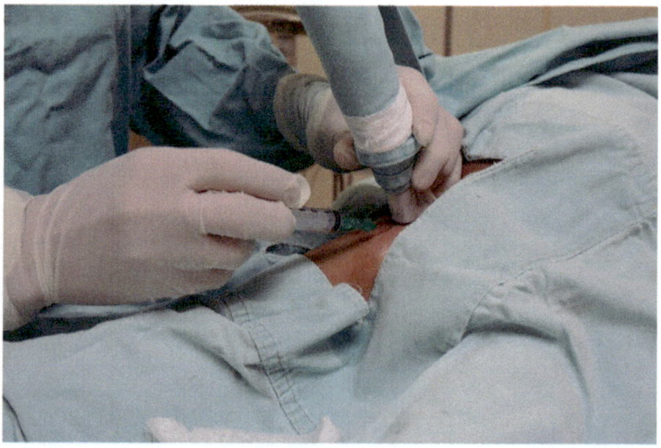

Fig. 18.26 Continue the puncture trajectory and cannulate the RBCV

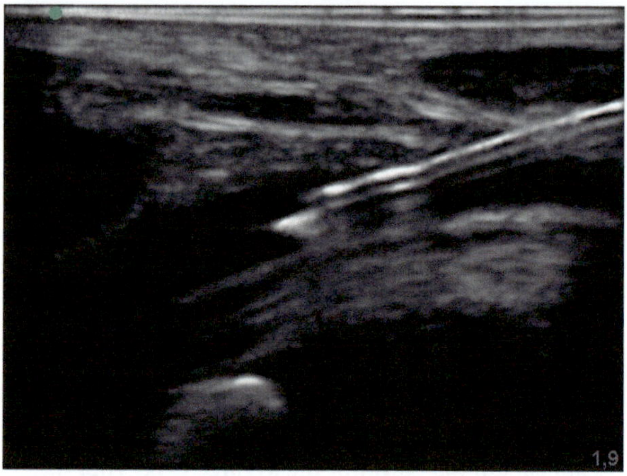

Fig. 18.27 LAX view of the cannulation of the RFV

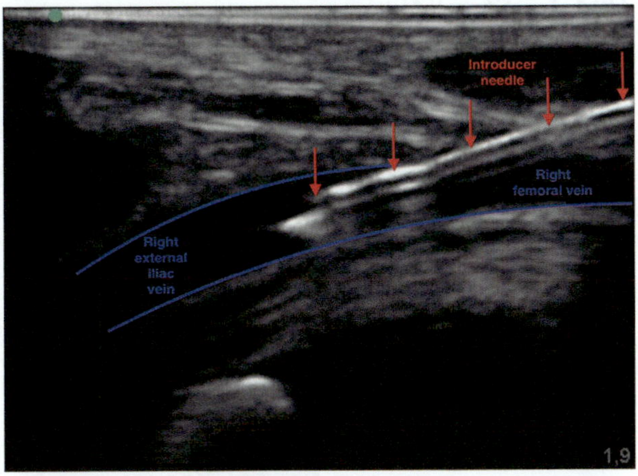

Fig. 18.28 Identifying structures

- The introducer needle is cannulating the RFV

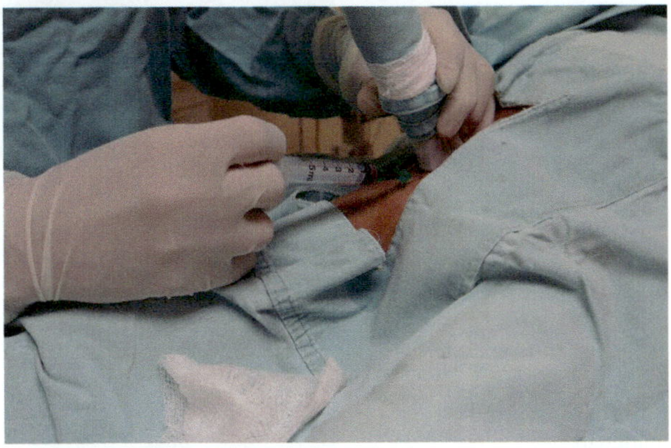

Fig. 18.29 Apply gentle negative pressure and check for blood return in the barrel of the syringe

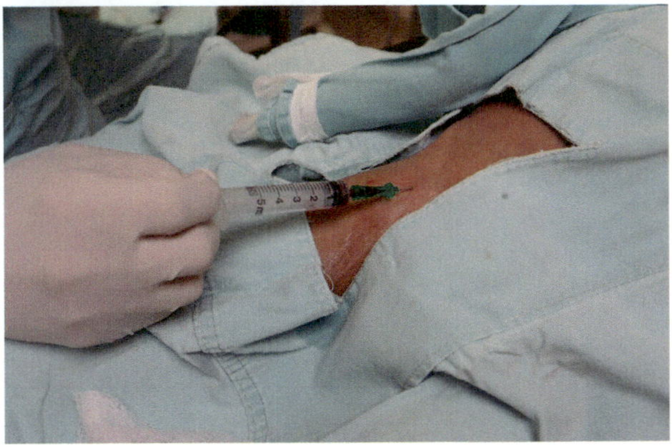

Fig. 18.30 Check for free blood flow

18.4.4 Step 04

- Hold the hub of the introducer needle firmly and remove the syringe (Fig. 18.31).
- Insert the 0.018" guidewire through the introducer needle (Fig. 18.32).
- It should easily pass through the J-tip end of the guide. If it does not, you can try passing through the straight end. If it still does not pass, the needle may have accidentally slipped out of the RFV.
- Place the transducer longitudinally over the inguinal ligament, like the puncture was performed (Fig. 18.33).
- Scan the location of the guidewire in the venous lumen in LAX (Figs. 18.34 and 18.35) or SAX view.

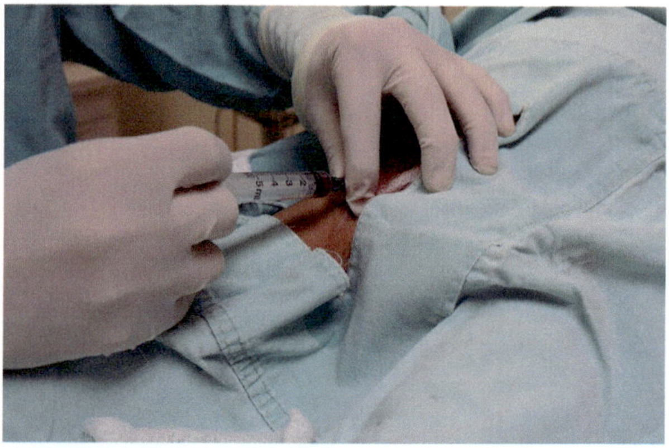

Fig. 18.31 Remove the syringe

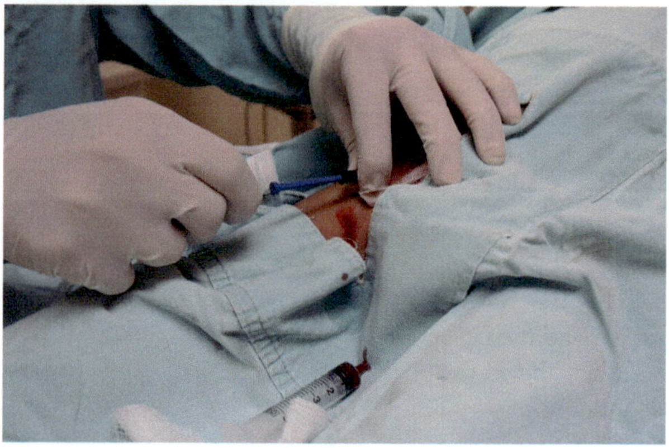

Fig. 18.32 Insert the guidewire

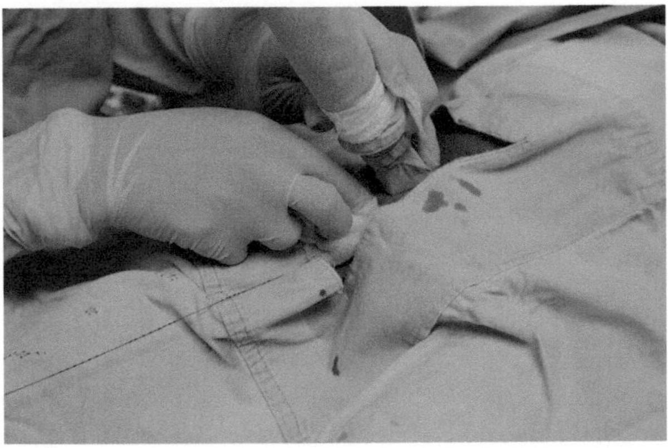

Fig. 18.33 Scan the inguinal region to verify the intravascular location of the guidewire

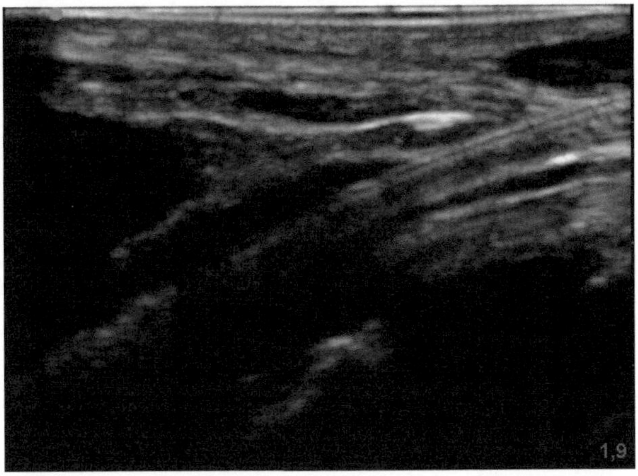

Fig. 18.34 LAX view of the guidewire in the RFV

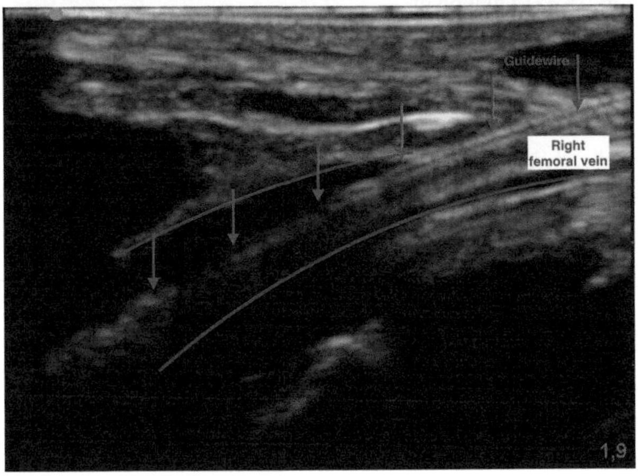

Fig. 18.35 Identifying structures

- Guidewire in the RFV

18.4.5 Step 05

- Once you have identified the guidewire inside the vein, the path will be dilated. This safety measure avoids dilation in case of incidental puncture of the femoral artery.
- Occlude the exit of the guide with your left hand and hold the guidewire with the same hand to help you introduce the dilator over the guidewire (Fig. 18.36).
- Dilate the path between the skin and the RFV.
- Insert the dilator. If you do it carefully, you will not need a skin incision (Fig. 18.37).
- When you are withdrawing, the dilator occludes the exit of the skin with your left hand and gauze, so it does not bleed (Fig. 18.38).

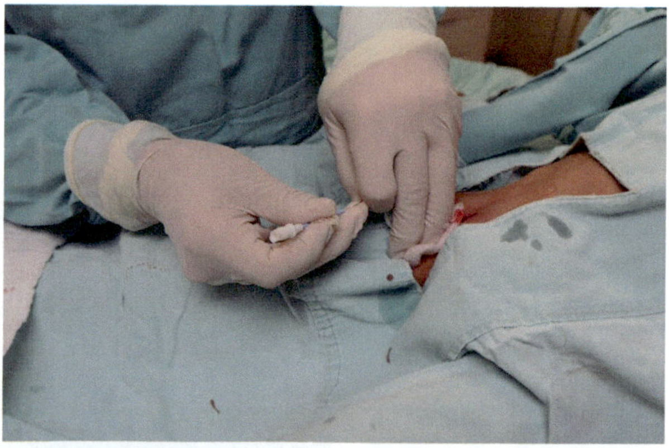

Fig. 18.36 Introduce the dilator over the guidewire

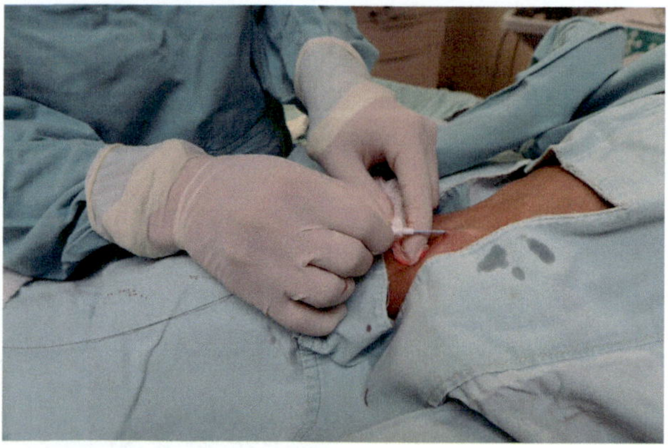

Fig. 18.37 Dilation of the skin

18.4.6 Step 06

- With the index finger of the left hand, occlude the entry of the guide into the skin and expose the distal tip of the guidewire to pass the catheter (Fig. 18.39).
- Advance the catheter over the guidewire (Seldinger's technique) (Fig. 18.40).
- Enter the desired catheter length.
- Remove the guidewire.
- Scan the intravenous location of the catheter (Fig. 18.41).
- LAX view of the catheter inside the RFV (Figs. 18.42 and 18.43).

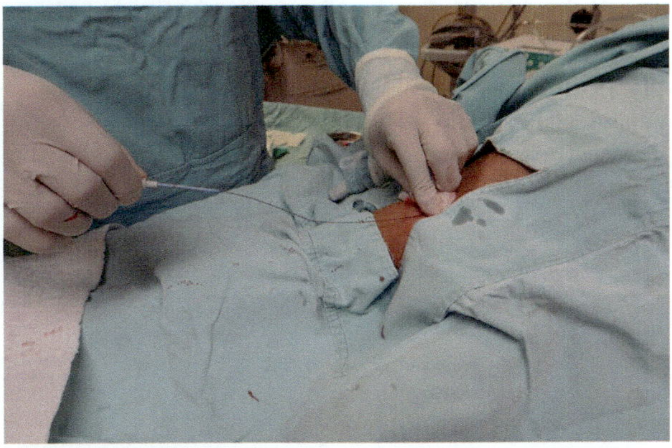

Fig. 18.38 Remove the dilator

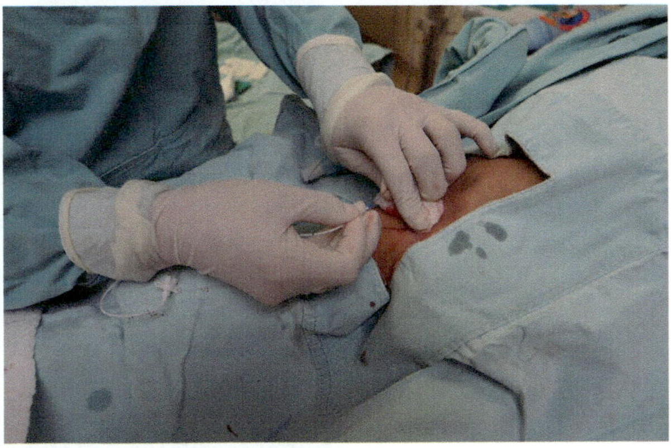

Fig. 18.39 Expose the distal tip of the guidewire to pass the catheter over the guidewire

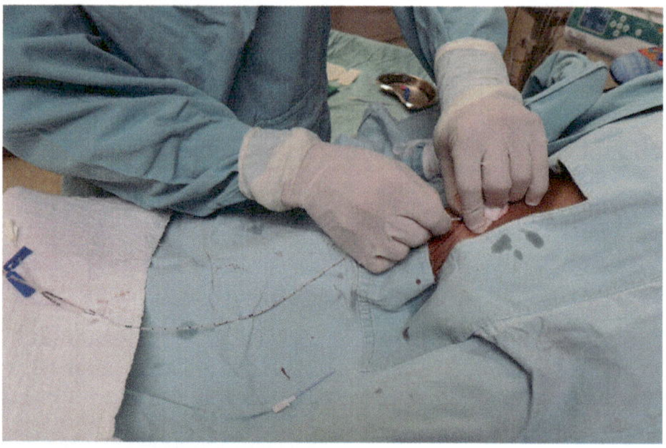

Fig. 18.40 Seldinger's technique: advance the catheter over the guidewire

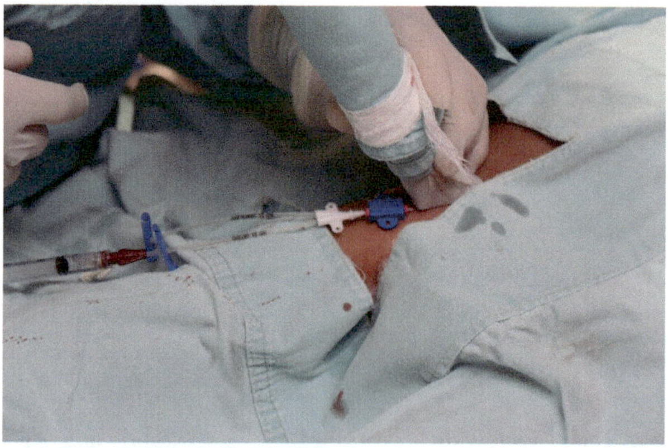

Fig. 18.41 Scan the intravascular location of the catheter

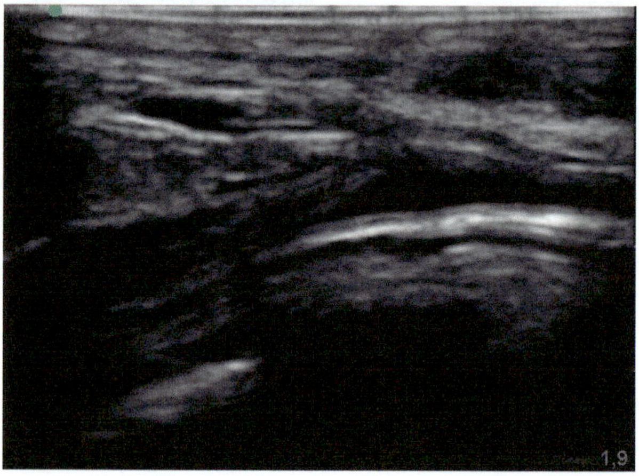

Fig. 18.42 LAX view of the catheter inside the RFV

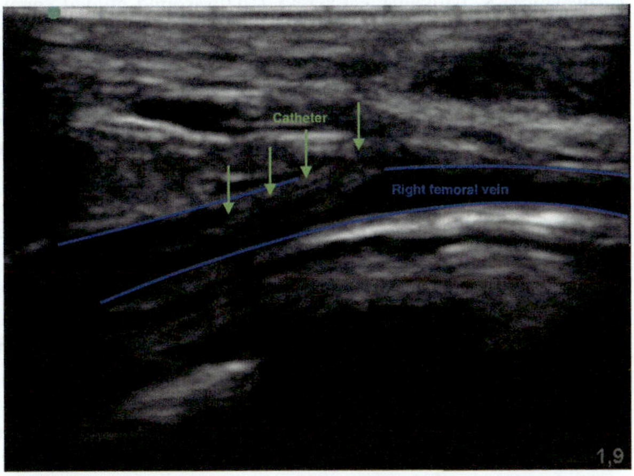

Fig. 18.43 Identifying structures
- The 4 Fr double-lumen catheter inside the RFV

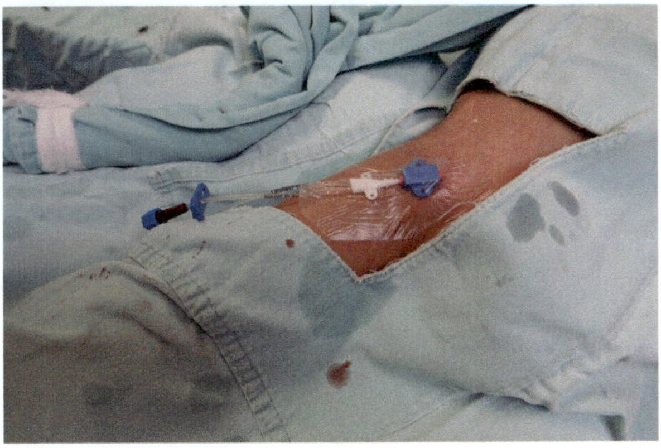

Fig. 18.44 Dressing according to the institutional protocol

18.4.7 Step 07

- Secure the catheter and place a sterile occlusive dressing according to the institutional protocol (Fig. 18.44).

Sources

1. Warkentine FH, Clyde Pierce M, Lorenz D, Kim IK. The anatomic relationship of femoral vein to femoral artery in euvolemic pediatric patients by ultrasonography: implications for pediatric femoral central venous access. Acad Emerg Med. 2008;15(5):426–30. https://doi.org/10.1111/j.1553-2712.2008.00087.x.

2. Iwashima S, Ishikawa T, Ohzeki T. Ultrasound-guided versus landmark-guided femoral vein access in pediatric cardiac catheterization. Pediatr Cardiol. 2008;29(2):339–42. https://doi.org/10.1007/s00246-007-9066-2.
3. Aouad MT, Kanazi GE, Abdallah FW, Moukaddem FH, Turbay MJ, Obeid MY, Siddik-Sayyid SM. Femoral vein cannulation performed by residents: a comparison between ultrasound-guided and landmark technique in infants and children undergoing cardiac surgery. Anesth Analg. 2010;111(3):724–8. https://doi.org/10.1213/ANE.0b013e3181e9c475. Epub 2010 Jul 2
4. Al Sofyani K, Julia G, Abdulaziz B, Yves CJ, Sylvain R. Ultrasound guidance for central vascular access in the neonatal and pediatric intensive care unit. Saudi J Anaesth. 2012;6(2):120–4. https://doi.org/10.4103/1658-354X.97023. Erratum in: Saudi J Anaesth. 2012 Oct-Dec;6(4):372. Khouloud, Al Sofyani [corrected to Al Sofyani, Khouloud]
5. Alten JA, Borasino S, Gurley WQ, Law MA, Toms R, Dabal RJ. Ultrasound-guided femoral vein catheterization in neonates with cardiac disease*. Pediatr Crit Care Med. 2012;13(6):654–9. https://doi.org/10.1097/PCC.0b013e318250af0c.
6. Ahn JH, Park J, Song IS, Kim KA, Park J, Min JJ, Kim CS, Lee JH. The angle range of leg abduction with external hip rotation which can minimize femoral artery and vein overlap in pediatric patients. Paediatr Anaesth. 2019;29(4):361–7. https://doi.org/10.1111/pan.13603. Epub 2019 Mar 21
7. Liu WL, Lin MC, Chan SC, Chen SN, Lin TY, Jan SL. Ultrasonographic measurements of femoral vessel diameter in neonates weighing less than 2.5 kg. Echocardiography. 2021;38(10):1741–6. https://doi.org/10.1111/echo.15203. Epub 2021 Sep 23

Chapter 19
Right Femoral/Iliac Vein in Neonates

19.1 Patient Positioning

- The patient is a premature patient weighing 1175 g.
- Position the patient with the feet near the border of the heating cradle.
- Position the patient supine with the legs extended, separated from the midline, and with gentle restraint at the ankles (Fig. 19.1).
- Place a roll under the hip. We do this with the diaper (Fig. 19.2).

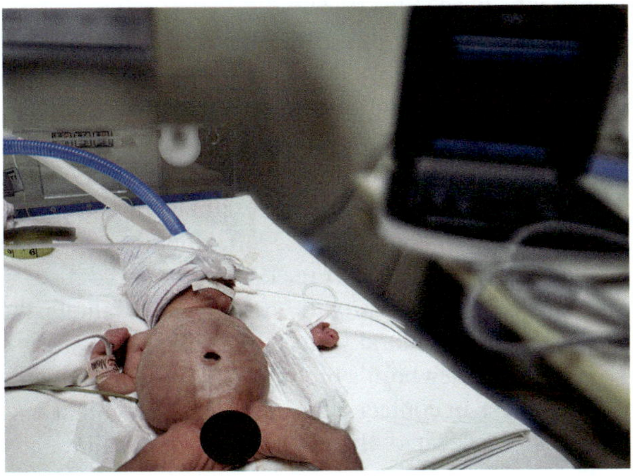

Fig. 19.1 Patient position

F. Montes-Tapia, *Atlas of Ultrasound-Guided Central Venous Catheter Placement*, https://doi.org/10.1007/978-3-031-61887-1_19

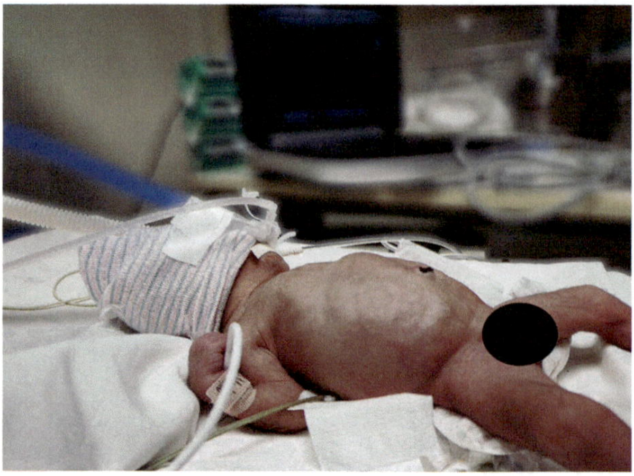

Fig. 19.2 Place a roll under the hip

19.2 Scanning Technique

- Do a preliminary vascular assessment (non-sterile), known as rapid femoral vein assessment (RaFeVA).
- The operator stands at the patient's feet.
- The ultrasound is placed at the level of the right or left shoulder or above the patient's head (Fig. 19.3).
- A high-frequency linear transducer (13–6 MHz) with a hockey stick transducer is used.
- The patient's leg at this age is so small in diameter that the transducer must be well positioned.
- The transducer is placed at the level of the inguinal ligament with the tip toward the patient's right side, which will be marked on the screen as the left side, corresponding to the operator's left. This is done to correlate the operator's movements with the screen (Fig. 19.3).
- Scan in SAX to identify the arteriovenous bundle, the right femoral artery (RFA), and the right femoral vein (RFV) (Figs. 19.4 and 19.5).
- Elevate the newborn's hip with a roll (in this patient, with the diaper) to keep the transducer in contact with the lower abdominal wall and inguinal region. If the hip is not elevated, the inguinal region would be in a depression, and contact of the transducer with this region could not occur.
- Position the inguinal ligament at half the length of the transducer and scan from lateral to medial (Fig. 19.6).
- Then scan in long-axis (LAX) view from lateral to medial to identify the RFA and then the RFV (Figs. 19.7, 19.8, 19.9 and 19.10).

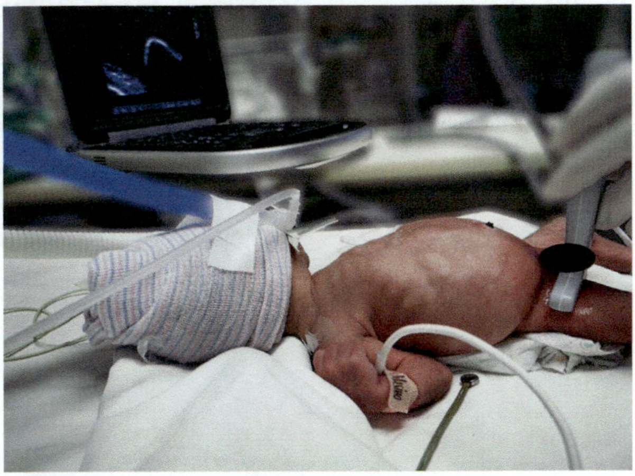

Fig. 19.3 The ultrasound is placed at the level of the left shoulder. The transducer is placed at the level of the inguinal ligament with the tip toward the patient's right side

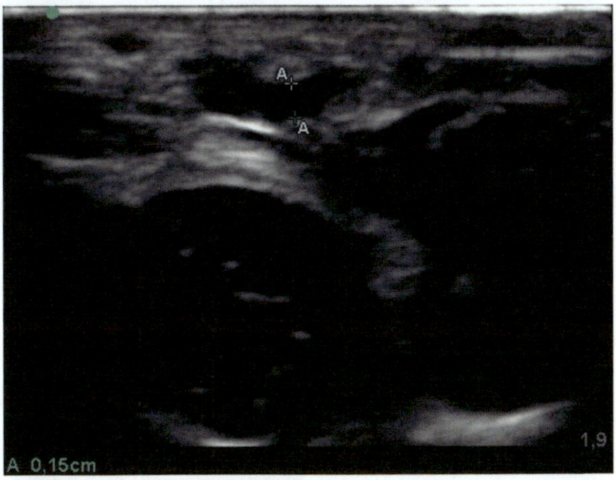

Fig. 19.4 SAX view of the right femoral bundle

- The right RFV measures 0,15 cm in the anteroposterior plane
- The scan depth of 1,9 cm

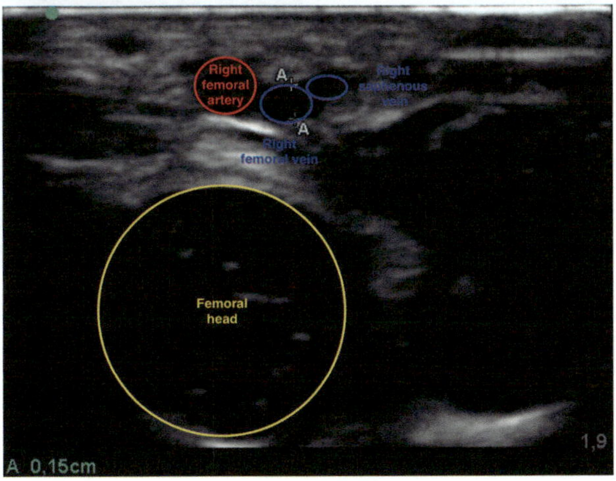

Fig. 19.5 Identifying structures

- Mickey Mouse sign, composed from medial to lateral of the saphenous vein draining into the RFV and RFA
- The femoral head of the femur is also seen

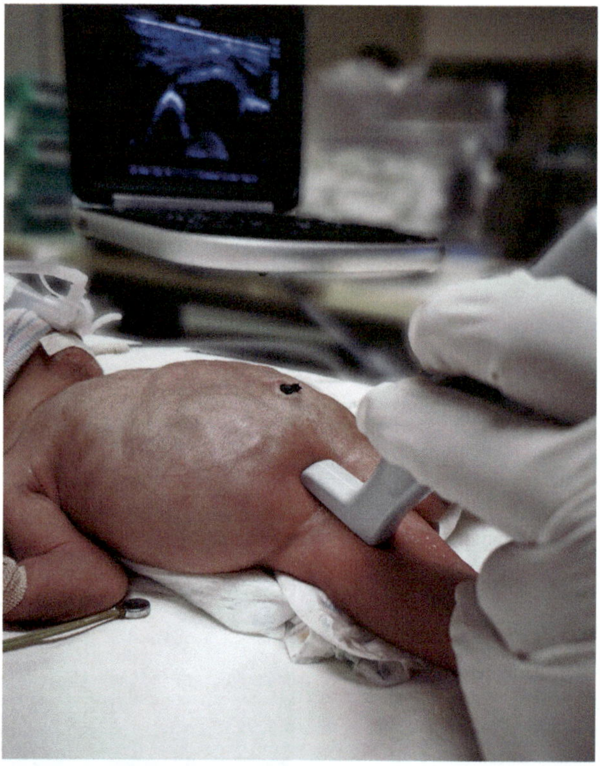

Fig. 19.6 Position the inguinal ligament at half the length of the transducer and scan from lateral to medial in LAX view

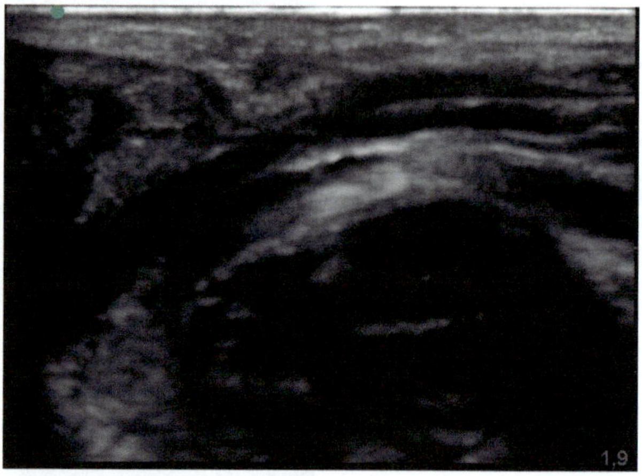

Fig. 19.7 Lateral scan at the level of the right inguinal ligament. LAX view of the RFA
- Scan depth at 1,9 cm

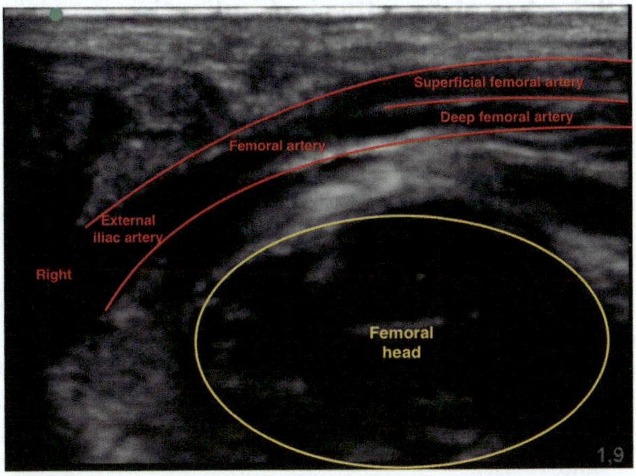

Fig. 19.8 Identifying structures

- The right external iliac artery that continues with the common femoral artery is seen in LAX, which divides into the superficial and deep femoral arteries
- The femoral head of the femur is identified

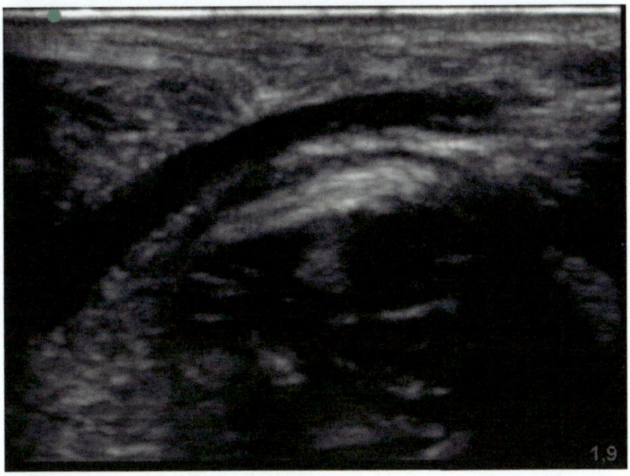

Fig. 19.9 Medial scan of the leg at the level of the right inguinal ligament. LAX view of the common RFV

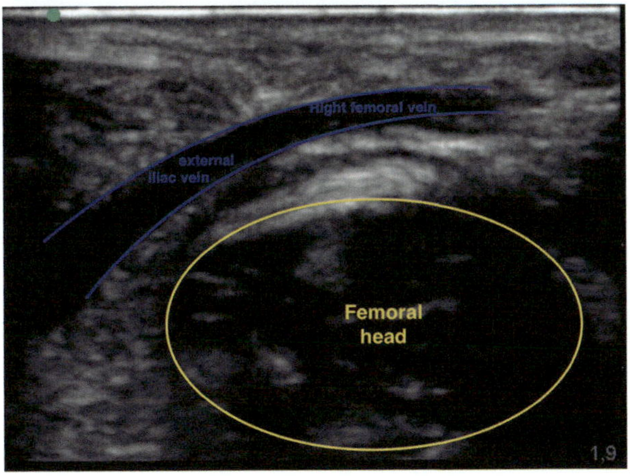

Fig. 19.10 Identifying structures

- The femoral veins continue with the external iliac vein, which begins behind the inguinal ligament

19.3 Local Anesthesia Application

- The sterile field only leaves the lower right abdomen, inguinal, and anterior thigh regions uncovered (Fig. 19.11).
- Position the patient with leg extension. You can do this with good sedation and restraint. You can also have an assistant keep the leg extended by holding it at the ankle.
- Real-time ultrasound-guided lidocaine infiltration.
- For infiltration, use a small infiltration needle 25 to 27 G.
- Use lidocaine 1%.
- Subcutaneous infiltration with lidocaine in the puncture tract 1–1,5 cm before the site chosen for RFV puncture and the catheter fixation area (Fig. 19.12).
- LAX view of lidocaine infiltration in the subcutaneous tissue (Figs. 19.13 and 19.14).

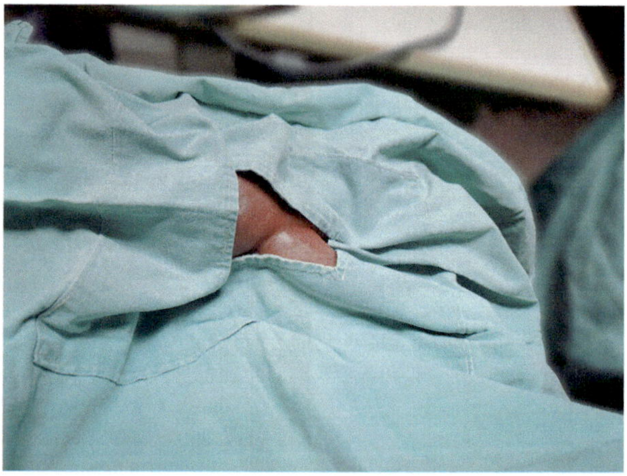

Fig. 19.11 The sterile field only leaves the lower right abdomen, inguinal, and anterior thigh regions uncovered

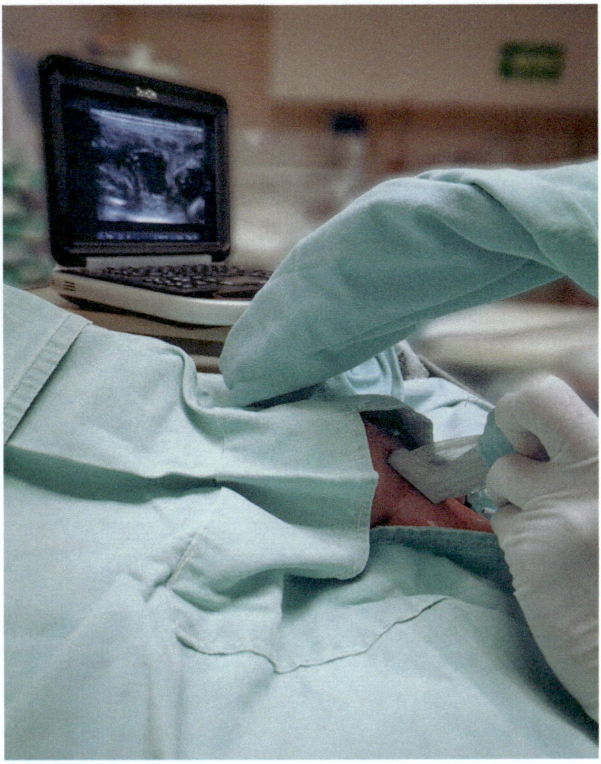

Fig. 19.12 Real-time ultrasound-guided lidocaine infiltration

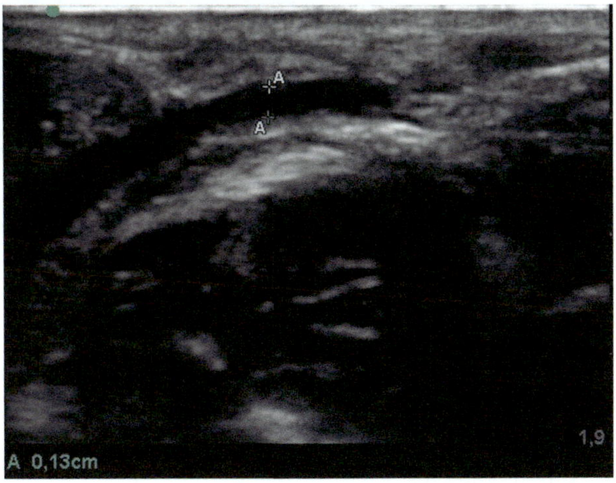

Fig. 19.13 Scan of the abdominal and inguinal region. LAX view of local anesthesia

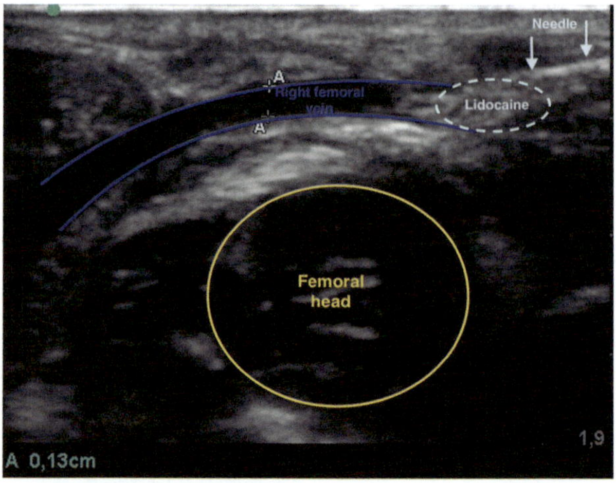

Fig. 19.14 Identifying structures
- The infiltration needle (25 G) is identified in the subcutaneous tissue
- Lidocaine will form a hyperechoic area
- This moment of the procedure can be used to determine if the site of choice for the puncture is in the plane of the RFV

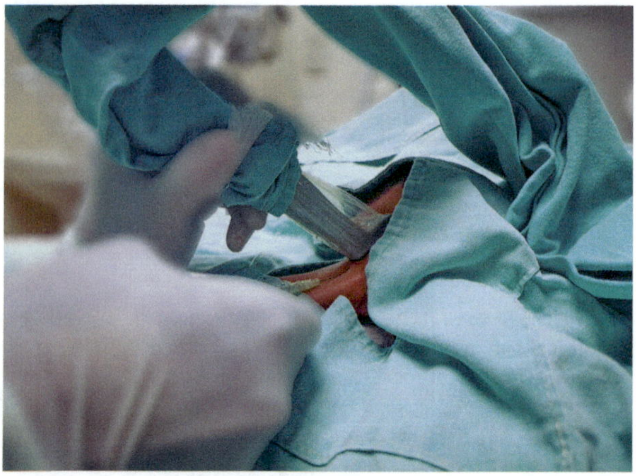

Fig. 19.15 Start the puncture at an angle of less than 10°, almost parallel to the skin

19.4 Steps for Real-Time Ultrasound-Guided Access to the Right Femoral/Iliac Vein in Neonates

19.4.1 Step 01

- We will use a 10-cm, double-lumen Vygon® 3 Fr catheter.
- Perform the puncture in LAX, below the inguinal ligament, using a 24-G intravenous catheter.
- Begin the ultrasound-guided dynamic needle tracking (DNT) to guide the puncture in real time.
- Start the puncture with an angle of less than 10°, almost parallel to the skin. The objective is to penetrate under the skin and first identify the location of the intravenous catheter and then over the vein (Fig. 19.15).

  - Puncture in the middle of the thickness of the transducer so that the intravenous catheter can be visualized along the path aligned with the vein (Figs. 19.16 and 19.17).

- Once the intravenous catheter is visible on the screen, redirect the puncture path into the vein.
- Remember, these premature patients have little subcutaneous tissue. A higher puncture angle can cause you to penetrate more deeply or incidentally puncture or traverse the vein or artery.
- Scan lateral or medial to locate the vein and redirect the intravenous catheter puncture to the path of the RFV.
- Once the RFV is located, restart the puncture, increasing the puncture angle to 10–20° to follow the path of the vein (Fig. 19.18).
- LAX view of the correct direction of the puncture (Figs. 19.19 and 19.20).

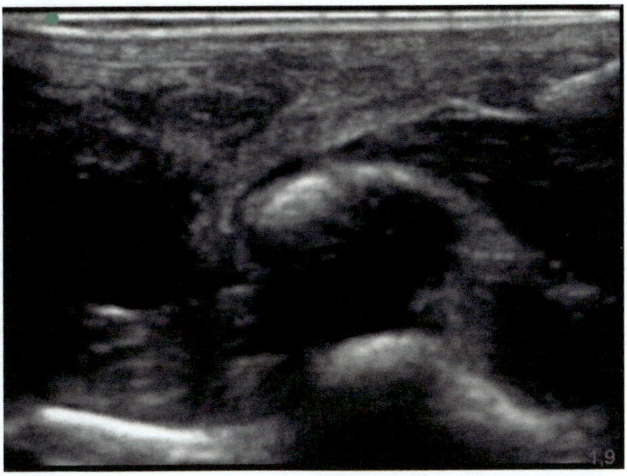

Fig. 19.16 LAX view of the entry of the intravenous catheter into the subcutaneous tissue

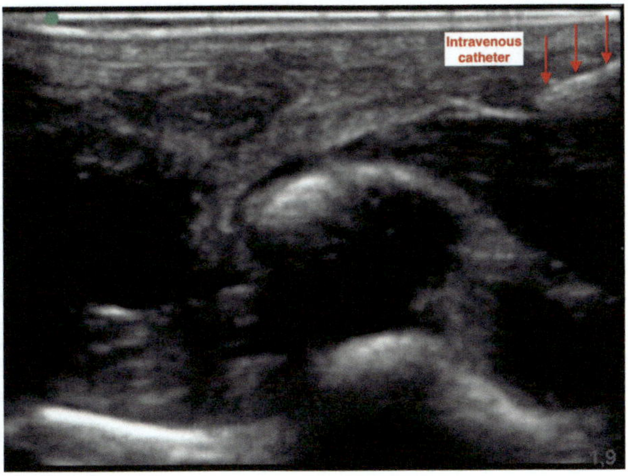

Fig. 19.17 Identifying structures

- Introduction of the intravenous catheter with a puncture angle of less than 10°; however, at this moment, it is not aligned with the RFV

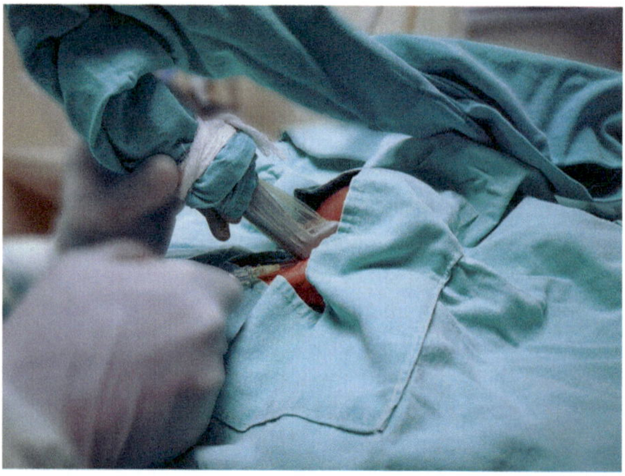

Fig. 19.18 Increase the puncture angle to 10–20° to follow the path of the vein

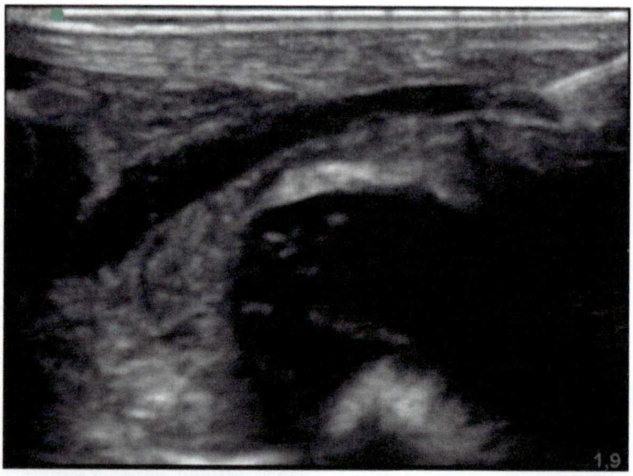

Fig. 19.19 LAX view of the correct direction of the puncture

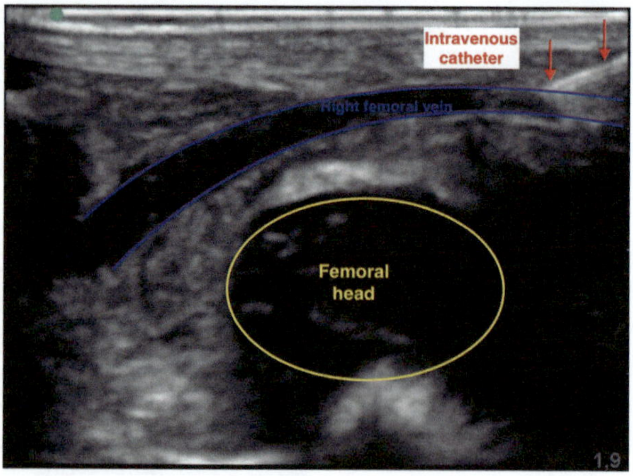

Fig. 19.20 Identifying structures

- It is seen that with the modification of the puncture direction and an increase in the puncture angle to 10–20°, there is correct alignment of the intravenous catheter with the RFV

19.4.2 Step 02

- Continue with the puncture since the puncture angle and the RFV are aligned (Fig. 19.21).
- LAX view of the intravenous catheter is reaching the anterior wall of the RFV (Figs. 19.22 and 19.23).
- Advance the intravenous to cannulate the RFV (Fig. 19.24).
- LAX view of the beginning of cannulation of the RFV (Figs. 19.25 and 19.26).

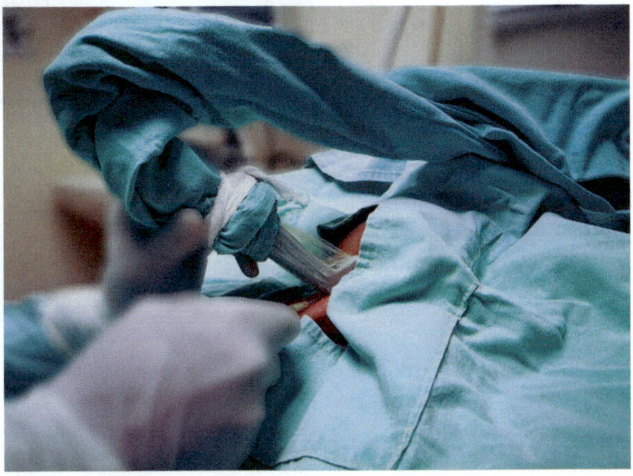

Fig. 19.21 Continue with the path of the puncture

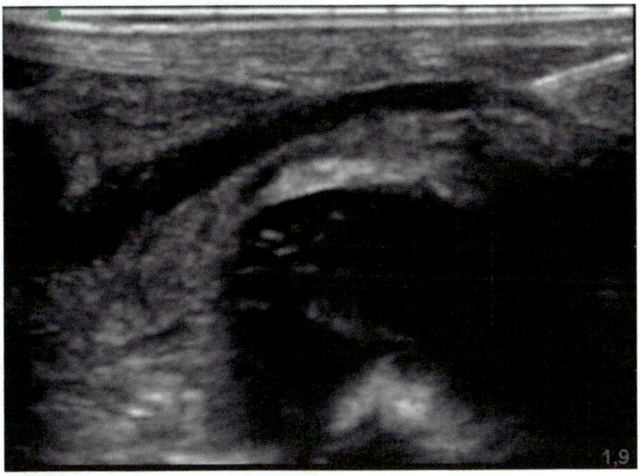

Fig. 19.22 LAX view of the puncture progression

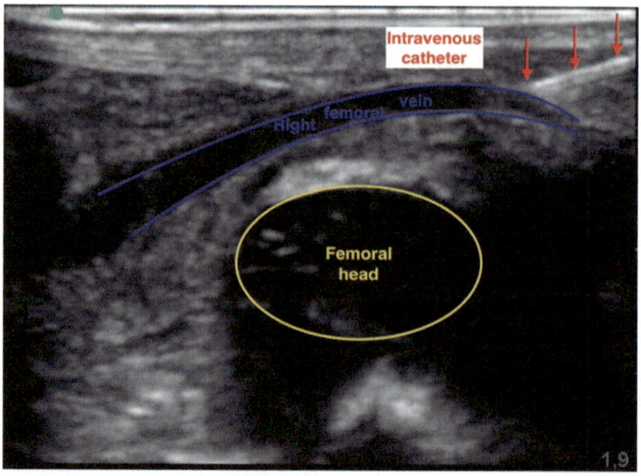

Fig. 19.23 Identifying structures

- The intravenous catheter reaches the anterior wall of the RFV

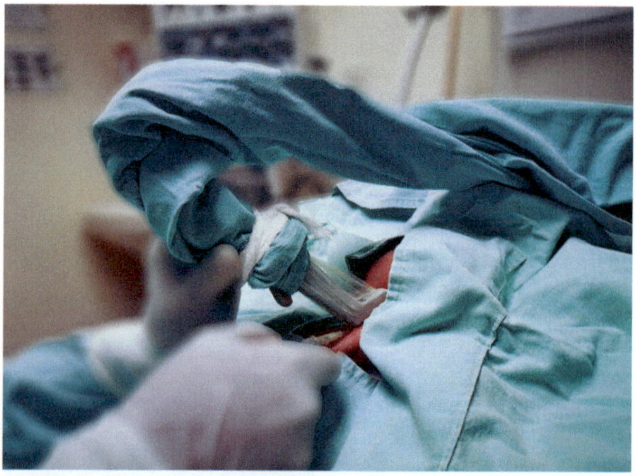

Fig. 19.24 Advance the intravenous catheter in DNT to cannulate the RFV

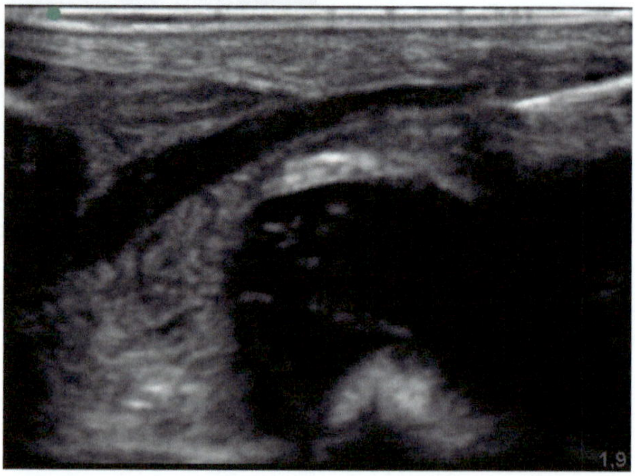

Fig. 19.25 LAX view of the beginning of cannulation of the RFV

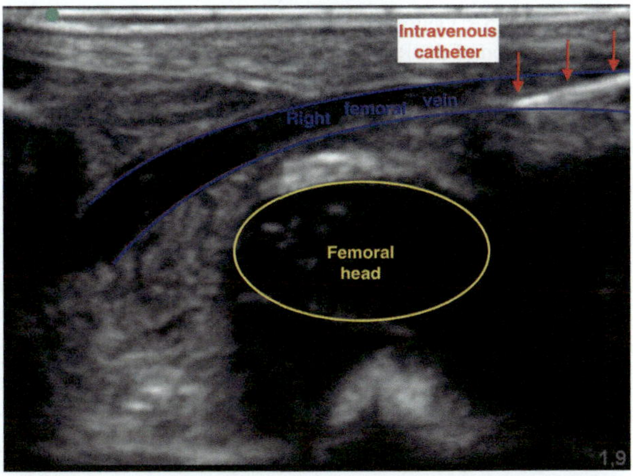

Fig. 19.26 Identifying structures

- The intravenous catheter enters the RFV

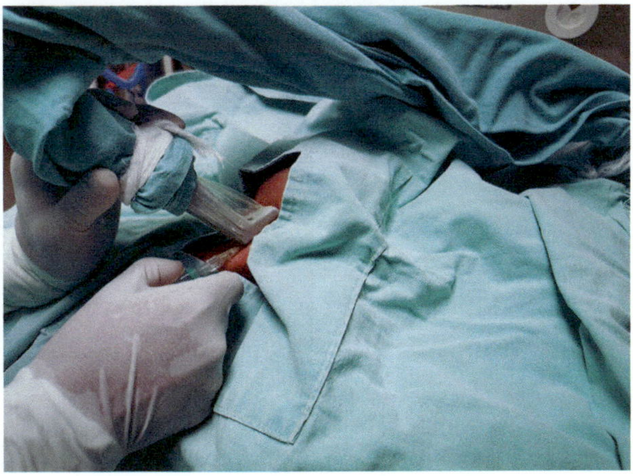

Fig. 19.27 Cannulation of the RFV

19.4.3 Step 03

- Once the intravenous catheter is identified as entering the lumen of the vein, the intravenous catheter is introduced further to completely cannulate the RFV with the catheter. This procedure is done in DNT (Fig. 19.27).
- LAX view of the complete cannulation of the RFV (Figs. 19.28, 19.29, 19.30 and 19.31).
- After visualizing complete cannulation of the RFV through the intravenous catheter, set the transducer aside.
- Remove the puncture needle.
- Leave only the intravenous tube cannulating the vein.

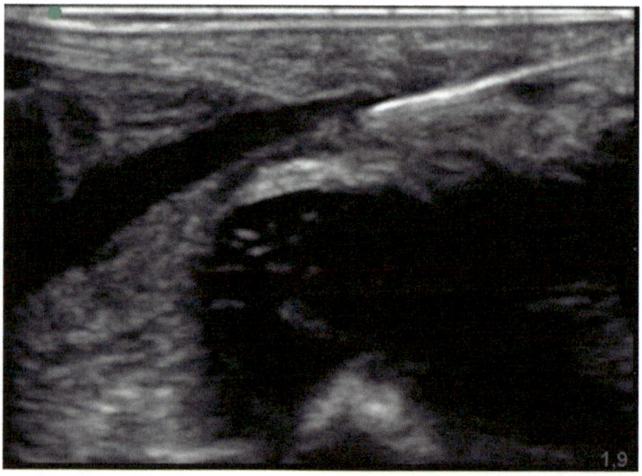

Fig. 19.28 LAX view of the cannulation of the RFV

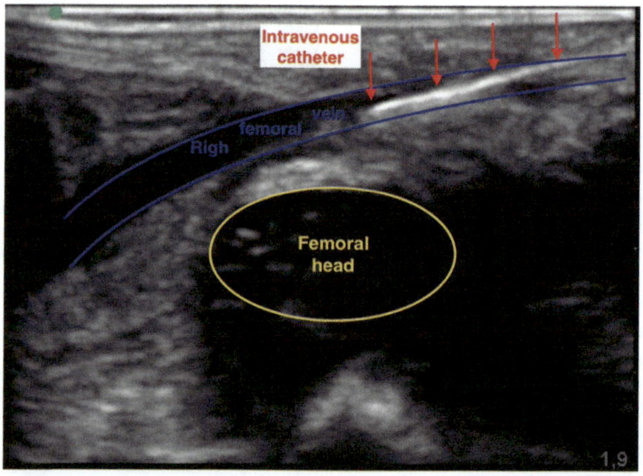

Fig. 19.29 Identifying structures
- Progression of RFV cannulation with the intravenous catheter

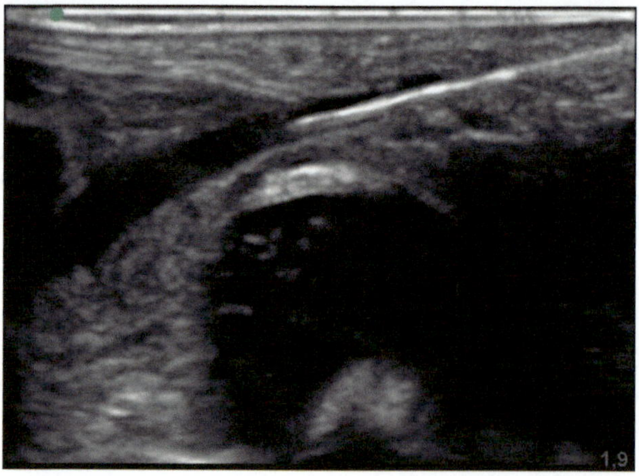

Fig. 19.30 LAX view of the complete cannulation of the RFV

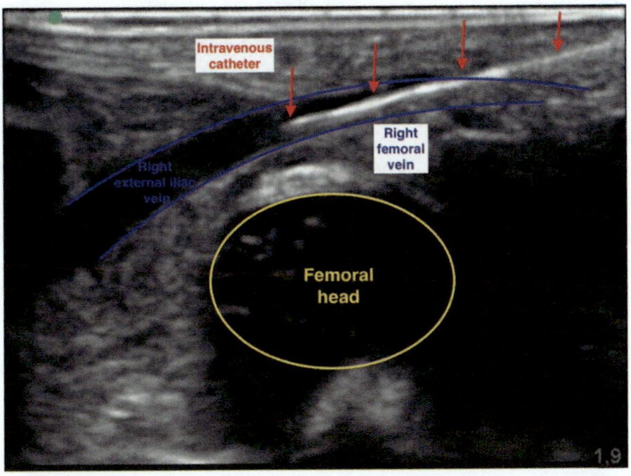

Fig. 19.31 Identifying structures
- The RFV is cannulated with the entire intravenous catheter without penetrating the posterior wall

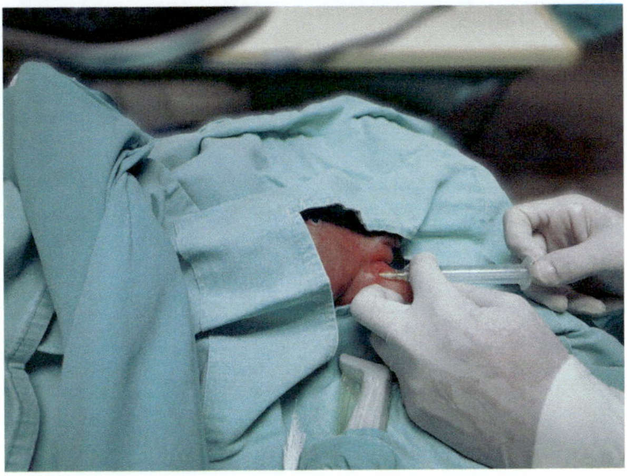

Fig. 19.32 Apply gentle negative pressure and check for return of blood

- Put a syringe and maintain gentle negative pressure on the syringe plunger until a flash of blood appears through the catheter tube that cannulates the RFV (Fig. 19.32).
- Or sometimes just remove the syringe from the intravenous catheter and blood coming out through the 24-G catheter (Fig. 19.33).

19.4.4 Step 04

- Insert the 0,3-mm nitinol guidewire, which should pass easily (Fig. 19.34).
- This type of guidewire is marked every 10 cm.
- The location of the guidewire can be checked in the venous lumen in SAX or LAX; one or the other is not necessary.

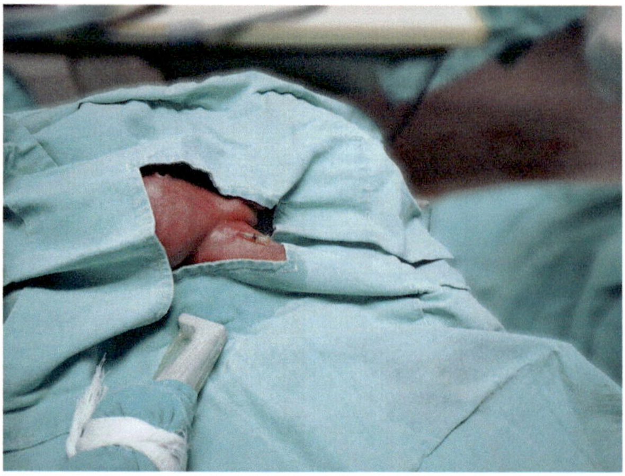

Fig. 19.33 Remove the syringe from the intravenous catheter to check the spontaneous outflow of blood

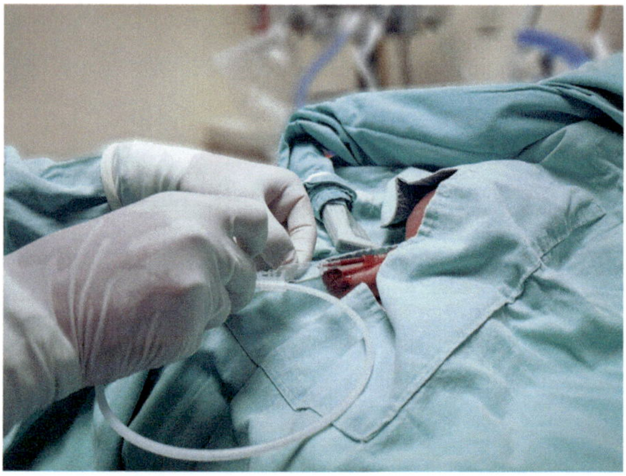

Fig. 19.34 Insert the guidewire

- Place the transducer transversely, above the inguinal ligament, and locate the arteriovenous bundle to locate the guidewire within the RFV (Fig. 19.35).
- SAX view of the guidewire in the RFV (Figs. 19.36 and 19.37).
- Place the transducer longitudinally over the inguinal ligament, like the puncture was performed (Fig. 19.38).
- LAX view of the guidewire in the RFV (Figs. 19.39 and 19.40).

19.4.5 Step 05

- Once you have identified the guidewire inside the vein, the path is dilated. This is a safety measure to avoid dilation in case of incidental puncture of the femoral artery (Fig. 19.41).

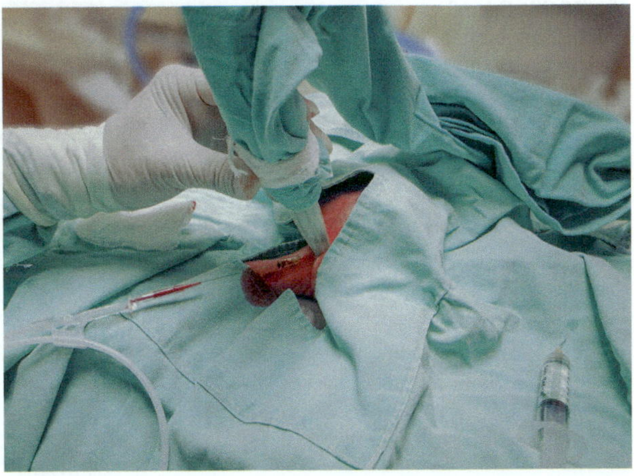

Fig. 19.35 Scan the inguinal region in SAX view to verify the intravascular location of the guidewire

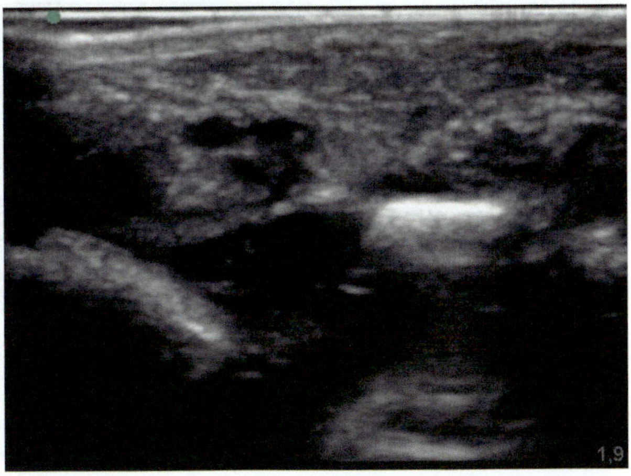

Fig. 19.36 SAX view of the guidewire in the RFV

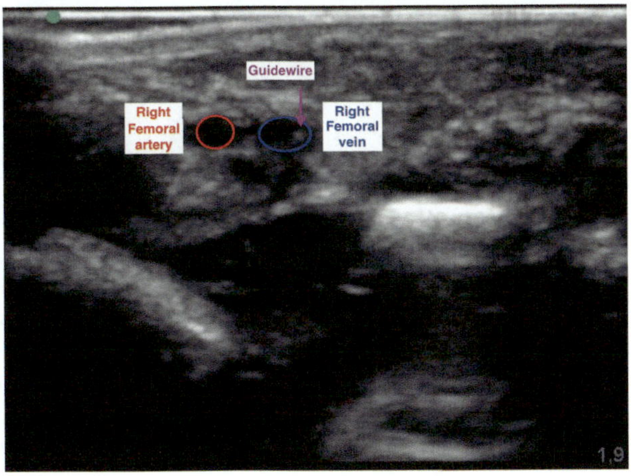

Fig. 19.37 Identifying structures

- A hyperechogenic dot image can be seen within the RFV

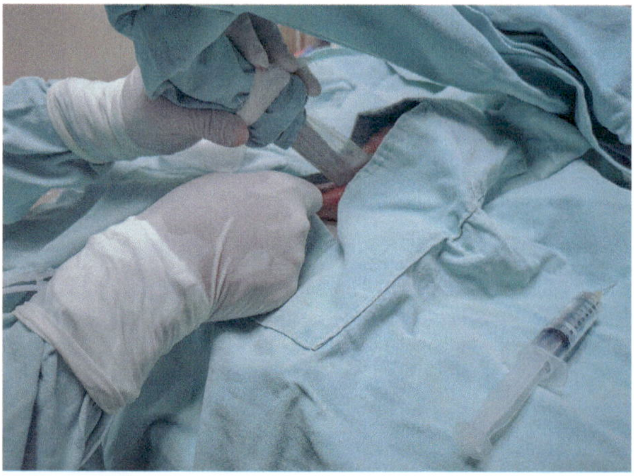

Fig. 19.38 Scan the inguinal region in LAX view to verify the intravascular location of the guidewire

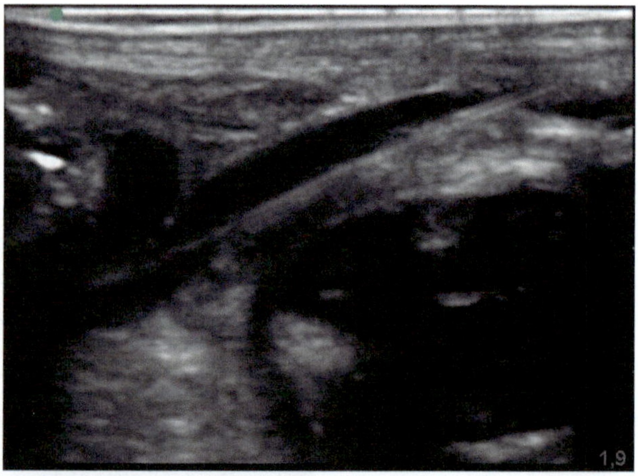

Fig. 19.39 LAX view of the guidewire in the RFV

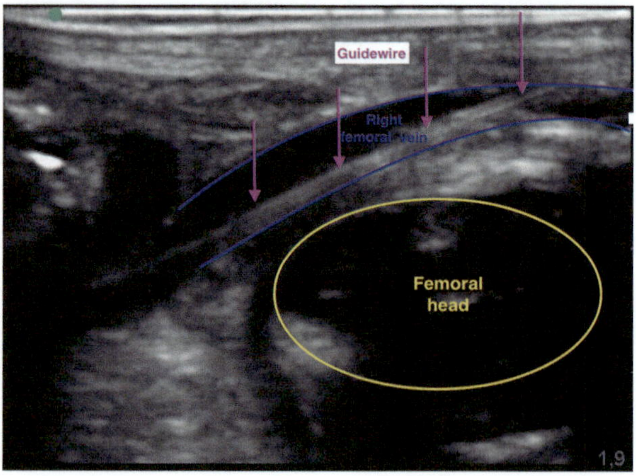

Fig. 19.40 Identifying structures
- Guidewire in the RFV

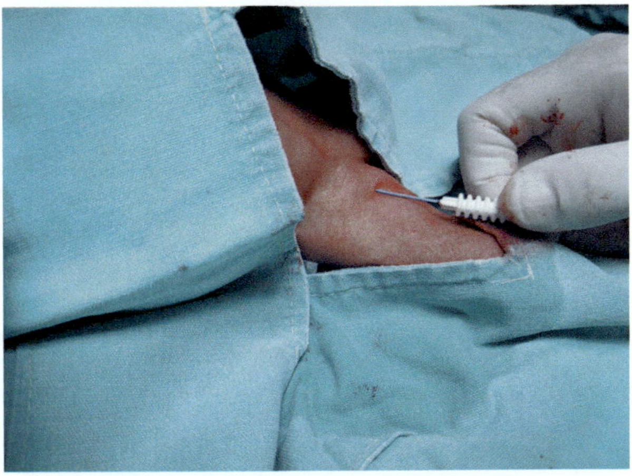

Fig. 19.41 Introduce the dilator over the guidewire

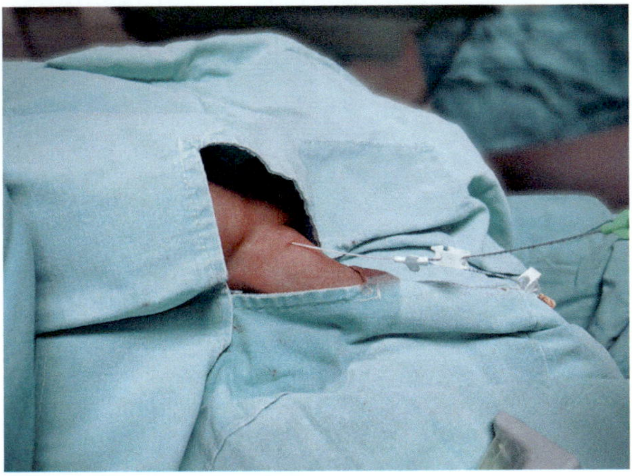

Fig. 19.42 Seldinger's technique: advance the catheter over the guidewire

- Dilate the path between the skin and the RFV delicately because the tissues are fragile.

19.4.6 Step 06

- Insert the 3 Fr double-lumen catheter using Seldinger's technique (Fig. 19.42).
- Introduce the desired catheter length (Fig. 19.43).
- Remove the guidewire.
- Scan the intravenous location of the catheter in LAX (Fig. 19.44).
- LAX view of the catheter inside the RFV (Figs. 19.45 and 19.46).

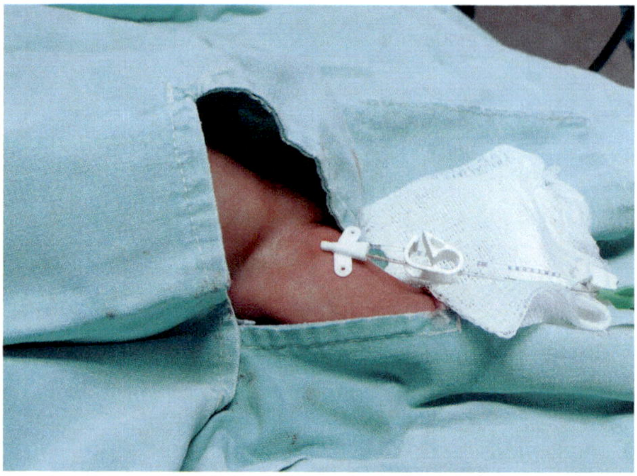

Fig. 19.43 Introduce the desired catheter length

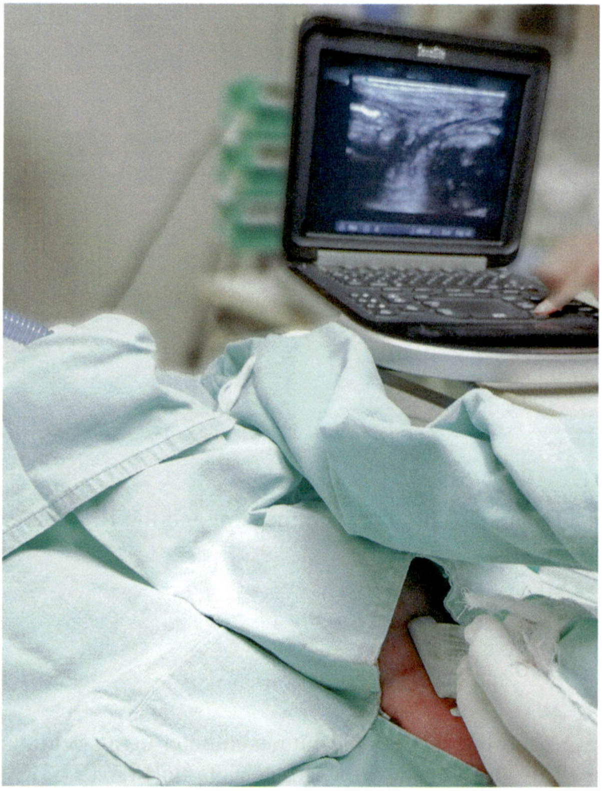

Fig. 19.44 Scan the intravenous location of the catheter

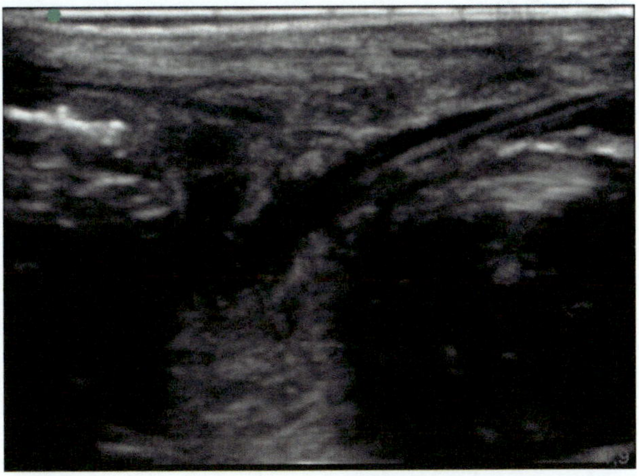

Fig. 19.45 LAX view of the catheter inside the RFV

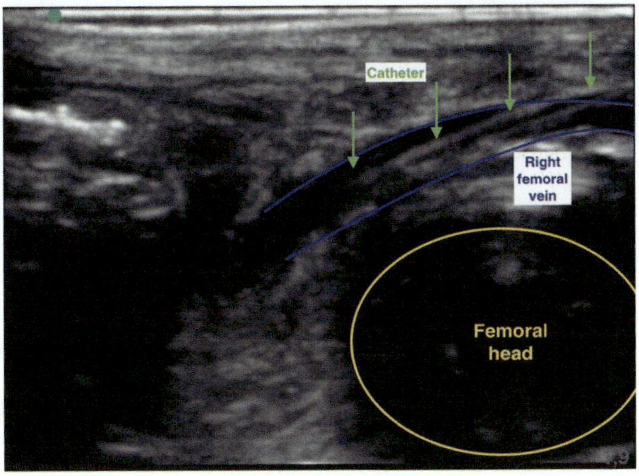

Fig. 19.46 Identifying structures
- The 3 Fr double-lumen catheter inside the RFV

19.4.7 Step 07

- Secure the catheter and place a sterile occlusive dressing according to the institutional protocol (Fig. 19.47).

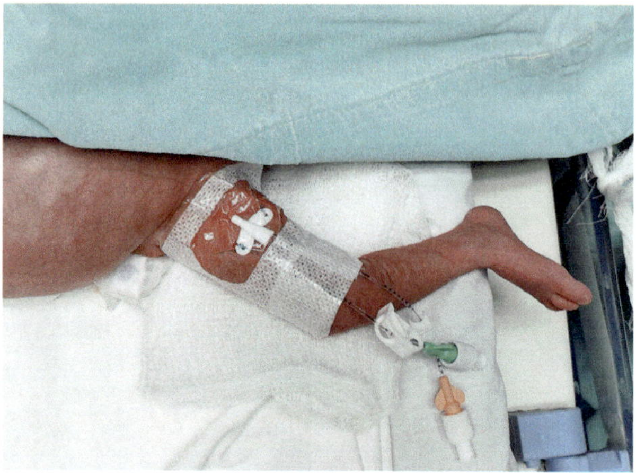

Fig. 19.47 Dressing according to the institutional protocol

Sources

1. Warkentine FH, Clyde Pierce M, Lorenz D, Kim IK. The anatomic relationship of femoral vein to femoral artery in euvolemic pediatric patients by ultrasonography: implications for pediatric femoral central venous access. Acad Emerg Med. 2008;15(5):426–30. https://doi.org/10.1111/j.1553-2712.2008.00087.x.
2. Iwashima S, Ishikawa T, Ohzeki T. Ultrasound-guided versus landmark-guided femoral vein access in pediatric cardiac catheterization. Pediatr Cardiol. 2008;29(2):339–42. https://doi.org/10.1007/s00246-007-9066-2.
3. Aouad MT, Kanazi GE, Abdallah FW, Moukaddem FH, Turbay MJ, Obeid MY, Siddik-Sayyid SM. Femoral vein cannulation performed by residents: a comparison between ultrasound-guided and landmark technique in infants and children undergoing cardiac surgery. Anesth Analg. 2010;111(3):724–8. https://doi.org/10.1213/ANE.0b013e3181e9c475. Epub 2010 Jul 2
4. Al Sofyani K, Julia G, Abdulaziz B, Yves CJ, Sylvain R. Ultrasound guidance for central vascular access in the neonatal and pediatric intensive care unit. Saudi J Anaesth. 2012;6(2):120–4. https://doi.org/10.4103/1658-354X.97023. Erratum in: Saudi J Anaesth. 2012 Oct-Dec;6(4):372. Khouloud, Al Sofyani [corrected to Al Sofyani, Khouloud]
5. Alten JA, Borasino S, Gurley WQ, Law MA, Toms R, Dabal RJ. Ultrasound-guided femoral vein catheterization in neonates with cardiac disease*. Pediatr Crit Care Med. 2012;13(6):654–9. https://doi.org/10.1097/PCC.0b013e318250af0c.
6. Ahn JH, Park J, Song IS, Kim KA, Park J, Min JJ, Kim CS, Lee JH. The angle range of leg abduction with external hip rotation which can minimize femoral artery and vein overlap in pediatric patients. Paediatr Anaesth. 2019;29(4):361–7. https://doi.org/10.1111/pan.13603. Epub 2019 Mar 21
7. Liu WL, Lin MC, Chan SC, Chen SN, Lin TY, Jan SL. Ultrasonographic measurements of femoral vessel diameter in neonates weighing less than 2.5 kg. Echocardiography. 2021;38(10):1741–6. https://doi.org/10.1111/echo.15203. Epub 2021 Sep 23

Chapter 20
Left Femoral Vein in Pediatrics

20.1 Patient Positioning

- The patient is a 6-month-old weighing 3,7 kg.
- Position the patient on the left side with the feet near the edge of the bed.
- Position the patient supine with the legs extended, separated from the midline, and with gentle restraint at the ankles.
- Place a small roll below the hip (Fig. 20.1).

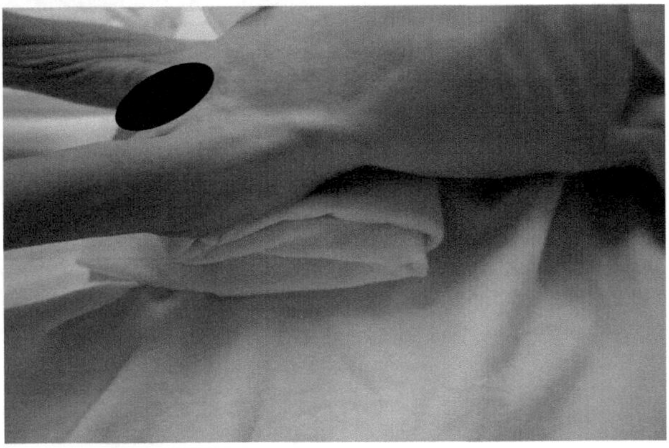

Fig. 20.1 Place a roll under the hip

F. Montes-Tapia, *Atlas of Ultrasound-Guided Central Venous Catheter Placement*, https://doi.org/10.1007/978-3-031-61887-1_20

20.2 Scanning Technique

- Do a preliminary vascular assessment (non-sterile), known as rapid femoral vein assessment (RaFeVA).
- The operator stands on the left side of the bed.
- The ultrasound is placed at the level of the right or left shoulder or above the patient's head.
- A high-frequency linear transducer (13–6 MHz) with a hockey stick transducer can be used.
- The transducer is placed transversely at the level of the inguinal ligament with the tip toward the patient's right side, which will be marked on the screen as the left side, corresponding to the operator's left. This correlates the operator's movements with those on the screen (Fig. 20.2).
- Short-axis (SAX) view of the femoral bundle (Figs. 20.3 and 20.4).

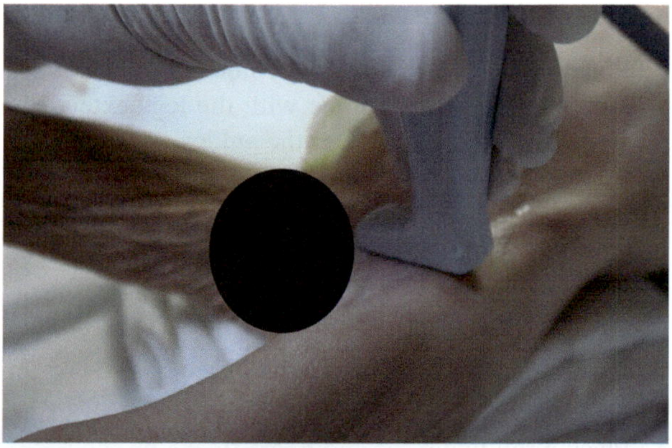

Fig. 20.2 Scan in SAX view

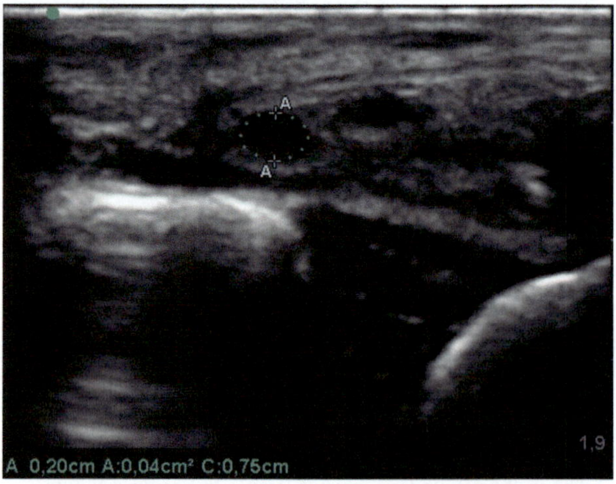

Fig. 20.3 SAX view of the femoral bundle
- Scan depth is 1,9 cm

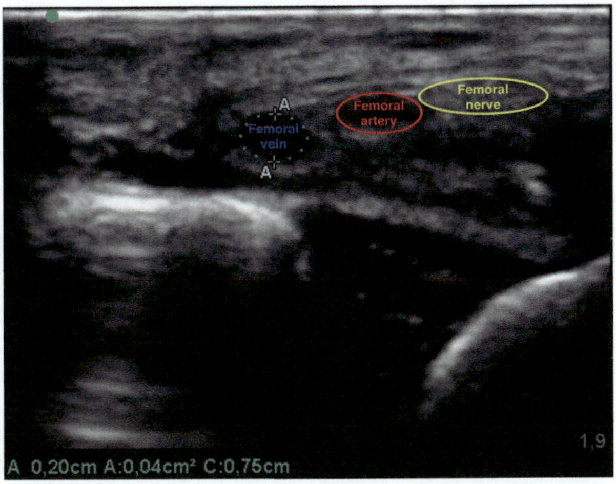

Fig. 20.4 Identifying structures

- Lateral to medial: femoral nerve, left femoral artery (LFA), and left femoral vein (LFV)
- The LFV measures 0,2 cm in the anteroposterior direction; the area of 0,04 cm^2 can also be calculated

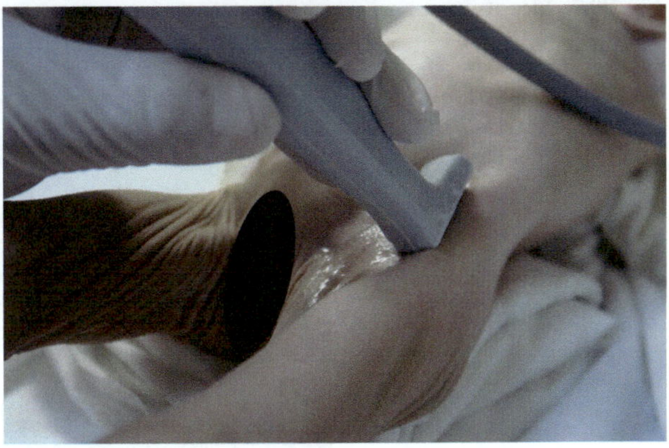

Fig. 20.5 Scan in LAX view

- Elevate the patient's hip with a roll to keep the transducer in contact with the lower abdominal wall and inguinal region. If the hip is not elevated, the inguinal region would be in a depression, and contact of the transducer with this region could not occur.
- Position the inguinal ligament at half the length of the transducer and scan from lateral to medial (Fig. 20.5).
- Then, scan in LAX from lateral to medial to identify the LFA and the LFV (Figs. 20.6, 20.7, 20.8 and 20.9).

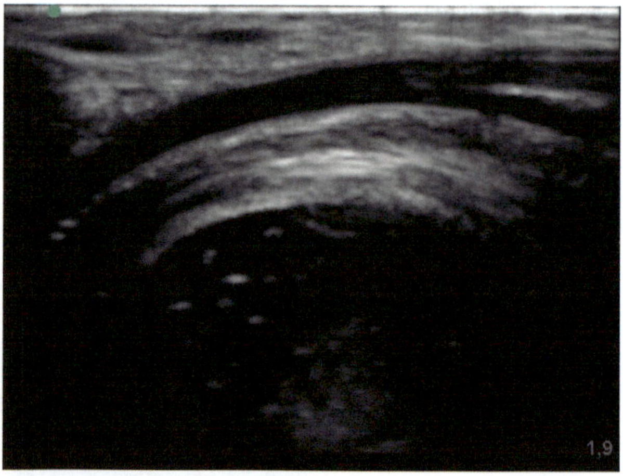

Fig. 20.6 Lateral scan of the left leg. LAX view of the LFA

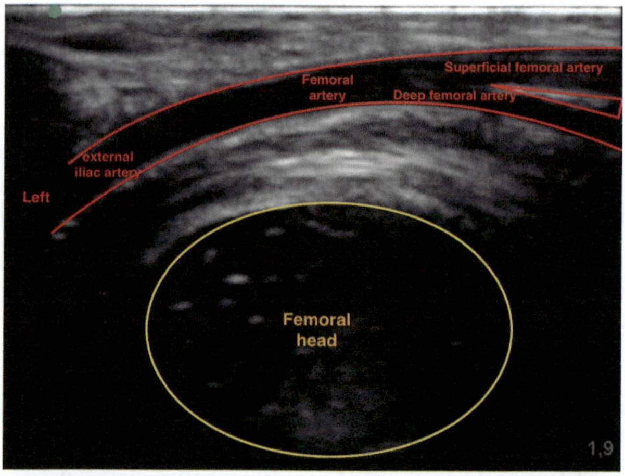

Fig. 20.7 Identifying structures
- The LFA divides into the superficial and deep left femoral arteries
- The femoral head is identified

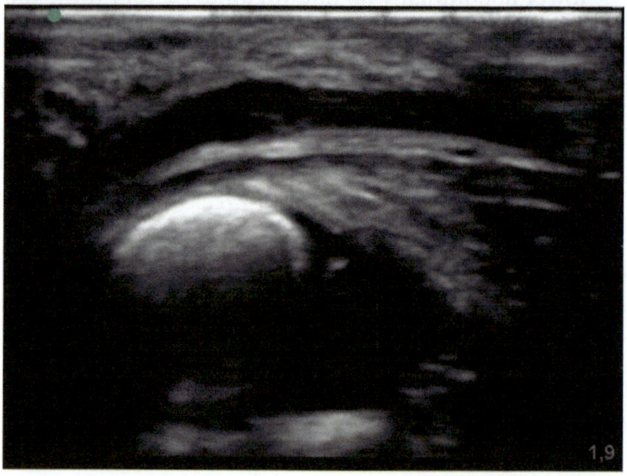

Fig. 20.8 Medial scan of the left leg. LAX view of the LFV

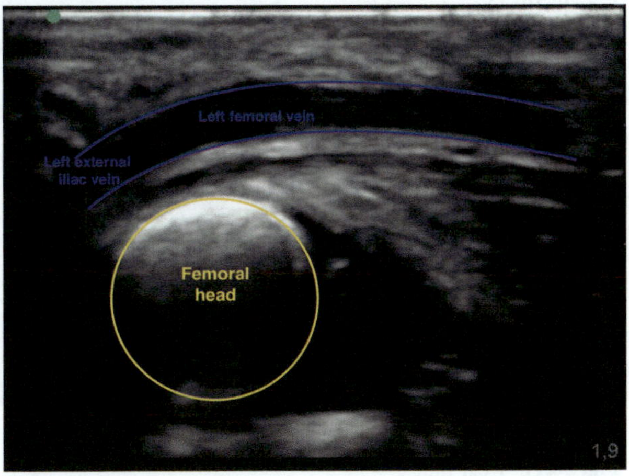

Fig. 20.9 Identifying structures
- The femoral vein above the femoral head

20.3 Local Anesthesia Application

- The sterile field only leaves the left inguinal and anterior thigh regions uncovered (Fig. 20.10).
- Position the patient with leg extension. You can do this with good sedation and restraint. You can also have an assistant keep the leg extended, holding it by the ankle.
- Real-time ultrasound-guided lidocaine infiltration.
- For infiltration, use a small needle 25–27 G.
- Use lidocaine 1%.
- Subcutaneous infiltration with lidocaine in the puncture tract 1,5–2 cm before the site chosen for LFV puncture and the catheter fixation area (Fig. 20.11).
- SAX view of lidocaine infiltration in the subcutaneous tissue (Figs. 20.12 and 20.13).

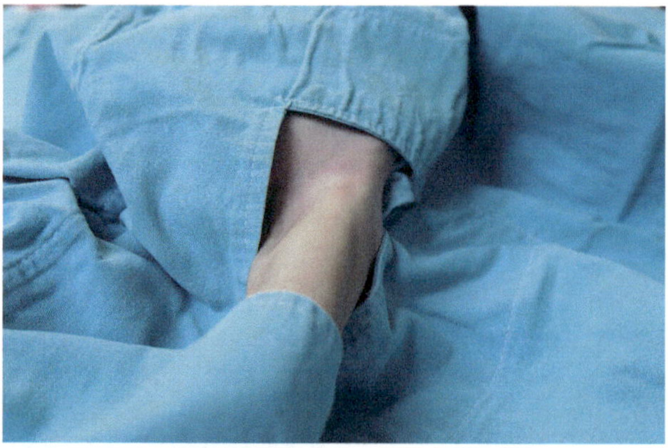

Fig. 20.10 Operator view

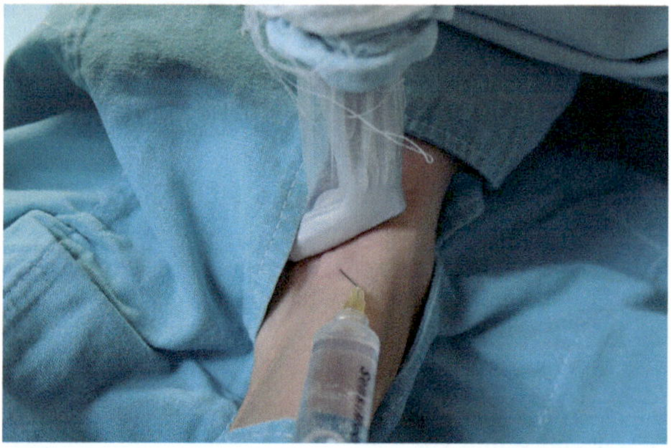

Fig. 20.11 Real-time ultrasound-guided lidocaine infiltration

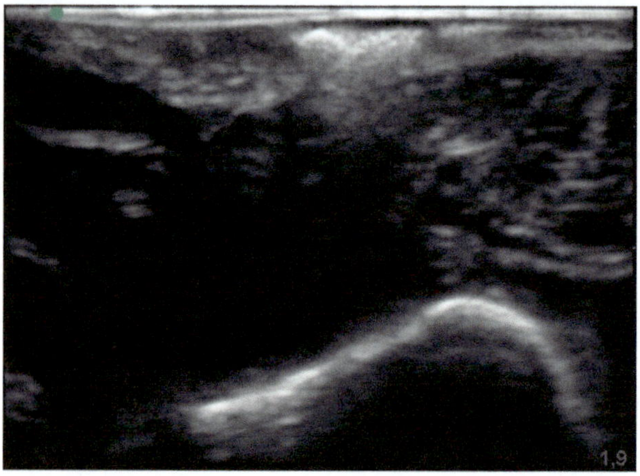

Fig. 20.12 SAX view of lidocaine infiltration

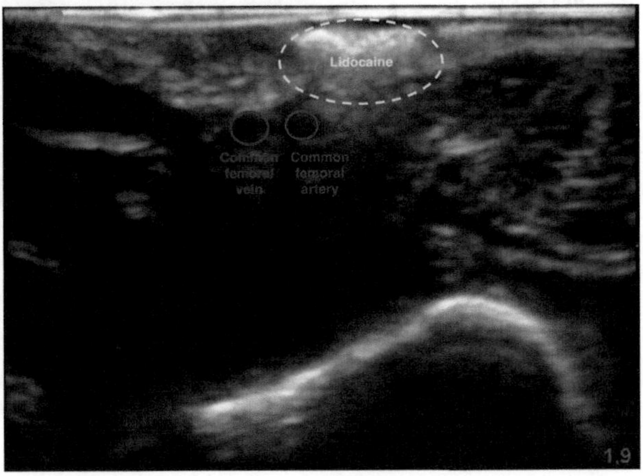

Fig. 20.13 Identifying structures
- Lidocaine will form a hyperechoic area that can opacify structures below the subcutaneous tissue

20.4 Steps for Real-Time Ultrasound-Guided Access to Left Femoral Vein in Pediatrics

20.4.1 Step 01

- We will use a 30-cm, double-lumen Arrow® 4 Fr catheter.
- Perform the puncture in SAX view, 2 or 3 cm below the inguinal ligament.
- Identify and place the vein in the middle part of the length of the transducer. It will also be displayed in the middle of the screen.
- Start the puncture by going to the middle part of the length of the transducer with an angle of less than 10°, almost parallel to the skin. The objective is to penetrate under the skin (Fig. 20.14).
- First, identify the location of the intravenous catheter (22G) and then over the vein (Figs. 20.15 and 20.16).
- Begin the ultrasound-guided dynamic needle tip positioning (DNTP) to guide the puncture in real time.
- Once the needle tip of the intravenous catheter is visible on the screen, redirect the puncture path into the vein.

20.4.2 Step 02

- Redirect the puncture medially and continue advancing at the same puncture angle (Fig. 20.17).
- SAX view of puncture redirection (Figs. 20.18 and 20.19).

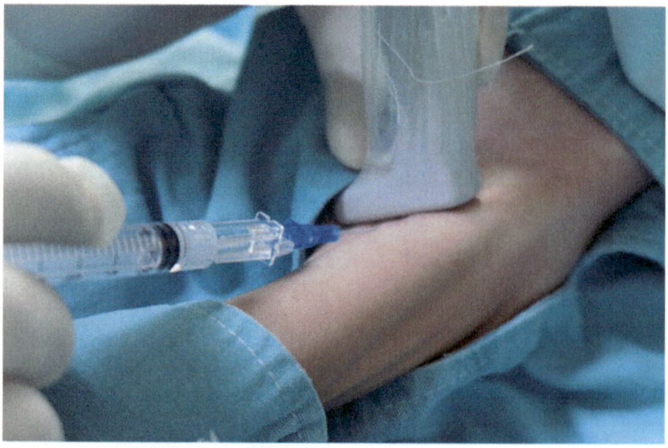

Fig. 20.14 Start the puncture at an angle of less than 10°

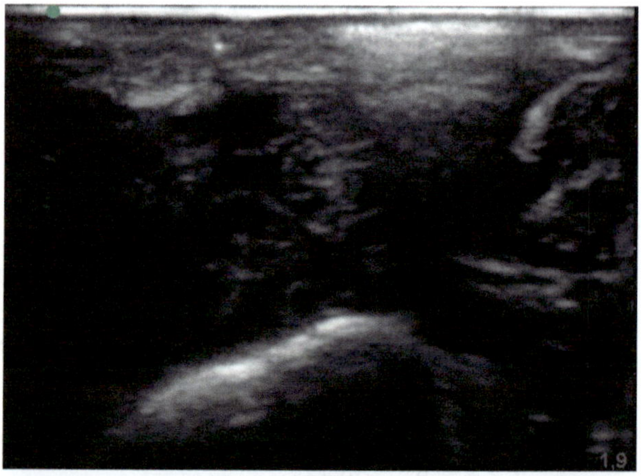

Fig. 20.15 SAX view of the beginning of the puncture

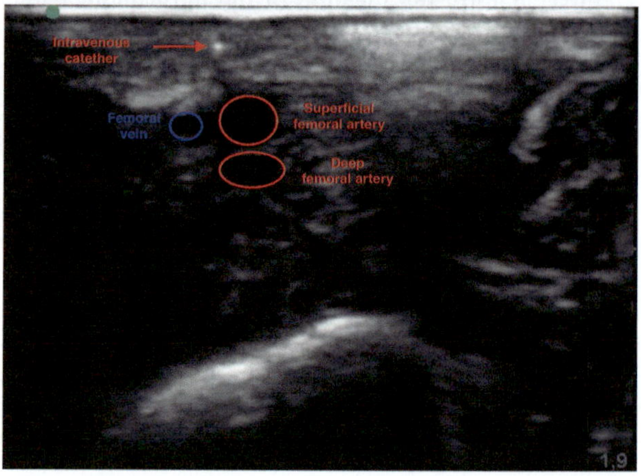

Fig. 20.16 Identifying structures

- The tip of the intravenous catheter is seen as a bright hyperechoic (white) dot in the subcutaneous tissue, in a direction between the arteries and the LFV

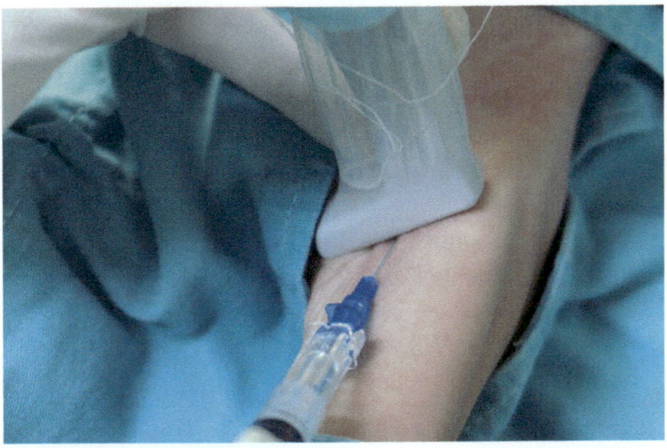

Fig. 20.17 Redirect the puncture medially

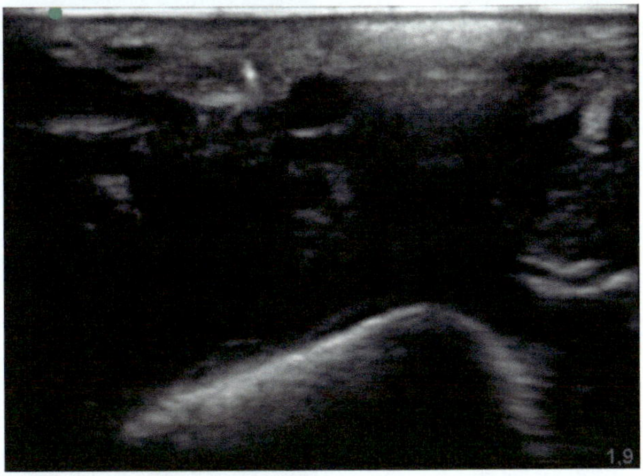

Fig. 20.18 Puncture redirection. SAX view of DNTP is now aligned in the direction of the vein

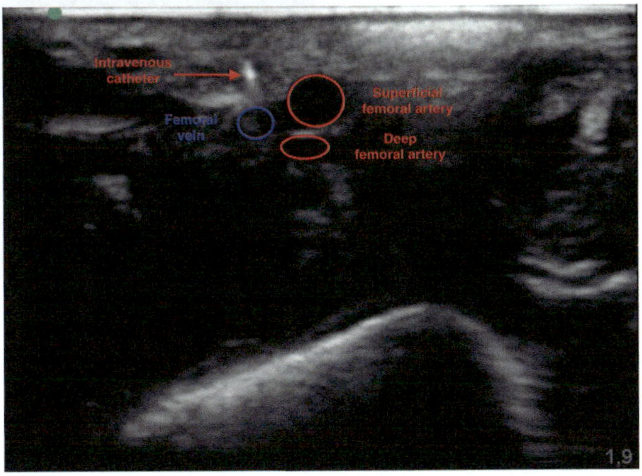

Fig. 20.19 Identifying structures

- The intravenous catheter is already in the direction of the LFV, which is smaller in diameter due to the compression made in that direction by the intravenous catheter
- The division of the two arteries can still be seen, indicating that a more proximal puncture is required

- The objective is to canalize the common LFV near the inguinal ligament or the external iliac vein above the inguinal ligament, which has a greater caliber.
- Sweep the transducer proximal to continuing with the DNTP, following the tip of the intravenous catheter (Fig. 20.20).
- SAX view of the progress of the puncture along the path of the LFV (Figs. 20.21 and 20.22).
- Follow the same direction because an adequate trajectory toward the LFV is already evident (Figs. 20.23 and 20.24).

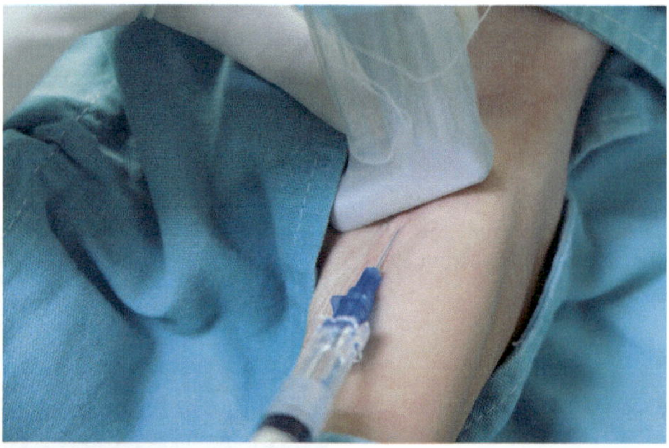

Fig. 20.20 Sweep the transducer proximally (toward the inguinal ligament) to perform the DNTP

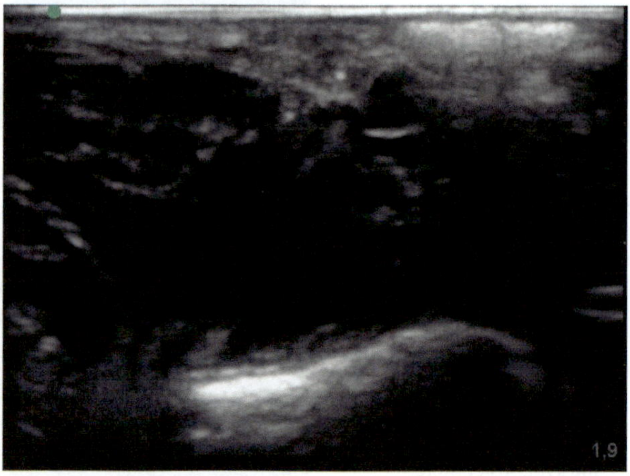

Fig. 20.21 SAX view of the progress of the puncture along the path of the LFV is visualized

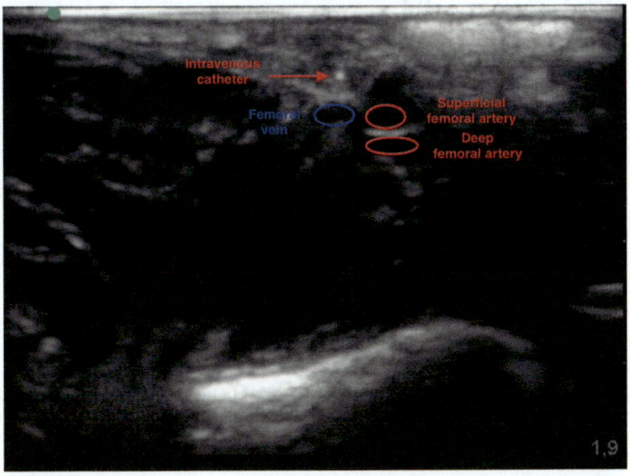

Fig. 20.22 Identifying structures

- Intravenous catheter approaching the LFV
- The vein is deforming to an oval due to the compression exerted on the tissues by the intravenous catheter
- The femoral arteries now share only one wall to become the common LFA later proximally

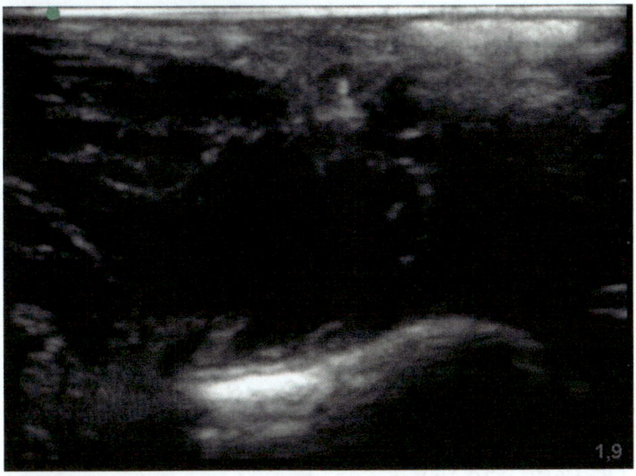

Fig. 20.23 SAX view of the intravenous catheter reaching the LFV and collapsing it

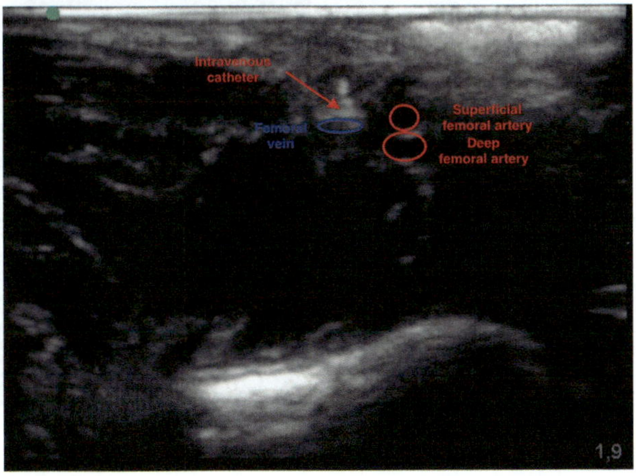

Fig. 20.24 Identifying structures

- The intravenous catheter has reached the LFV and is almost completely compressing it to begin cannulation of the vein
- The superficial and deep femoral arteries join to form the common LFA artery

20.4.3 Step 03

- Continue the puncture of less than 10° (because the patient has little subcutaneous tissue) to cannulate the LFV. DNPT is making us arrive at the inguinal ligament level with the transducer (Fig. 20.25).
- SAX view of the intravenous catheter cannulating the LFV (Figs. 20.26 and 20.27).
- Once you see the cannulation of the LFV on the screen (Fig. 20.27), set the transducer aside.
- Hold the catheter hub firmly. Aspirate the syringe to check the blood return in the flashback chamber or up to the syringe (Fig. 20.28).
- Hold the flange of the catheter hub and insert the intravenous catheter, moving it through the needle to cannulate the vein (Fig. 20.29).

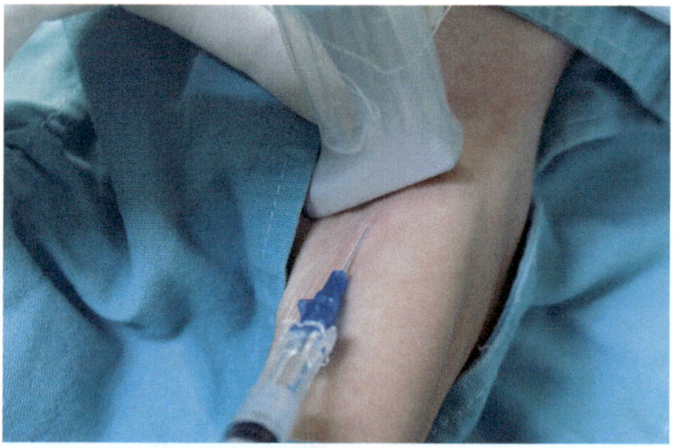

Fig. 20.25 The transducer is already over the inguinal ligament

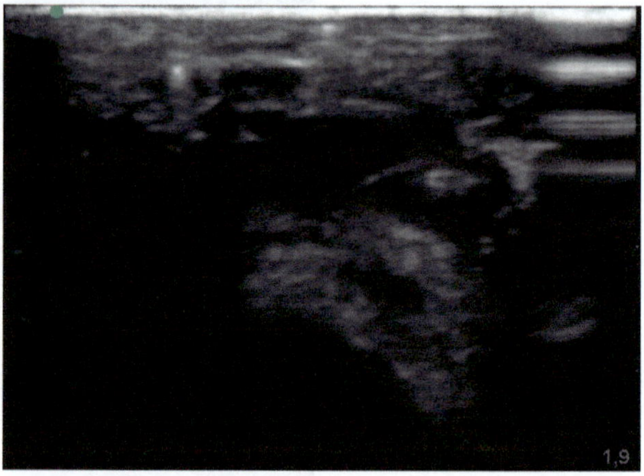

Fig. 20.26 SAX view of the intravenous catheter cannulating the LFV

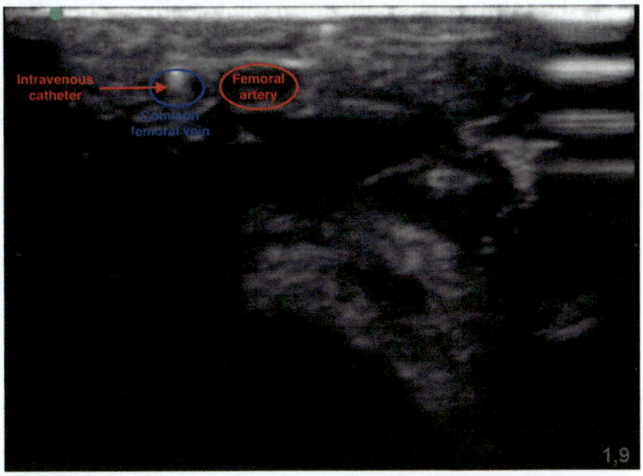

Fig. 20.27 Identifying structures
- The tip of the intravenous catheter needle is within the lumen of the LFV and has not passed through the posterior wall

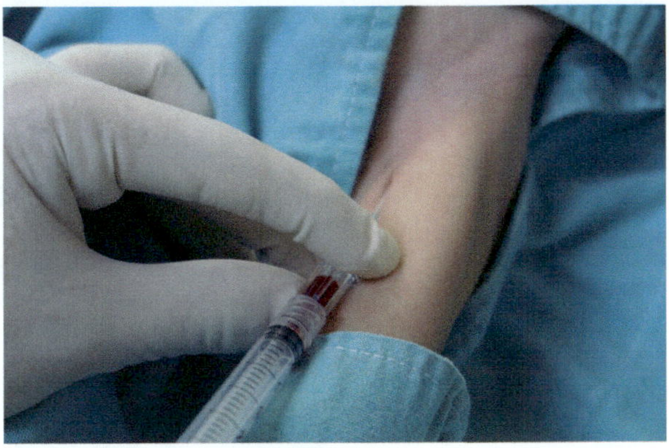

Fig. 20.28 Check for free blood flow

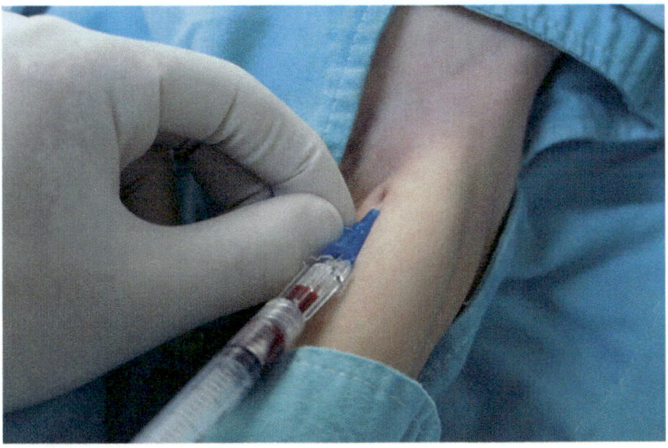

Fig. 20.29 Hold the flange of the catheter hub and insert the intravenous catheter, moving it through the needle to cannulate the vein

- If the intravenous catheter moves easily within the vein, withdraw the puncture needle in the opposite direction, leaving only the catheter tube cannulating the vein (Fig. 20.30).
- Once you have inserted the entire intravenous catheter, place a syringe and check for free blood flow through the catheter tube, cannulating the LFV (Fig. 20.31).

20.4.4 Step 04

- Hold the catheter hub firmly and remove the syringe (Fig. 20.32).
- Sometimes, when removing the syringe, some blood returns through the catheter tube (Fig. 20.33).
- Insert the 0.018" guide through the intravenous catheter (Fig. 20.34).

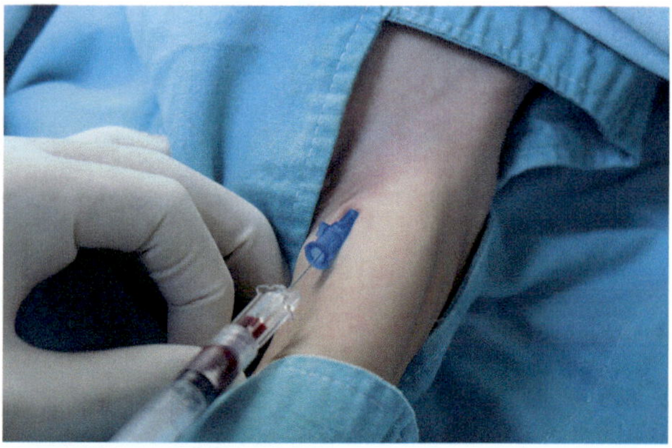

Fig. 20.30 Withdraw the puncture needle and leave only the catheter tube cannulating the vein

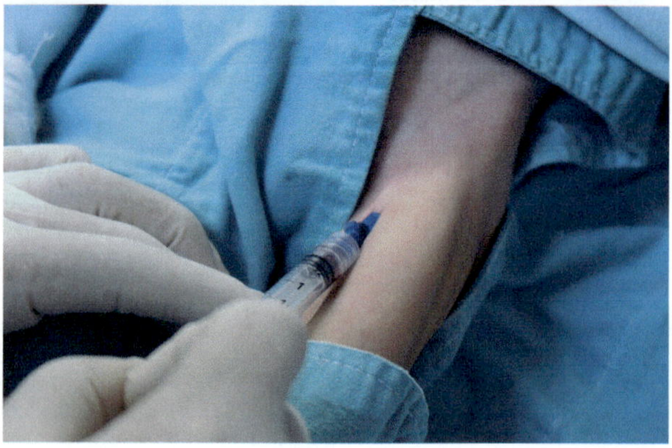

Fig. 20.31 Check for free blood flow through the catheter tube

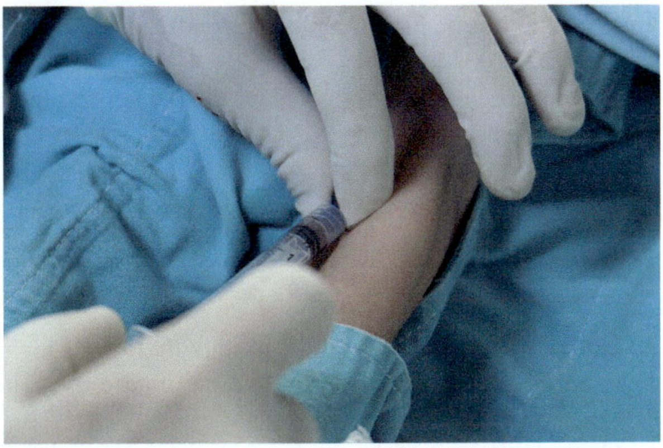

Fig. 20.32 Remove the syringe

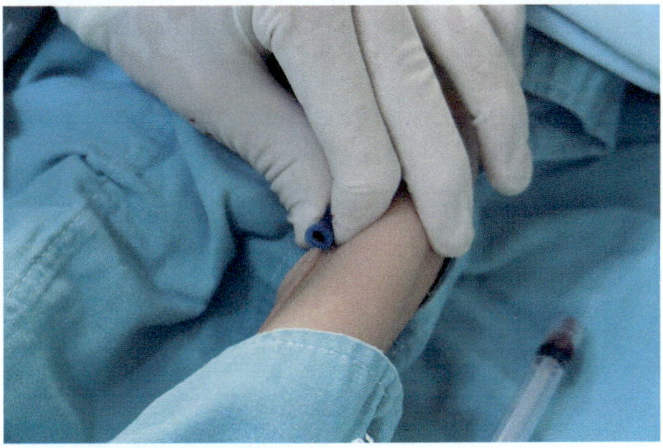

Fig. 20.33 Blood returns through the catheter tube

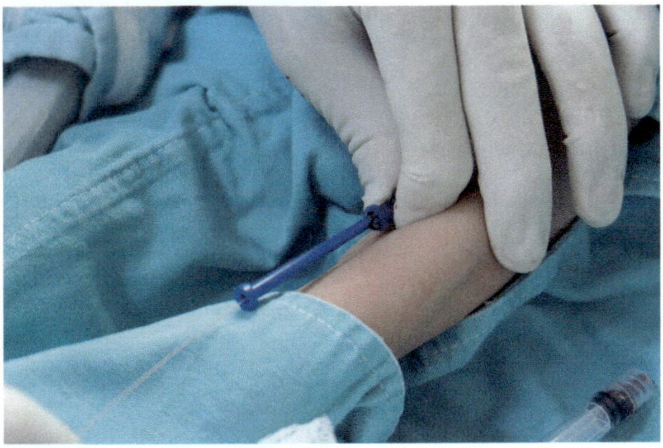

Fig. 20.34 Insert the guidewire

- It should easily pass through the J-tip end of the guide. If it does not, you can try passing through the straight end. If it still does not pass, the catheter may have accidentally slipped out of the LFV.

- With the left hand and a piece of gauze, occlude the exit if there is blood return (Fig. 20.35).
- Scan the location of the guidewire in the venous lumen in SAX view (Figs. 20.36 and 20.37).

20.4.5 Step 05

- Once you have identified the guidewire inside the vein, the path is dilated. This is a safety measure to avoid dilation in case of incidental puncture of the femoral artery.
- Occlude the exit of the guide with your left hand and hold the guidewire with the same hand to help you introduce the dilator over the guidewire (Fig. 20.38).
- Dilate the path between the skin and the LFV.

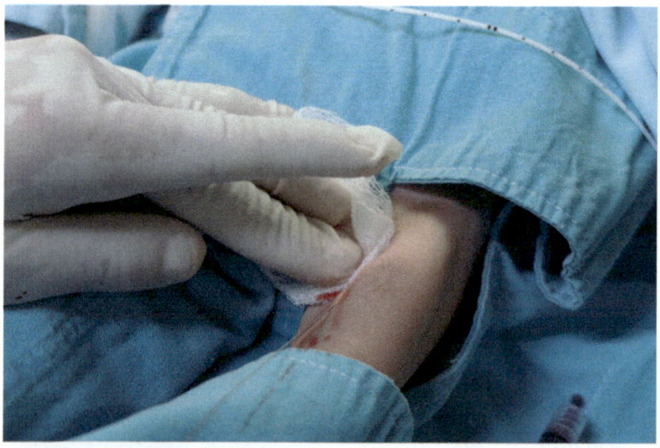

Fig. 20.35 Occlude the exit if there is blood return

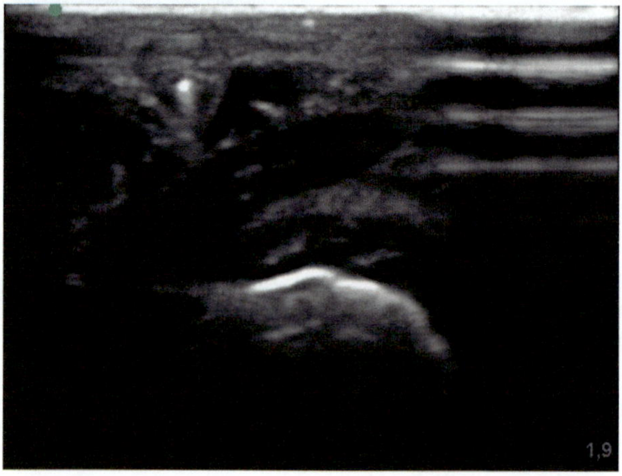

Fig. 20.36 SAX view of the guidewire within the LFV

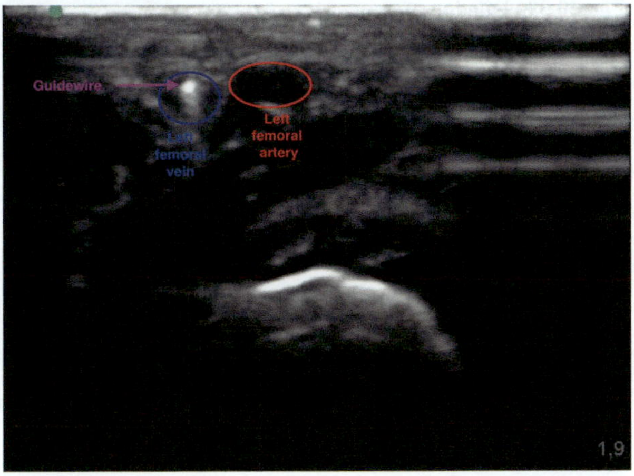

Fig. 20.37 Identifying structures

- The guidewire can be seen within the LFV. It is more echogenic than the intravenous catheter and has the comet tail sign

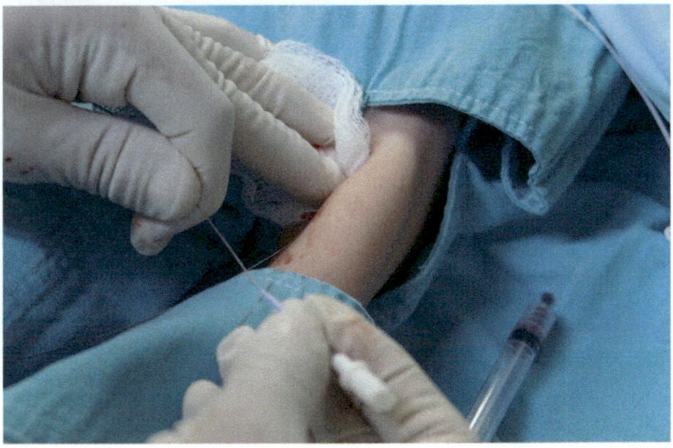

Fig. 20.38 Introduce the dilator over the guidewire

- Insert the dilator. If you do it carefully, you will not need a skin incision (Fig. 20.39).
- When you are withdrawing, the dilator occludes the exit of the skin with your left hand and gauze, so it does not bleed (Fig. 20.40).

20.4.6 Step 06

- Advance the catheter over the guidewire (Seldinger's technique) (Fig. 20.41).
- Enter the desired catheter length.
- Remove the guidewire.
- Scan the intravenous location of the catheter (Fig. 20.42).
- SAX view of the catheter inside the LFV (Figs. 20.43 and 20.44).

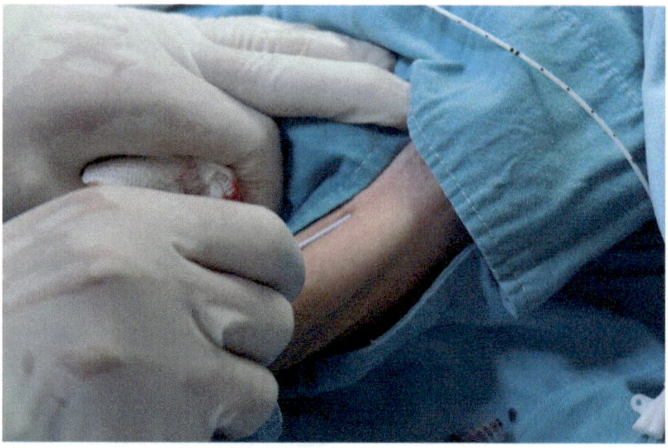

Fig. 20.39 Dilation of the skin

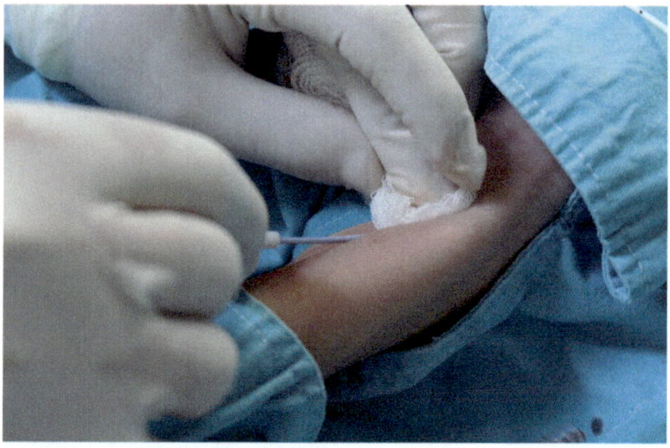

Fig. 20.40 Remove the dilator

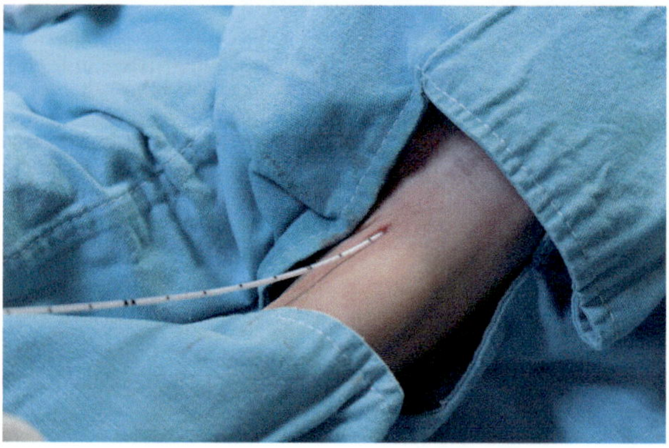

Fig. 20.41 Seldinger's technique: advance the catheter over the guidewire

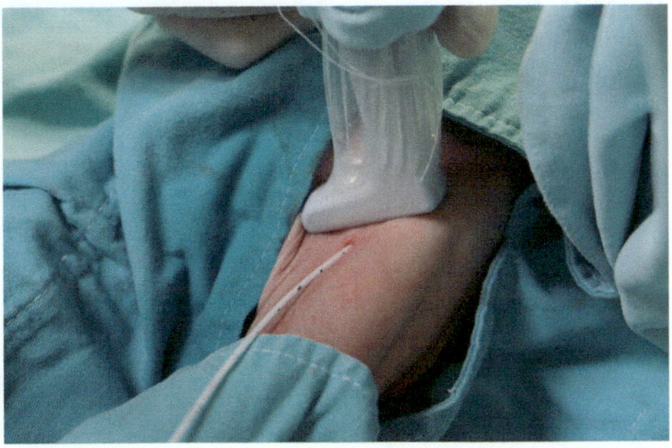

Fig. 20.42 Scan the intravascular location of the catheter

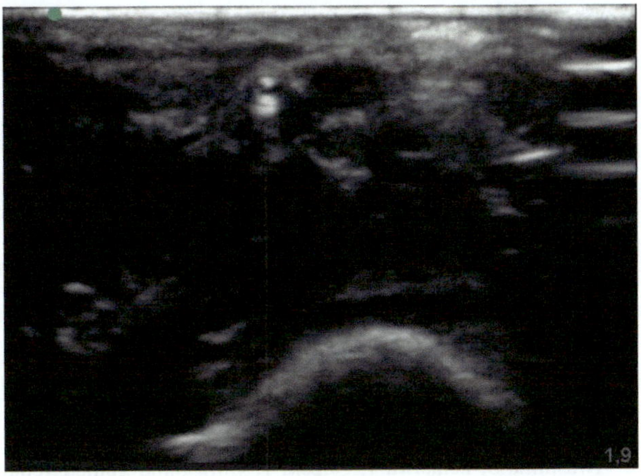

Fig. 20.43 SAX view of the catheter inside the LFV

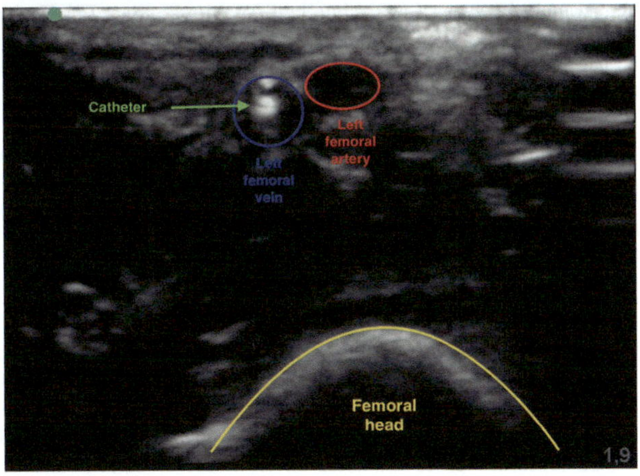

Fig. 20.44 Identifying structures

- The double-lumen catheter is visualized within the LFV

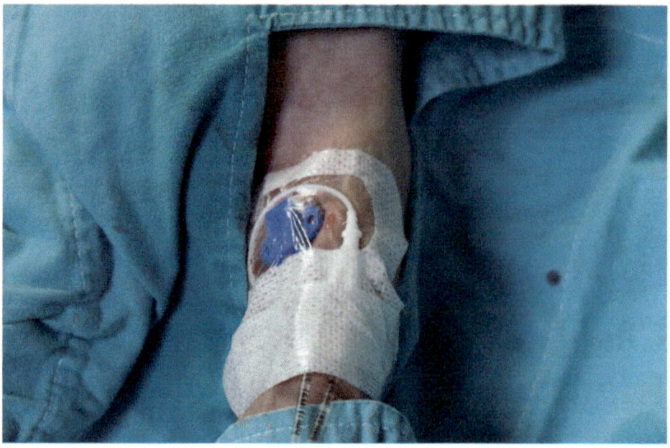

Fig. 20.45 Dressing according to the institutional protocol

20.4.7 Step 07

- Secure the catheter and place a sterile occlusive dressing according to the institutional protocol (Fig. 20.45).

Sources

1. Warkentine FH, Clyde Pierce M, Lorenz D, Kim IK. The anatomic relationship of femoral vein to femoral artery in euvolemic pediatric patients by ultrasonography: implications for pediatric femoral central venous access. Acad Emerg Med. 2008;15(5):426–30. https://doi.org/10.1111/j.1553-2712.2008.00087.x.
2. Iwashima S, Ishikawa T, Ohzeki T. Ultrasound-guided versus landmark-guided femoral vein access in pediatric cardiac catheterization. Pediatr Cardiol. 2008;29(2):339–42. https://doi.org/10.1007/s00246-007-9066-2.
3. Aouad MT, Kanazi GE, Abdallah FW, Moukaddem FH, Turbay MJ, Obeid MY, Siddik-Sayyid SM. Femoral vein cannulation performed by residents: a comparison between ultrasound-guided and landmark technique in infants and children undergoing cardiac surgery. Anesth Analg. 2010;111(3):724–8. https://doi.org/10.1213/ANE.0b013e3181e9c475. Epub 2010 Jul 2
4. Al Sofyani K, Julia G, Abdulaziz B, Yves CJ, Sylvain R. Ultrasound guidance for central vascular access in the neonatal and pediatric intensive care unit. Saudi J Anaesth. 2012;6(2):120–4. https://doi.org/10.4103/1658-354X.97023. Erratum in: Saudi J Anaesth. 2012 Oct-Dec;6(4):372. Khouloud, Al Sofyani [corrected to Al Sofyani, Khouloud]
5. Alten JA, Borasino S, Gurley WQ, Law MA, Toms R, Dabal RJ. Ultrasound-guided femoral vein catheterization in neonates with cardiac disease*. Pediatr Crit Care Med. 2012;13(6):654–9. https://doi.org/10.1097/PCC.0b013e318250af0c.
6. Ahn JH, Park J, Song IS, Kim KA, Park J, Min JJ, Kim CS, Lee JH. The angle range of leg abduction with external hip rotation which can minimize femoral artery and vein overlap in pediatric patients. Paediatr Anaesth. 2019;29(4):361–7. https://doi.org/10.1111/pan.13603. Epub 2019 Mar 21
7. Liu WL, Lin MC, Chan SC, Chen SN, Lin TY, Jan SL. Ultrasonographic measurements of femoral vessel diameter in neonates weighing less than 2.5 kg. Echocardiography. 2021;38(10):1741–6. https://doi.org/10.1111/echo.15203. Epub 2021 Sep 23

Chapter 21
Left Femoral/Iliac Vein in Neonates

21.1 Patient Positioning

- The patient is a premature infant weighing 750 g.
- Place the patient with the feet near the border of the heating cradle.
- Position the patient supine with the legs extended, separated from the midline, and with gentle restraint at the ankles (Fig. 21.1).
- Place a roll under the hip to slightly elevate the leg.

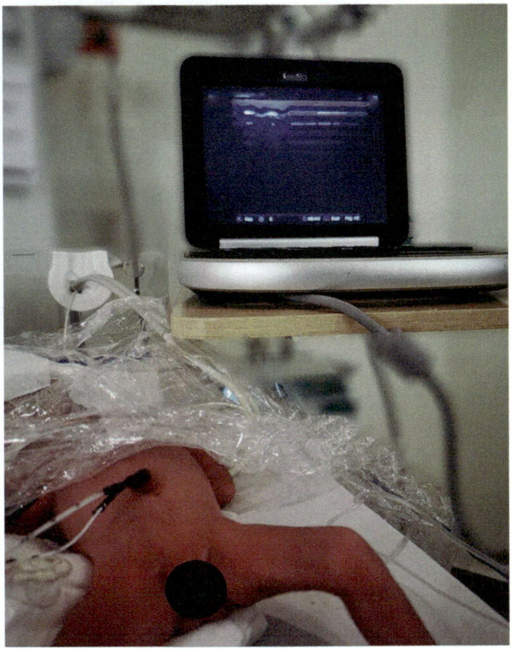

Fig. 21.1 Patient position

F. Montes-Tapia, *Atlas of Ultrasound-Guided Central Venous Catheter Placement*, https://doi.org/10.1007/978-3-031-61887-1_21

21.2 Scanning Technique

- Do a preliminary vascular assessment (non-sterile), known as rapid femoral vein assessment (RaFeVA).
- The operator stands at the patient's feet.
- The ultrasound is placed at the level of the left (Fig. 21.1) or right shoulder or above the patient's head.
- A high-frequency linear transducer (13–6 MHz) with a hockey stick transducer can be used.
- This procedure is performed with zoom mode to facilitate the visibility of the left femoral vein (LFV).
- The patient's leg at this age is so small in diameter that the transducer must be well positioned.
- Place the transducer at the level of the inguinal ligament with the tip of the hockey stick transducer toward the patient's right side, which will be marked on the monitor as the left side, corresponding to the operator's left. This is done to correlate the operator's movements with those of the monitor (Fig. 21.2).
- Scan in short-axis (SAX) view to identify the arteriovenous bundle (Figs. 21.3 and 21.4).
- The small roll made with a diaper is visible under the hip (Fig. 21.5).

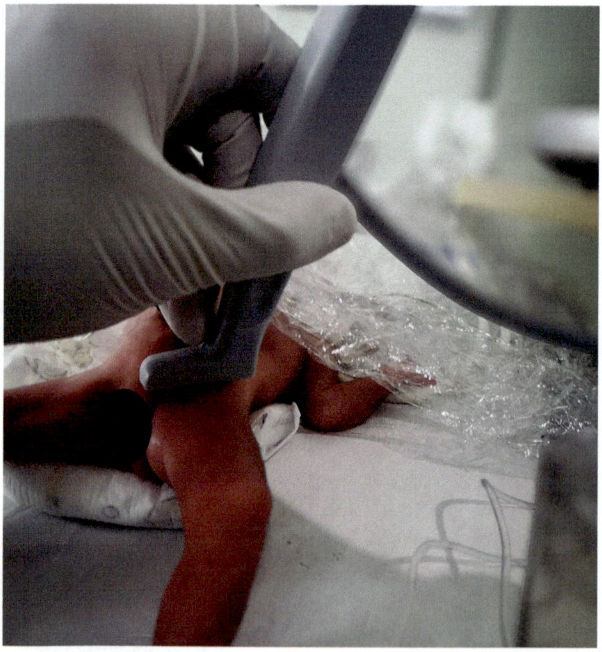

Fig. 21.2 Tip of the hockey stick transducer toward the patient's right side

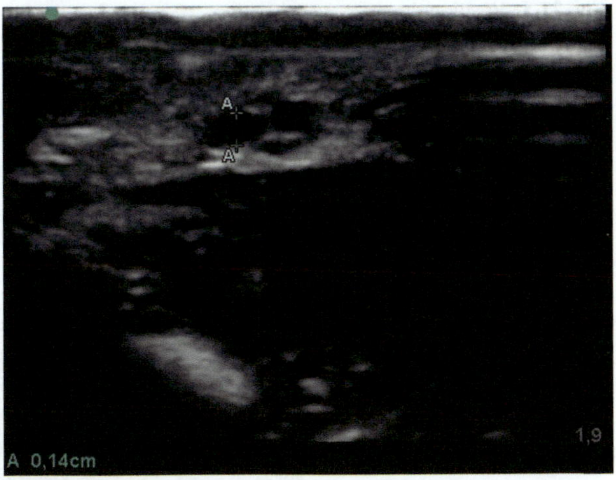

Fig. 21.3 SAX view of the left femoral bundle
- The LFV measures 0.14 cm in the anteroposterior plane
- The scan depth is 1.9 cm

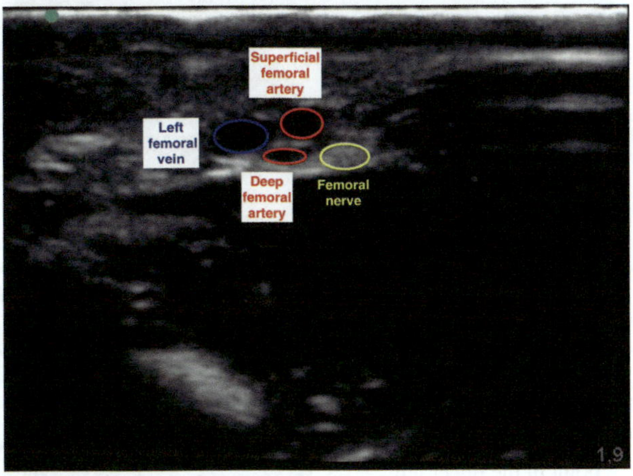

Fig. 21.4 Identifying structures
- From medial to lateral, the left femoral vein (LFV) and the left femoral artery (LFA)
- The femoral nerve is inferior and lateral to the LFA

- Elevate the newborn's hip with a roll to keep the transducer in contact with the lower abdominal wall and inguinal region. If the hip is not elevated, the inguinal region will be in a depression, and contact of the transducer with this region cannot occur.
- The tip of the transducer is proximal.
- Position the inguinal ligament at half the length of the transducer.
- Then scan in long-axis (LAX) view, zoom mode, from lateral to medial to identify the LFA and then the LFV (Figs. 21.6, 21.7, 21.8 and 21.9).

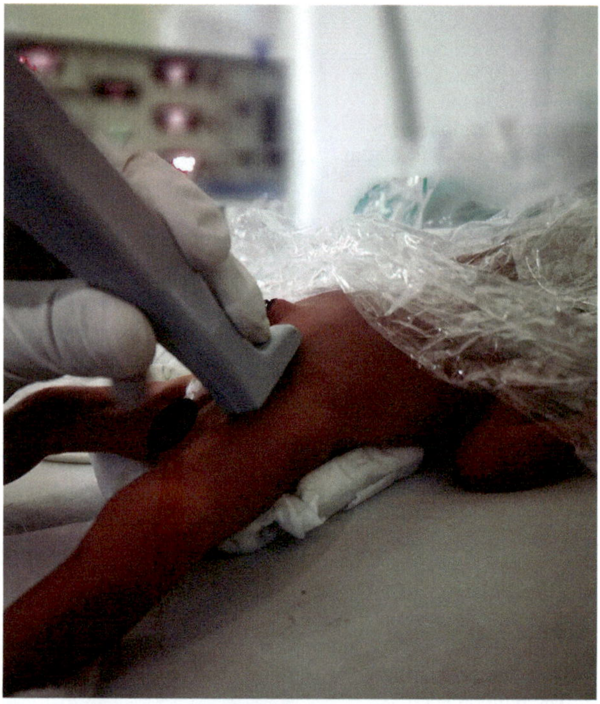

Fig. 21.5 Position the inguinal ligament at half the length of the transducer and scan from lateral to medial in LAX view

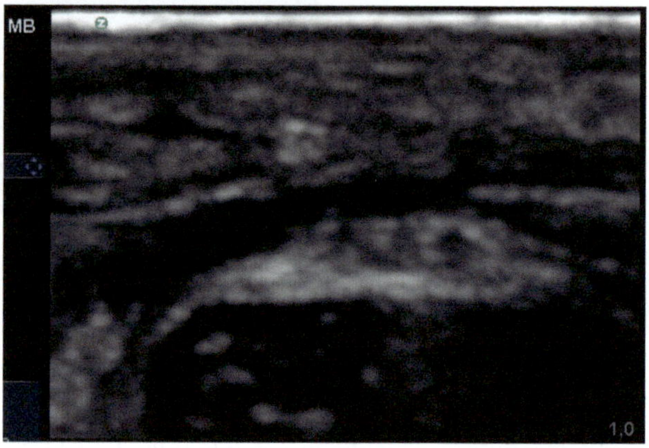

Fig. 21.6 Lateral scan of the left leg. LAX view of the LFA

- Now, the scan is in zoom mode. That mode is shown because there is a "Z" inside the aqua point in the upper left
- The scanning in zoom mode has a depth of 1.0 cm

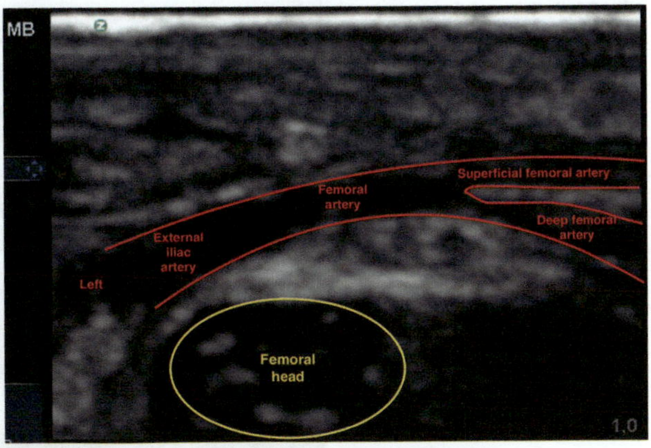

Fig. 21.7 Identifying structures
- The LFA divides into the superficial and deep femoral arteries
- The femoral head is identified

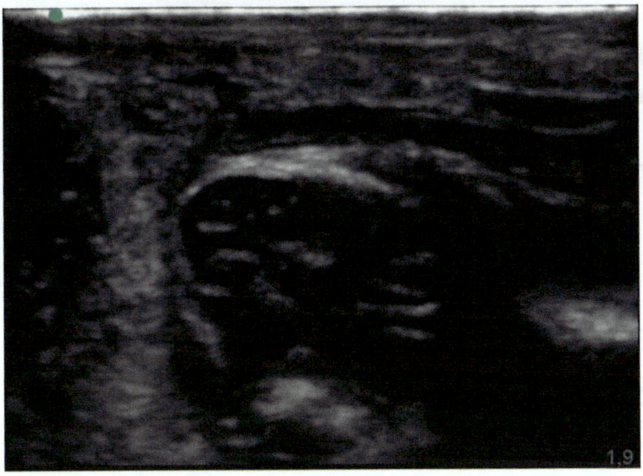

Fig. 21.8 Medial scan of the left leg. LAX view of the LFV
- The LFV is visualized in LAX medial to the artery
- Now, the image is in normal mode with a scanning depth of 1.9 cm; therefore, the "Z" is not displayed within the aqua point on the upper left of the monitor
- This scan is performed to see the differences in the visualization of the two types of depths: zoom mode (Figs. 21.6 and 21.7) and normal mode (Figs. 21.7 and 21.8)

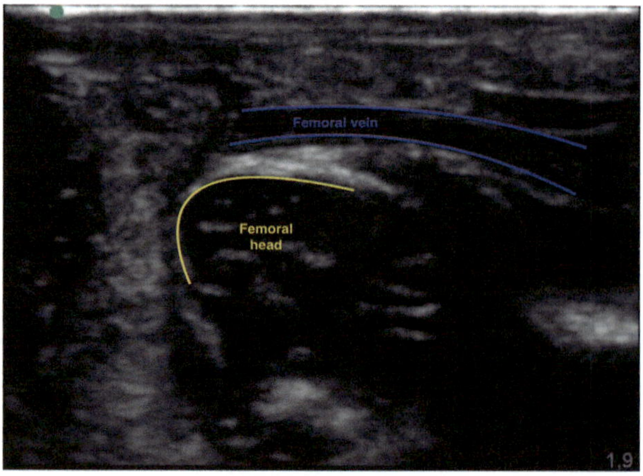

Fig. 21.9 Identifying structures
- The LFV in LAX
- The femoral head is visualized
- The distance from the skin to the vein is less than 0.5 cm

21.3 Steps for Real-Time Ultrasound-Guided Access to Left Femoral/Iliac Vein in Neonates

21.3.1 Step 01

- We will use a 10-cm, double-lumen Vygon® 3 Fr catheter.
- The sterile field only leaves the left abdomen, inguinal, and anterior thigh regions uncovered (Fig. 21.10).
- The patient has flexed the hip. Correct the position to maintain leg extension.
- Leg extension can be achieved by improving sedation and restraint. You can also have an assistant keep the leg extended, holding it by the ankle.
- Once you have positioned the extended leg, you will note that this maneuver improves full support of the hockey stick transducer in the inguinal-abdominal region (Fig. 21.11).
- Scan from lateral to medial and locate the LFV.
- Perform the puncture in LAX, below the inguinal ligament, using a 24-G intravenous catheter.
- Begin the puncture by going to the middle part of the length of the transducer with an angle of less than 10°, almost parallel to the skin (Fig. 21.12). The objective is to penetrate under the skin. First identify the location of the intravenous catheter and then over the vein.
  - Puncture in the middle of the thickness of the transducer so that the intravenous catheter can be visualized along the path aligned with the vein (Figs. 21.13 and 21.14).
- Once the intravenous catheter is visible on the screen, redirect the puncture path into the vein.

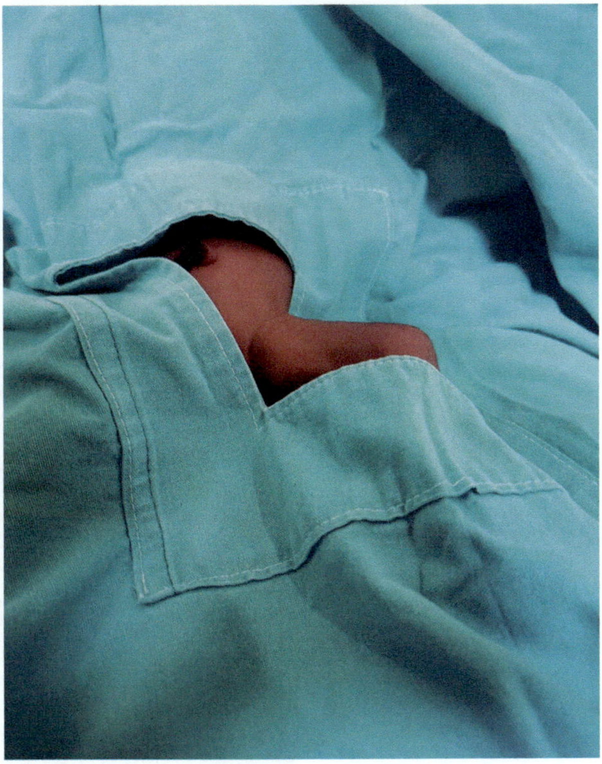

Fig. 21.10 The sterile field only leaves the left abdomen, inguinal, and anterior thigh regions uncovered

- Begin the ultrasound-guided dynamic needle tracking (DNT) to guide the puncture in real time.
- Remember, these premature patients have little subcutaneous tissue. A higher puncture angle can cause you to penetrate more deeply or incidentally puncture or traverse the vein or artery.

21.3.2 Step 02

- Redirect the scan (medial or lateral) to fully visualize the LFV and continue the puncture.
- Once the LFV is completely displayed, increase the puncture angle to 10–20° so the intravenous catheter is directed to the vein (Fig. 21.15).
- Continue with the new puncture direction, inserting the intravenous catheter more deeply and following the ultrasound puncture in LAX in DNT in the path of the footprint (Figs. 21.16 and 21.17).

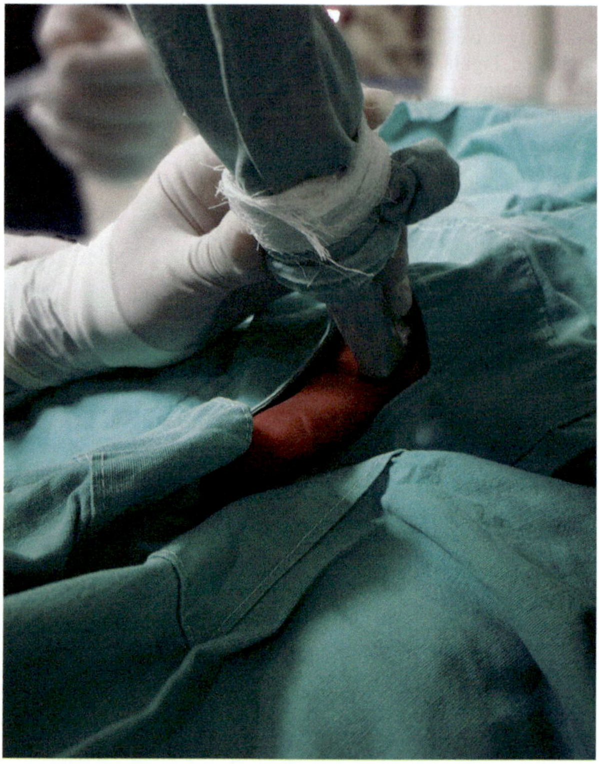

Fig. 21.11 Scan the LFV in LAX view

21.3.3 Step 03

- Once you have identified the canalization of the vein on the ultrasound monitor (Figs. 21.18 and 21.19), set the transducer aside.
- Aspirate the syringe to check the blood return in the flashback chamber or up to the syringe.
- Hold the flange of the hub of the intravenous catheter and insert it, displacing it from the needle to cannulate the vein (Fig. 21.20).
- If the intravenous catheter moves easily within the vein, withdraw the needle in the opposite direction, leaving only the intravenous tube cannulating the vein.

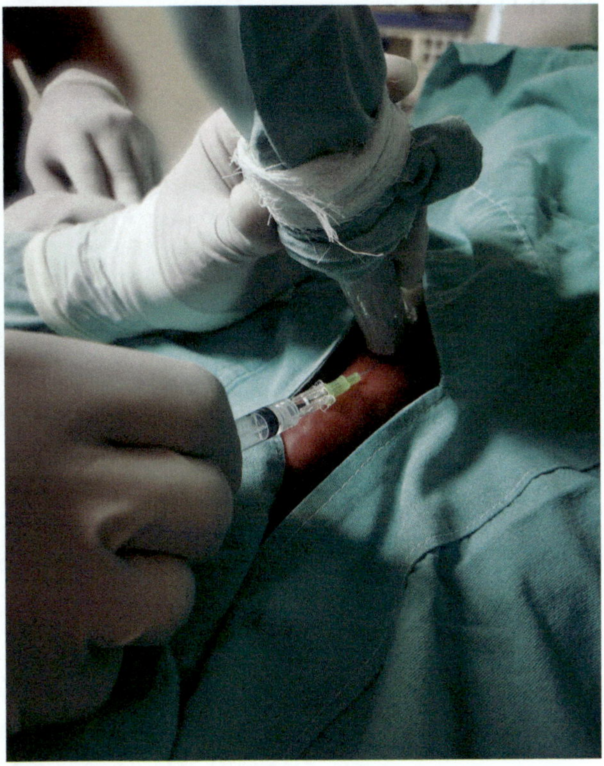

Fig. 21.12 Start the puncture at an angle of less than 10°, almost parallel to the skin

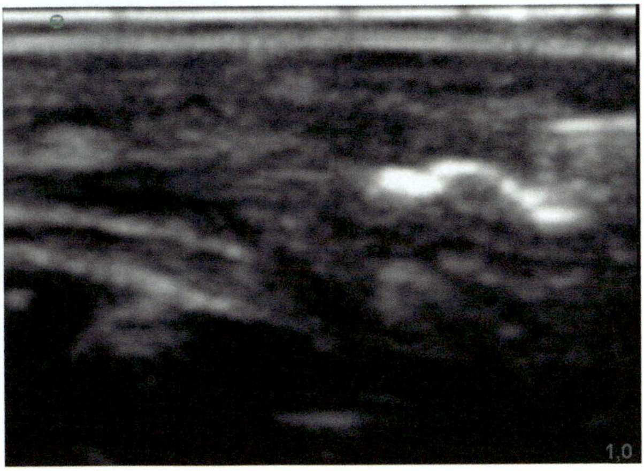

Fig. 21.13 Redirect the scan and increase the puncture angle to 10–20°

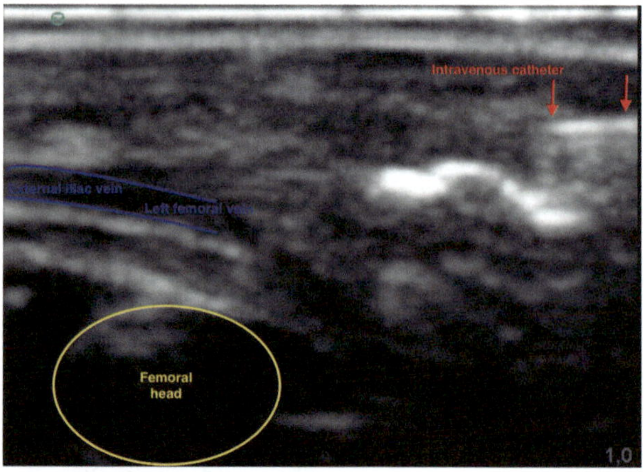

Fig. 21.14 LAX view in zoom mode of the beginning of the puncture

- Puncture depth 1,0 cm

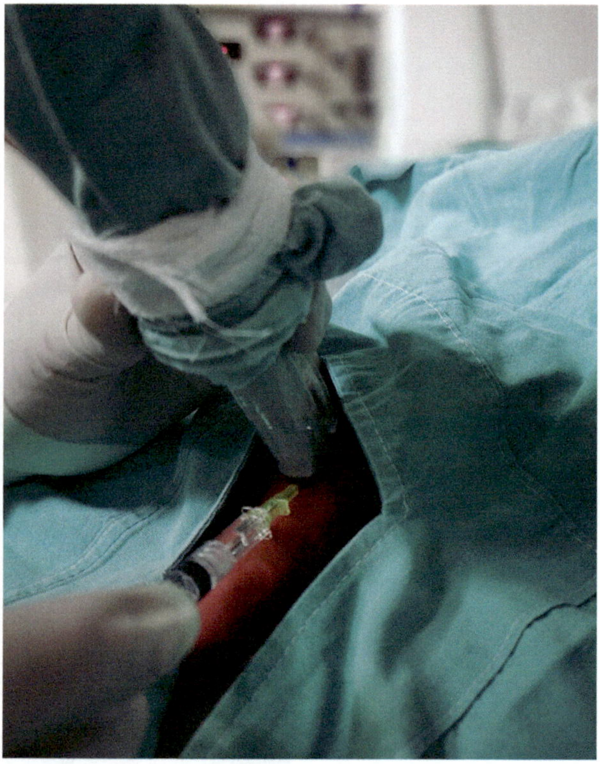

Fig. 21.15 Identifying structures

- Introduction of the intravenous catheter with a puncture angle of less than 10°; however, at this moment, it is not aligned with the LFV

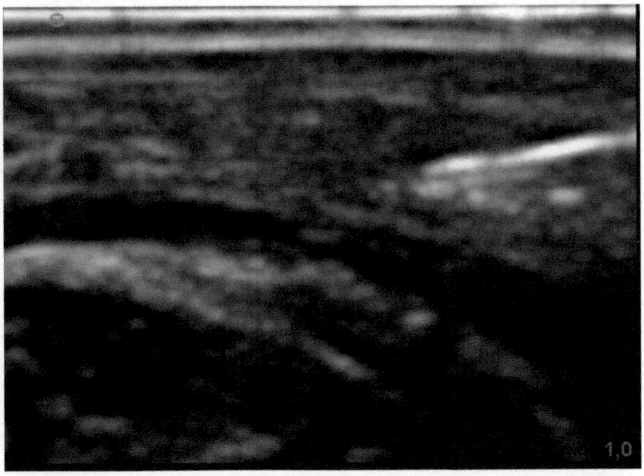

Fig. 21.16 LAX view of the increased puncture angle to 10°–20°. The LFV is now fully displayed

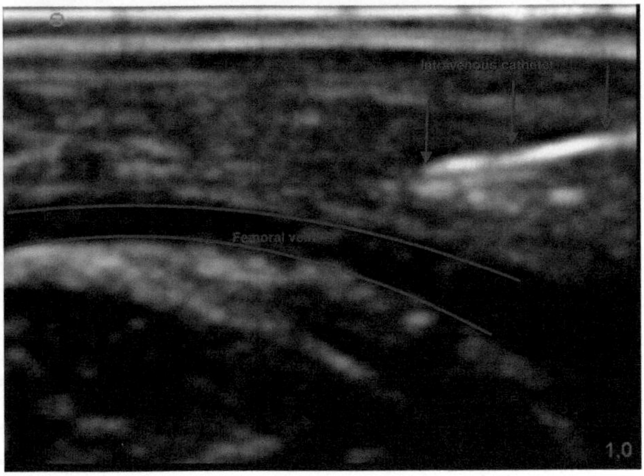

Fig. 21.17 Identifying structures

- It is seen that with the modification of the puncture angle to 20°, the intravenous catheter is in the trajectory of the LFV, so the puncture continues

21.3.4 Step 04

- Hold the hub of the catheter tube firmly with your left hand.
- Insert the 0,3-mm nitinol guidewire, which should pass easily (Fig. 21.21).
- This type of guidewire is marked every 10 cm.
- Scan the guidewire in LAX view.
- Place the transducer longitudinally over the inguinal ligament as the puncture was performed (Fig. 21.22).
- LAX view of the guidewire within the lumen of the LFV (Figs. 21.23 and 21.24).
- You can scan the guidewire in SAX view.
- Place the transducer transversely, above the inguinal ligament, and locate the arteriovenous bundle (Fig. 21.25).
- Scan the location of the guidewire in the LFV in SAX (Figs. 21.26 and 21.27).

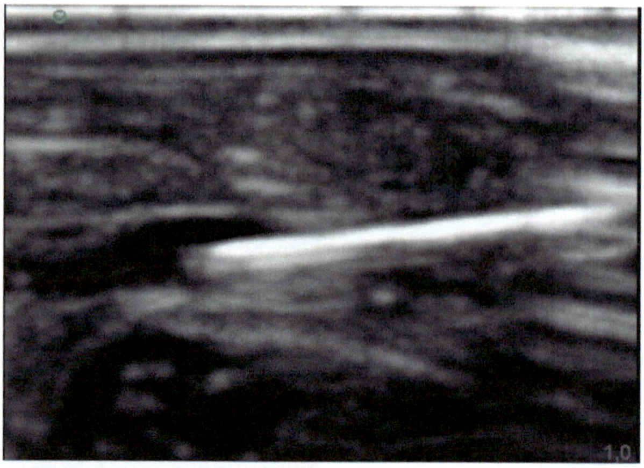

Fig. 21.18 LAX view of cannulation of the LFV

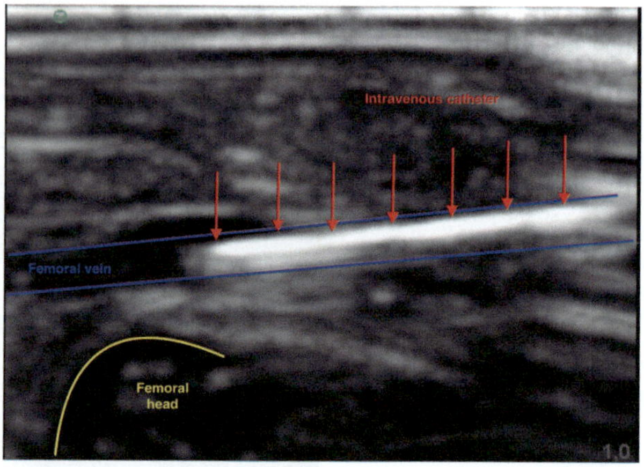

Fig. 21.19 Identifying structures
- The LFV is being cannulated with the entire intravenous catheter without penetrating the posterior wall

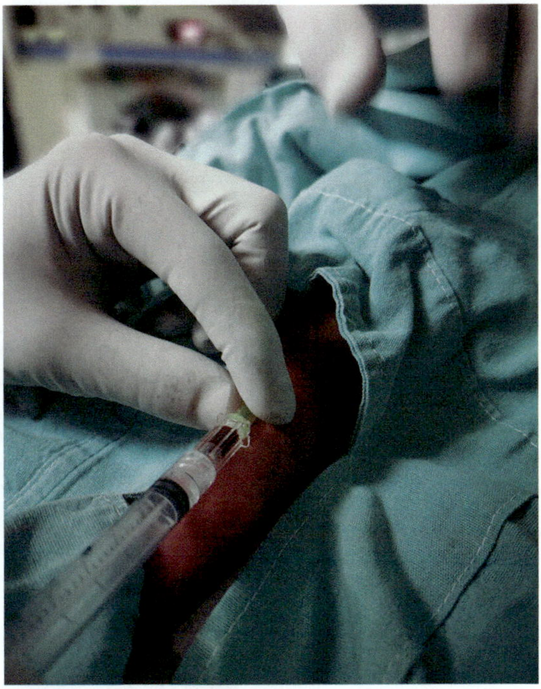

Fig. 21.20 Cannulates the LFV by inserting the intravenous catheter and withdrawing the puncture needle in the opposite direction

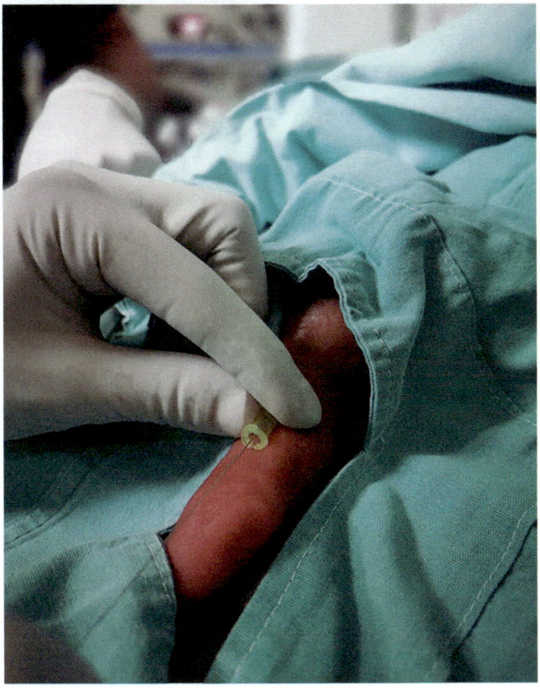

Fig. 21.21 Insert the guidewire

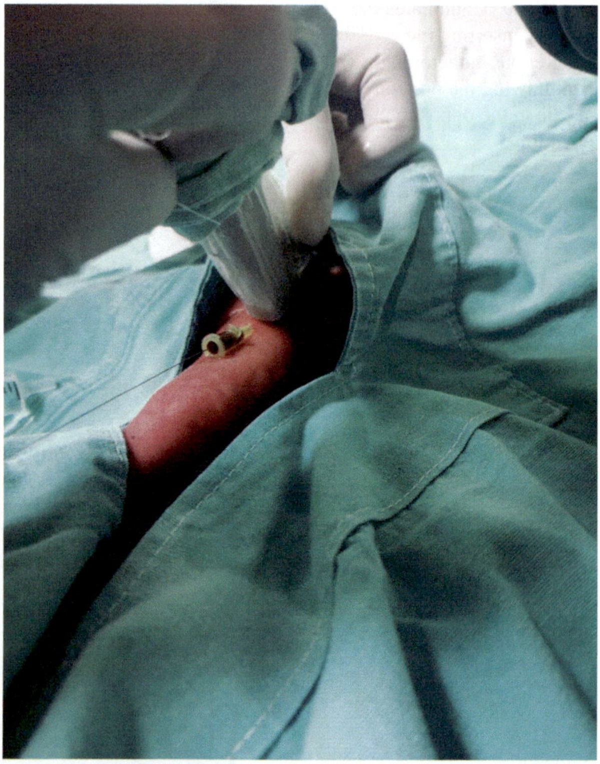

Fig. 21.22 Place the transducer longitudinally over the inguinal ligament

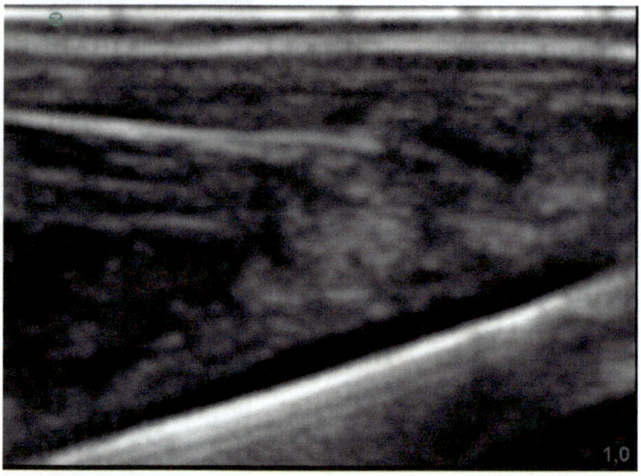

Fig. 21.23 LAX view of the guidewire in the LFV

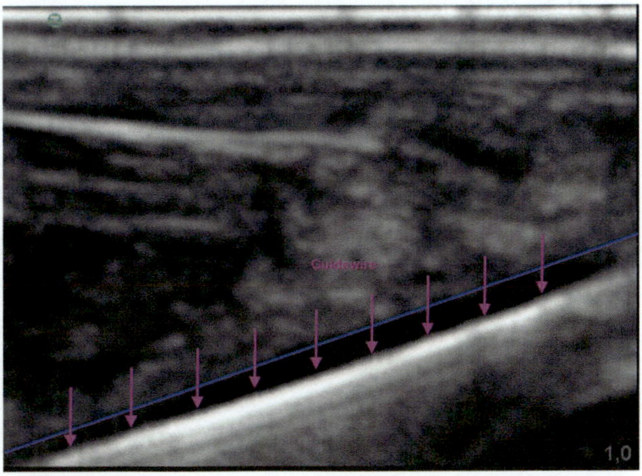

Fig. 21.24 Identifying structures

- Guidewire that hides the posterior wall of the vein due to the artifact caused by the guidewire

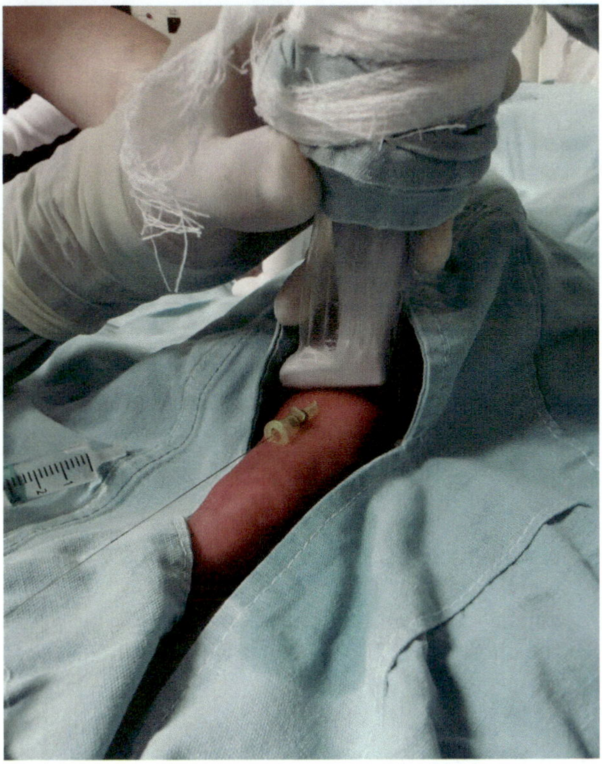

Fig. 21.25 Scan the location of the guidewire in the venous lumen in SAX view

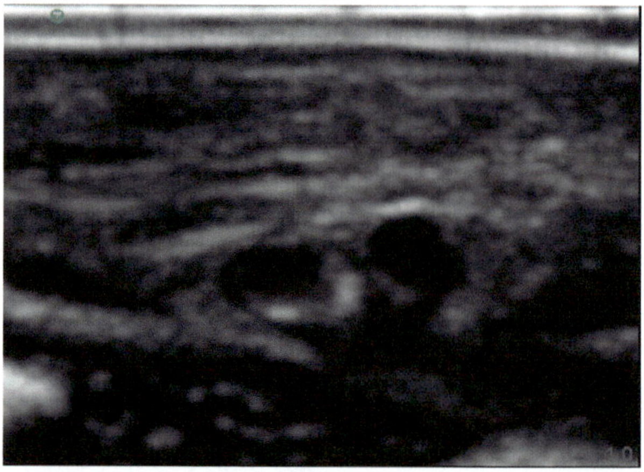

Fig. 21.26 SAX view of the guidewire within the lumen of the LFV

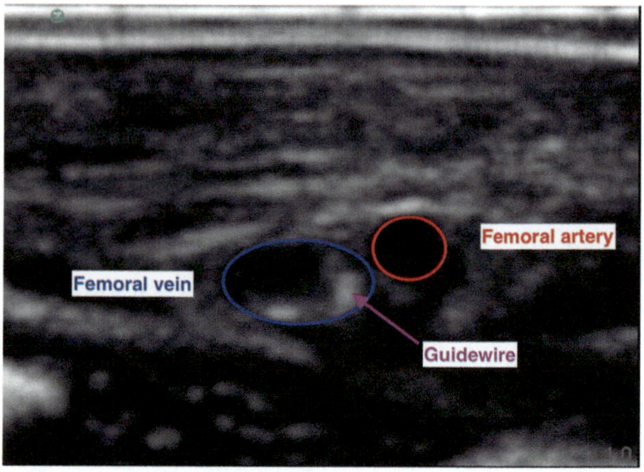

Fig. 21.27 Identifying structures

- A hyperechoic image, the guidewire, with its respective comet tail, can be seen within the LFV

21.3.5 Step 05

- For infiltration, use a small needle 25 to 27 G.
- Use lidocaine 1%.
- Subcutaneous infiltration with lidocaine in the puncture tract 1,5–2 cm before the site chosen for LFV puncture and the catheter fixation area (Fig. 21.28).

21.3.6 Step 06

- Dilate the path between the skin and the LFV delicately because the tissues are fragile.
- Insert the dilator. If you do it carefully, you will not need a skin incision (Fig. 21.29).

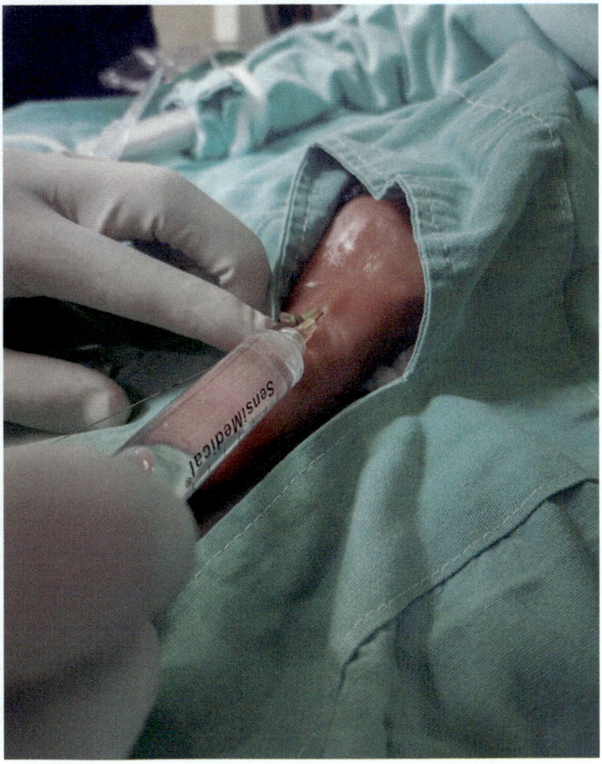

Fig. 21.28 Lidocaine infiltration

21.3.7 Step 07

- Advance the catheter over the guidewire (Seldinger's technique) (Fig. 21.30).
- Enter the desired catheter length.
- Remove the guidewire.
- Scan the intravenous location of the catheter.
- LAX view of the catheter inside the LFV (Figs. 21.31 and 21.32).

21.3.8 Step 08

- Secure the catheter and place a sterile occlusive dressing according to the institutional protocol (Fig. 21.33).

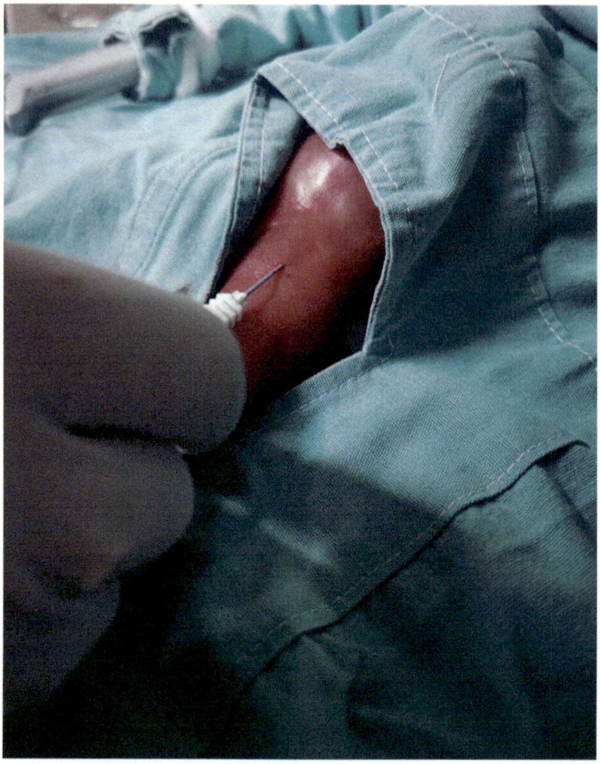

Fig. 21.29 Dilation of the skin

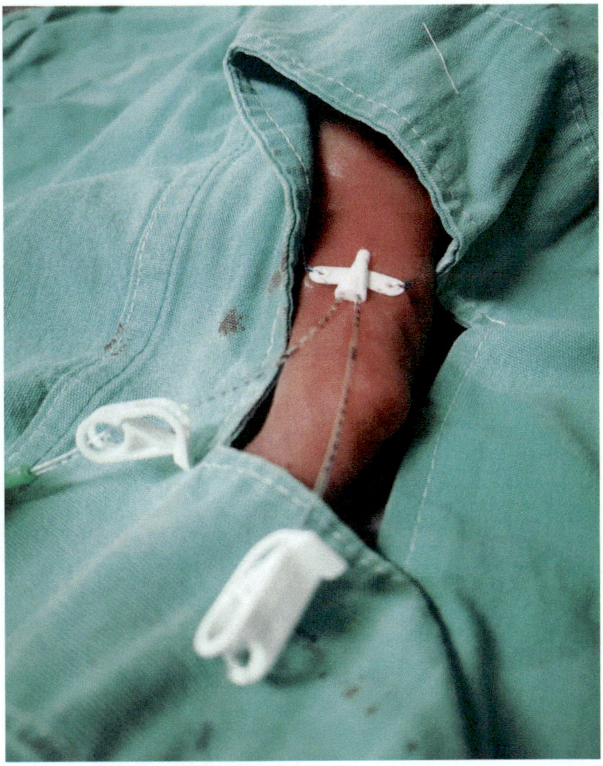

Fig. 21.30 Seldinger's technique: advance the catheter over the guidewire

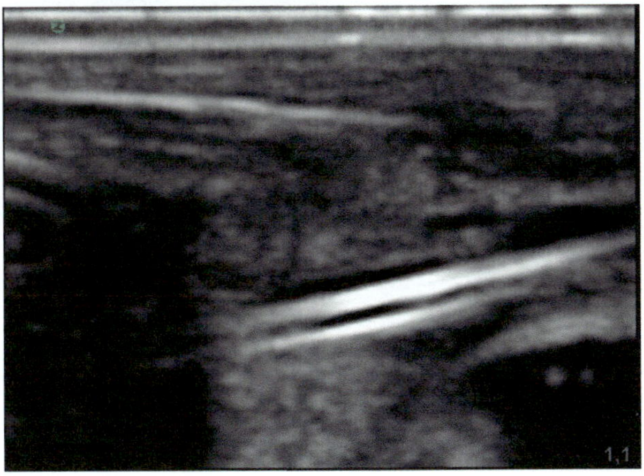

Fig. 21.31 LAX view of the catheter inside the LFV

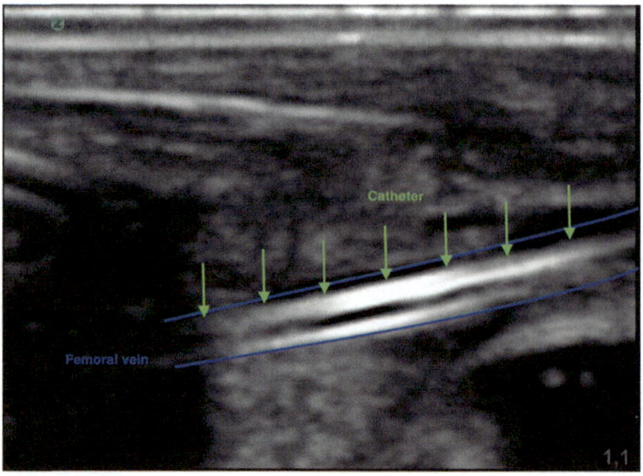

Fig. 21.32 Identifying structures

- The 3 Fr double-lumen catheter within the LFV

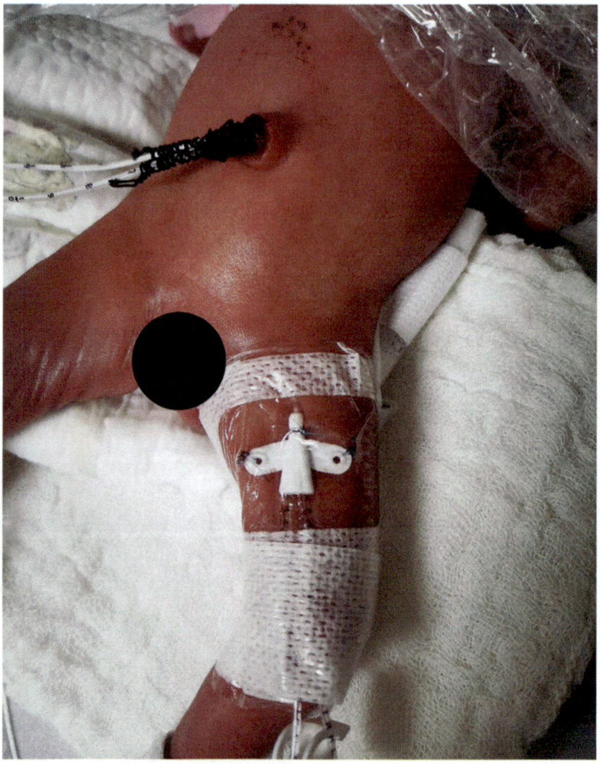

Fig. 21.33 Dressing according to the institutional protocol

Sources

1. Warkentine FH, Clyde Pierce M, Lorenz D, Kim IK. The anatomic relationship of femoral vein to femoral artery in euvolemic pediatric patients by ultrasonography: implications for pediatric femoral central venous access. Acad Emerg Med. 2008;15(5):426–30. https://doi.org/10.1111/j.1553-2712.2008.00087.x.
2. Iwashima S, Ishikawa T, Ohzeki T. Ultrasound-guided versus landmark-guided femoral vein access in pediatric cardiac catheterization. Pediatr Cardiol. 2008;29(2):339–42. https://doi.org/10.1007/s00246-007-9066-2.
3. Aouad MT, Kanazi GE, Abdallah FW, Moukaddem FH, Turbay MJ, Obeid MY, Siddik-Sayyid SM. Femoral vein cannulation performed by residents: a comparison between ultrasound-guided and landmark technique in infants and children undergoing cardiac surgery. Anesth Analg. 2010;111(3):724–8. https://doi.org/10.1213/ANE.0b013e3181e9c475. Epub 2010 Jul 2
4. Al Sofyani K, Julia G, Abdulaziz B, Yves CJ, Sylvain R. Ultrasound guidance for central vascular access in the neonatal and pediatric intensive care unit. Saudi J Anaesth. 2012;6(2):120–4. https://doi.org/10.4103/1658-354X.97023. Erratum in: Saudi J Anaesth. 2012 Oct-Dec;6(4):372. Khouloud, Al Sofyani [corrected to Al Sofyani, Khouloud]
5. Alten JA, Borasino S, Gurley WQ, Law MA, Toms R, Dabal RJ. Ultrasound-guided femoral vein catheterization in neonates with cardiac disease*. Pediatr Crit Care Med. 2012;13(6):654–9. https://doi.org/10.1097/PCC.0b013e318250af0c.
6. Ahn JH, Park J, Song IS, Kim KA, Park J, Min JJ, Kim CS, Lee JH. The angle range of leg abduction with external hip rotation which can minimize femoral artery and vein overlap in pediatric patients. Paediatr Anaesth. 2019;29(4):361–7. https://doi.org/10.1111/pan.13603. Epub 2019 Mar 21
7. Liu WL, Lin MC, Chan SC, Chen SN, Lin TY, Jan SL. Ultrasonographic measurements of femoral vessel diameter in neonates weighing less than 2.5 kg. Echocardiography. 2021;38(10):1741–6. https://doi.org/10.1111/echo.15203. Epub 2021 Sep 23

Chapter 22
Brachial Vein in Pediatrics

22.1 Patient Positioning

- The patient is a 10-year-old weighing 30 kg.
- Position the patient supine.
- Place the extended left arm at shoulder level at a 90° angle (Fig. 22.1).
- The head may be centered or turned to the right.
- Place a tourniquet close to the armpit.

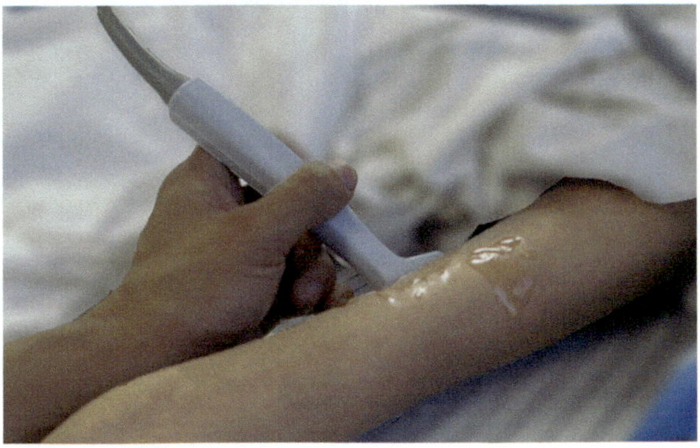

Fig. 22.1 Patient position and LAX view scan

F. Montes-Tapia, *Atlas of Ultrasound-Guided Central Venous Catheter Placement*, https://doi.org/10.1007/978-3-031-61887-1_22

22.2 Scanning Technique

- Do a preliminary vascular assessment (non-sterile).
- The operator sits at the end of the left outstretched arm.
- The ultrasound can be placed above the left shoulder or head or in front of the operator.
- A high-frequency linear transducer (13–6 MHz) with a hockey stick-type or 5-cm footprint probe can be used.
- Divide the arm into three segments and scan the middle third on the medial side.
- Start scanning the arm in long-axis (LAX) view by placing the transducer longitudinal to the arm and with the tip of the transducer directed to proximal (Fig. 22.1).
- LAX view of the left brachial vein (LBrV) (Figs. 22.2 and 22.3).

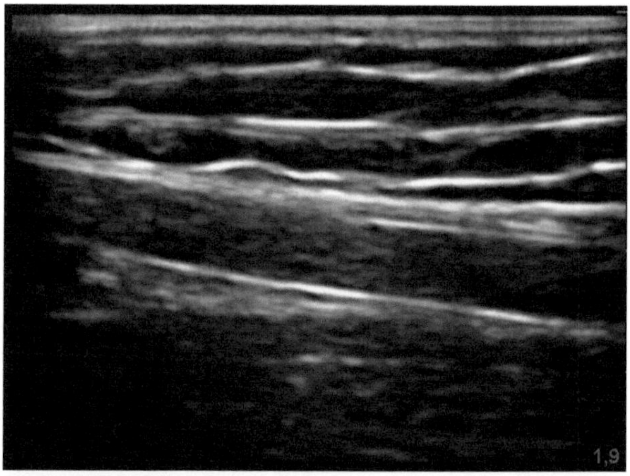

Fig. 22.2 LAX view of the LBrV

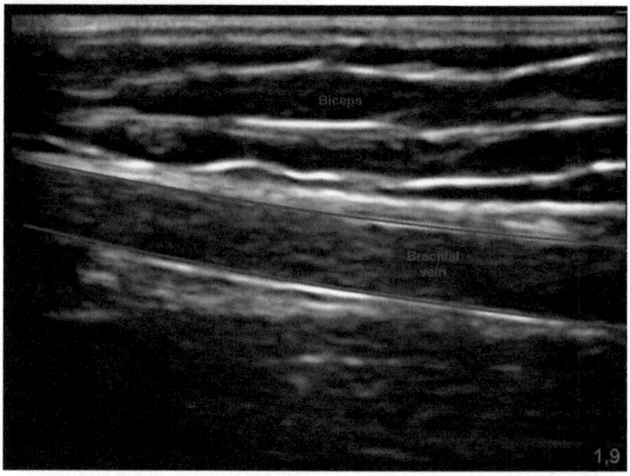

Fig. 22.3 Identifying structures
- Longitudinal view of the LBrV below the biceps muscle

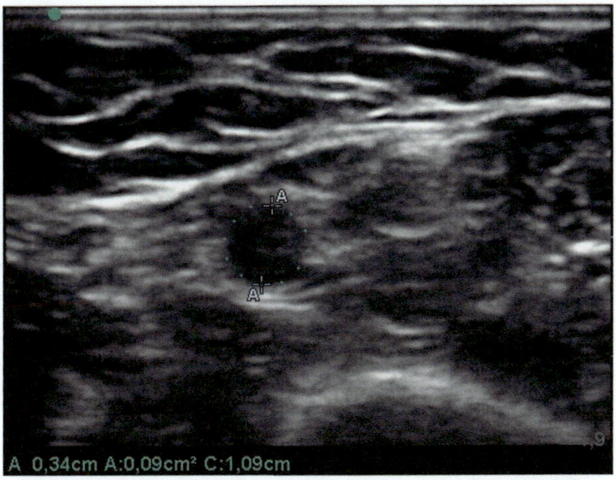

Fig. 22.4 SAX view of the brachial bundle
- The scan depth is 1,9 cm

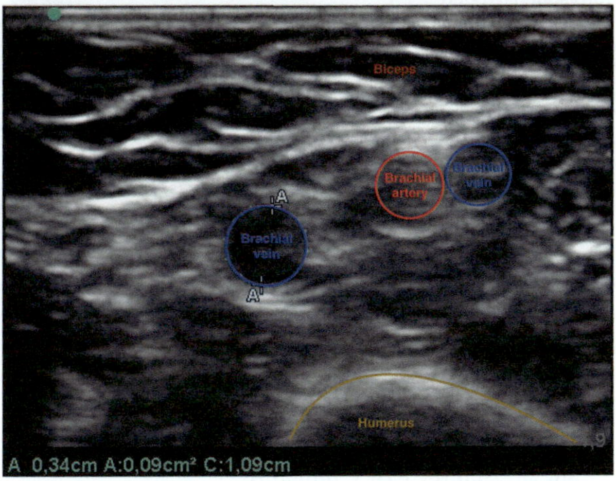

Fig. 22.5 Identifying structures
- The diameter of the left medial brachial vein with tourniquet is 0,34 cm, with an area of 0,09 cm^2
- The humerus is at the base of the image

- Now scan in short-axis (SAX) view (at the same level where scanning is done in LAX view), review the vein depth and arrangement, and verify the vein diameter at this level.
- SAX view of the LBrV (Figs. 22.4 to 22.5).

22.3 Local Anesthesia Application

- The sterile field only leaves the middle and proximal third of the left arm uncovered (Fig. 22.6).
- Real-time ultrasound-guided lidocaine infiltration in LAX view (Fig. 22.7).
- For infiltration, use a small needle 25- 27-G.
- Use 1% lidocaine.

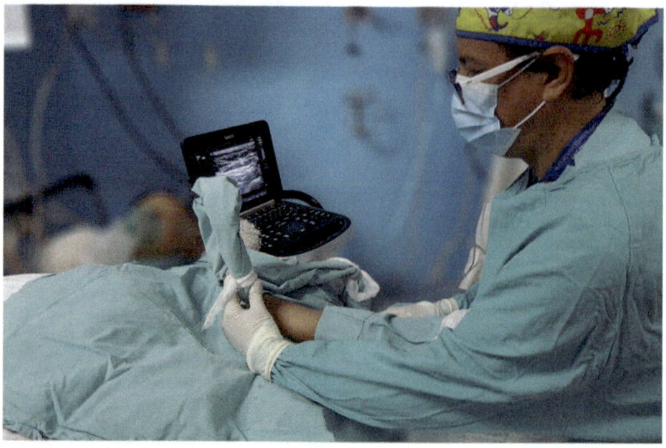

Fig. 22.6 Operator position

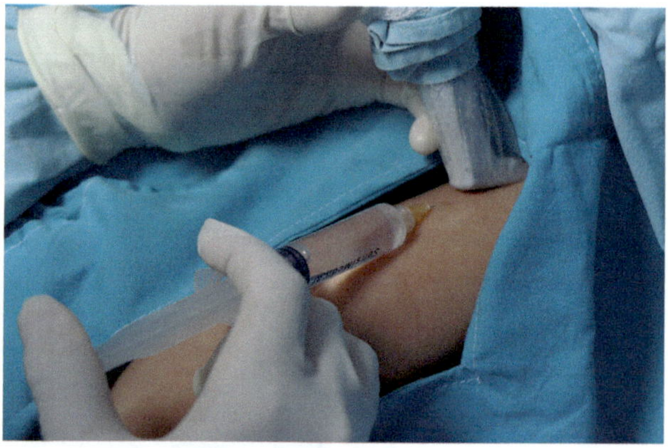

Fig. 22.7 Real-time ultrasound-guided lidocaine infiltration

- Subcutaneous infiltration with lidocaine in the puncture tract 1,5–2 cm before the site chosen for LBrV puncture.
- You can use the lidocaine infiltration puncture to guide where to perform the puncture with the introducer needle.

22.4 Steps for Real-Time Ultrasound-Guided Access to Left Brachial Vein

22.4.1 Step 01

- We will use a 4 Fr single-lumen PowerPICC™.
- Measure the distance from the entry site in the left arm to the central location site using the measuring tape of the Power PICC™ and section the catheter to the appropriate length (Fig. 22.8).

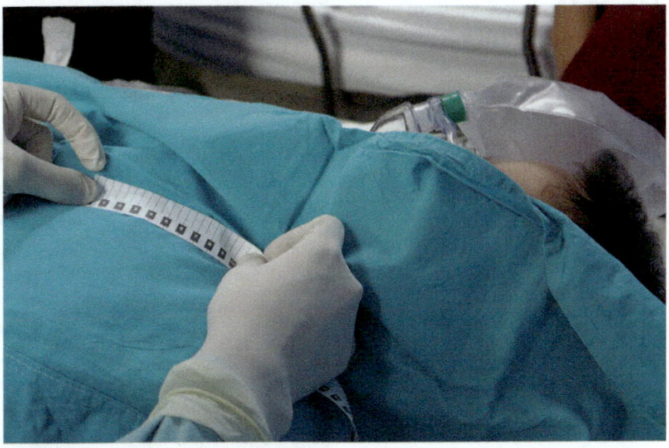

Fig. 22.8 Measure the distance from the entry site in the left arm to the central location

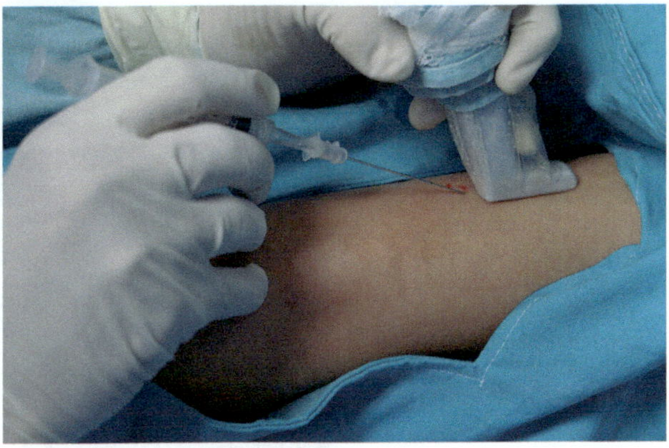

Fig. 22.9 Start the puncture with an angle of 20–30°

- Start scanning the left arm in LAX view of the middle third on the medial side.
- Puncture with a 21-G introducer needle at an angle of 20–30° (Fig. 22.9).
- LAX view of the start of the puncture (Figs. 22.10 and 22.11).
- Begin the ultrasound-guided dynamic needle tracking (DNT) to guide the puncture in real time.

22.4.2 Step 02

- Redirect the scan (medial or lateral) to visualize the LBrV fully and continue the puncture (Fig. 22.12).
- Once the LBrV is completely displayed, continue inserting the introducer needle more deeply following the ultrasound puncture in LAX in DNT in the footprint path (Figs. 22.13 and 22.14).

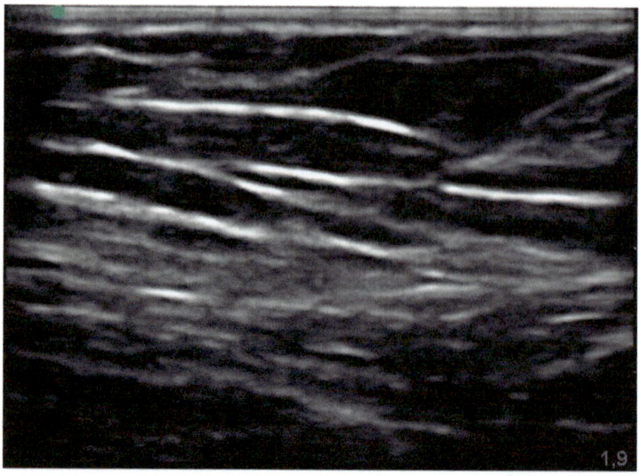

Fig. 22.10 LAX view of the start of the LBrV puncture

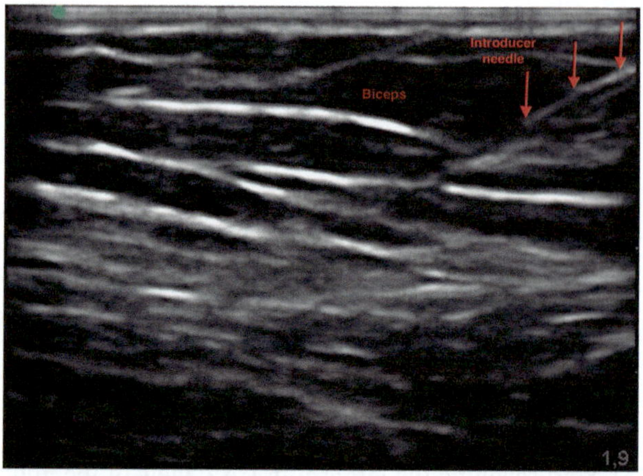

Fig. 22.11 Identifying structures

- The introducer needle is recognized in a longitudinal view
- The introducer needle passes the skin and begins to penetrate the biceps muscle; however, the path is not yet related to the LBrV

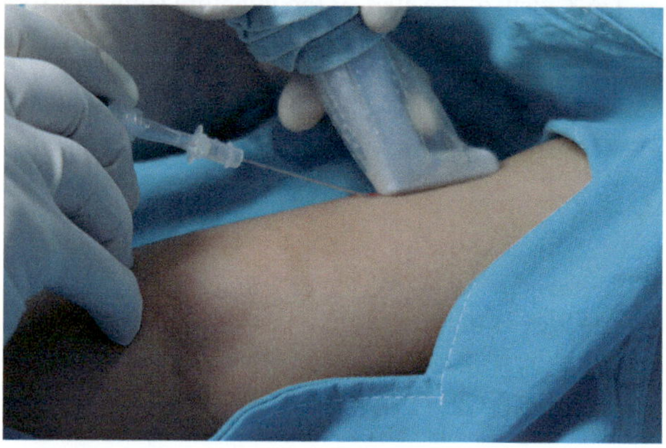

Fig. 22.12 Redirect the scan medial or lateral

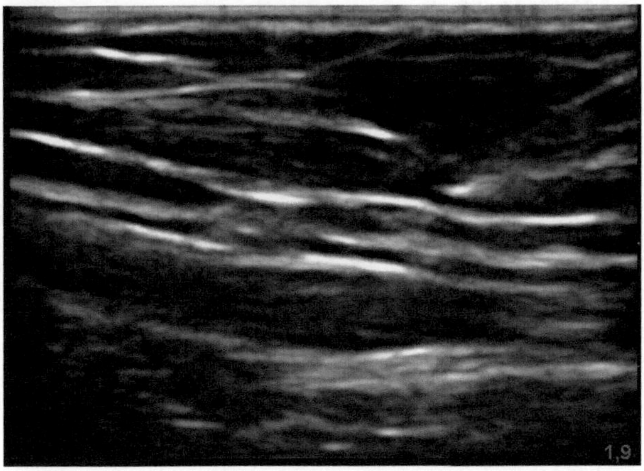

Fig. 22.13 LAX view of the puncture progression

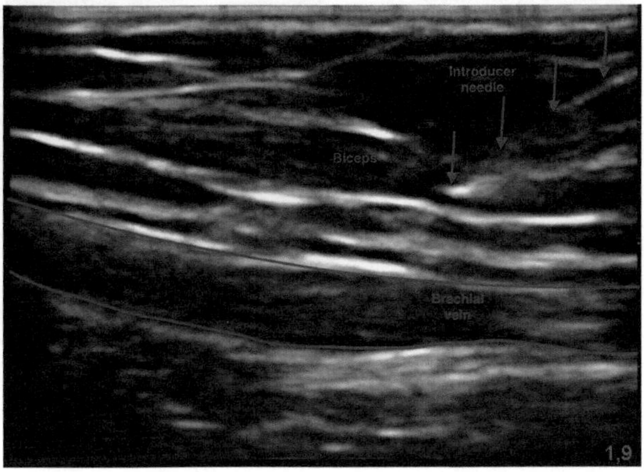

Fig. 22.14 Identifying structures
- Progress has been made with deep insertion of the introducer needle; now, the puncture is in the correct path to the LBrV

- Modify the puncture angle between 10° and 20° and continue with the introduction of the introducer needle (Fig. 22.15).
- LAX view of the arrival of the needle to the anterior wall of the LBrV (Figs. 22.16 and 22.17).

22.4.3 Step 03

- Since the puncture is in the correct direction, insert the introducer needle more deeply to cannulate the vein, making sure not to penetrate the posterior wall (Fig. 22.18).

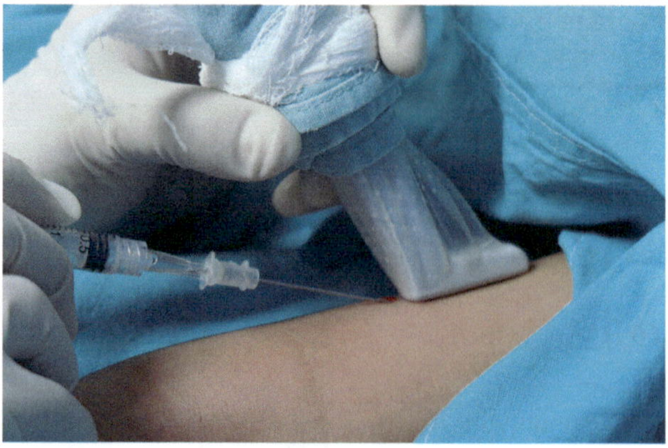

Fig. 22.15 Modify the puncture angle to 10–20° to redirect toward the vein

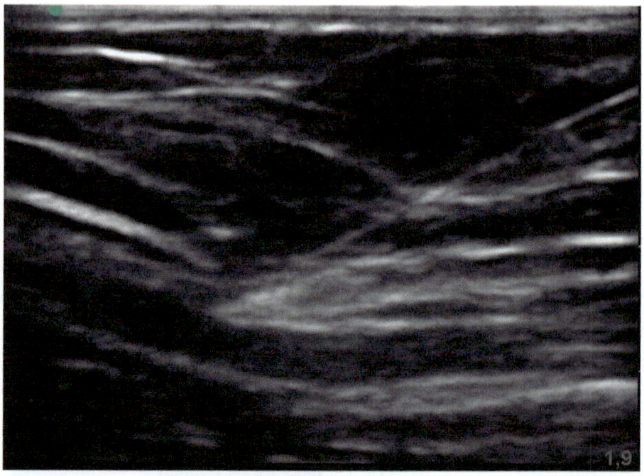

Fig. 22.16 LAX view of the arrival of the needle to the anterior wall of the LBrV

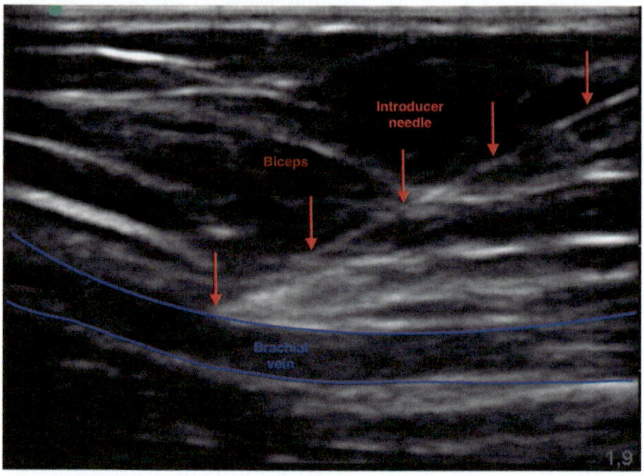

Fig. 22.17 Identifying structures

- The introducer needle is visualized in the anterior wall of the LBrV before penetrating it

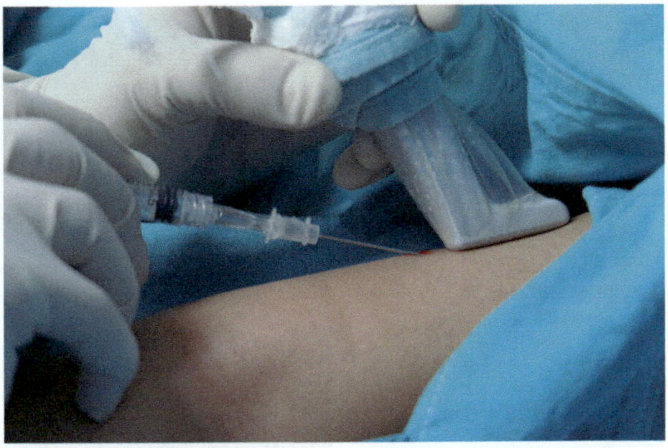

Fig. 22.18 Progression of the puncture in DNT with proximal advancement of the transducer

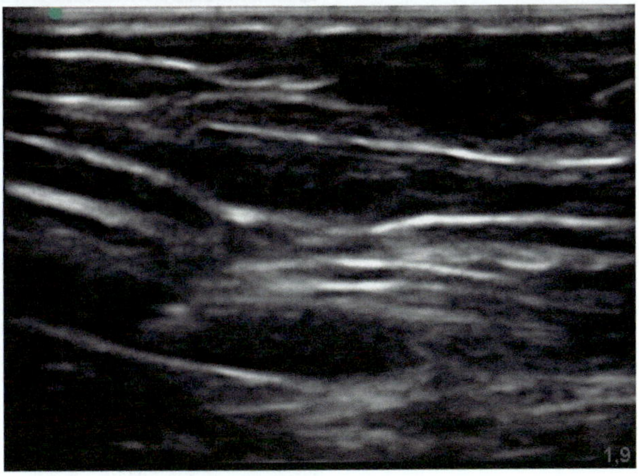

Fig. 22.19 LAX view of the penetration of the introducer needle into the LBrV

- LAX view of the penetration of the LBrV by the introducer needle (Figs. 22.19 and 22.20).
- Immediately after the lumen of the LBrV is penetrated, blood is noticed in the flashback chamber; stop advancing the introducer needle (Fig. 22.21).
- LAX view of the LBrV cannulation (Figs. 22.22 and 22.23).
- Set the transducer aside.
- Hold the hub of the introducer needle.
- There are three ways to identify that you cannulated the vein:
  - Identify vein cannulation on the screen.
  - Loss of resistance when advancing the introducer needle.
  - Spontaneous return of blood in the flashback chamber due to tourniquet compression.
- Hold the hub of the introducer needle.
- Maintain gentle negative pressure on the syringe plunger until a flash of blood appears in the barrel of the syringe, and check for free flow (Fig. 22.24).

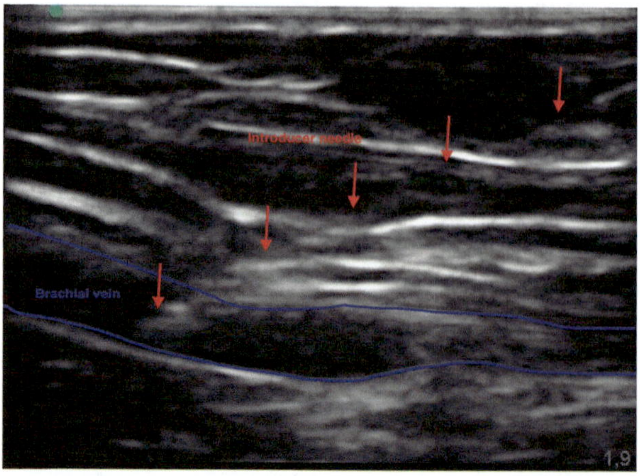

Fig. 22.20 Identifying structures

- The introducer needle exerts pressure on the anterior wall when penetrating the vein without passing to the posterior wall. You can see anterior wall depression due to compression

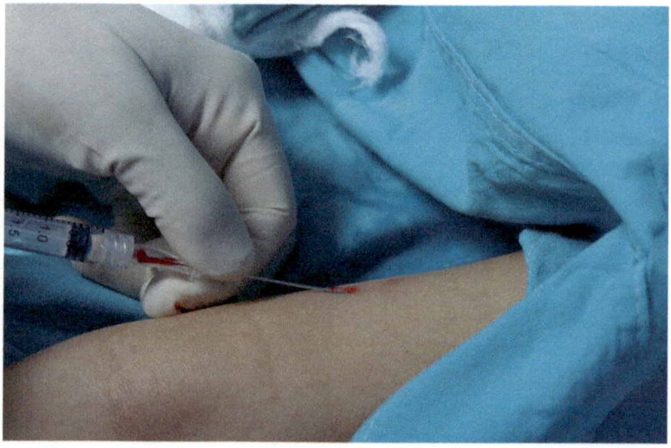

Fig. 22.21 Blood is noticed in the flashback chamber; stop advancing the introducer needle

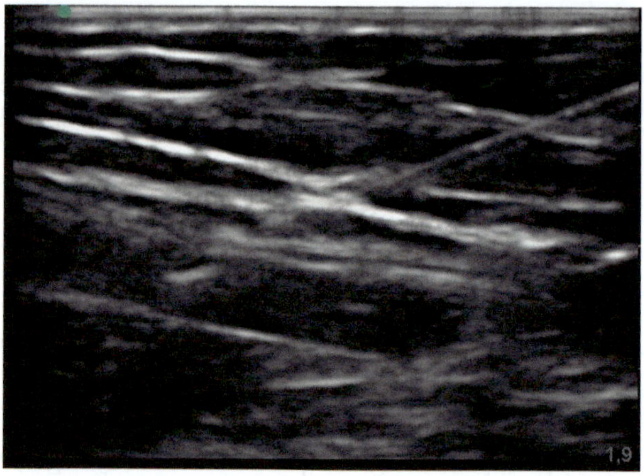

Fig. 22.22 LAX view of the LBrV cannulation before setting the transducer aside

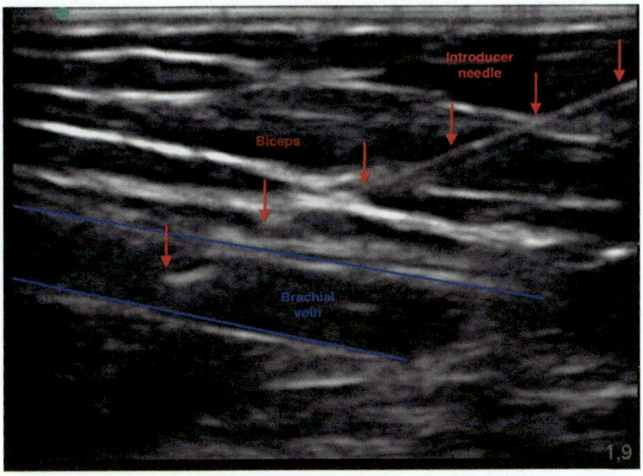

Fig. 22.23 Identifying structures
- The introducer needle cannulates the LBrV, and by not exerting puncture pressure, the vein has recovered its caliber without anterior wall deformities, as in Fig. 22.20
- The introducer needle has not penetrated the posterior wall and remains in the lumen of the vein

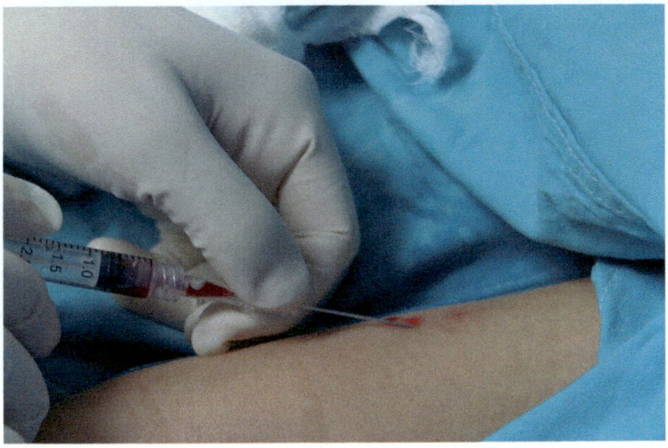

Fig. 22.24 Maintain gentle negative pressure on the syringe plunger

22.4.4 Step 04

- Once cannulated, the vein with the introducer needle.
- Introduce the 0.018" guidewire of the PowerPICC™ equipment in the introducer needle (Fig. 22.25).
- Check the location of the intravascular guidewire, especially if it is not easily inserted into the vein (Fig. 22.26).
- LAX view of the intravenous guidewire (Figs. 22.27 and 22.28).

22.4.5 Step 05

- Place the vascular micro-introducer over the guidewire (Fig. 22.29).
- Carefully insert the micro-introducer.

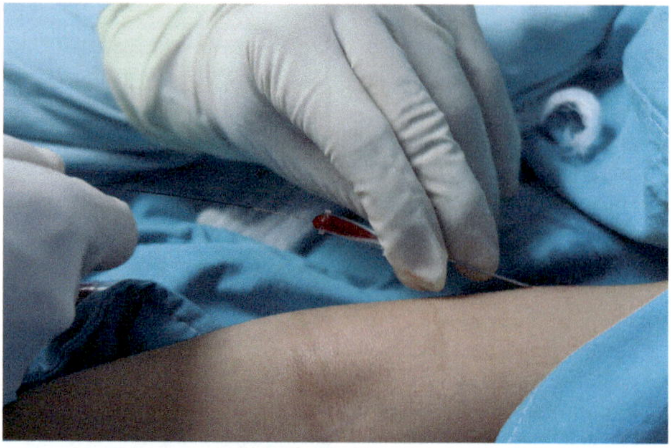

Fig. 22.25 Insert the guidewire

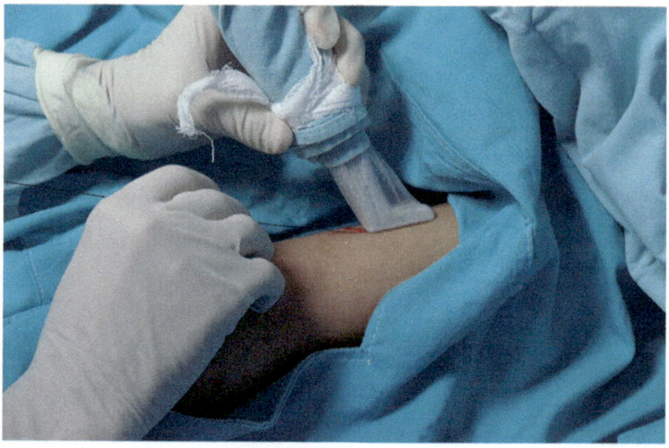

Fig. 22.26 Scan the intravascular location of the guidewire

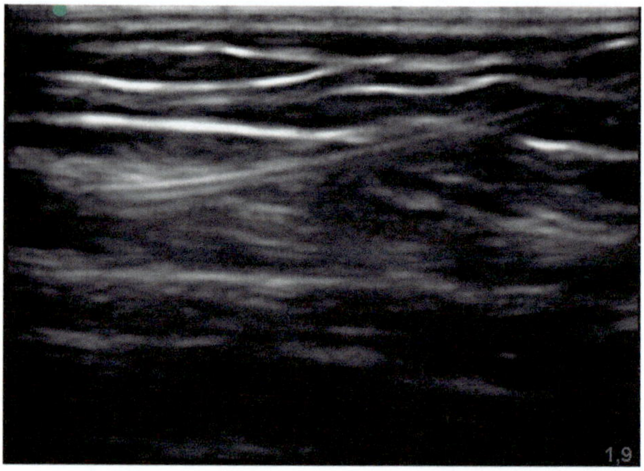

Fig. 22.27 LAX view of the intravascular guidewire

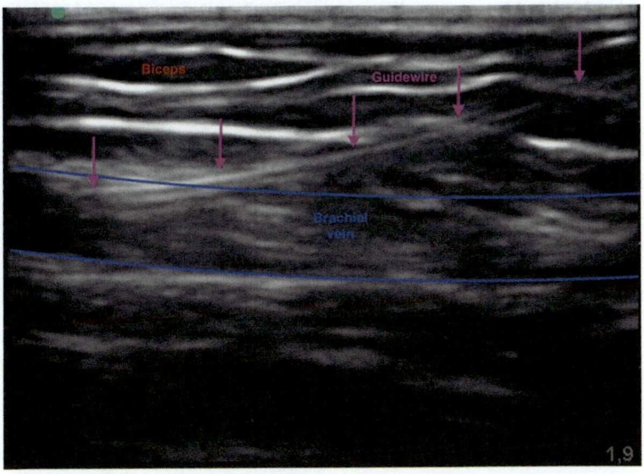

Fig. 22.28 Identifying structures
- The guidewire inside the LBrV

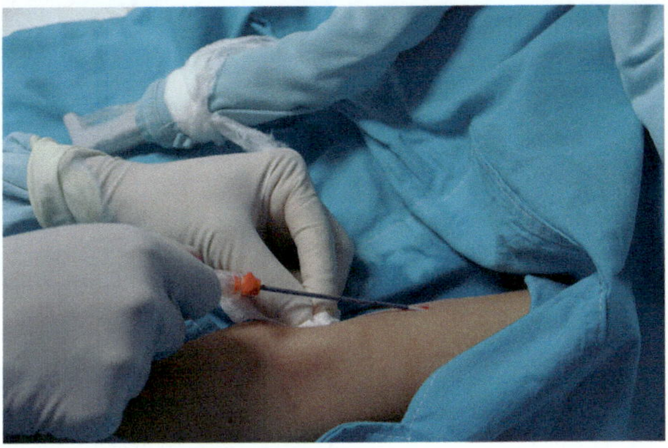

Fig. 22.29 Insert the vascular micro-introducer over the guidewire

- If the micro-introducer cannot be inserted, make a small incision in the upper part of the skin with a #11 scalpel blade so that it passes easily (Fig. 22.30).
- Do not make the incision too large because blood may leak more easily.
- Introduce the micro-introducer without bending the guidewire (Fig. 22.31). Dilate the path from the skin to the vein and cannulate the vein with the micro-introducer using Seldinger's maneuver (Fig. 22.32).

22.4.6 Step 06

- Remove the guidewire with the inner dilator and leave only the peel-away sheath (Fig. 22.33).
- Using the modified Seldinger's technique, introduce the catheter through the peel-away sheath (Figs. 22.34 and 22.35).

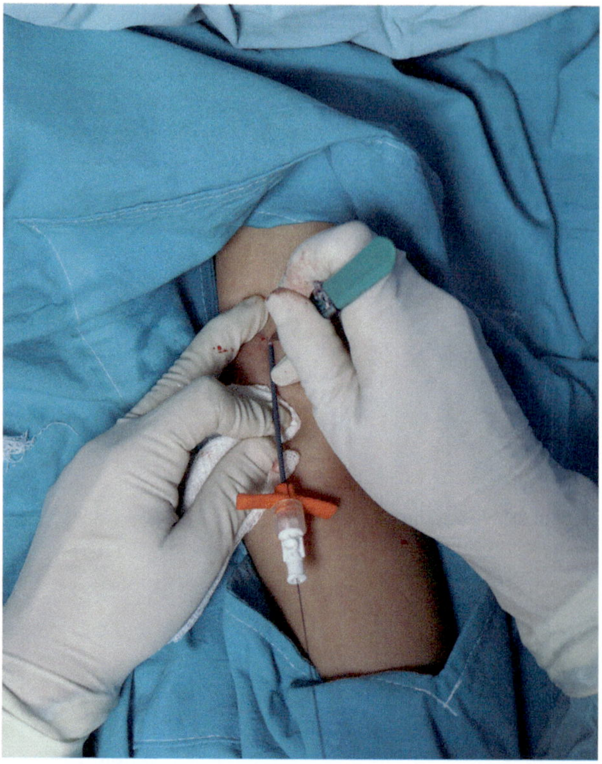

Fig. 22.30 Make a small incision in the upper part of the skin

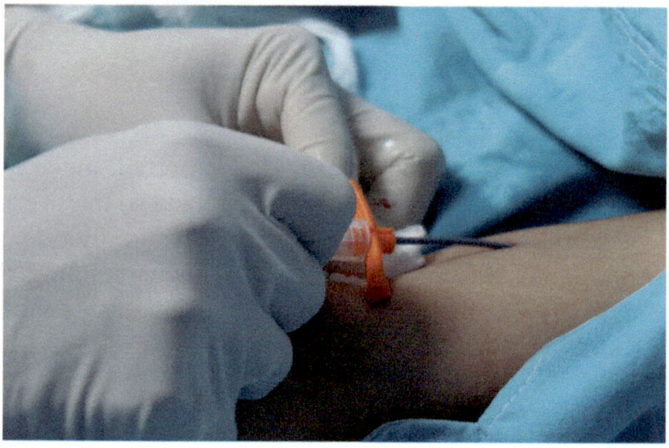

Fig. 22.31 Insert the micro-introducer

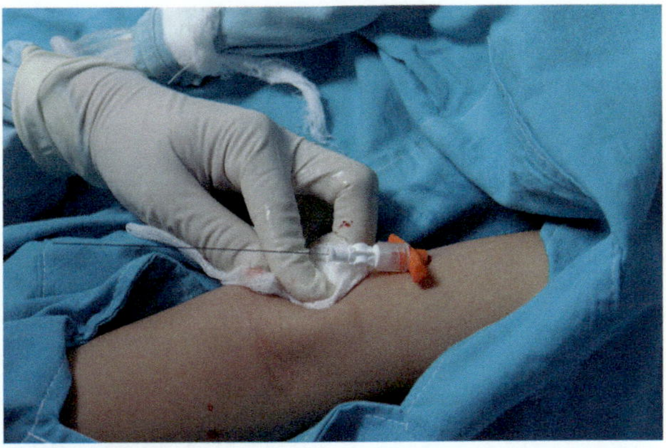

Fig. 22.32 Insert the entire micro-introducer

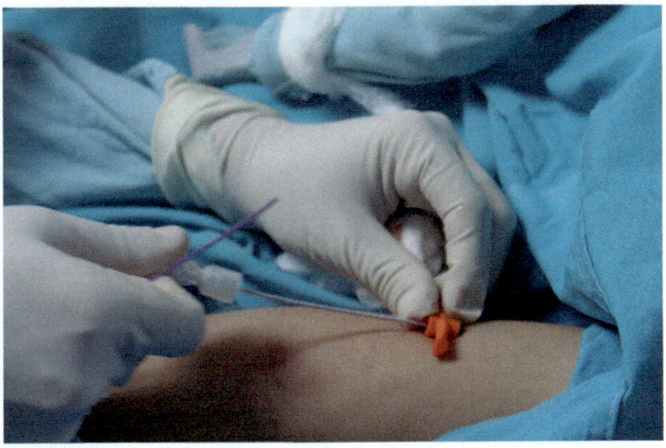

Fig. 22.33 Remove the guidewire with the inner dilator

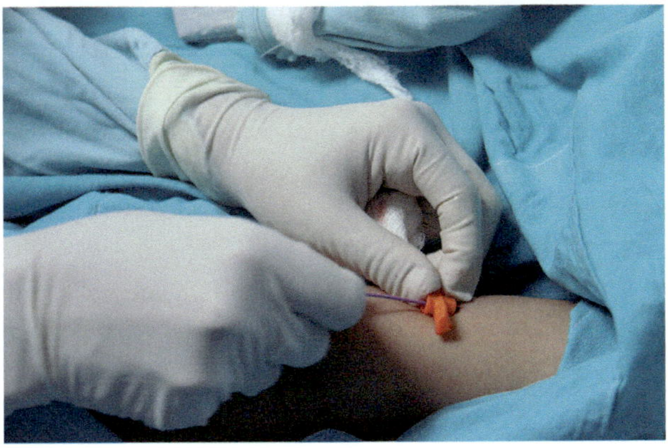

Fig. 22.34 Introduce the catheter through the peel-away sheath

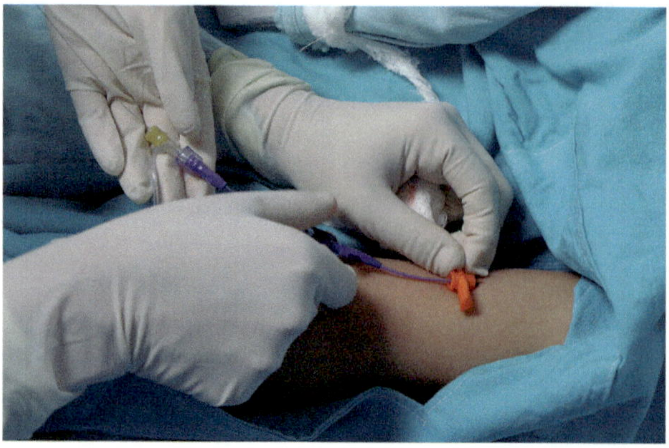

Fig. 22.35 Insert the previously measured catheter length

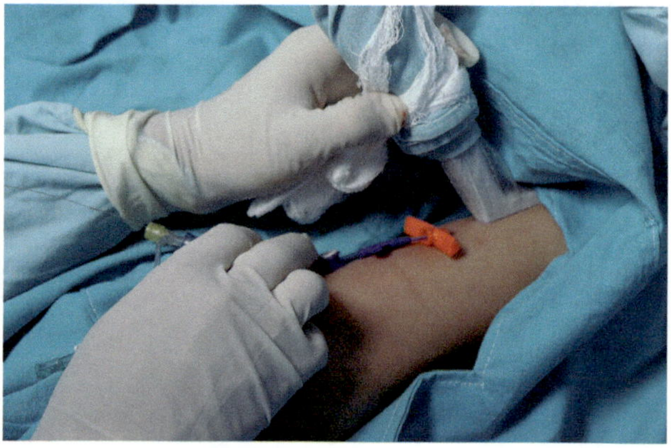

Fig. 22.36 Scan the location of the catheter in LAX view

- Scan the intravenous location of the catheter before removing the peel-away sheath (Fig. 22.36).
- LAX view of the intravascular 4 Fr PICC (Figs. 22.37 and 22.38).
- Before you remove the peel-away sheath, scan the cervicothoracic region (red arrowhead) (Fig. 22.39) to confirm that the catheter has not lodged in the left internal jugular vein and is in the left brachiocephalic vein (LBCV) in the way to the superior vena cava.
  - If the catheter is found in the left internal jugular vein, you need to realize maneuvers to redirect the catheter toward the LBCV.
- LAX view of the LBCV (Figs. 22.40 and 22.41).
- Remove the peel-away sheath (Fig. 22.42).

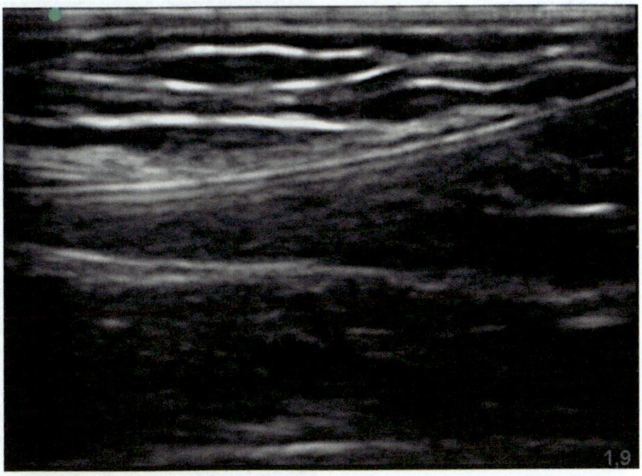

Fig. 22.37 LAX view of the intravascular PICC

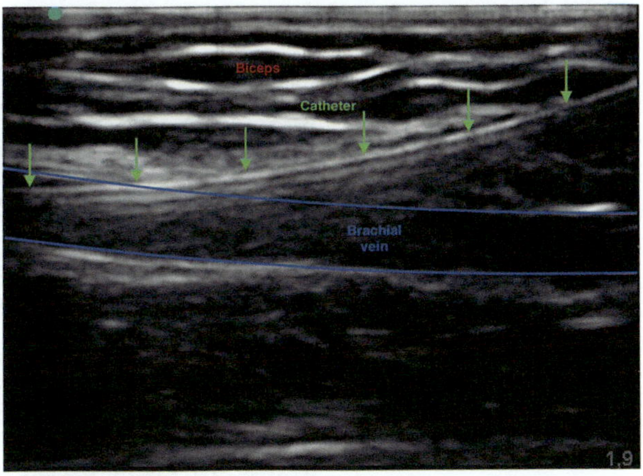

Fig. 22.38 Identifying structures
- The 4 Fr PICC in the lumen of the LBrV

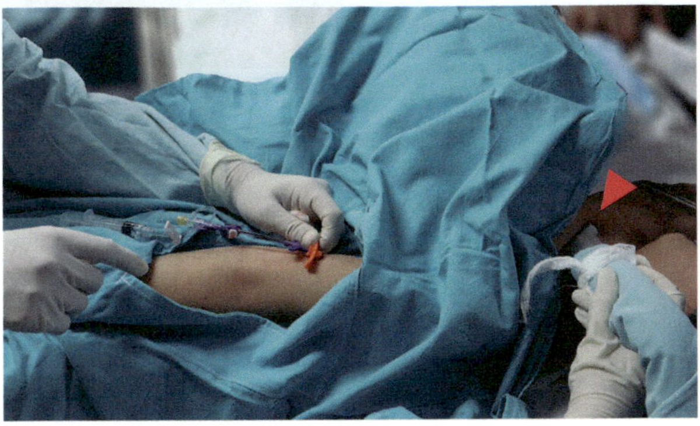

Fig. 22.39 Scan the cervicothoracic region

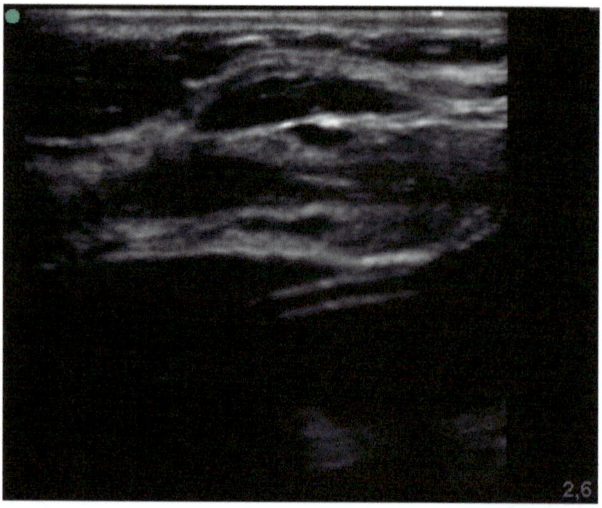

Fig. 22.40 Scan of the left supraclavicular fossae

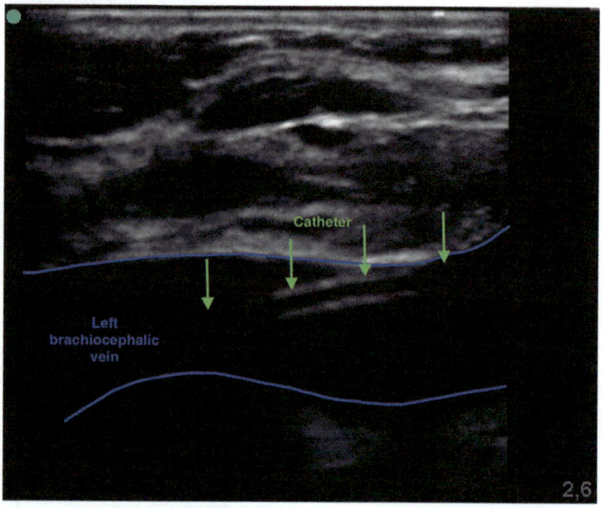

Fig. 22.41 Identifying structures
- LAX view of the LBCV
- The PICC is in the LBCV, a good position indicating that it is in the direction of the superior vena cava

22.4.7 Step 07

- Place the StatLock® catheter stabilization device system (Fig. 22.43).
- Place a sterile dressing (Fig. 22.44).

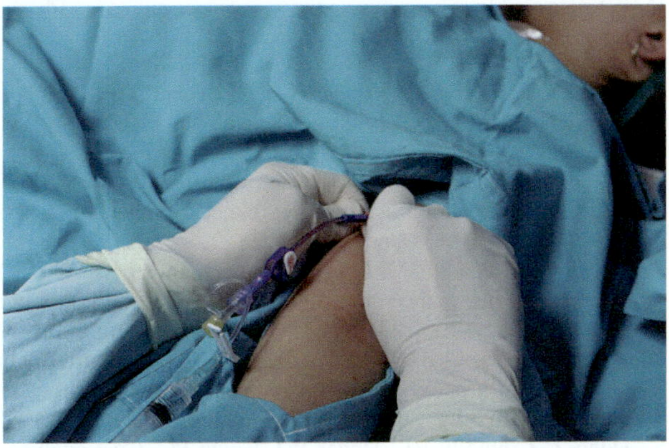

Fig. 22.42 Remove the peel-away sheath

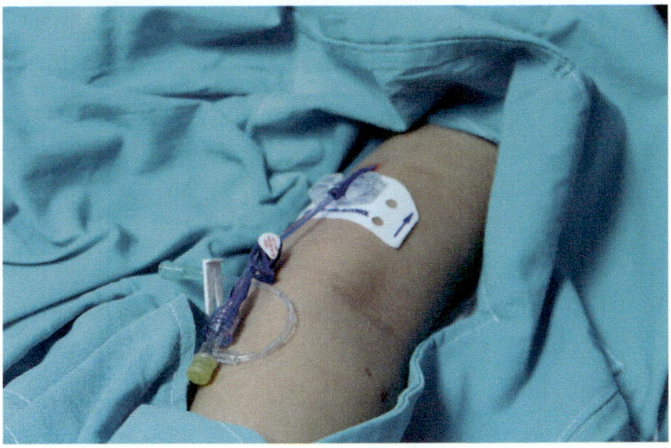

Fig. 22.43 Place the StatLock system sterile

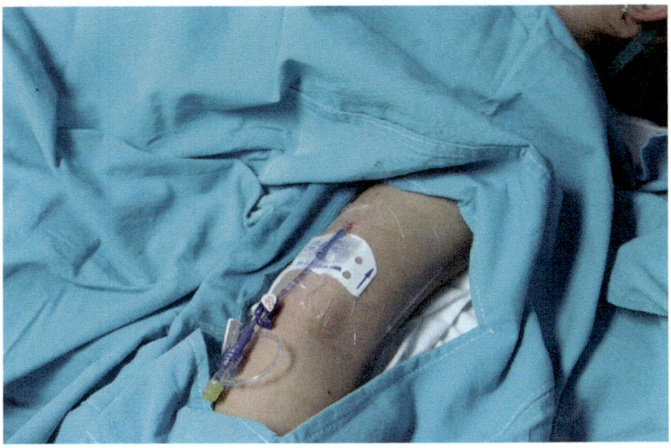

Fig. 22.44 Place a sterile patch over the StatLock® system

Sources

1. Crowley JJ, Pereira JK, Harris LS, Becker CJ. Peripherally inserted central catheters: experience in 523 children. Radiology. 1997;204(3):617–21. https://doi.org/10.1148/radiology.204.3.9280234.
2. Racadio JM, Doellman DA, Johnson ND, Bean JA, Jacobs BR. Pediatric peripherally inserted central catheters: complication rates related to catheter tip location. Pediatrics. 2001;107(2):E28. https://doi.org/10.1542/peds.107.2.e28.
3. Fricke BL, Racadio JM, Duckworth T, Donnelly LF, Tamer RM, Johnson ND. Placement of peripherally inserted central catheters without fluoroscopy in children: initial catheter tip position. Radiology. 2005;234(3):887–92. https://doi.org/10.1148/radiol.2343031823.
4. Tran HS, Burrows BJ, Zang WA, Han DC. Brachial arteriovenous fistula as a complication of placement of a peripherally inserted central venous catheter: a case report and review of the literature. Am Surg. 2006;72(9):833–6. https://doi.org/10.1177/000313480607200914.
5. Dong Z, Connolly BL, Ungar WJ, Coyte PC. Cost analysis of peripherally inserted central catheter in pediatric patients. Int J Technol Assess Health Care. 2018;34(1):38–45. https://doi.org/10.1017/S026646231700109X.

Chapter 23
Cephalic Vein in Pediatrics

23.1 Patient Positioning

- The patient is a 12-year-old adolescent weighing 86 kg.
- Position the patient supine.
- Place the extended arm at shoulder level at a 90° angle (Fig. 23.1).

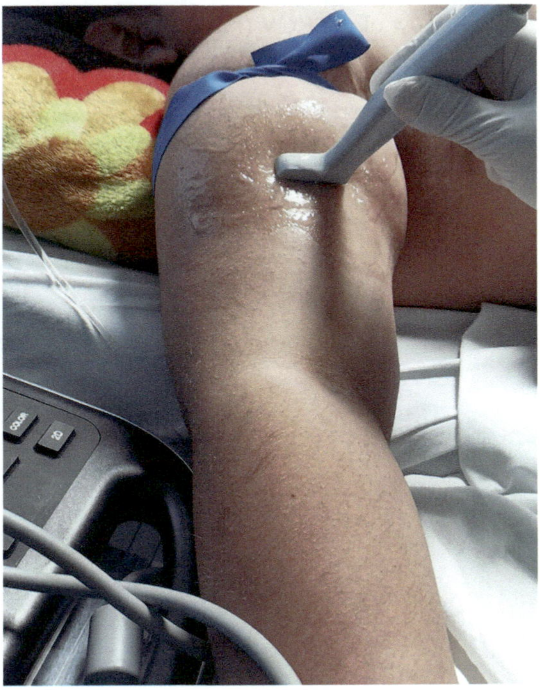

Fig. 23.1 Patient position and scan in SAX view

F. Montes-Tapia, *Atlas of Ultrasound-Guided Central Venous Catheter Placement*, https://doi.org/10.1007/978-3-031-61887-1_23

- The head may be centered or turned to the right.
- Place a tourniquet close to the armpit.

23.2 Scanning Technique

- Do a preliminary vascular assessment (non-sterile).
- The operator stands at the end of the outstretched arm.
- The ultrasound can be placed on the right side of the arm, but the best position is above the right shoulder.
- A high-frequency linear transducer (13–6 MHz), with a hockey stick-type or 5-cm footprint probe, can be used.
- Divide the arm into three segments and scan the proximal third on the lateral face.
- Start scanning the arm in short-axis (SAX) view by placing the transducer transverse to the arm and with the tip of the transducer directed to the patient's right side (Fig. 23.1).
- SAX view of the right cephalic vein (RCV) (Figs. 23.2 and 23.3).
- Now scan in long-axis (LAX) view (at the same level where scanning is done in SAX view), review the vein depth and arrangement, and verify the vein diameter at this level (Fig. 23.4).
- LAX view of the RCV (Figs. 23.5 and 23.6).

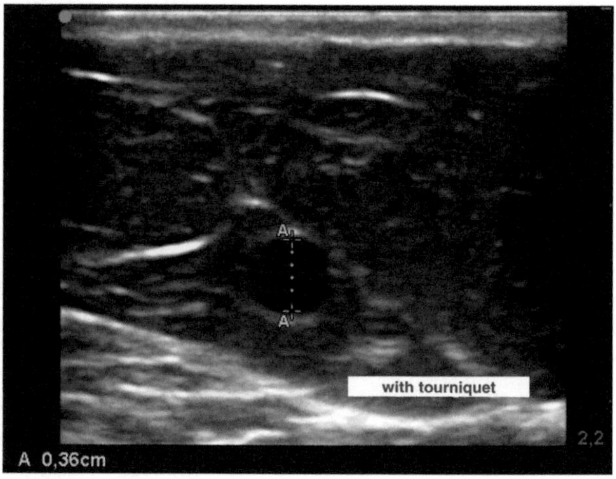

Fig. 23.2 SAX view of the RCV

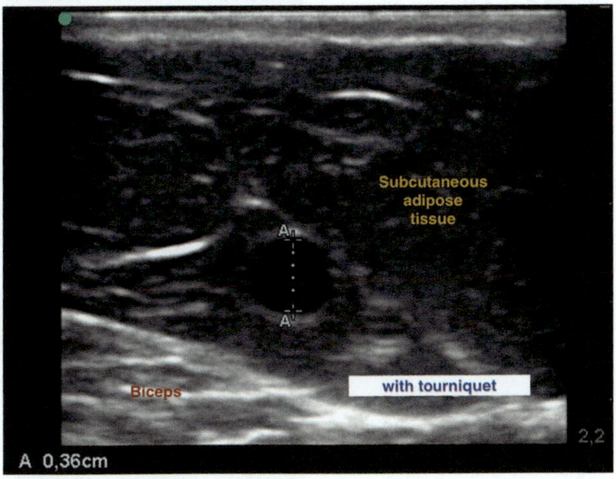

Fig. 23.3 Identifying structures
- The RCV measures 0,36 cm in diameter, with the tourniquet placed at the armpit level
- Thick subcutaneous adipose tissue (SAT)
- The biceps muscle lies below the RCV
- Scanning is done at a depth of 2,2 cm

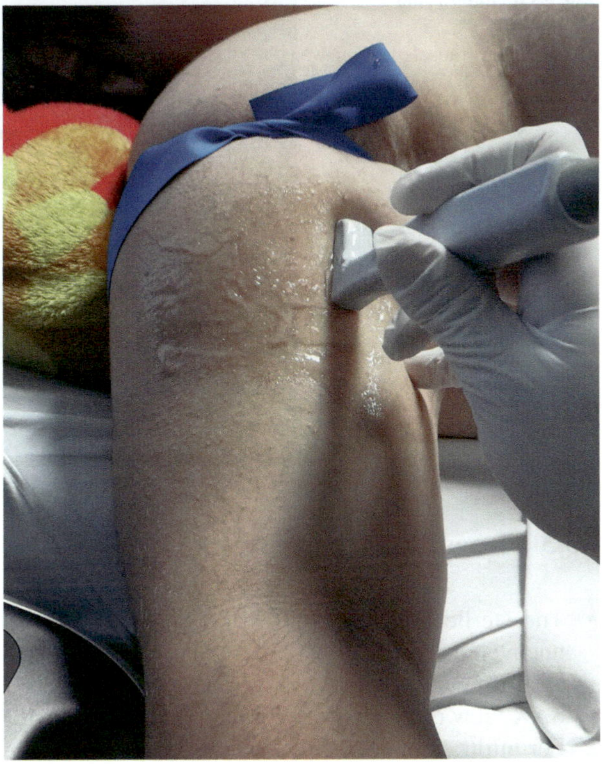

Fig. 23.4 Scan the RCV in LAX view

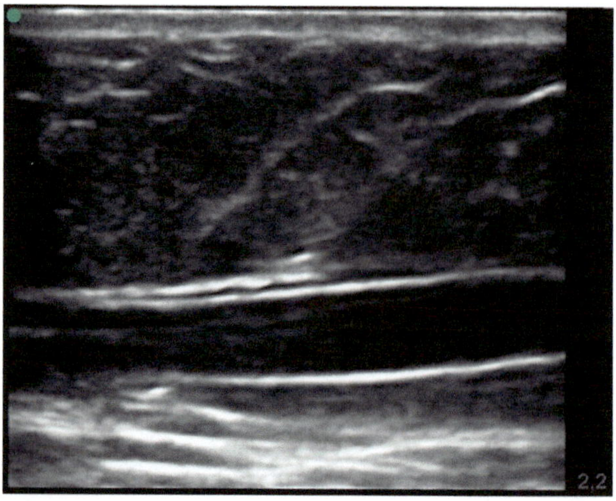

Fig. 23.5 LAX view of the RCV

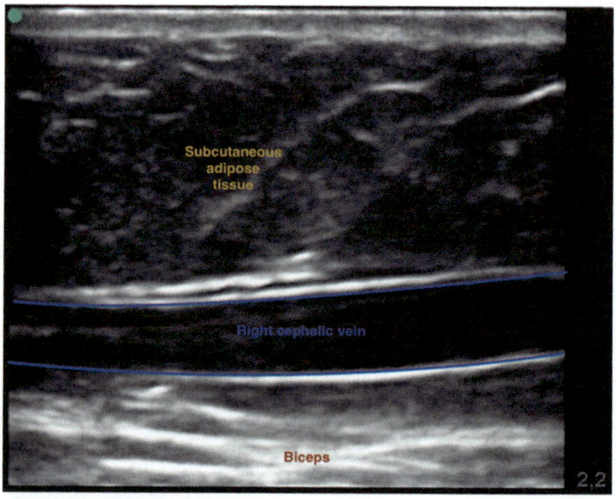

Fig. 23.6 Identifying structures
- The biceps muscle lies below the RCV

23.3 Local Anesthesia Application

- The sterile field only leaves the middle and proximal third of the right arm uncovered.
- Real-time ultrasound-guided lidocaine infiltration (Fig. 23.7).
- SAX view of lidocaine infiltration (Figs. 23.8 and 23.9).
- For infiltration, use a small needle 25–27 G.
- Use lidocaine 1%.
- Subcutaneous infiltration with lidocaine in the puncture tract 1,5–2 cm before the site chosen for RCV puncture.
- You can use the lidocaine infiltration puncture to guide where to perform the puncture with the introducer needle.

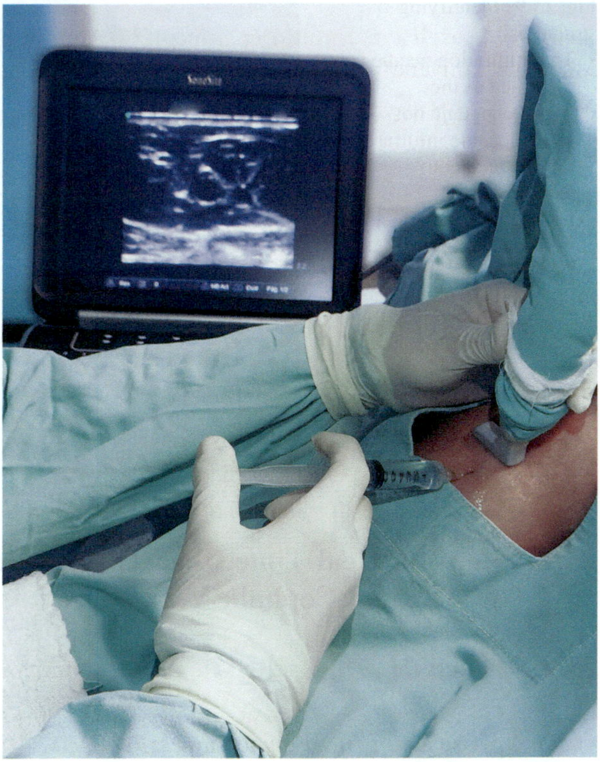

Fig. 23.7 Real-time ultrasound-guided lidocaine infiltration

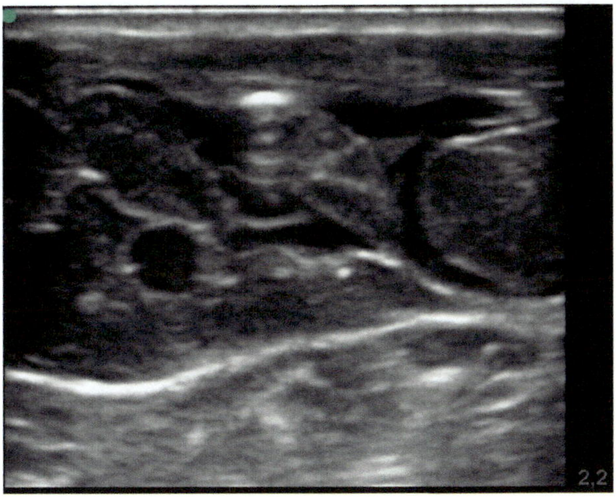

Fig. 23.8 SAX view of lidocaine infiltration

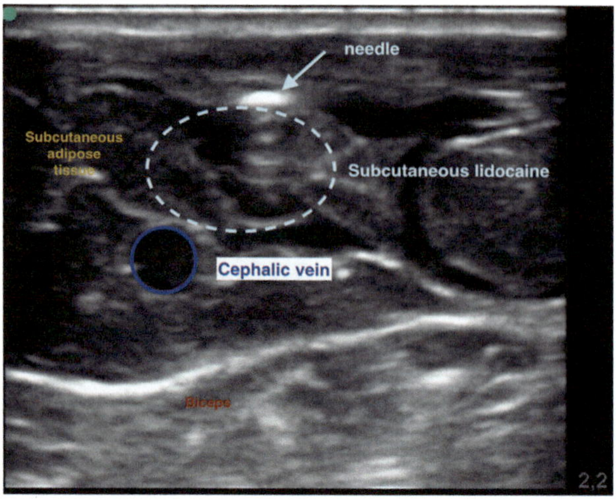

Fig. 23.9 Identifying structures
- The infiltration needle is identified as the hyperechogenic dot
- The lidocaine infiltrates the subcutaneous adipose tissue
- Lidocaine will form a hyperechoic area
- RCV is above the biceps

23.4 Steps for Real-Time Ultrasound-Guided Access to the Right Cephalic Vein

23.4.1 Step 01

- We will use a 4 Fr single-lumen PowerPICC™.
- Measure the distance from the entry site in the arm to the central location site using the measuring tape of the PowerPICC™ and section the catheter to the appropriate length.
- Start scanning the arm in SAX view between the middle and proximal thirds on the lateral side.
- Puncture with a 21-G introducer needle at an angle of 20–30° (Fig. 23.10).
- SAX view of the start of the puncture (Figs. 23.11 and 23.12).
- Begin the ultrasound-guided dynamic needle tip positioning (DNTP) to guide the puncture in real time.

23.4.2 Step 02

- Increase the puncture angle to 30–40°, advancing toward the RCV (Fig. 23.13).
- SAX view of the progress of the LCV puncture (Figs. 23.14 and 23.15).

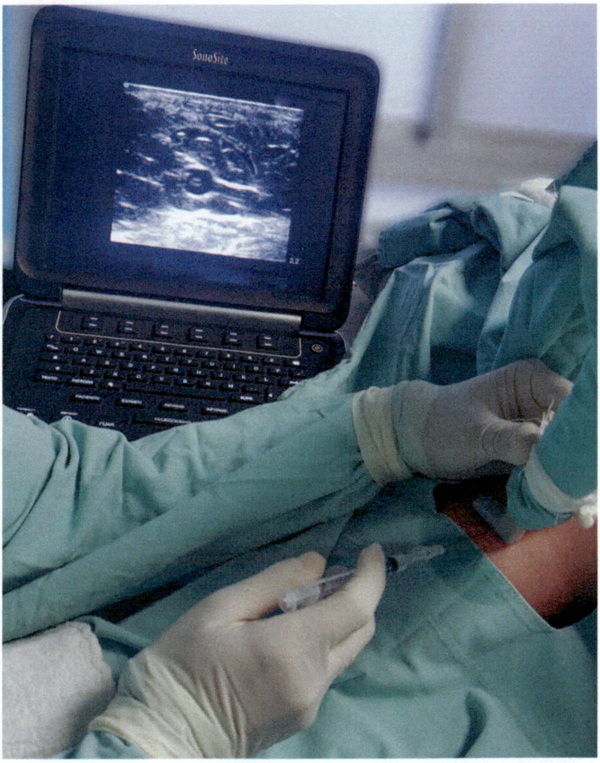

Fig. 23.10 Start the puncture with an angle of 20–30°

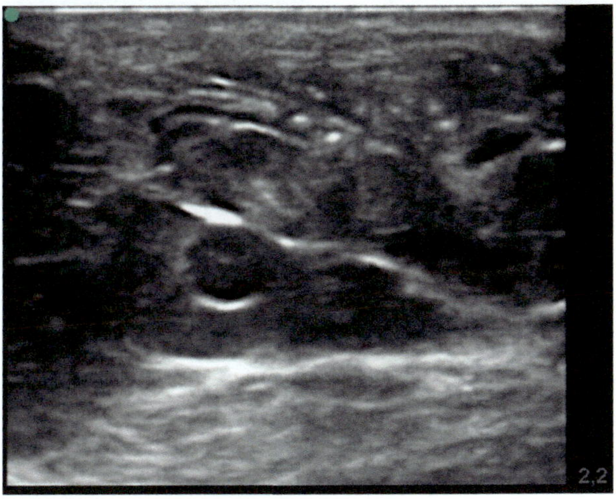

Fig. 23.11 SAX view of the start of the puncture

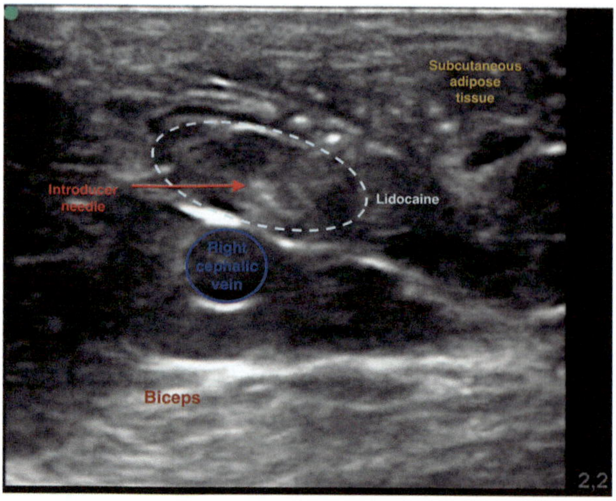

Fig. 23.12 Identifying structures

- The tip of the introducer needle is recognized in real time by a bright hyperechoic (white) dot that moves through the tissues
- It also helps to recognize the tip of the introducer needle by the movements of the surrounding tissue when the needle is penetrating; hence, dynamic needle tip positioning is the basis for successful SAX punctures
- At this moment, the direction of the needle is the outer edge of the RCV

Fig. 23.13 Increase the puncture angle to 30–40° to redirect toward the vein

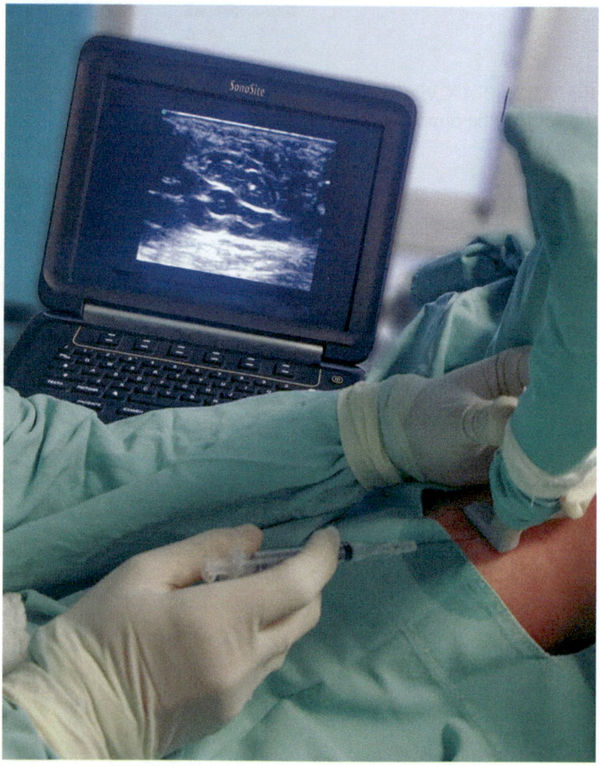

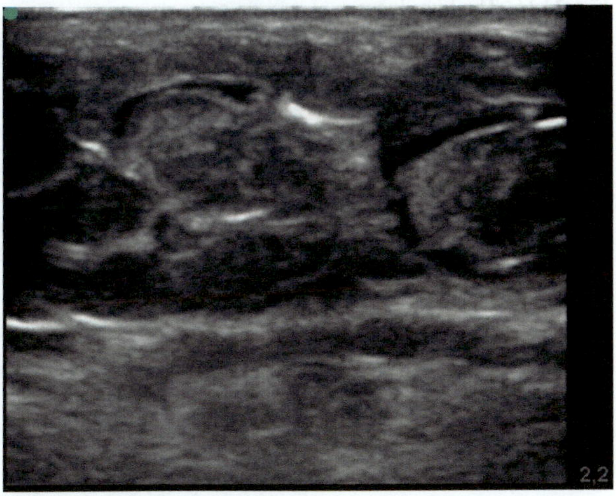

Fig. 23.14 SAX view of the progress of the RCV LBV puncture with the introducer needle

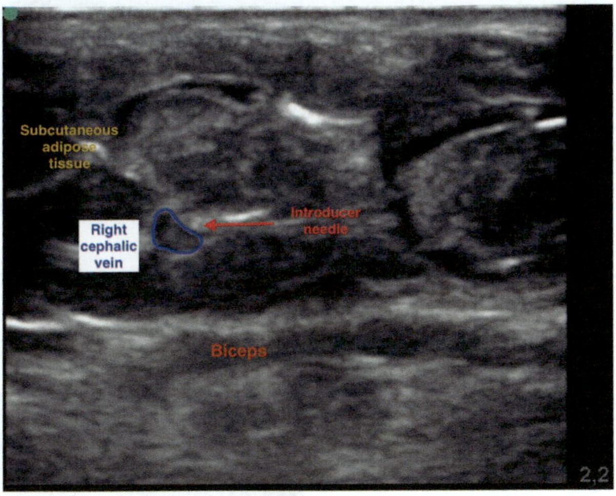

Fig. 23.15 Identifying structures
- The introducer needle reaches the anterior wall of the RCV and deforms the anterior wall of the vein

23.4.3 Step 03

- Continue the introduction of the introducer needle after the puncture in the DNTP, and sweep the transducer proximally to follow the needle as it advances toward the vein until cannulated (Fig. 23.16).
- SAX view of the progression of RCV puncture and cannulation (Figs. 23.17, 23.18, 23.19 and 23.20).
- Immediately after visualizing the RCV cannulation, maintain a gentle negative pressure on the syringe plunger until a flash of blood appears in the barrel of the syringe (Fig. 23.21).

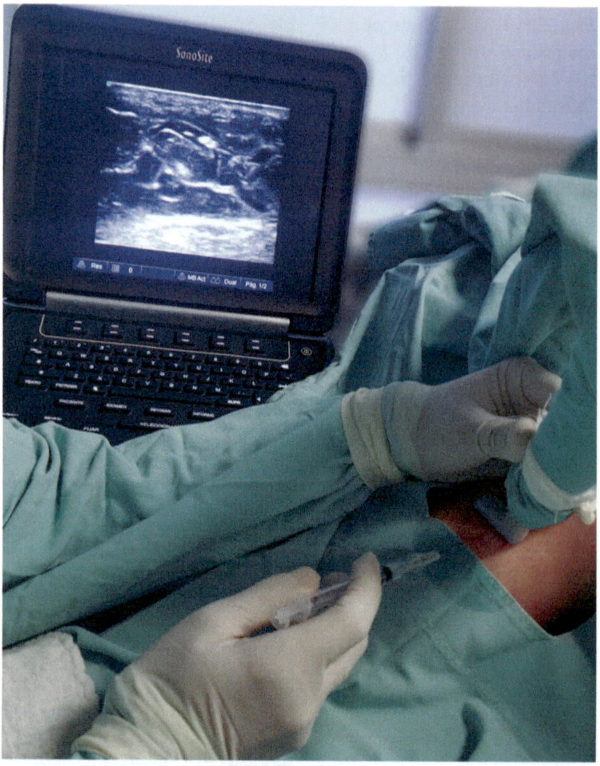

Fig. 23.16 The introducer needle advances following the path to cannulate the vein, so the transducer is advanced proximally to follow the tip of the needle

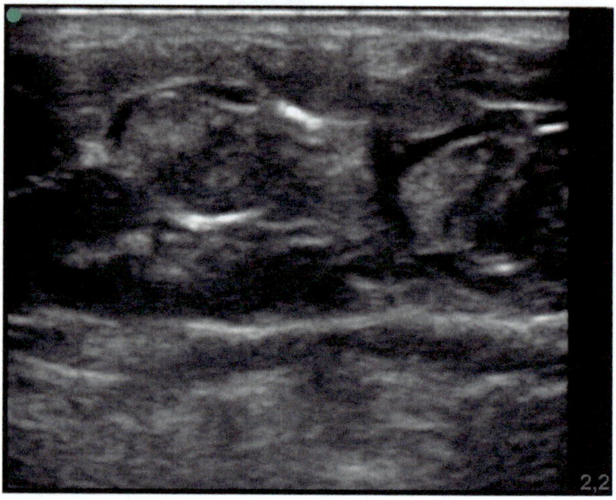

Fig. 23.17 SAX view of the start of the RCV canalization

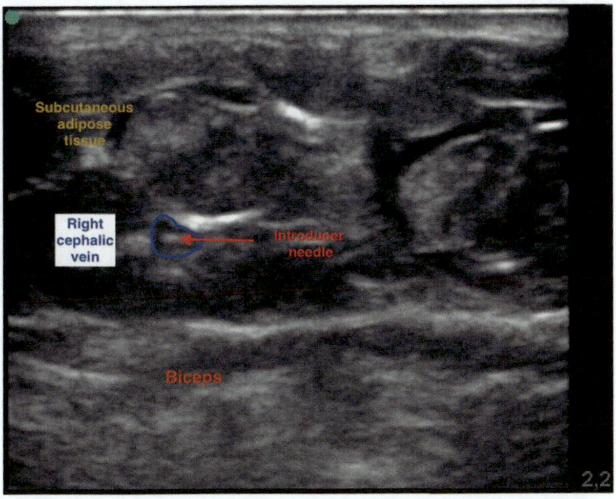

Fig. 23.18 Identifying structures
- The tip of the introducing needle is visualized entering the lumen of the RCV
- Due to the pressure exerted by the puncture, the RCV is small and has a deformity of the anterior wall

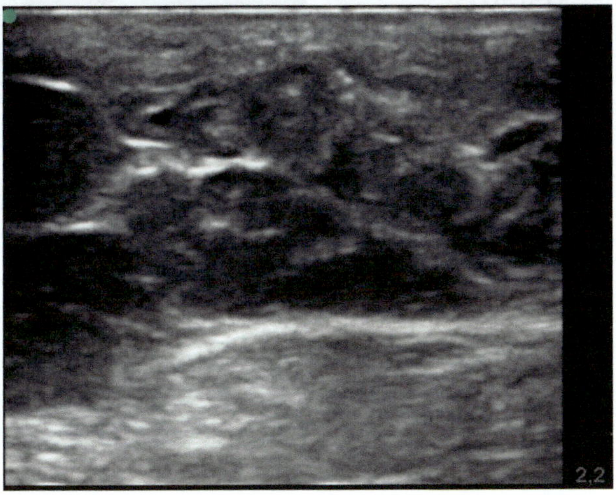

Fig. 23.19 SAX view of the canalization of the RCV

- Set the transducer aside.
- Stop advancing with the puncture to not perforate the posterior wall.
- Patients with a tourniquet bruise more easily, hence the importance of not perforating the posterior wall.

23.4.4 Step 04

- Introduce the 0.018" guidewire of the PowerPICC™ equipment in the introducer needle (Fig. 23.22).

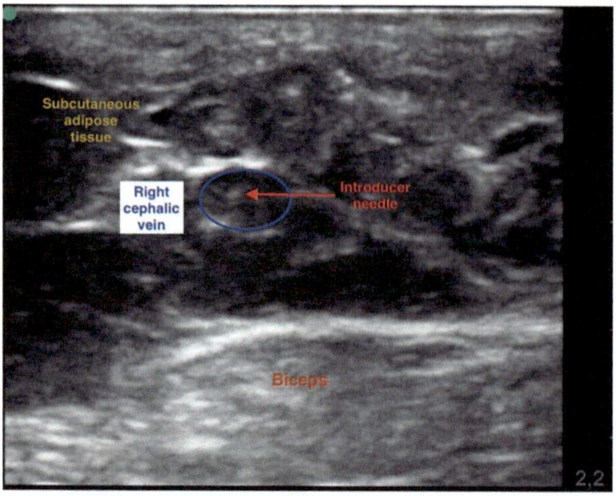

Fig. 23.20 Identifying structures
- Once the RCV is canalized, and by not exerting more pressure on it, it returns to its original diameter

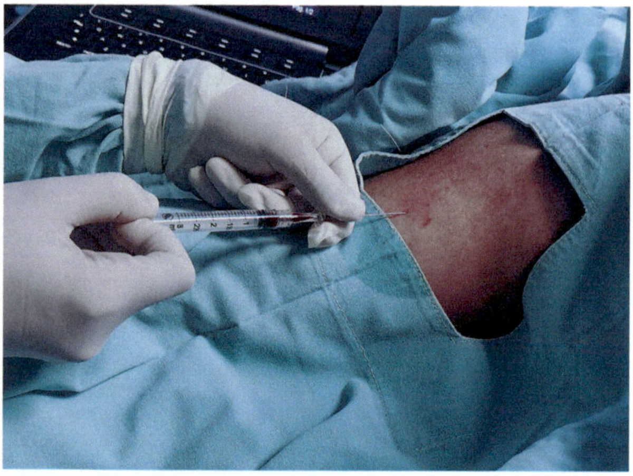

Fig. 23.21 Maintain gentle negative pressure on the syringe plunger

- Check the location of the intravascular guidewire, especially if it is not easily inserted into the vein (Fig. 23.23).
- SAX view of the intravenous guidewire (Figs. 23.24 and 23.25).

23.4.5 Step 05

- Place the vascular micro-introducer over the guidewire (Fig. 23.26).
- Carefully insert the micro-introducer.
- If the micro-introducer cannot be inserted, make a small incision in the upper part of the skin with a #11 scalpel blade so it passes easily (Fig. 23.27).

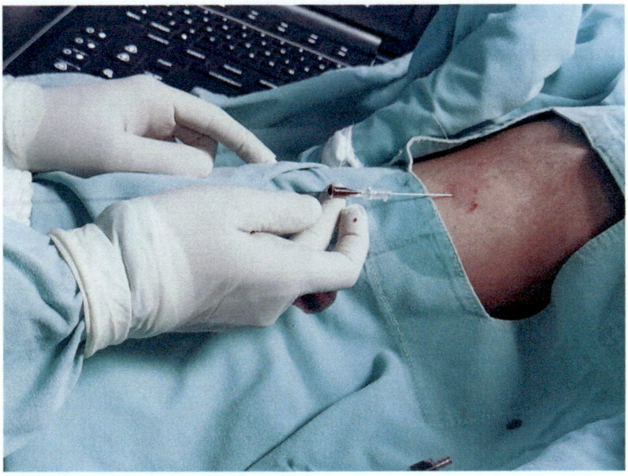

Fig. 23.22 Insert the guidewire

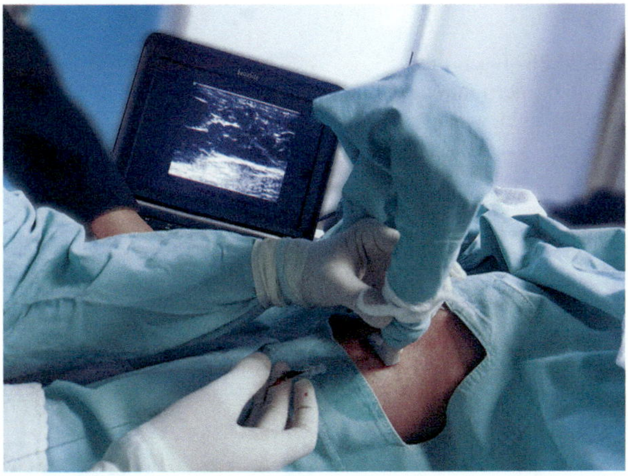

Fig. 23.23 Scan the intravascular location of the guidewire

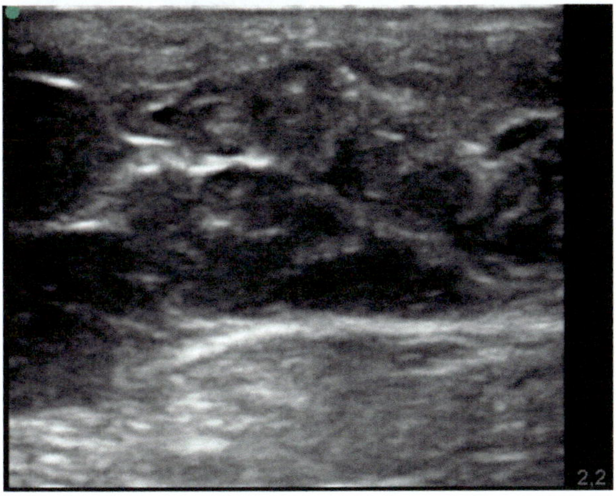

Fig. 23.24 SAX view of the intravenous guidewire

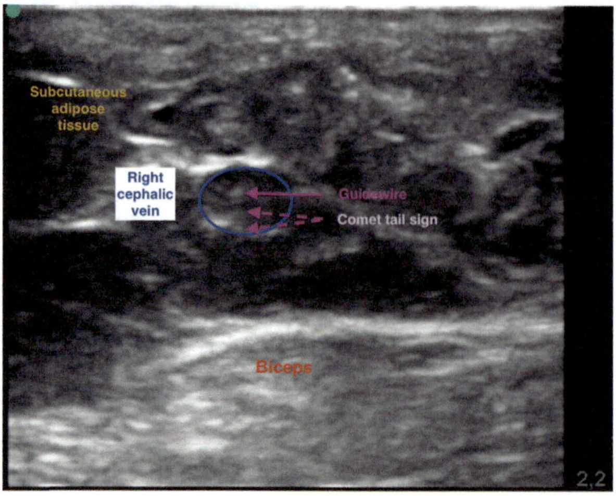

Fig. 23.25 Identifying structures
- The guidewire is inside the RCV
- The guidewire causes the comet tail sign

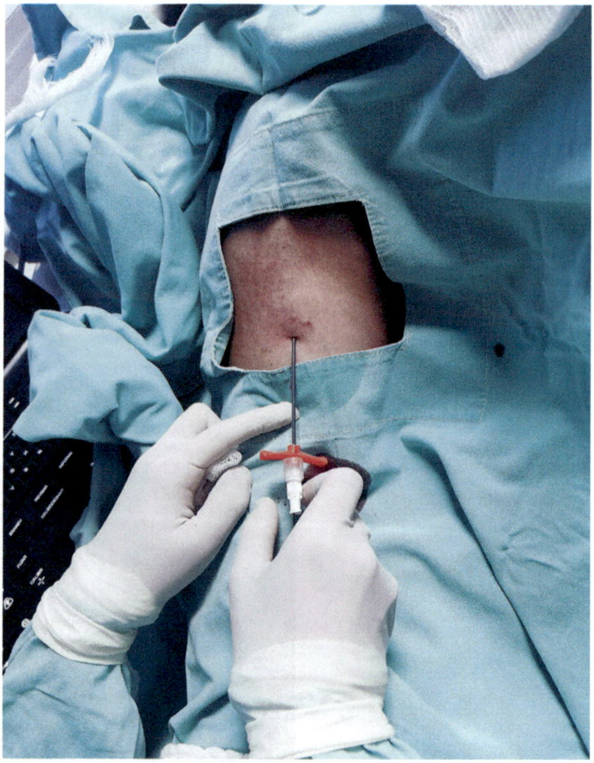

Fig. 23.26 Insert the vascular micro-introducer over the guidewire

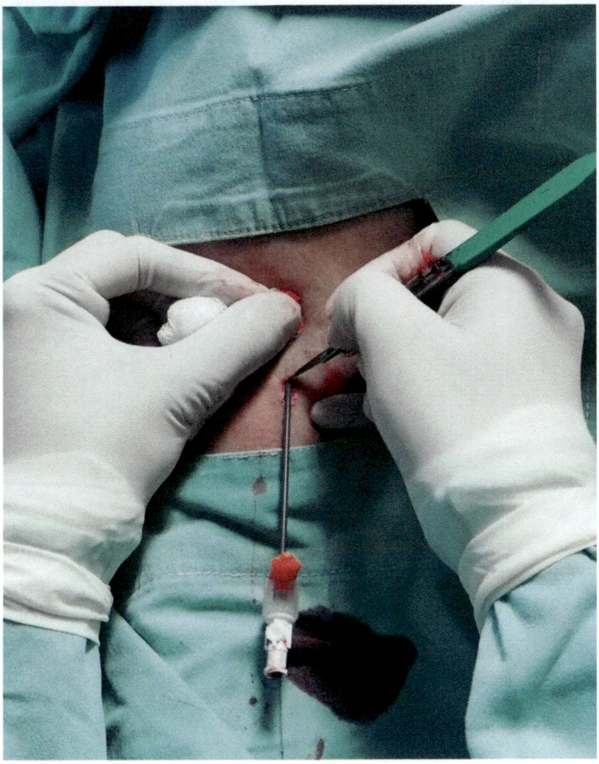

Fig. 23.27 Make a small incision in the upper part of the skin

- Do not make the incision too large because blood may leak more easily.
- Introduce the micro-introducer without bending the guidewire. Dilate the path from the skin to the vein and cannulate the vein with the micro-introducer using Seldinger's maneuver (Fig. 23.28).

23.4.6 Step 06

- Remove the guidewire with the inner dilator and leave only the peel-away sheath.
- Using the modified Seldinger's technique, introduce the catheter through the peel-away sheath (Fig. 23.29).
- Remove the peel-away sheath (Fig. 23.30).
- SAX view of the intravascular 4 Fr peripherally inserted central catheter (PICC) (Figs. 23.31 and 23.32).

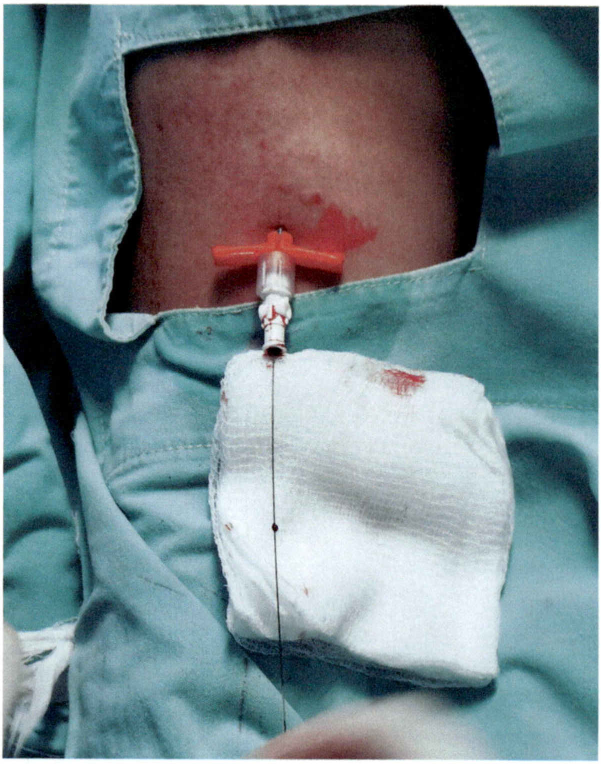

Fig. 23.28 Insert the micro-introducer

23.4.7 Step 07

- Place the StatLock® catheter stabilization device system and the sterile dressing (Fig. 23.33).

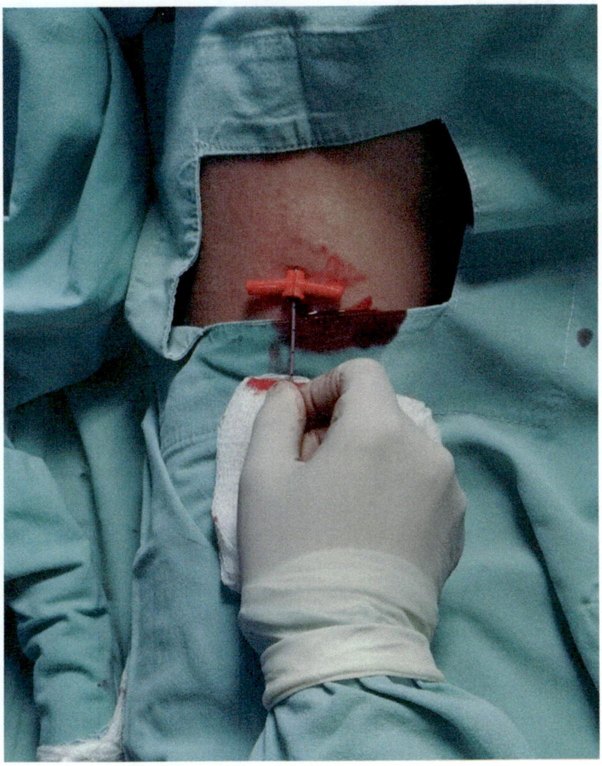

Fig. 23.29 Introduce the catheter through the peel-away sheath

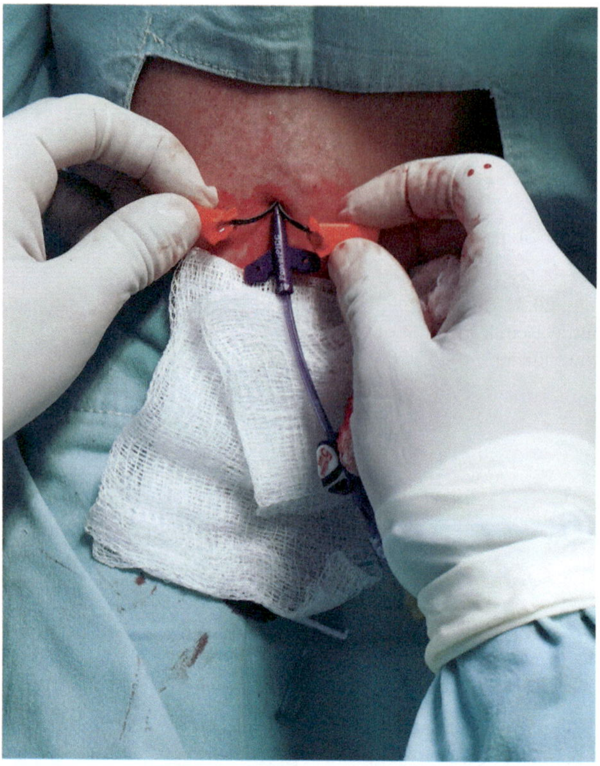

Fig. 23.30 Remove the peel-away sheath

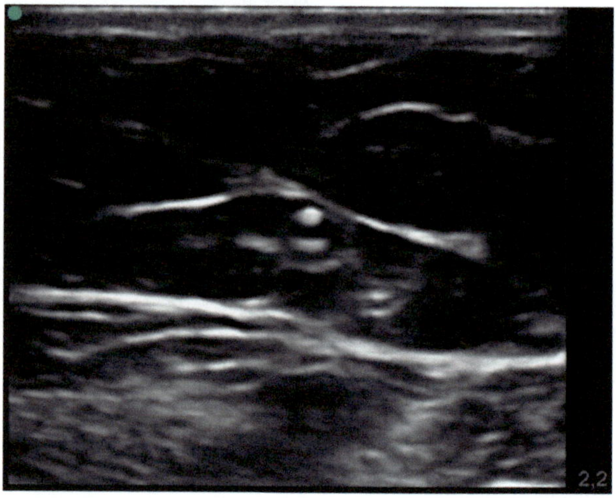

Fig. 23.31 SAX view of the intravascular PICC

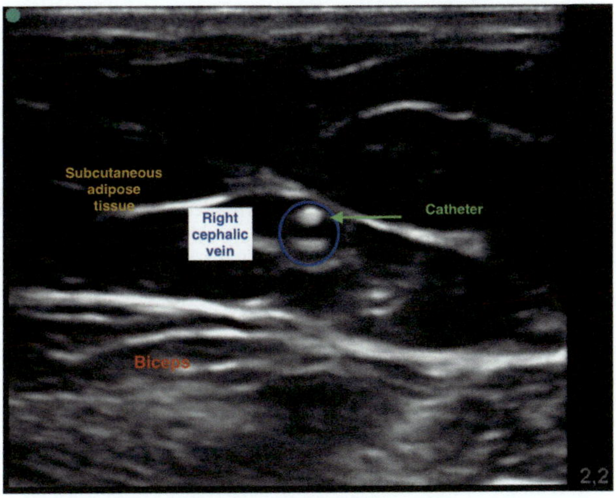

Fig. 23.32 Identifying structures
- The PICC is identified as a hyperechogenic dot with a larger diameter than the introducer needle

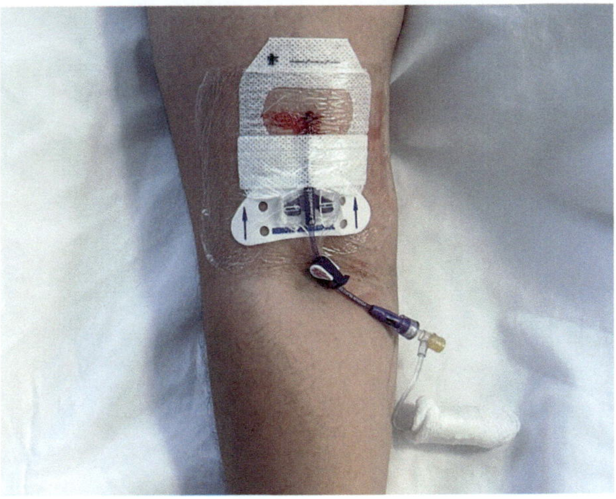

Fig. 23.33 Place the StatLock and the sterile dressing

Sources

1. Crowley JJ, Pereira JK, Harris LS, Becker CJ. Peripherally inserted central catheters: experience in 523 children. Radiology. 1997;204(3):617–21. https://doi.org/10.1148/radiology.204.3.9280234.
2. Racadio JM, Doellman DA, Johnson ND, Bean JA, Jacobs BR. Pediatric peripherally inserted central catheters: complication rates related to catheter tip location. Pediatrics. 2001;107(2):E28. https://doi.org/10.1542/peds.107.2.e28.
3. Fricke BL, Racadio JM, Duckworth T, Donnelly LF, Tamer RM, Johnson ND. Placement of peripherally inserted central catheters without fluoroscopy in children: initial catheter tip position. Radiology. 2005;234(3):887–92. https://doi.org/10.1148/radiol.2343031823.
4. Tran HS, Burrows BJ, Zang WA, Han DC. Brachial arteriovenous fistula as a complication of placement of a peripherally inserted central venous catheter: a case report and review of the literature. Am Surg. 2006;72(9):833–6. https://doi.org/10.1177/000313480607200914.
5. Dong Z, Connolly BL, Ungar WJ, Coyte PC. Cost analysis of peripherally inserted central catheter in pediatric patients. Int J Technol Assess Health Care. 2018;34(1):38–45. https://doi.org/10.1017/S026646231700109X.

Chapter 24
Basilic Vein in Pediatrics

24.1 Patient Positioning

- The patient is a 12-year-old adolescent weighing 80 kg.
- Position the patient supine.
- Place the extended arm at shoulder level at a 90° angle (Fig. 24.1).
- The head may be centered or turned to the left.
- Place a tourniquet close to the armpit.

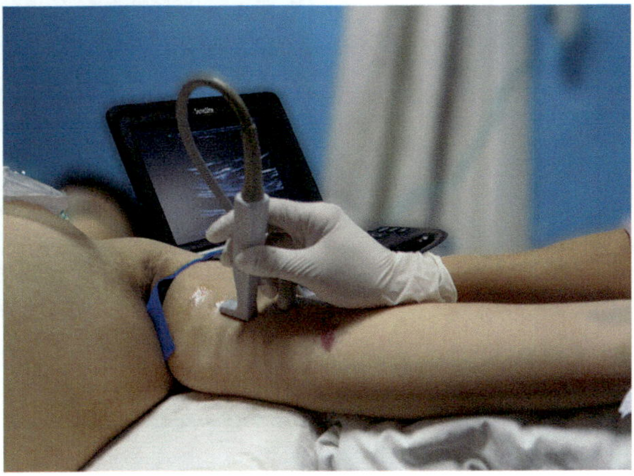

Fig. 24.1 Patient position

F. Montes-Tapia, *Atlas of Ultrasound-Guided Central Venous Catheter Placement*, https://doi.org/10.1007/978-3-031-61887-1_24

24.2 Scanning Technique

- Do a preliminary vascular assessment (non-sterile).
- The operator stands at the end of the outstretched arm.
- Place the ultrasound in any of the following positions: above the left shoulder or in front of the operator (Fig. 24.1).
- A high-frequency linear transducer (13–6 MHz) with a hockey stick-type or 5-cm footprint probe can be used.
- Divide the arm into three segments and scan the middle third on the medial side.
- Start scanning the arm in long-axis (LAX) view by placing the transducer longitudinally to the arm and with the tip of the transducer directed toward the patient's head.
- LAX view of the left basilic vein (LBV) (Figs. 24.2 and 24.3).
- Now, scan the middle third of the arm in short-axis (SAX) view (at the same level where scanning is done in LAX view), review the vein depth and arrangement, and verify the vein diameter at this level (Fig. 24.4).
- SAX view of the LBV without and with a tourniquet to compare the increase in diameter and better visualize the vein to perform venipuncture (Figs. 24.5, 24.6, 24.7 and 24.8).

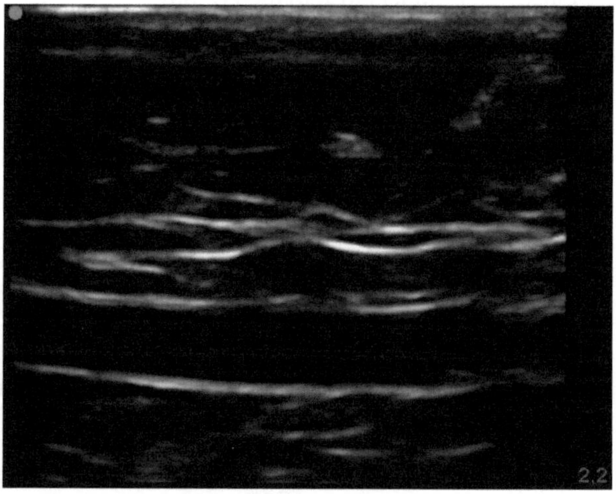

Fig. 24.2 LAX view of the left basilic vein

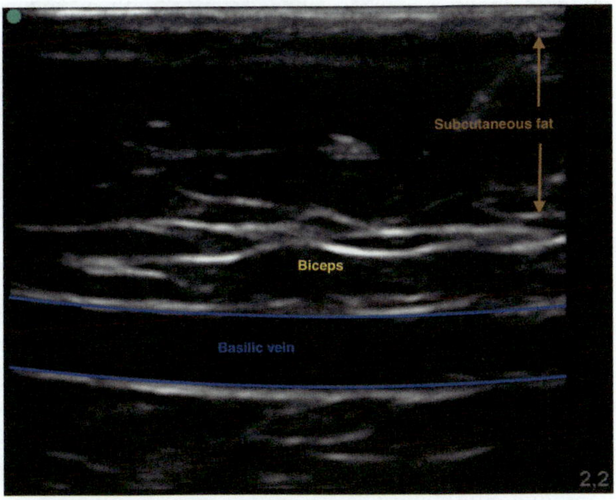

Fig. 24.3 Identifying structures
- Scan depth is 2,2 cm
- Prominent subcutaneous fatty tissue
- Biceps muscle over the basilic vein

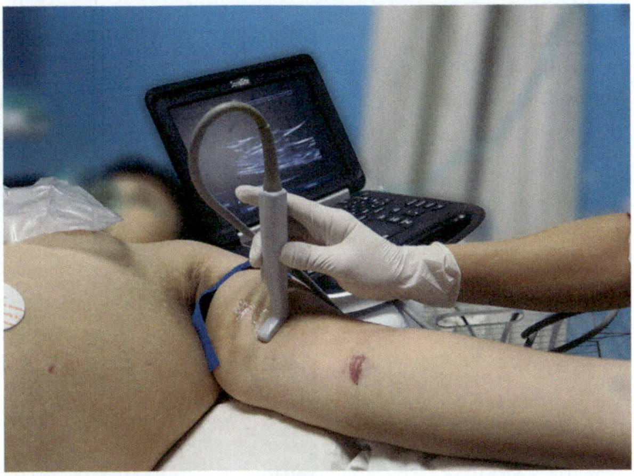

Fig. 24.4 Scanning in the middle third of the arm with the transducer in a transverse position (to perform the SAX view)

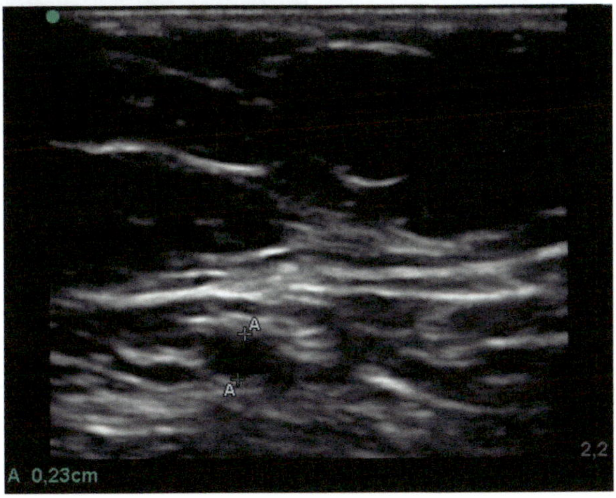

Fig. 24.5 LAX view of the basilic vein without the tourniquet

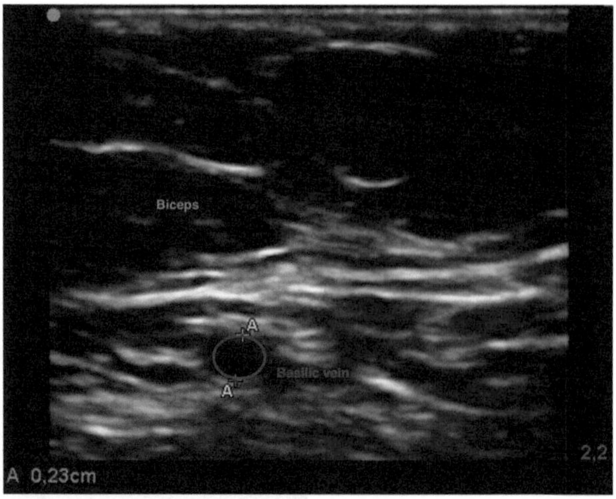

Fig. 24.6 Identifying structures

- The diameter of the basilic vein without the tourniquet is 0,23 cm

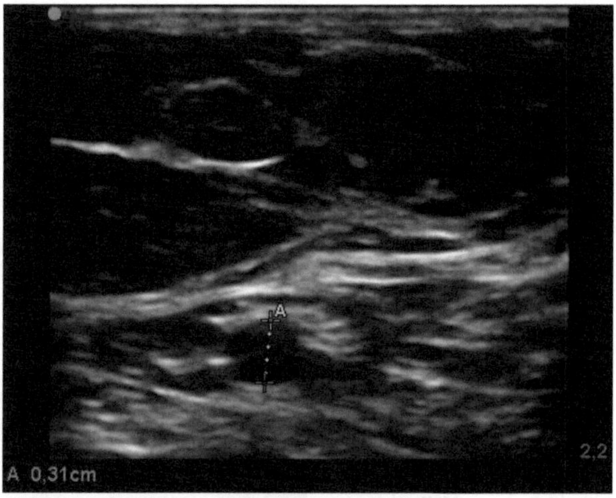

Fig. 24.7 LAX view of the basilic vein with the tourniquet

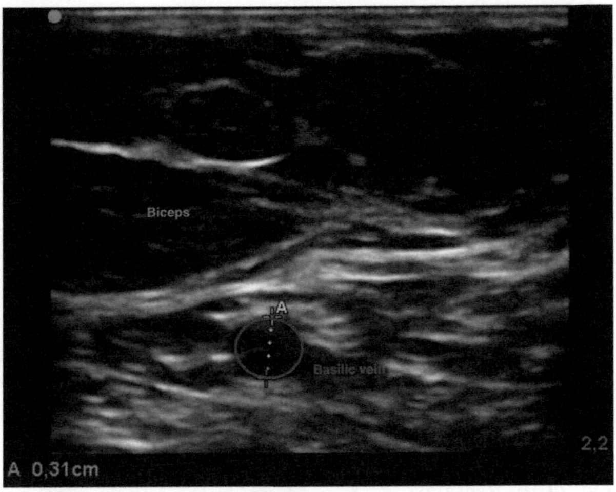

Fig. 24.8 Identifying structures
- The basilic vein with the tourniquet increases the diameter to 0,31 cm

24.3 Local Anesthesia Application

- The sterile field only leaves the middle and distal third of the left arm uncovered (Fig. 24.9).
- Real-time ultrasound-guided lidocaine infiltration (Fig. 24.10).
- For infiltration, use a small needle 25- 27-G.
- Use 1% lidocaine.
- Subcutaneous infiltration with lidocaine in the puncture tract 1,5–2 cm before the site chosen for LBV puncture.
- You can use the lidocaine infiltration puncture to guide where to perform the puncture with the intravenous catheter.

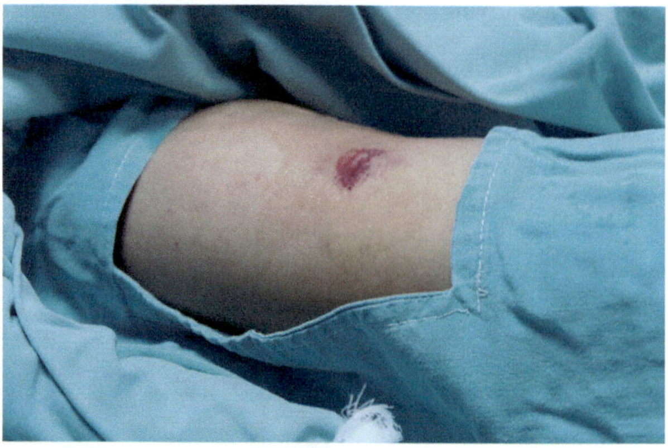

Fig. 24.9 Prepare the middle and distal third of the arm

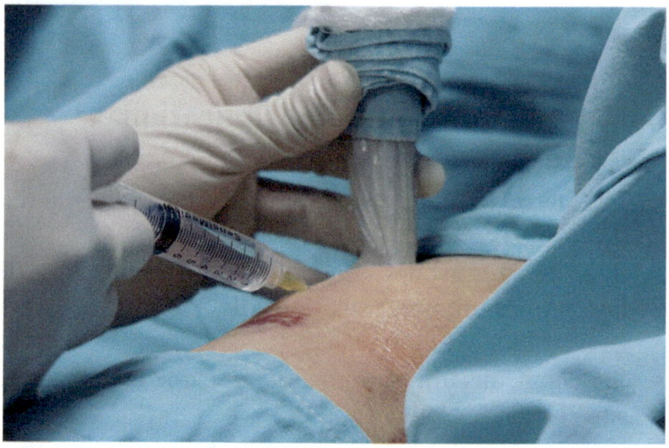

Fig. 24.10 Real-time ultrasound-guided lidocaine infiltration

24.4 Steps for Real-Time Ultrasound-Guided Access to Left Basilic Vein

24.4.1 Step 01

- We will use a 4 Fr single-lumen PowerPICC™.
- Measure the distance from the entry site in the arm to the central location site using the measuring tape of the PowerPICC ™ and section the catheter to the appropriate length.
- Start scanning the arm in LAX view of the middle third on the medial side.
- Puncture with a 20-G intravenous catheter at an angle of 20–30° (Fig. 24.11).
- LAX view of the start of the puncture (Figs. 24.12 and 24.13).
- Always perform the puncture with dynamic needle tracking (DNT).

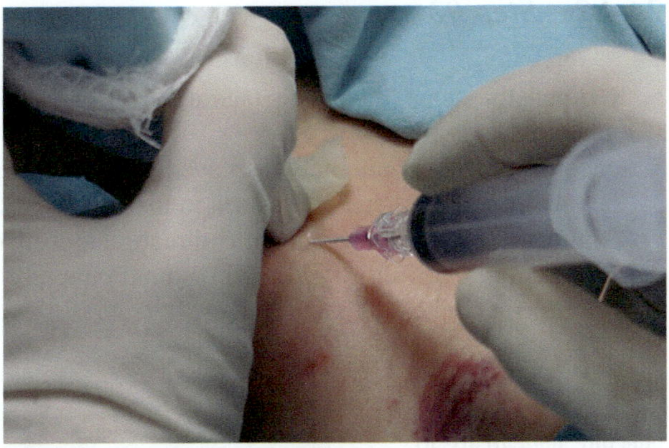

Fig. 24.11 Start the puncture with an angle of 20–30°

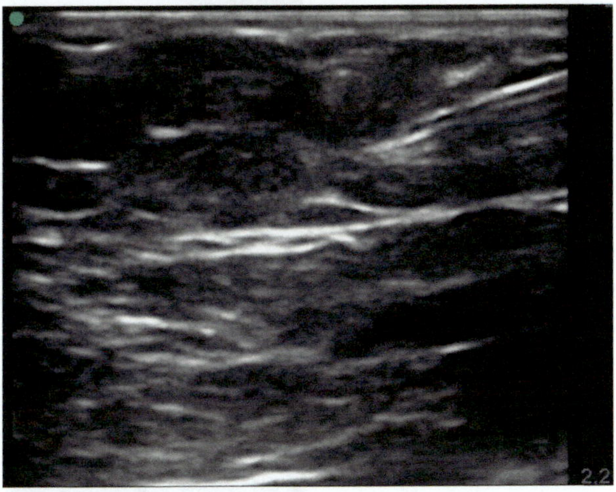

Fig. 24.12 LAX view of the start of the puncture

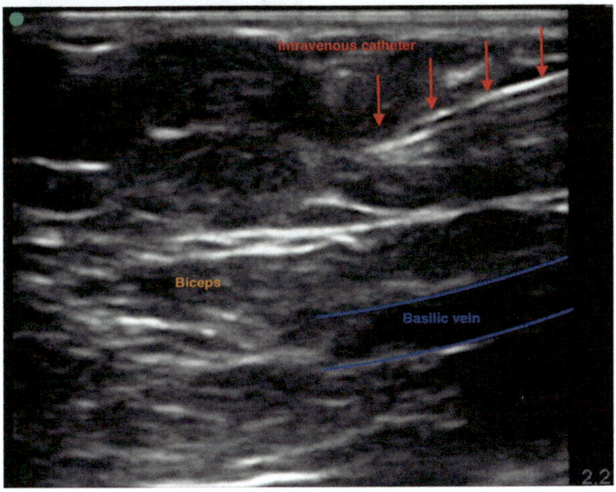

Fig. 24.13 Identifying structures

- The intravenous catheter is identified in the subcutaneous fatty tissue almost parallel to the vein
- The basilic vein is not yet centered. Only the distal half is seen
- Redirect the transducer

24.4.2 Step 02

- Redirect the scan (medial or lateral) to fully visualize the LBV and continue puncture.
- Once the LBV is completely displayed, increase the puncture angle to 40–50° so the intravenous catheter is directed to the vein (Fig. 24.14).
- Continue with the new puncture direction, inserting the intravenous catheter more deeply and following the ultrasound puncture in LAX in DNT in the path of footprint (Figs. 24.15 and 24.16).

Fig. 24.14 Increase the puncture angle to 40–50° to redirect toward the vein

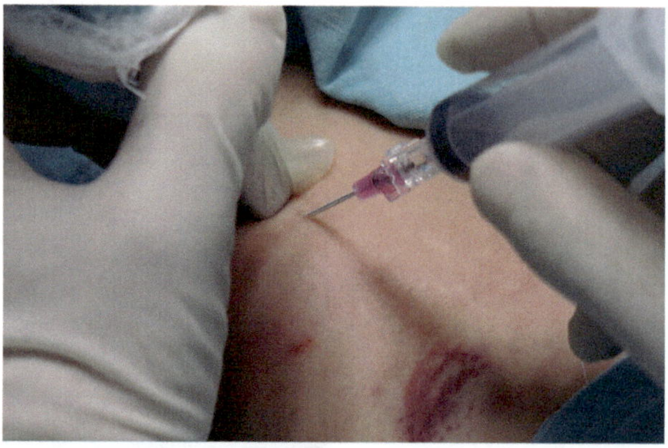

Fig. 24.15 LAX view of the puncture angle modification

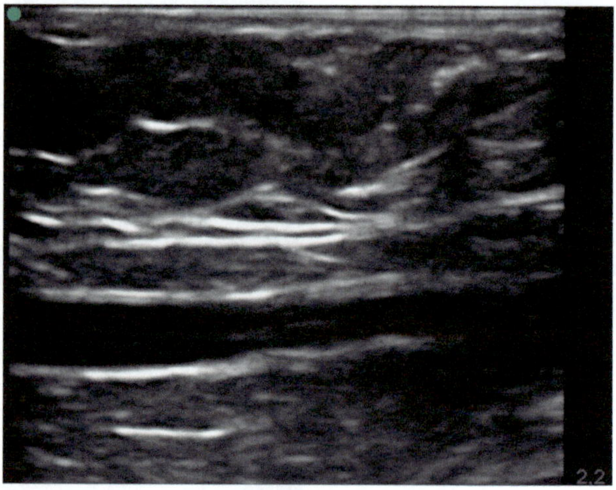

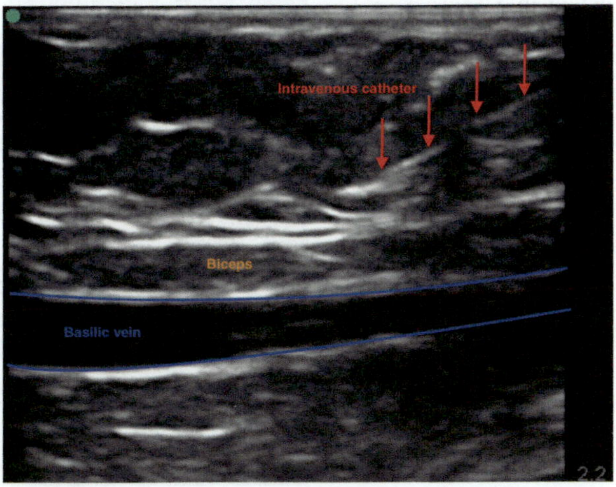

Fig. 24.16 Identifying structures
- Intravenous catheter with puncture angle modification (40–50°)
- The intravenous catheter is still in the subcutaneous fatty tissue but with a better direction toward the vein

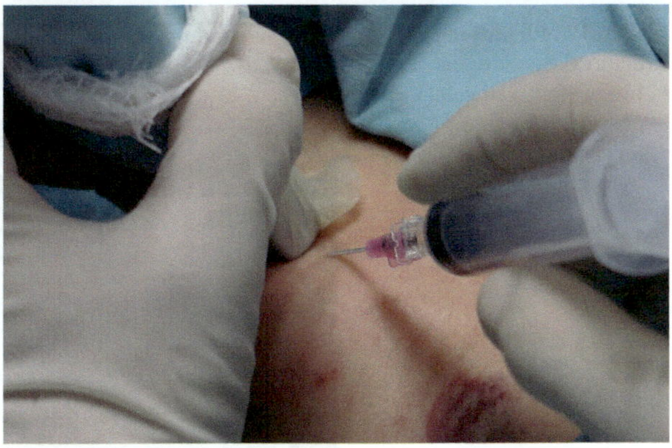

Fig. 24.17 Advance the transducer proximally as more intravenous catheter penetrates to visualize it (DNT) fully

24.4.3 Step 03

- Continue with the introduction of the intravenous catheter following the puncture in DNT, which requires advancing the transducer proximally and lateral or medial movements to fully visualize the intravenous catheter as it advances toward the vein (Fig. 24.17).
- LAX view of the approach of the intravenous catheter to the LBV (Figs. 24.18 and 24.19).
- LAX view of the continuation of the puncture, now cannulating the LBV (Figs. 24.20 and 24.21).

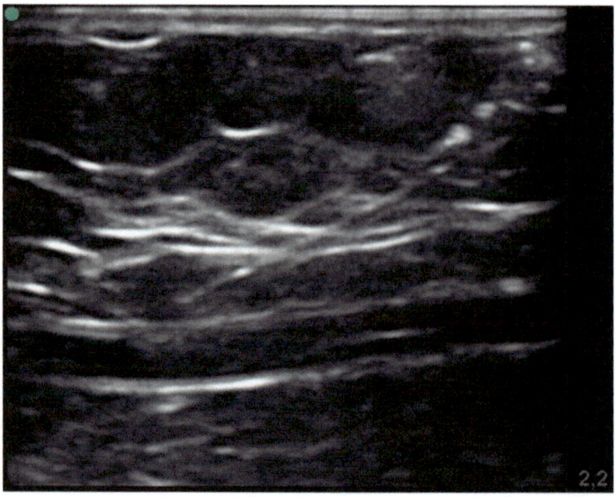

Fig. 24.18 LAX view of the progress of the LBV puncture with the intravenous catheter

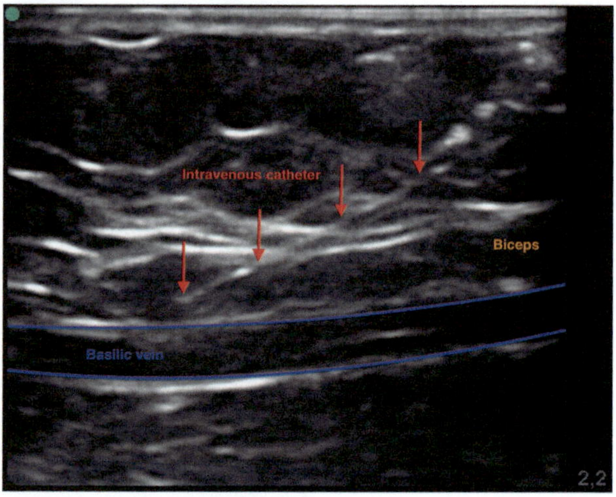

Fig. 24.19 Identifying structures

- Intravenous catheter passing through the biceps muscle and close to reaching the vein

- There are three ways to identify that you cannulated the vein:
  - Identify cannulation of the vein on the screen.
  - There is a loss of resistance when the intravenous catheter is being advanced.
  - The spontaneous return of blood in the flashback chamber due to compression generated by the tourniquet.
- Then, the operator sets the transducer aside and aspirates the syringe to check the blood flow (Fig. 24.22).

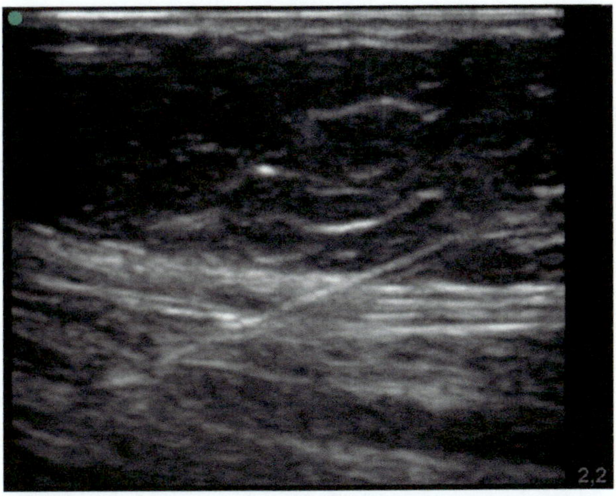

Fig. 24.20 LAX view of the LBV being cannulated by the intravenous catheter

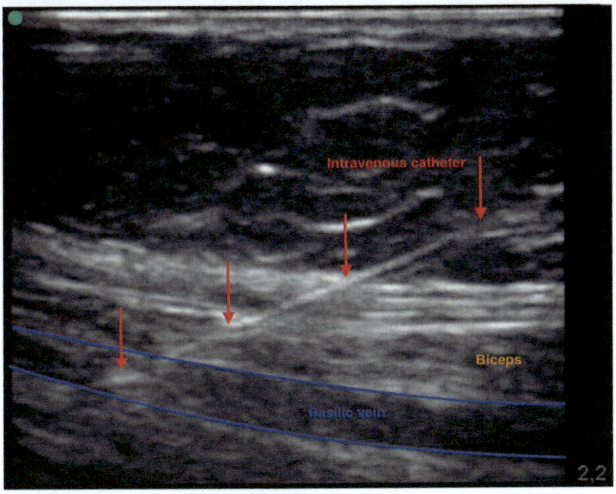

Fig. 24.21 Identifying structures

- The intravenous catheter penetrates the anterior wall of the LBV, which is cannulated without crossing the posterior wall

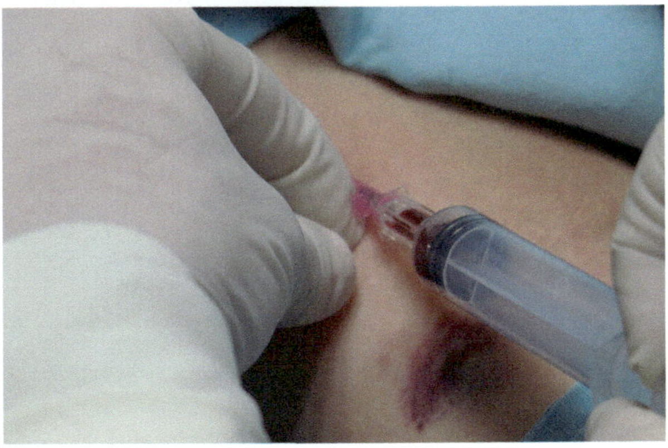

Fig. 24.22 Maintain gentle negative pressure on the syringe plunger

24.4.4 Step 04

- Once cannulated the vein with the intravenous catheter, withdraw the puncture needle.
- Introduce the 0.018" guidewire of the PowerPICC™ equipment in the intravenous cannula (Fig. 24.23).

24.4.5 Step 05

- Place the vascular micro-introducer over the guidewire (Fig. 24.24).
- Carefully insert the micro-introducer without bending the guidewire (Fig. 24.25).

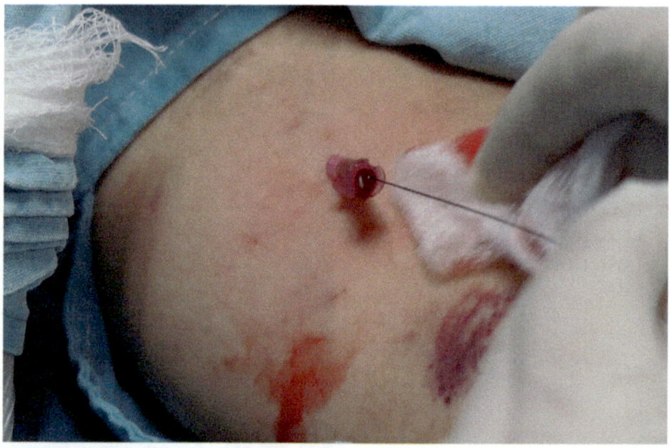

Fig. 24.23 Insert the guidewire

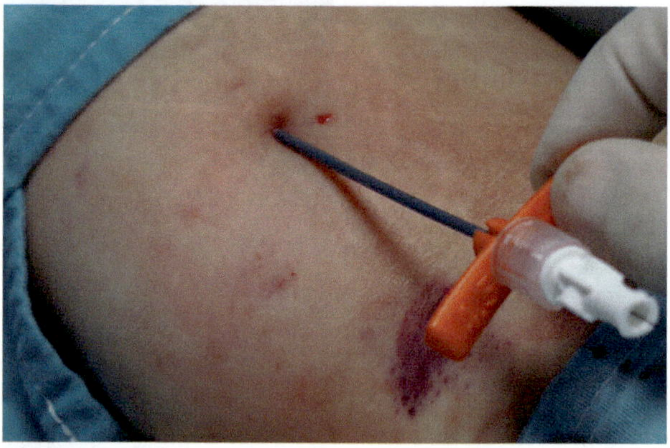

Fig. 24.24 Insert the vascular micro-introducer over the guidewire

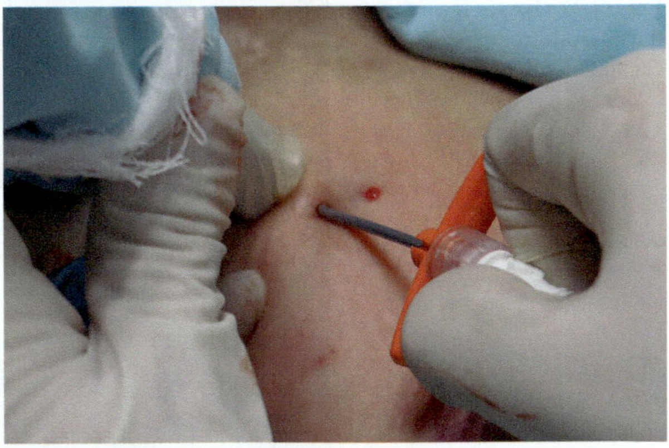
Fig. 24.25 Insert the micro-introducer

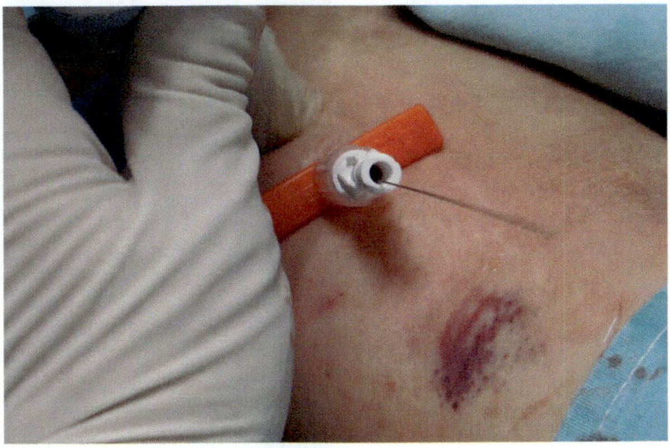
Fig. 24.26 Place the transducer longitudinally over the LBV

- Dilate the path from the skin to the vein and cannulate the vein with the micro-introducer using Seldinger's maneuver.
- Sometimes, you need to make a small incision in the skin with a scalpel, so it passes easily. It was not necessary for this patient.
- Once you insert the micro-introducer, place the transducer longitudinally and scan the vein (Fig. 24.26).
- LAX view to confirm that the micro-introducer is cannulating the LBV (Figs. 24.27 and 24.28).

24.4.6 Step 06

- Remove the guidewire with the inner dilator and leave only the peel-away sheath.
- Using the modified Seldinger's technique, introduce the catheter through the peel-away sheath (Fig. 24.29).

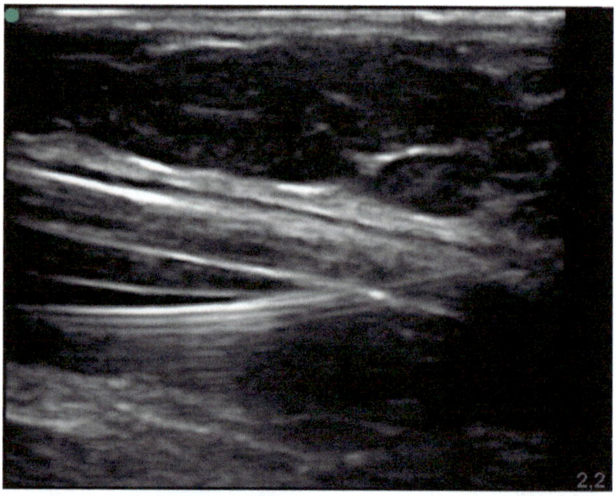

Fig. 24.27 LAX view of the micro-introducer cannulating the LBV

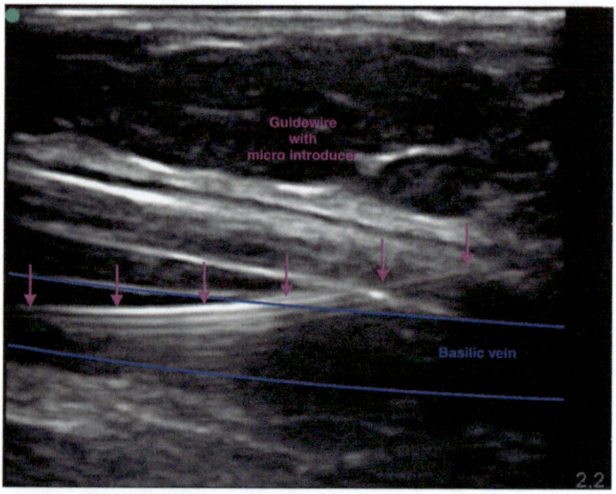

Fig. 24.28 Identifying structures
- Cannulation of the basilic vein with a micro-introducer on the guidewire

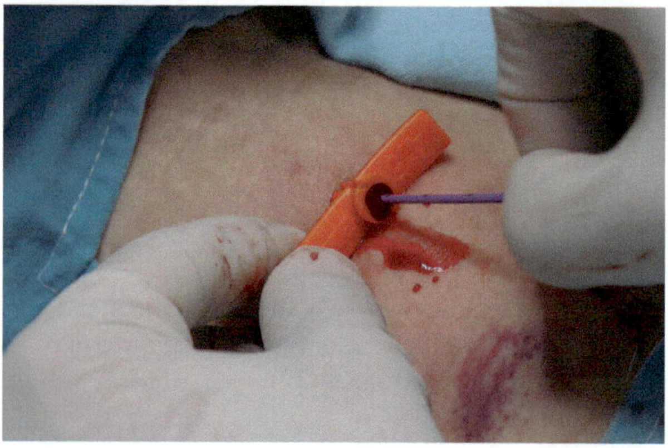

Fig. 24.29 Introduce the catheter through the peel-away sheath

- Scan the intravenous location of the catheter before removing the peel-away sheath (Fig. 24.30).
- LAX view of the intravascular 4 Fr PICC (Figs. 24.31 and 24.32).
- Remove the peel-away sheath (Figs. 24.33 and 24.34).

24.4.7 Step 07

- Place the StatLock® catheter stabilization device system and the sterile dressing (Fig. 24.35).

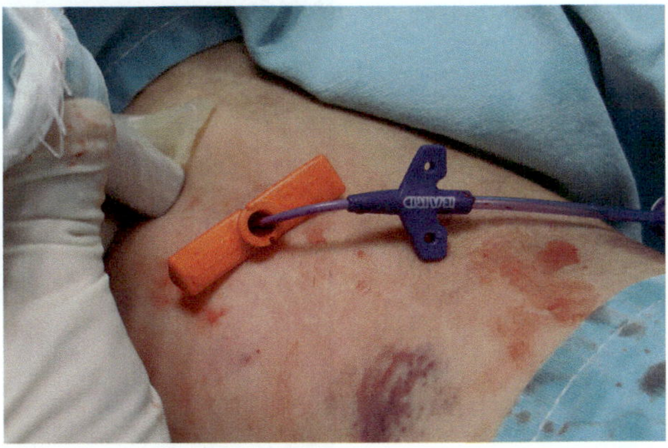

Fig. 24.30 Scan the location of the catheter in LAX view

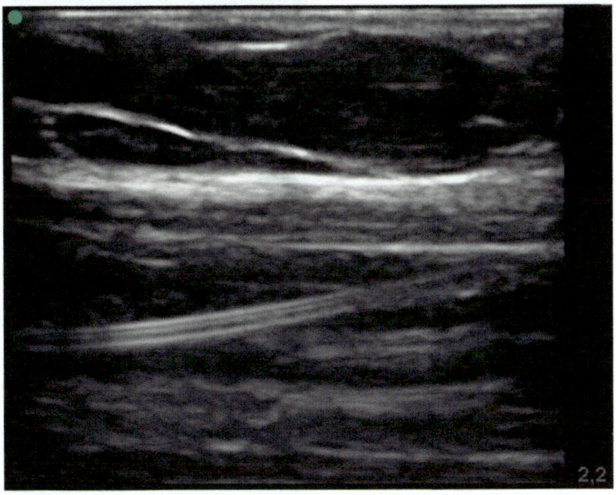

Fig. 24.31 LAX view of the intravascular PICC

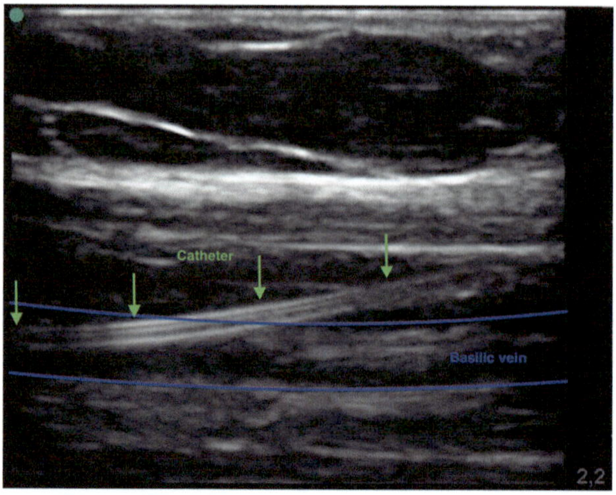

Fig. 24.32 Identifying structures

- The 4 Fr PICC in the lumen of the LBV

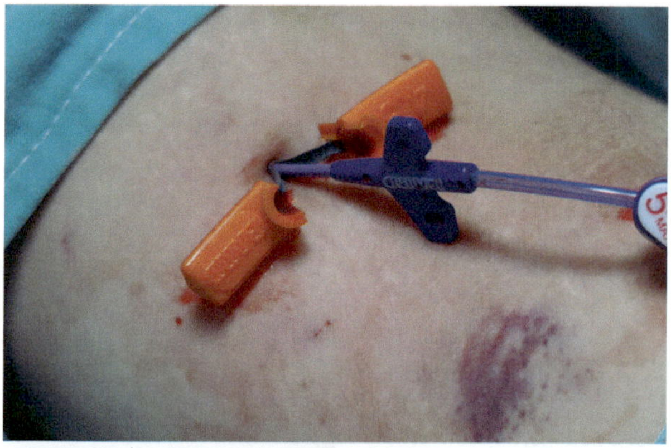

Fig. 24.33 Remove the peel-away sheath

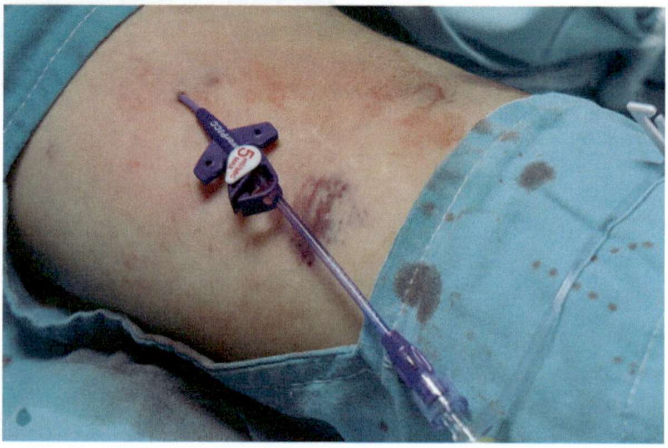

Fig. 24.34 Catheter entry into the skin without the peel-away sheath

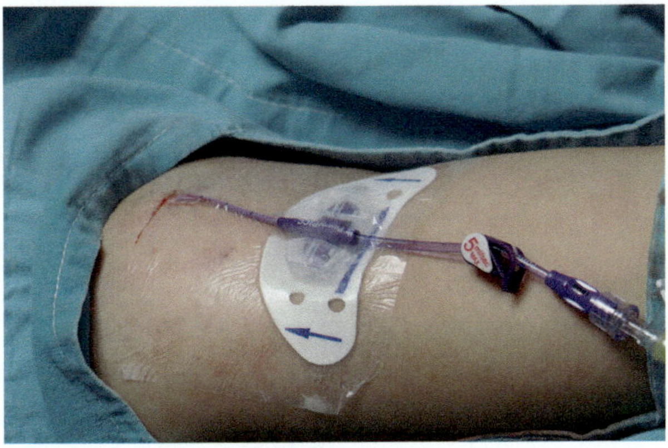

Fig. 24.35 Place the StatLock and the sterile dressing

Sources

1. Crowley JJ, Pereira JK, Harris LS, Becker CJ. Peripherally inserted central catheters: experience in 523 children. Radiology. 1997;204(3):617–21. https://doi.org/10.1148/radiology.204.3.9280234.
2. Racadio JM, Doellman DA, Johnson ND, Bean JA, Jacobs BR. Pediatric peripherally inserted central catheters: complication rates related to catheter tip location. Pediatrics. 2001;107(2):E28. https://doi.org/10.1542/peds.107.2.e28.
3. Fricke BL, Racadio JM, Duckworth T, Donnelly LF, Tamer RM, Johnson ND. Placement of peripherally inserted central catheters without fluoroscopy in children: initial catheter tip position. Radiology. 2005;234(3):887–92. https://doi.org/10.1148/radiol.2343031823.
4. Tran HS, Burrows BJ, Zang WA, Han DC. Brachial arteriovenous fistula as a complication of placement of a peripherally inserted central venous catheter: a case report and review of the literature. Am Surg. 2006;72(9):833–6. https://doi.org/10.1177/000313480607200914.
5. Dong Z, Connolly BL, Ungar WJ, Coyte PC. Cost analysis of peripherally inserted central catheter in pediatric patients. Int J Technol Assess Health Care. 2018;34(1):38–45. https://doi.org/10.1017/S026646231700109X.

Index

F. Montes-Tapia, *Atlas of Ultrasound-Guided Central Venous Catheter Placement*, https://doi.org/10.1007/978-3-031-61887-1

S

GPSR Compliance

The European Union's (EU) General Product Safety Regulation (GPSR) is a set of rules that requires consumer products to be safe and our obligations to ensure this.

If you have any concerns about our products, you can contact us on ProductSafety@springernature.com

In case Publisher is established outside the EU, the EU authorized representative is:

Springer Nature Customer Service Center GmbH
Europaplatz 3
69115 Heidelberg, Germany

Batch number: 10726133

Printed by Printforce, the Netherlands